ESSENTIALS OF *Ophthalmology*

Edited by

George B. Bartley, M.D.

Consultant, Department of Ophthalmology, Mayo Clinic and Mayo Foundation; Associate Professor of Ophthalmology, Mayo Medical School; Rochester, Minnesota

Thomas J. Liesegang, M.D.

Head, Section of Ophthalmology, Mayo Clinic Jacksonville, Jacksonville, Florida; Professor of Ophthalmology, Mayo Medical School; Rochester, Minnesota

With Eleven Contributors

ESSENTIALS OF
Ophthalmology

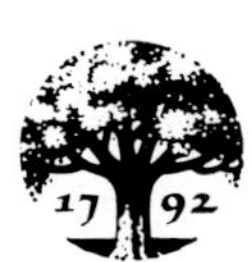

J.B. Lippincott Company PHILADELPHIA
NEW YORK   LONDON   HAGERSTOWN

*We dedicate this book to our residents,
from whom we continue to learn much.*

Assistant Production Manager: Lori J. Bainbridge
Production: Barbara A. Conover, Publications Management
Compositor: Capital City Press
Printer/Binder: Printed and bound by Impresora Donneco Internacional
S.A. de C.V., a division of R. R. Donnelley & Sons Company.

Manufactured in Mexico

6 5 4 3 2 1

Library of Congress Cataloging-in-Publication Data

Essentials of opthalmology/[edited by] George B. Bartley,
   Thomas J. Liesegang ; with contributors.
      p. cm.
   Includes index.
   ISBN 0-397-51142-6
   1. Ophthalmology.   I. Bartley, George B.   II. Liesegang, Thomas J.
   [DNLM: 1. Eye Disease. 2. Ophthalmology. WW 100 E78]
   RE46.E87   1992
   617.7—dc20
   DNLM/DLC
   for Library of Congress   91-35011
                                                           CIP

   Every effort has been made to ensure drug selections and dosages are in accordance
with current recommendations and practice. Because of ongoing research, changes in
government regulations, and the constant flow of information on drug therapy, reactions,
and interactions, the reader is cautioned to check the package insert for each drug
for indications, dosages, warnings, and precautions, particularly if the drug is new or
infrequently used.

CONTRIBUTORS

James P. Bolling, M.D.
Consultant, Section of Ophthalmology, Mayo Clinic Jacksonville, Jacksonville, Florida; Assistant Professor of Ophthalmology, Mayo Medical School; Rochester, Minnesota

Richard F. Brubaker, M.D.
Chair, Department of Ophthalmology, Mayo Clinic and Mayo Foundation; Professor of Ophthalmology, Mayo Medical School; Rochester, Minnesota

John D. Bullock, M.D.
Professor and Chairman, Department of Ophthalmology; Professor of Surgery, Wright State University; Dayton, Ohio

R. Jean Campbell, M.B.,Ch.B.
Consultant, Department of Ophthalmology and Consultant, Section of Surgical Pathology, Mayo Clinic and Mayo Foundation; Professor of Pathology, Mayo Medical School; Rochester, Minnesota

Jay C. Erie, M.D.
Consultant, Department of Ophthalmology, Mayo Clinic and Mayo Foundation; Assistant Professor of Ophthalmology, Mayo Medical School; Rochester, Minnesota

James A. Garrity, M.D.
Consultant, Department of Ophthalmology, Mayo Clinic and Mayo Foundation; Assistant Professor of Ophthalmology, Mayo Medical School; Rochester, Minnesota

David C. Herman, M.D.
Consultant, Department of Ophthalmology, Mayo Clinic and Mayo Foundation; Assistant Professor of Ophthalmology, Mayo Medical School; Rochester, Minnesota

George G. Hohberger, M.D.
Consultant, Department of Ophthalmology, Mayo Clinic and Mayo Foundation; Instructor in Ophthalmology, Mayo Medical School; Rochester, Minnesota

Douglas H. Johnson, M.D.
Consultant, Department of Ophthalmology, Mayo Clinic and Mayo Foundation; Associate Professor of Ophthalmology, Mayo Medical School; Rochester, Minnesota

Thomas J. McPhee, M.D.
Consultant, Section of Ophthalmology, Mayo Clinic Scottsdale, Scottsdale, Arizona; Assistant Professor of Ophthalmology, Mayo Medical School; Rochester, Minnesota

John M. Pach, M.D.
Consultant, Department of Ophthalmology, Mayo Clinic and Mayo Foundation; Instructor in Ophthalmology, Mayo Medical School; Rochester, Minnesota

PREFACE

The transition from intern to first-year ophthalmology resident is arguably the most diverse in medicine. As the eye in large measure is physically delineated from the rest of the body by the bony orbit, likewise ophthalmology is separated from the mainstream of medicine by its unique vocabulary, anatomy, and equipment. The young physician well versed in the management of A-V (atrioventricular) block must become facile in recognizing A and V patterns of strabismus; the doctor familiar with PVCs (premature ventricular contractions) must learn how to diagnose a PVC (posterior vitreous collapse).

To ease this transition, several years ago we had the idea of asking our staff members to compile a handout of information that he or she considered essential knowledge for matriculating residents. The project burgeoned into an introductory textbook that we hope will be helpful not only to new residents in ophthalmology but also to medical students and physicians in primary care. We asked our contributors to summarize what they thought was essential clinical knowledge, information that they wished our new residents knew the first day of residency to allow them to "hit the ground running." The focus of the book, therefore, is clinical; we have deliberately not emphasized embryology, pharmacology, and advanced anatomy. These important topics can be studied in the excellent loose-leaf volumes of *Duane's Foundations of Clinical Ophthalmology*, edited by William Tasman, M.D., and Edward A. Jaeger, M.D. Current in-depth clinical information is also available in *Duane's Clinical Ophthalmology*, for which we believe our book will be a useful primer.

We wish to express our appreciation to our colleagues who gave freely of their time to contribute chapters, to Marlene M. Spencer for superb secretarial work, to LeAnn M. Stee for editorial guidance, to Dianne F. Kemp, Dorothy Tienter, and Ginny A. Dunt for manuscript production, to the Section of Visual Information for the artwork, and to Darlene Cooke and Lisa McAllister at J.B. Lippincott Company for their encouragement and support.

George B. Bartley, M.D.
Thomas J. Liesegang, M.D.

CONTENTS

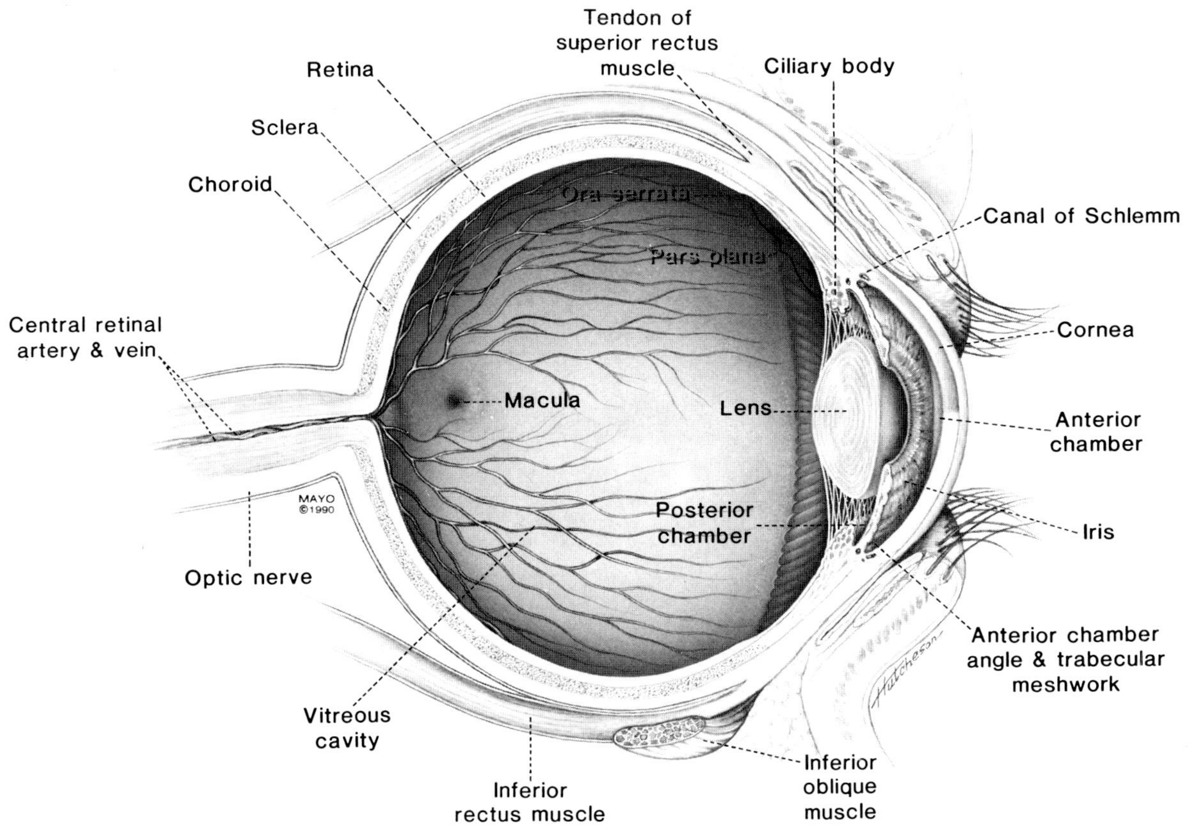

Retina
Sclera
Choroid
Central retinal artery & vein
Optic nerve
MAYO ©1990
Macula
Vitreous cavity
Inferior rectus muscle
Tendon of superior rectus muscle
Ora serrata
Pars plana
Posterior chamber
Ciliary body
Canal of Schlemm
Cornea
Lens
Anterior chamber
Iris
Anterior chamber angle & trabecular meshwork
Inferior oblique muscle
Hutcheson

INTRODUCTION TO OPHTHALMOLOGY

Richard F. Brubaker

In 1835 when Charles Darwin gazed from the gunwales of the *Beagle* as it lay at anchor off the Galapagos Archipelago, he was at the brink of discovery of the forces of nature that have permitted biologic diversity to occur. Given Darwin's seminal work and that virtually all extant animals that live in lighted environments have evolved a visual system, one can deduce immediately the importance of vision to survival.

In higher animals, the visual system is exquisite, and its secrets have piqued the interest of some of the world's most outstanding scientists. Since 1895 when Alfred Nobel scribed in his own hand the famous will establishing the Nobel Prizes, no fewer than seven visual scientists have been recipients of the award in physiology and medicine. The first was Allvar Gullstrand in 1911 for his work on the optics of the eye, followed in 1967 by Ragnar Granit, H. Keffer Hartline, and George Wald for their discoveries of the chemistry and physiology of signal transduction and the retinal processing of vision. In 1981, Roger W. Sperry, David H. Hubel, and Torsten N. Wiesel received the Nobel Prize for their research on the signal processing and development of the visual system in the brain.

It is no wonder that physicians and scientists have held such fascination for the visual system. The human eye gathers and transmits to the brain information about the environment equally well from arm's length or from distant galaxies. These data are collected from nearly 30 million receptor rods and cones, processed, and transmitted to the central nervous system over 3 million separate channels. The rate of data transfer from eye to brain is equivalent to more than a billion bits per second, enough to transmit as many as 15,000 individual telephone conversations at once.

In darkness, the sensitivity of the eye permits it to detect objects so dim that only a few photons enter the pupil every second. The amplification of such a system is truly remarkable. If one could convert into photons the energy necessary to evaporate a mere 10 drops of water (130 calories), one would have a sufficient number of photons to stimulate every eye of every human being who has ever lived for his or her entire lifetime at the threshold rate of stimulation! Despite this incredible sensitivity, the retina can function well when bombarded with tens of billions of photons per second, giving it a dynamic range of 9 orders of magnitude!

Under optimal conditions, the visual system can detect the disalignment of less than 10 seconds of arc between two lines or can discriminate a change in hue or brightness of less than 1%. Yet these benchmarks are simple compared with the tracking and catching of a fly ball in center field or the identification of a specific human face, feats that are beyond the capabilities of the largest and fastest computers.

Given the complexity of the visual system,

it is no wonder that it sometimes fails. For every function or process, there is a disease that is characterized by its dysfunction. Ophthalmologists are concerned with the maintenance and repair of this myriad of conditions, a role they share with other health professionals. Anyone who wants to master the subject can begin with Hermann von Helmholtz's 3-volume *Physiological Optics* and then for light reading tackle Sir Stewart Duke-Elder's 15-volume *System of Ophthalmology*. The task is herculean. Yet, all health professionals must have at least a working knowledge of the commonest ailments of the eye.

In this textbook, *Essentials of Ophthalmology*, the editors and authors have attempted to summarize the most common and important problems encountered in clinical practice. The book can be useful to medical students as an introduction to the subject or to general practitioners as a refresher. This text is given to all men and women before their commencement as residents in ophthalmology at the Mayo Clinic. The material herein is the foundation on which the residency begins and builds.

Dealing with the visual system can only instill a sense of awe in one of nature's marvels. What is more, practitioners who apply their knowledge and skill to assuage failing vision will find themselves revered by grateful patients. As Sir Arthur Conan Doyle put it, "A man grudges a half-crown to cure his chest or his throat, but he'd spend his last dollar over his eye" (Doyle, A.C. [ed.]: *The Stark Munro Letters*. Second edition. New York, D. Appleton and Company, 1895, p. 379).

2

OPHTHALMIC HISTORY AND EXAMINATION

Jay C. Erie

The basic eye examination consists of 10 steps.

The basic ophthalmic examination consists of a careful patient history, an assessment of visual function, and a physical examination of the eyes. Examination of the eyes and surrounding tissues not only yields valuable information for the diagnosis and treatment of primary ocular disease but also can provide clues about systemic conditions. A systematic routine must be adopted to ensure that an important sign is not overlooked. A nonemergency ophthalmic examination can be accomplished in 10 steps:

History
Visual acuity
Pupillary reactions
External examination
Ocular motility
Confrontation visual fields
Slit-lamp biomicroscopy
Intraocular pressures
Direct ophthalmoscopy
Indirect ophthalmoscopy

In addition, supplementary diagnostic tests as indicated by the history and results of prior examination include the following:

Exophthalmometry
Tear film evaluation
Corneal sensation test
Keratometry
Gonioscopy
Perimetry
Color vision test
Stereopsis
Amsler grid test
Transillumination
Tonography
Lancaster red/green test
Double Maddox rod test
Ultrasonography
Fluorescein angiography
Magnetic resonance imaging/computed tomography
Electrophysiologic studies (dark adaptation, electroretinography, electro-oculography)

Blurred vision is the most common chief concern elicited during the history taking.

The history should include not only the patient's chief concern but also general information about the patient's age, occupation, past and present medical and ocular problems, systemic and ocular medications, and drug allergies and any family history of eye disease.

Visual blurring is the most frequent chief concern, and it requires careful consideration. Some of the important features of this complaint that need to be determined include whether one or both eyes are involved and whether near or distance vision is preferentially affected. The duration and the course of the visual loss (acute or chronic) are essential details. It is not uncommon for the patient to discover visual defects accidentally by covering one eye.

The nature of the decreased vision may suggest causes. If the patient complains that objects that should be straight appear bent or wavy (*metamorphopsia*), in most cases this distortion is due to macular pathology. Blind spots in the normal visual field (visual field defects or *scotomas*) may result from disorders of the media, retina, optic nerve, or brain. Useful tests to detect scotomas are the Amsler grid and formal perimetry. Halos, or rainbow-like fringes seen around a point source of light, may be a symptom of corneal edema, often resulting from an abrupt rise in intraocular pressure. Overwearing of contact lenses may also cause corneal edema and halos around lights. In both cases, the halos are accompanied by pain. Media opacities, such as cataracts, can also cause halos. In this case, however, pain is absent. Sudden, complete loss of vision is an ocular emergency. The loss may be permanent or momentary (*amaurosis fugax*). Amaurosis fugax, in most cases, implies an embolic cause, usually due to ipsilateral carotid disease or cardiac disease. Visualizing the embolus during ophthalmoscopy or finding asymmetric retinal artery pressures helps one to make the diagnosis.

Ocular pain is the second most frequent ocular complaint.

As with pain elsewhere in the body, ocular discomfort requires further definition. One should carefully elicit the onset of the pain, its severity, and location. Headache is a frequent ophthalmic complaint, but it rarely relates to a disturbance within the visual system. The chief exception to this rule is *asthenopia* (eye strain), which refers to vague ocular discomfort associated with near work. *Presbyopia*, uncorrected hyperopia, uncorrected *astigmatism*, and decompensated *phorias* may all cause asthenopia. A general medical evaluation may be indicated in a patient with headaches and a normal eye examination.

A *foreign body sensation* usually indicates irritation of the corneal or conjunctival epithelium. This may be mild and due to a dry eye syndrome or to inflammation of the lids or conjunctiva (*blepharitis*). This must be distinguished from itching, which is a symptom of ocular allergy. Acute, localized pain that is intensified by movement of the eyelids suggests a corneal abrasion or a foreign body located on the cornea or upper tarsal conjunctiva. The use of fluorescein in the tear film identifies the location of the corneal epithelial defect.

Photophobia (an increased sensitivity to light) and glare should be distinguished from ocular pain because these symptoms relate to disturbances within the visual system. Corneal edema or inflammation, iritis, posterior subcapsular cataracts, and ocular albinism frequently give rise to such symptoms.

Diplopia refers to the simultaneous perception of two separate images.

The most important determination in the evaluation of diplopia is whether the double vision disappears when one eye is covered. Monocular diplopia is usually due to abnormalities of the media, usually corneal or lenticular changes, such as keratoconus or cataracts. Binocular diplopia is almost always due to abnormal alignment of the eyes, from either a neurogenic or a myogenic cause. In patients with long-standing strabismus, however, double vision is usually not a problem because of foveal suppression. The nature of the diplopia (whether horizontal or vertical) should be noted. This is a clue as to which extraocular muscle (or muscles) is involved. It is also important to know whether the separation of images changes in various gaze positions; the degree of diplopia often increases in the field of action of a paretic muscle.

Abnormal ocular secretion refers either to lacrimation or to discharge.

The chronicity, severity, and laterality of any ocular drainage should be noted. Acute onset of tearing (*epiphora*) and the presence of ocular discomfort suggest an irritative cause with reflex *lacrimation*. A corneal foreign body, corneal abrasion, blepharitis, or even dry eyes may cause reflex tearing. Causes of chronic epiphora are usually due to obstruction within the nasolacrimal system and are not usually associated with ocular discomfort. The initial office evaluation of the patency of the drainage system involves inspection of the puncta and irrigation of the canaliculi and nasolacrimal ducts.

Ocular discharge (mattering) is almost always a result of allergic or infectious external disease. If the discharge is watery and associated with burning, conjunctival injection, and an enlarged preauricular lymph node, then viral conjunctivitis should be suspected. A purulent discharge without a preauricular node usually indicates a bacterial infection. A mucous discharge accompanied by itching is a common sign of allergic conjunctivitis, a disorder that may be associated with seasonal rhinitis or hay fever.

Other visual disturbances include the perception of floaters, flashing lights (photopsia), and visual hallucinations.

Floaters resulting from posterior vitreous detachment are usually not significant unless their frequency or severity has increased dramatically. Floaters, however, may indicate a vitreous hemorrhage, and this symptom warrants a thorough examination.

Photopsia refers to the perception of flashing lights. It is usually the result of direct retinal stimulation from a retinal tear or vitreous traction. This symptom frequently precedes the onset of retinal detachment. Patients with photopsia should have a careful peripheral retinal examination, including indirect ophthalmoscopy with scleral depression.

Cerebral cortex disturbances may give rise to *visual hallucinations* as a result of a seizure disorder, migraine, or drug toxicity. Formed hallucinations localize to the temporal lobe, whereas unformed hallucinations originate in the occipital lobe.

The past ocular history may yield several clues.

The patient should be specifically questioned about previous cataract, extraocular muscle, glaucoma, retinal, eyelid, and orbital operations or laser treatments. Previous episodes of significant ocular injury should be noted. Of particular importance is a history of an intraocular hemorrhage. It is important to know whether the patient has been previously diagnosed as having, or been treated for, the following: glaucoma, amblyopia, or episodes of ocular inflammation. A complete list of past and present eye medications, including the dosage and frequency of administration, is needed. Several ophthalmic medications have systemic side effects.

The past medical history may explain the ocular symptoms and signs.

The eyes are frequently involved in diseases affecting the rest of the body. The ocular manifestations in certain multisystem disorders may allow confirmation of the systemic disease. In some instances, eye involvement may be subtle enough to avoid detection unless the clinician knows to look for it. Specifically, the patient should be questioned for a history of diabetes, hypertension, stroke, cancer, thyroid disease, renal insufficiency, collagen vascular diseases, disorders of the skin and mucous membranes, and metabolic diseases.

A limited history of previous surgical procedures may be helpful. In particular, one should note procedures that may be a clue to associated ocular conditions. For example, cardiac valve replacement and carotid artery operations are frequently associated with embolic disease of the retinal circulation or with visual field defects due to embolic disease to the brain. A complete list of medications that are being used is necessary for the evaluation of possible ophthalmic side effects. A complete list of drug allergies is appropriate.

The family history helps the physician to unravel the ocular symptoms and signs.

Because glaucoma has a strong hereditary component, each patient should be specifically questioned about the presence of glaucoma in family members. A specific history of retinal detachment, cataracts, or macular degeneration may be helpful to know. Because most causes of night blindness (*retinitis pigmentosa*) and color blindness (*achromatopsia*) are hereditary, it may be useful to obtain such a history in other family members.

The measurement of visual acuity should be part of every eye examination, regardless of symptoms.

The quantitative measurement of the distance vision of the eye is traditionally recorded as a *Snellen fraction*. The numerator is the testing distance. The denominator is the distance at which the smallest letter or object that can be seen subtends an angle of 5 minutes of arc at the nodal point of the eye (or, in simpler terms, the distance at which a normal eye can see the 20/20 letter). To see a letter of this size, however, the eye must be capable of resolving differences of 1 minute of arc (Fig. 2–1). The Snellen chart is made up of letters of graduated sizes, and the distance at which each letter subtends an angle of 5 minutes of arc is indicated along the side of the chart (Fig. 2–2).

The Snellen chart is situated 20 feet (6

meters) from the patient under adequate, diffuse illumination without glare. Each eye is examined separately. If the patient normally wears glasses, the test should be done both without and with the corrective lenses and recorded as "uncorrected" ("sc") and "corrected" ("cc"), respectively.

A common misconception is that 20/40 vision is "twice as bad" as 20/20 vision. In fact, in terms of visual efficiency, 20/40 is only 85% of normal. Visual efficiency estimates were adapted from a report by the Council on Eye

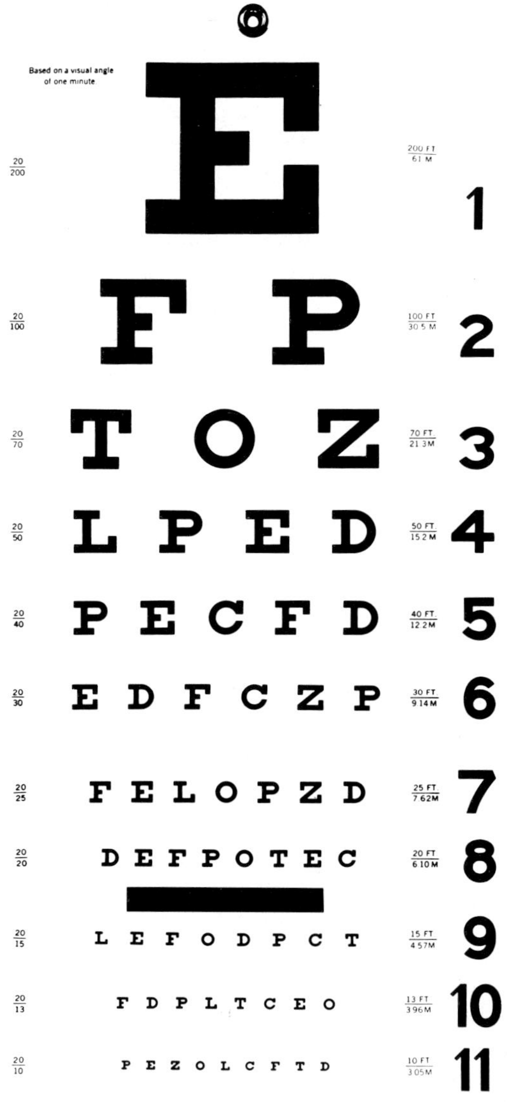

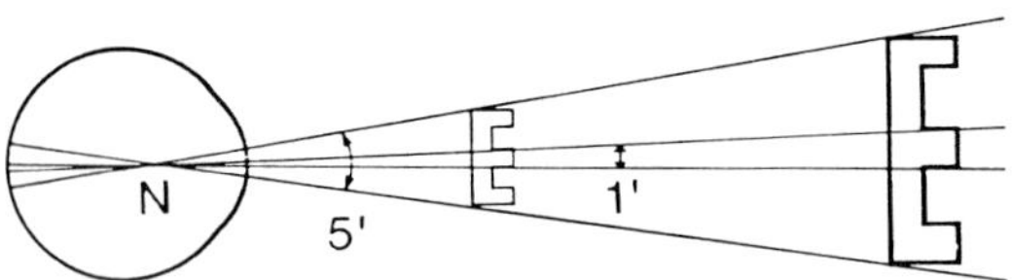

Fig. 2–1. Snellen distance acuity. Each letter subtends an angle of 5 minutes at a specific distance. Each detail of the letter subtends an angle of 1 minute. N is the nodal point.

TABLE 2–1 Distance Central Visual Acuity Notations

Snellen		Loss of central vision, %
English	*Metric*	
20/20	6/6	0
20/25	6/7.5	5
20/30	6/9	10
20/40	6/12	15
20/50	6/15	25
20/60	6/18	30
20/70	6/21	35
20/80	6/24	40
20/100	6/30	50
20/200	6/60	80
20/300	6/90	85
20/400	6/120	90

From Basic and Clinical Science Course 1987–1988. Section 2: Optics, Refraction, and Contact Lenses. San Francisco, American Academy of Ophthalmology, 1987. By permission of the publisher.

Health (Tables 2–1 and 2–2). Although 20/20 has arbitrarily been chosen as "normal" acuity, many persons have vision better than 20/20 (recorded as 20/15, 20/12, or 20/10).

If the patient is able to read all the letters on the 20/20 line, the vision is recorded as 20/20 (or 6/6 in metric measurement). If the patient sees all but two of the letters on the 20/20 line, it is recorded as 20/20−2. The notation 20/60+2 means that all of the 20/60 letters were read correctly in addition to two letters on the 20/50 line.

If the patient is unable to read the top "E" on the chart (20/400), the patient is moved closer to the chart until it can be read. The distance from the chart to the patient is recorded as the numerator in the Snellen fraction. The visual acuity would be 5/400, for example, if the patient was able to read the large "E" at 5 feet from the chart.

If the patient is unable to leave the examining chair, the distance at which the patient is able to count fingers is recorded. The examiner's fingers are approximately the size of the 20/200 letter. If, for example, the patient was able to count fingers at 5 feet, the recorded vision would be 5/200 or count fingers (CF) at 5 feet. If the patient is unable to count fingers, then the examiner should determine at what distance the patient is able to perceive hand motion (HM). For example, HM 3 feet means that the patient can accurately perceive hand motions at a distance no greater than 3 feet.

If the patient is unable to see hand motion, then it is necessary to determine whether the patient can perceive light. This testing is done by covering the fellow eye completely and holding a bright light in front of the eye in question. A convenient light source is the intense light of the indirect ophthalmoscope. If an eye is unable to perceive light, the examiner should record this as "no light perception" (NLP). If the patient is able to perceive light, it is recorded as "LP."

If the patient can perceive light, one should determine whether the patient is able to perceive the direction from which the light is being projected. This is done by covering the fellow eye completely and holding a light source in one of the quadrants in front of the eye to be examined. The patient is asked to identify the direction from which the light is entering the eye. If all the answers are consistently correct, the vision may be recorded as "light perception with accurate projection."

TABLE 2–2 Near Central Visual Acuity Notations

Type size		Near point	Loss of central vision, %
Snellen	*Jaeger*		
14/14	1−	3	0
14/18	2−	4	0
14/21		5	5
14/28	3	6	10
14/35	6	8	50
14/45	7−	9+	60
14/56	8	12	80
14/70	11	14	85
14/112	14	22	95

From Basic and Clinical Science Course 1987–1988. Section 2: Optics, Refraction, and Contact Lenses. San Francisco, American Academy of Ophthalmology, 1987. By permission of the publisher.

The pinhole test helps to identify uncorrected refractive errors.

The *pinhole* vision is tested if the visual acuity is worse than 20/30 in an eye. A pinhole

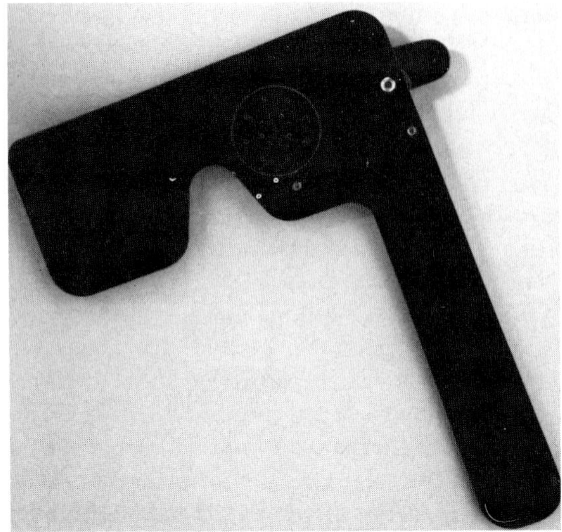

Fig. 2–3. Pinhole aperture used to test visual acuity. The optical diameter of the pinhole aperture for general clinical purposes (refractive errors from −5 D to +5 D) is 1.2 mm. For refractive errors greater than 5 diopters, a lens that corrects most of the refractive error, in addition to the pinhole, is necessary to obtain useful pinhole visions.

aperture is placed in front of the eye to ascertain any improvement in acuity (Fig. 2–3). The use of a pinhole compensates for any uncorrected refractive error, such as nearsightedness, farsightedness, or astigmatism. A patient with a refractive error, but without other abnormality, should have a visual acuity of 20/25 or better reading through the pinhole. The diffraction of light through the pinhole often prevents the 20/20 line from being seen. For example, a patient who has a visual acuity (Va) of 20/40 improves the acuity to 20/25 with the pinhole (PH); this result should be recorded as Va 20/40, PH 20/25. If the visual acuity fails to improve with the pinhole, the examiner should suspect a cause other than refractive error for the reduced vision, such as media opacities, retinal disorders, or optic nerve disease.

Occasionally, a patient may have extremely poor vision due to the presence of an opaque media that prevents the examiner from viewing the retina. In this case, the examiner can demonstrate retinal function if the patient can project light. Accurate light projection, unfortunately, does not predict the presence or absence of macular function. Macular function, however, may be tested in the presence of opaque media by using *entoptic phenomenon*. To do this, the patient sits with the eyes closed as the examiner massages the eyeball gently with the lighted end of a small flashlight. The patient is then asked to describe what is seen. If the macula is functioning properly, the patient will see a red central area surrounded by retinal blood vessels; this is often described as "cracked mud" or "veins in a leaf." If macular function is impaired, the central area will be dark rather than red, and no blood vessels will be seen. Disadvantages of this test are that it is highly subjective and it is difficult for some elderly people to comprehend.

The visual acuity of preschool children or patients who are unable to read may be tested with the illiterate *E chart*, consisting entirely of the letter E facing in different directions (Fig. 2–4). In this test, the child is taught to point a finger in the same direction as the bars of the E. The average 3- to 4-year-old child can cooperate satisfactorily with this test. For children younger than this, Allen cards may be used (Fig. 2–5). Identification of the various pictures on the Allen cards allows quantification of acuity to the level of 20/30.

Fig. 2–4. Snellen letter E. The letter is presented in different directions and sizes. The patient is asked to point a finger in the same direction as the bars of the E.

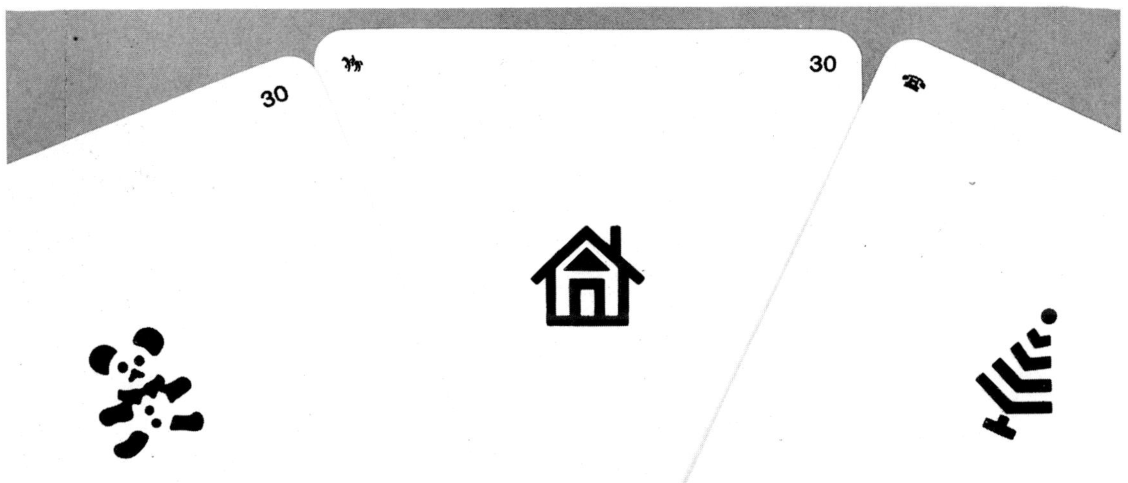

Fig. 2–5. Allen picture cards. This test comes in several formats: distance projection, near card, or separate cards to be used at various distances.

Near vision should be tested with the patient's reading glasses or bifocals.

Near visual acuity is measured with the AMA reading card or other equivalent near cards. The patient should wear his or her reading glasses. The patient holds the card approximately 14 inches from the eye, and the vision is recorded for each eye separately. The vision can be recorded directly from the chart as 14/14, 14/24, or as Jaeger equivalent J-1, J-2. In patients older than 30 years, the distance at which the letters are seen most clearly should also be recorded. If a patient is unable to identify small letters at 14 inches (about 40 cm) but is able to read them better if the card is held farther away, then latent hyperopia or uncorrected presbyopia should be suspected.

Both pupils should constrict when light is shined into either eye.

The pupils should be inspected for size, shape, and reaction to direct and consensual light. If the light response is abnormal, then the pupillary reaction to accommodation should be examined.

The mechanics of testing are not difficult, but they must be scrupulously applied. The examiner should not stand in front of the patient, nor shine the light directly at the patient. He or she should stand with the light off to the side and have the patient look at a distant target to eliminate accommodation. The beam of light should be small enough that only one eye is stimulated at a time.

Normal pupil size ranges from 3 to 5 mm in room light. The pupils are larger in young, nearsighted, and blue-eyed people, and they are smaller in elderly persons and in persons with diabetes. Unequal pupil size (*anisocoria*) of up to 1 mm is a normal finding in 20% of the population, but it is abnormal if one or both pupils do not react promptly to light. If one is unsure of the anisocoria in bright illumination, one should test for it in semidarkness, observing the other conditions for correct testing of the pupils.

The pupil is normally round. In the absence of surgical manipulation, irregularity is almost always pathologic. The pupil may be irregular because of previous inflammation that has resulted in iris adhesions (posterior synechiae) to the lens. Irregularities due to colobomas of the iris are in the area of the fetal cleft, which is usually located inferonasally. Blunt trauma, iris tumors, syphilis, and surgical procedures can also distort the iris.

The afferent pupillary defect indicates optic nerve disease.

The speed and duration of the direct reaction to light of the two eyes are compared. Each pupil should contract to direct light and when light is shined in the pupil of the opposite side; the latter response is the consensual reaction to light.

The consensual response should be as brisk and as sustained as the response in the tested eye; if it is not, some degree of *afferent pupillary defect* (or *Marcus Gunn pupil*) is present, indicating damage to the optic nerve of the tested eye. This is most easily demonstrated by the *swinging flashlight test*, in which the light is rapidly alternated between the eyes and a paradoxic dilatation in the affected eye is observed (Fig. 2–6). The brain interprets the decrease in signals from the nerve with the conduction defect as it would if the intensity of the light were reduced, and thus both pupils dilate. The examiner must be careful not to elicit accommodation either by standing in front of the patient or by holding the light directly in front of the eye.

The afferent pupillary defect attests to the presence of a conduction defect, not to its time of onset. This defect lasts as long as there is a conduction difference between the two eyes.

The pupil constricts with the near response.

Reaction to accommodation is tested by holding a finger a few inches away from the eye being tested. The patient is then asked to look at a distant object and then directly at the finger. The pupil normally constricts when looking at the near object and dilates when looking at the distant object. Under normal

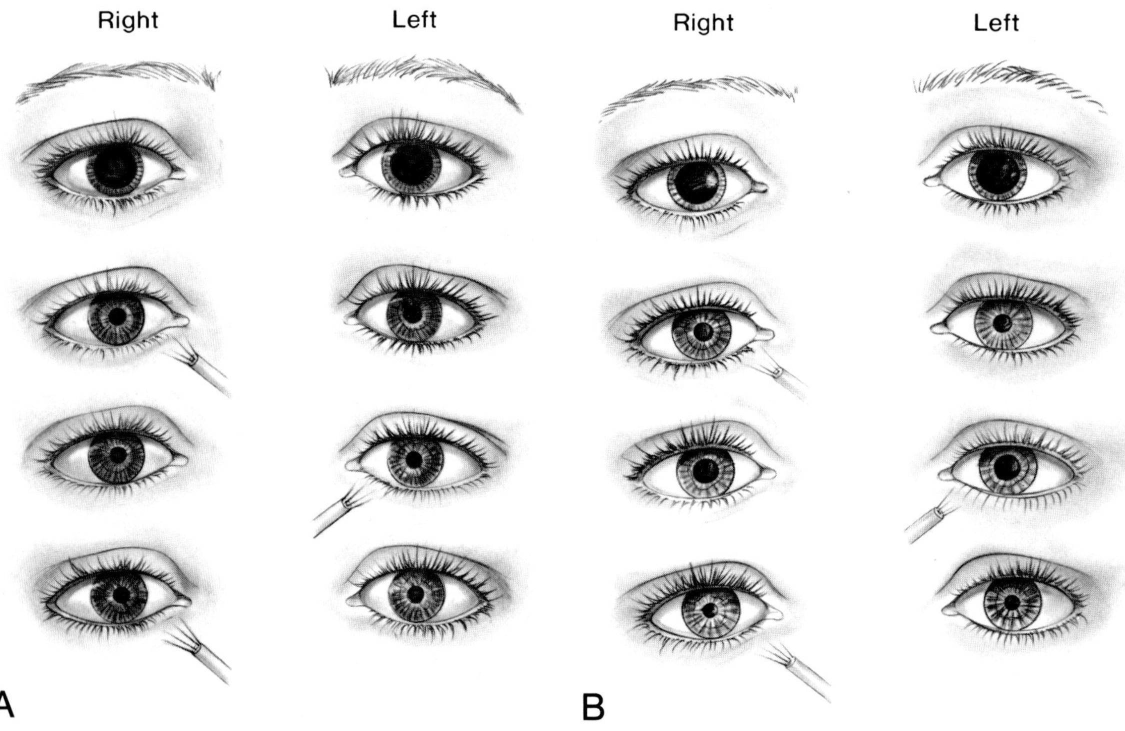

Fig. 2–6. Swinging flashlight test. *A*, Normal response to swinging flashlight test with no change in the size of the pupils. Note the consensual reaction to light. *B*, Afferent pupillary defect in the left eye. Both pupils constrict when light is shined in the right eye; however, when the flashlight is swung back to the left eye, both pupils dilate.

conditions, if the pupil reacts to light, it will react to accommodation also. Therefore, this does not need to be tested if the direct and consensual light responses are present. If the pupil does not react to light but does to accommodation, the condition is referred to as *light-near dissociation*. Light-near dissociation is found in Adie's pupil, Parinaud's syndrome, Argyll Robertson pupil, and bilateral optic neuropathy.

Careful examination of the external ocular structures may detect many important abnormalities.

Craniofacial abnormalities such as Down's syndrome or Crouzon's disease may be associated with ophthalmic findings. Any facial asymmetry, abnormal separation of the canthi (hypertelorism or hypotelorism) or abnormal inclination of the palpebral fissures (mongoloid or antimongoloid slant) should be noted.

Many craniofacial disorders are associated with ophthalmic findings.

Ptosis can be described as a condition in which the upper lid is at a lower position on the cornea than normal; it can be measured with the limbus or central light reflex used as reference points. The use of a straight edge is helpful to determine the difference between the two upper eyelid positions. In adults, the usual position of the upper eyelid margin is 1.5 mm below the upper limbus or 3 to 4 mm above the light reflex (the *margin reflex distance*). If the vertical distance from limbus to limbus is considered to be 11 mm, then 4 mm of ptosis would result in bisection of the center of the cornea or pupil by the lid margin.

The measurement of *levator function* is important in the evaluation of ptosis. The amount of excursion of the upper eyelid from maximal straight downgaze to maximal upgaze is determined with a millimeter rule (Fig. 2–7). A major error in evaluating the amount of

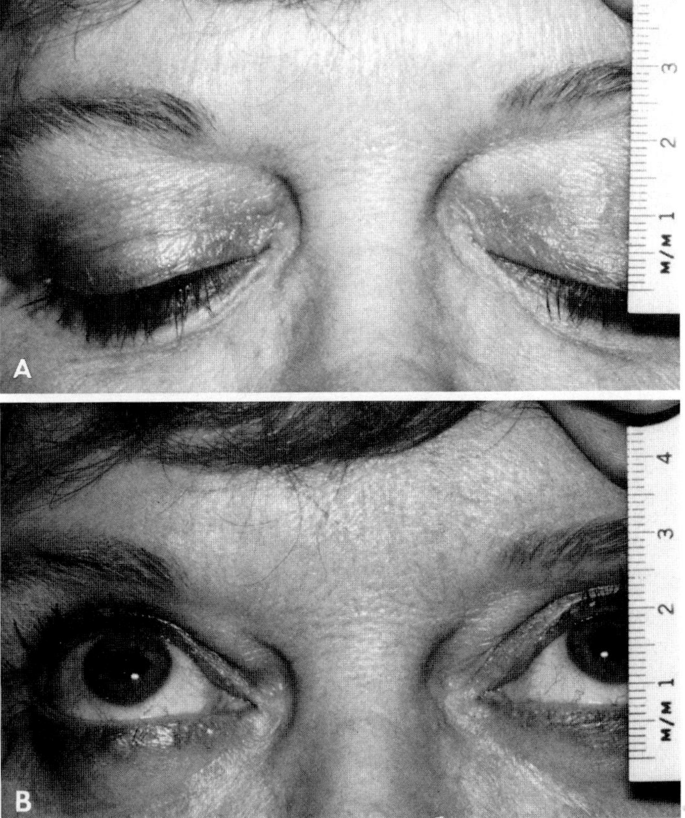

Fig. 2–7. Levator function (in this case, 20 mm) is measured by determining the excursion of the eyelid from downgaze (*A*) to upgaze (*B*).

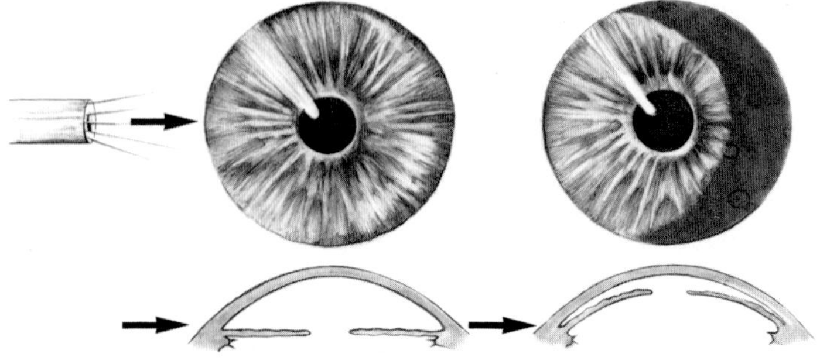

Fig. 2–8. Estimation of depth of anterior chamber by oblique illumination.

levator function occurs when the patient overcomes the ptosis by using the frontalis muscle. Contraction of the frontalis muscle adds 2 to 3 mm of lid elevation if the brow is uncontrolled. This error can be avoided if the examiner presses his or her thumb over the center of the patient's eyebrow while measuring. This method prevents the frontalis muscle action on the skin overlying the lid. The levator function is normally 10 mm or more.

Inversion (*entropion*) and eversion (*ectropion*) of the lids should be noted. Entropion should be distinguished from *trichiasis*; in the latter, the eyelid margin is properly positioned but ocular irritation occurs from misdirected eyelashes.

Proptosis refers to the forward displacement of the globe without regard to the width of the palpebral fissures. Quantitative measurements are made with an exophthalmometer (see page 203, Chapter 8), but an estimate can be made by comparing the corneal profiles from above the brow as the patient looks down. Asymmetry of more than 2 mm is clinically significant. Palpation and auscultation of the orbit are helpful in further diagnosis.

Opacity and clarity of the cornea are evaluated by examining the *corneal light reflex*. The reflex should be sharp and clear. A ground-glass appearance indicates diffuse corneal edema.

Anterior chamber depth is evaluated by projecting the beam of the light parallel to the iris plane from the temporal side (Fig. 2–8). If a shadow is cast on the nasal iris, some degree of anterior chamber narrowing is present. Caution should be used in dilating such eyes until gonioscopy (see pages 117 and 125, Chapter 5) is performed.

The conjunctiva and sclera are inspected for hyperemia, discharge, or abnormal pigmentation. The inferior cul-de-sac can be easily inspected by pressing down over the bony maxilla to pull the lid down with a finger and asking the patient to look up. The upper lid may be everted for inspection of the palpebral conjunctiva by having the patient look down while the examiner grasps the lashes, pulling down and out, and presses on the lid with a cotton-tipped applicator at the upper lid fold (that is, superior border of the tarsal plate) and

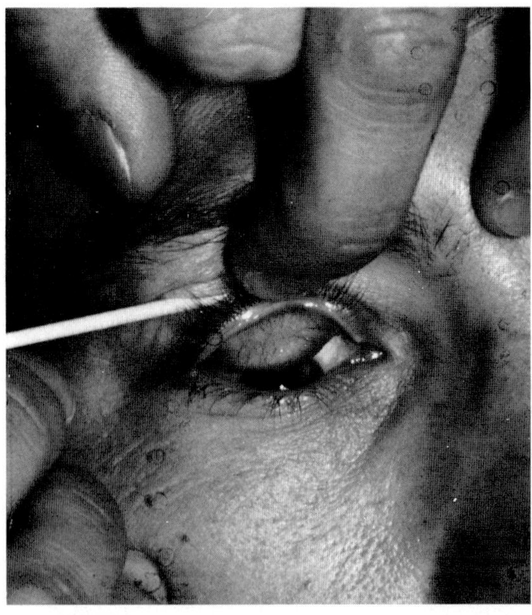

Fig. 2–9. Eversion of the upper eyelid; this may be done with or without topical anesthesia.

flips the lid over the applicator (Fig. 2–9). To restore the everted upper lid, the examiner simply asks the patient to look up and simultaneously pulls the lashes gently down.

The movement and alignment of the eyes, both individually and together, in all fields of gaze should be examined.

The *primary position of gaze* is the position assumed by the eyes when fixing at a distant object directly ahead. Secondary positions are any eye positions other than the primary; they include the six *cardinal positions* (Fig. 2–10).

The primary position of gaze may be ascertained by utilizing the corneal light reflex. The patient is asked to look directly at a hand light held in front of the eye. Normally, the corneal light reflex is slightly decentered nasally because the pupillary axis does not correspond to the visual axis. This angle between the visual and pupillary axis is referred to as the *angle kappa* (Fig. 2–11). Angle kappa is considered

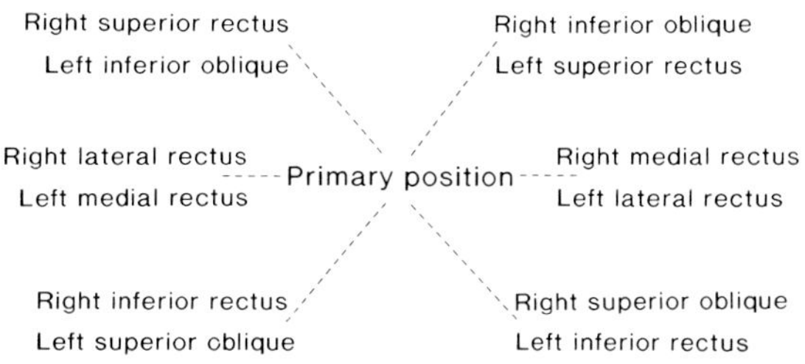

Fig. 2–10. The six cardinal positions of gaze and the yoke muscles in which primary actions are in that field of gaze. In each position, one muscle of each eye is the prime mover.

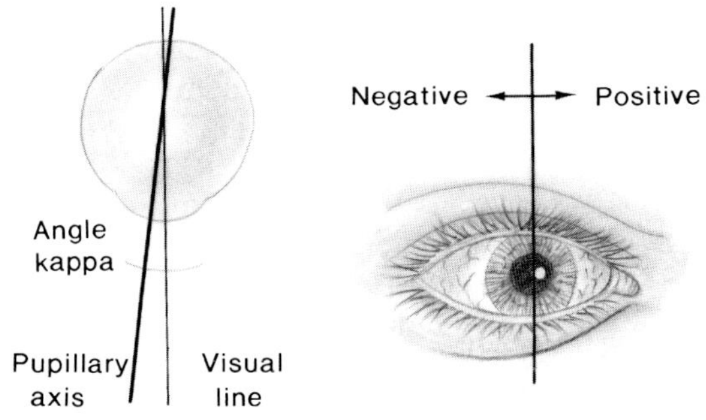

Fig. 2–11. Angle kappa (angle between visual and pupillary axis).

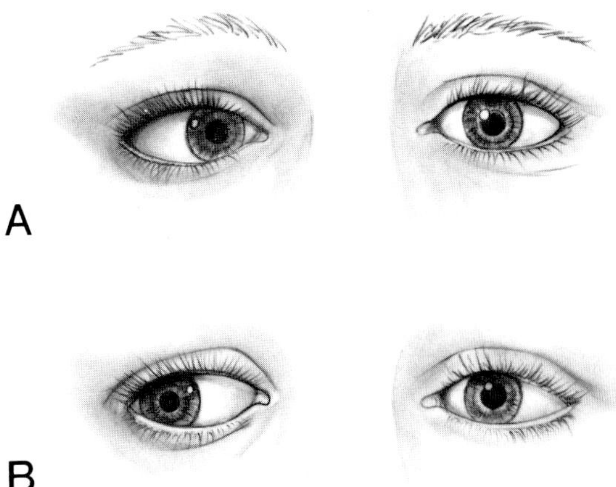

Fig. 2–12. Corneal light reflex. *A,* Esotropia. *B,* Exotropia.

positive if the corneal light reflex is nasal to the center of the cornea, and it is negative if the corneal light reflex is temporal to the center of the cornea. A positive angle kappa up to 5° is considered physiologic in orthophoric (straight) eyes.

Any gross asymmetry of light reflex in one eye will indicate deviation of that eye (Fig. 2–12). Location of the reflex on the nasal side of the cornea indicates that the eye is turned outward (*exotropia*); location of the reflex temporal to the central cornea indicates that the eye is deviated inward (*esotropia*). Each millimeter of deviation is equivalent to 7° or 15 Δ of deviation. One degree approximately equals 2 Δ.

Eyes that are perfectly aligned with no deviation even when fusion is artificially disrupted are *orthophoric*. *Heterophoria* is a misalignment in which fusion keeps the deviation latent. *Heterotropia*, however, is a manifest misalignment of the ocular axis. The presence or absence of heterophoria or heterotropia is best determined with the cover/uncover test.

In the *cover/uncover test*, each eye is covered and then uncovered to determine whether the fellow eye moves to refixate (Fig. 2–13). If the uncovered eye moves nasally to refixate, exotropia is present. If the uncovered eye moves temporally, esotropia is present. If the covered eye refixates as it is uncovered, then a phoria or latent deviation is present. If it moves nasally, exophoria is present; if it moves

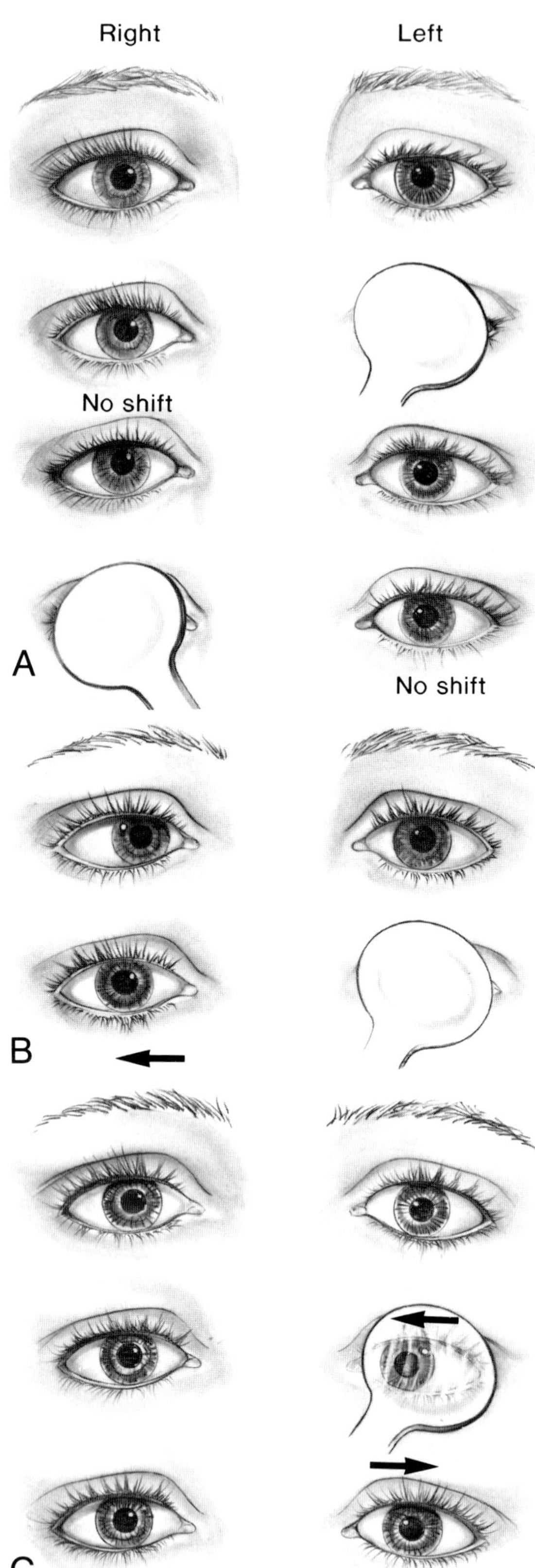

temporally, esophoria is present. The amount of vertical deviation (hyperphoria and hypophoria or hypertropia and hypotropia) is similarly noted.

The *alternate cover test* is used to measure the maximal deviation of a phoria or tropia by completely disrupting fixation. This is done by rapidly alternating the cover between the eyes. Small degrees of esodeviation and exodeviation can be detected by this method. A prism may then be used to neutralize the deviation, and a quantitative measurement of the strabismus can be obtained.

It is important to be aware that the alternate cover test does not distinguish between a phoria or tropia. Therefore, one must first perform the cover/uncover test to determine whether the deviation is a phoria or tropia. Then, the alternate cover test is performed to determine the amount of deviation, whether it be a phoria or tropia.

The *Maddox rod* test is another accurate method for measurement of a heterophoria or heterotropia. Like the alternate cover test, it does not distinguish between a phoria and a tropia. A Maddox rod consists of a series of thin, red glass cylinders placed side by side, usually mounted in a circular holder that is by convention held before the right eye (Fig. 2–14 *A*). A point source of light shined through this lens is seen as a red streak 90° away from the axis of the multiple cylinders of the rod. With the Maddox rod in front of the right eye, the left eye sees the white light directly, whereas the right eye views a red line. The Maddox rod disrupts fixation, and the separation of the red streak and the white light becomes a measurement of the deviation. Horizontal alignment can be checked by orientating the Maddox rod so that the red streak is vertical, and vertical alignment can be checked by orientating the rod so that the red streak is horizontal.

The patient views the fixating light with both eyes open. If the streak appears to run

Fig. 2–13. Cover/uncover test. *A*, Orthophoria: no movement is seen. *B*, Esotropia: the deviated right eye moves from adduction to primary (an outward shift). *C*, Esophoria: the newly uncovered eye makes a fusional divergence movement.

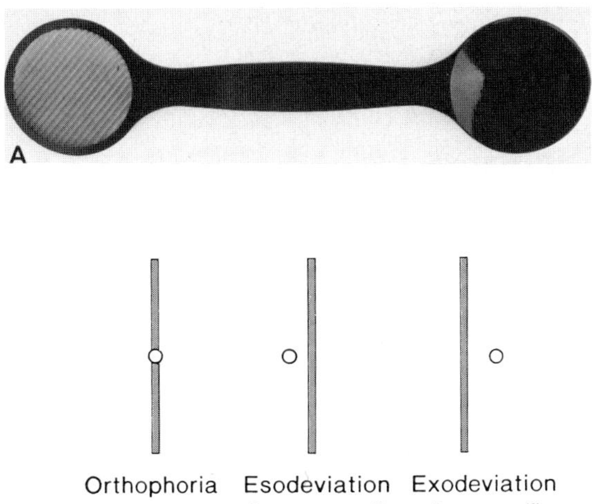

Fig. 2–14. *A*, Maddox rod. *B*, Maddox rod test. The left eye sees the white light directly, whereas the right eye sees a red line when the Maddox rod is held horizontally in front of the right eye.

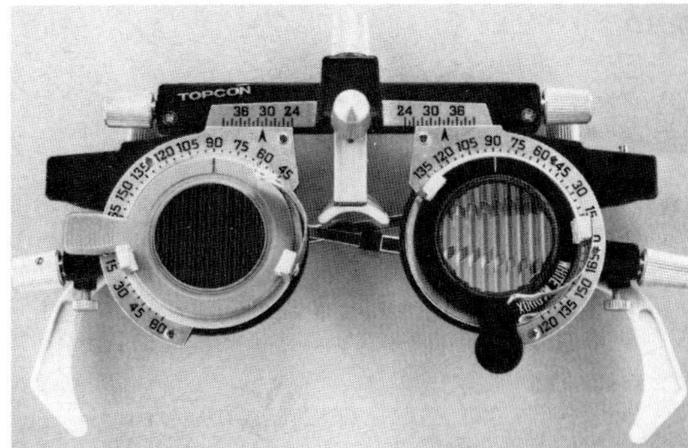

Fig. 2–15. Double Maddox rod.

through the center of the light both vertically and horizontally as the Maddox rod is turned, orthophoria is present in both directions. If the streak is displaced away from the light, either a phoria or tropia is present (Fig. 2–14 *B*). A prism can then be held in front of one eye and adjusted until the red line appears to pass through the white light. The power of such a prism reflects the angle of deviation.

With the Maddox rod held in front of the right eye, an esodeviation is present if the red streak is to the right of the white light, and an exodeviation is present if the red streak is to the left of the white light. The reasons for this effect are as follows. With the eye deviated nasally, as in an esodeviation, the image projects on a point nasal to the fovea. The visual direction of a point on the nasal retina, however, is temporal to the object of regard. Hence, with the Maddox rod in front of the right eye, an esodeviation is "uncrossed"; the red streak (right eye) is to the right of the white light (left eye). In an exodeviation the eye is deviated temporally and the image projects on a point temporal to fixation. The visual direction of this point, however, is nasal to the object of regard, and the resulting exodeviation is "crossed"; the red streak (right eye) is to the left of the white light (left eye).

The double Maddox rod test, in which a red Maddox rod is placed in front of one eye and a white Maddox rod is placed in front of the other eye, is useful to diagnose and to quantitate torsional diplopia from cyclodeviations (Fig. 2–15) (see page 257, Chapter 10).

Finally, the cardinal positions of gaze should be determined. The patient is asked to look in the six cardinal positions. The examiner should check for limitation of gaze in any direction or for double vision in any field of gaze due to limitation of one eye. Both monocular rotations (*ductions*) and the movement of both eyes together (*versions*) should be evaluated with particular attention to limitation or overaction in a gaze direction.

The normal peripheral visual field for each eye extends approximately 50° superiorly, 60° nasally, 70° inferiorly, and 90° temporally.

Confrontation peripheral field tests are a helpful technique if they are done properly and used when indicated. They are not a substitute for formal field tests, but they are helpful as a screening check or in bedside examinations. The examination is performed binocularly; the patient closes one eye and the examiner closes his or her own opposite eye. The patient is asked to fixate with one eye on the physician's

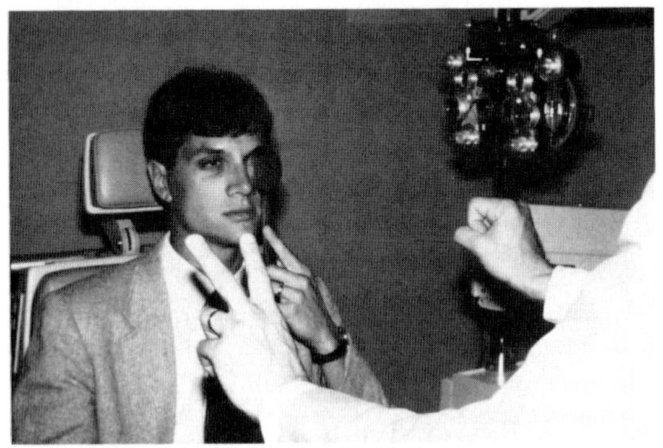

Fig. 2–16. Confrontation visual field test.

nose. The examiner then uses the field of his or her right eye as a standard for measuring the field in the patient's left eye and the field in his or her left eye for measuring the field in the patient's right eye. The examiner asks the patient to count the number of fingers on the hand that the physician presents successively to each of the four quadrants of the patient's eye (Fig. 2–16). If the patient is unable to count fingers, then the ability to perceive hand motion should be determined.

Next, the physician uses both hands simultaneously, presenting stimuli to both the nasal and temporal fields of an eye. Various combinations of fingers are presented. The patient is asked to indicate the number of fingers he or she sees. In addition to evaluating the fields, this also tests the patient's ability to calculate, which is a parietal lobe function, and the existence or absence of the extinction phenomenon. The patient with parietal lobe disease may miss half of the field because of the extinction phenomenon rather than a true field defect.

Finally, a more subtle confrontation test involves simultaneously presenting identically colored test objects to the patient's nasal and temporal fields. The red tops of two plastic tropicamide (Mydriacyl) or cyclopentolate (Cyclogyl) bottles can be used. The patient may say that the one cap is not colored or is a faded red or pink compared with the other cap. Such a response may indicate the presence of a subtle hemianopic defect.

Anyone with reduced central acuity has, by definition, a relative central scotoma or defect.

The *Amsler grid* can be used to detect central and paracentral defects encroaching on the central 10° of vision. The test is performed monocularly at 12 inches with the patient's attention directed to the central fixation point. The patient is asked whether any defect or distortion of the checkerboard pattern is present (see Fig. 7–5).

Formal visual field tests are performed with either a perimeter or a tangent screen.

Various sizes of test objects are presented from the nonseeing to the seeing areas. A focus of points describing the point at which the patient just detects the object is connected by lines. These concentric circles describe the field of vision. The field is always plotted "as the patient sees it." In the right eye, for example, the blind spot is located to the right of fixation because the optic nerve is located nasal to the fovea and projects temporally. Visual field testing is discussed in greater detail in Chapters 5 and 7.

The slit lamp allows a binocular, three-dimensional, magnified view of the anterior and posterior segments.

The slit-lamp biomicroscope consists of a microscope and special light source, both capable of rotating around a common axis (Fig. 2–17). The image view through the microscope can be kept in focus with the light source. Using the biomicroscope, one can examine the anterior ocular structures to the depth of the anterior vitreous. In addition, the fundus can be visualized binocularly with the Hruby lens or 90 D lens in conjunction with the slit lamp.

The slit-lamp light source can be gradually varied from a wide beam, flooding most of the corneal surface, to a narrow beam or an optical section. With an optical section, living tissue

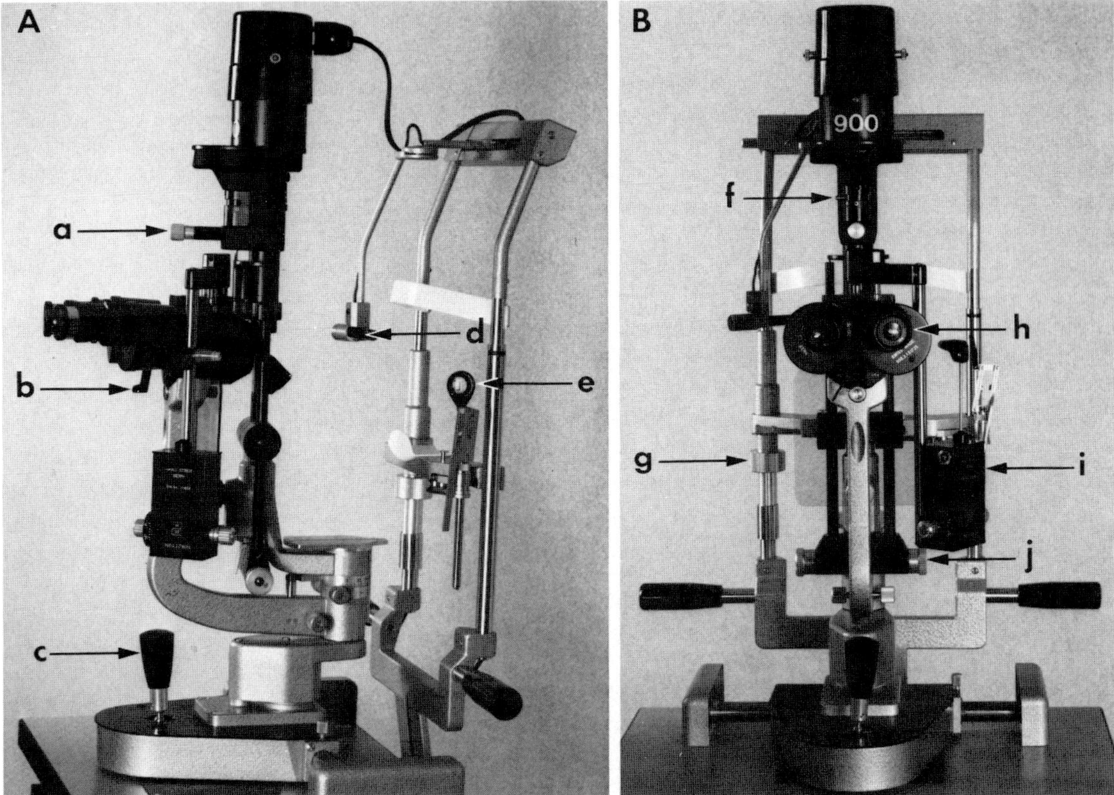

Fig. 2–17. Haag-Streit slit lamp. *A*, View of side. *a*, Control for rotation of slit and for varying the slit length. *b*, Lever for changing magnification. *c*, Control lever for horizontal and vertical adjustment. *d*, Fixation light. *e*, Hruby lens. *B*, View from front. *f*, Lever for three filters. *g*, Adjustment control for chin rest. *h*, Interchangeable eyepieces (10×, 16×). *i*, Goldmann tonometer. *j*, Control for setting slit width.

and the cornea-lens relationship can be examined as though being viewed in cross section.

There are six methods of illumination with the slit lamp.

Specific abnormal features are best revealed by certain types of illumination. For features to be detailed best, it is necessary to know the six various types of illumination and their uses. With *diffuse illumination*, the light is shown on the eye with a wide slit and the illuminated area is viewed through the microscope. This is most useful for gross examination of the cornea with microscopic magnification (Fig. 2–18 *A*). *Direct focal illumination* is a section method of illuminating individual layers of the anterior portion of the eye. The beam of light is focused

in the same way as the microscope-illuminated features of the cross-section studied. This is useful for detection of corneal staining, foreign bodies, and stromal and epithelial abnormalities (Fig. 2–18 *B*). With *indirect illumination* the slit is directed so that scattered light illuminates the area under examination. The operator can view objects not in the direct beam of light. By directing the light on the sclera, the examiner can evaluate pterygia involving the cornea (Fig. 2–18 *C*). It is the illumination of choice for detection of aqueous flare. Cells or increased protein in the aqueous (Tyndall phenomenon) is visible with ordinary illumination and magnification using the narrow beam of indirect light.

Retroillumination is used for examining a transparent structure against an illuminated

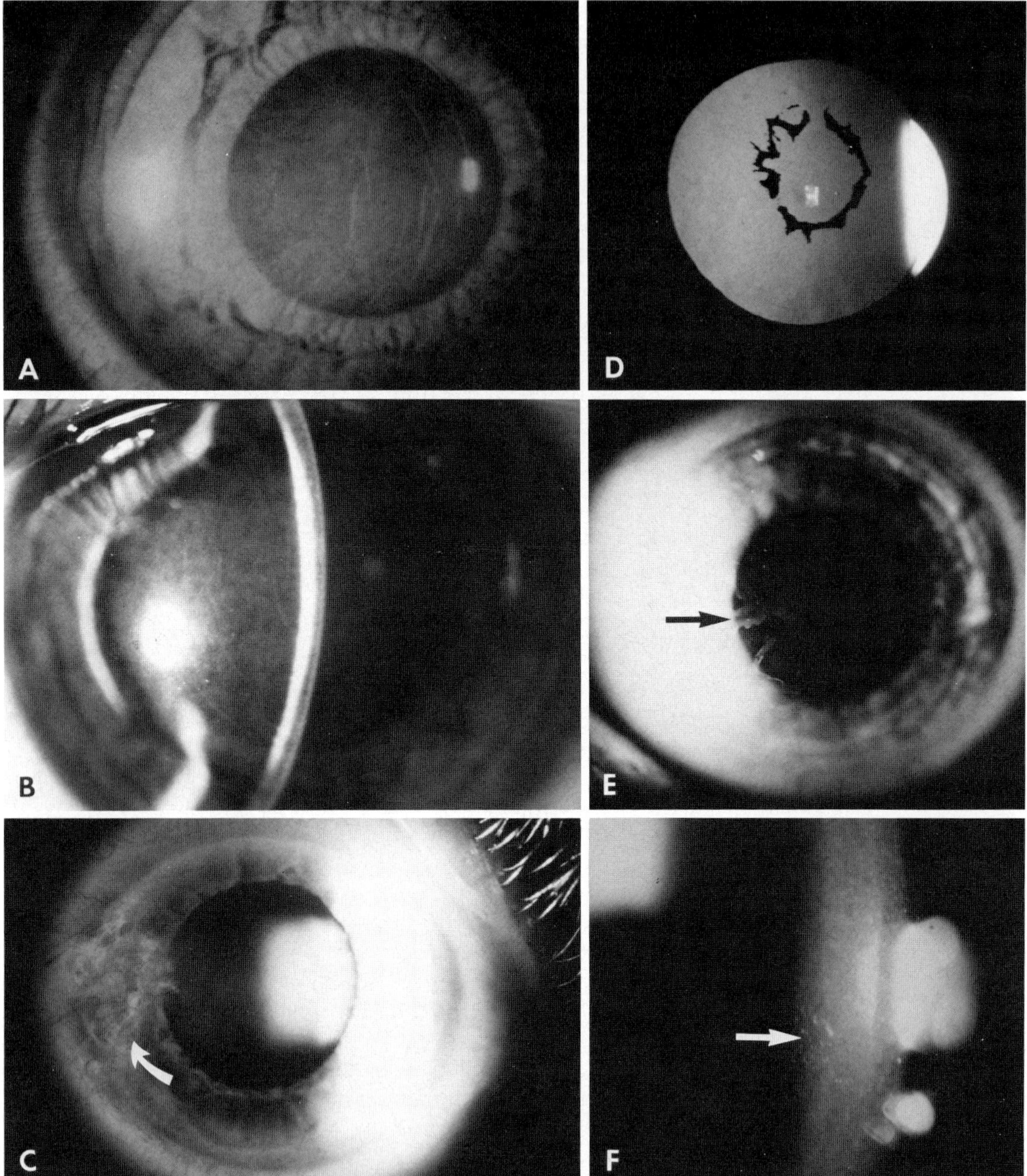

Fig. 2–18. Types of slit-lamp illumination. *A*, Diffuse illumination of interstitial keratitis. *B*, Direct focal illumination of interstitial keratitis. *C*, Indirect illumination of a pterygium (*arrow*). *D*, Retroillumination of a pigment ring on the anterior lens capsule. *E*, Sclerotic scatter of an anterior basement membrane dystrophy (*arrow*). *F*, Specular reflection of endothelial cells (*arrow*).

background. The light beam is reflected off a solid body with the eye (iris, retina) creating an effect of having the light source behind the object to be observed. This technique is invalu-able for observing lenticular opacities and iris transillumination defects (Fig. 2–18 *D*). With *sclerotic scatter illumination*, a wide beam of light is directed at the temporal limbus. Some of the light will be internally reflected in the substance of the cornea. Any deviation in transparency of the cornea will be seen by the observer. With this method, corneal edema is easily detected (Fig. 2–18 *E*). *Specular reflection* is a type of illumination useful for observing endothelial cells in a limited area. The light is directly reflected from the cornea and the microscope is focused on the area from which the light is being reflected so that the light that is directly reflected is viewed through the microscope. High magnification is necessary (Fig. 2–18 *F*).

Special dyes instilled in the tear film may be used to help detect ocular abnormalities with the slit lamp.

Fluorescein can be used to detect epithelial defects, and *rose bengal* can be used to detect dead and dying cells on the ocular surface. With fluorescein, a cobalt filter is used to delineate clearly the areas of epithelial absence. A white light is used for assessing rose-bengal staining.

The pressure inside the eye is most accurately measured by applanation tonometry.

Gross approximation of intraocular pressure may be made by palpation of the eyeball through closed lids (*tactile tension*). The patient is asked to look down, and the examiner places two forefingers on the upper lid over the globe, exerting pressure alternately with each forefinger while the other rests on the globe. Pressure just sufficient to indent the globe slightly should be applied. Only rough approximations such as soft, normal, or hard can be made. This method of determining intraocular pressure should be used only for persons who cannot cooperate for quantitative pressure measurement.

Accurate intraocular pressure may be determined with tonometers. All clinical tonometers measure the intraocular pressure by relating a deformation of the globe to the force responsible for the deformation. There are two basic types of tonometers, which differ according to the shape of the deformation: 1) indention tonometers (Schiøtz tonometer) and 2) applanation tonometers (Goldmann and Perkins tonometers).

The *Schiøtz tonometer* uses a weighted plunger that indents the cornea and displaces a volume of fluid within the eye (Fig. 2–19). The amount of indentation is measured on the tonometer's scale in twentieths of a millimeter. The scale reading is then converted to an estimation of intraocular pressure in millimeters of mercury according to tables supplied with the instrument. Schiøtz tonometry now is rarely used in ophthalmic practice, but it is important to understand the technique and its underlying principles.

After instillation of a local anesthetic, such as one drop of tetracaine, the patient is placed in the supine position and fixation is directed

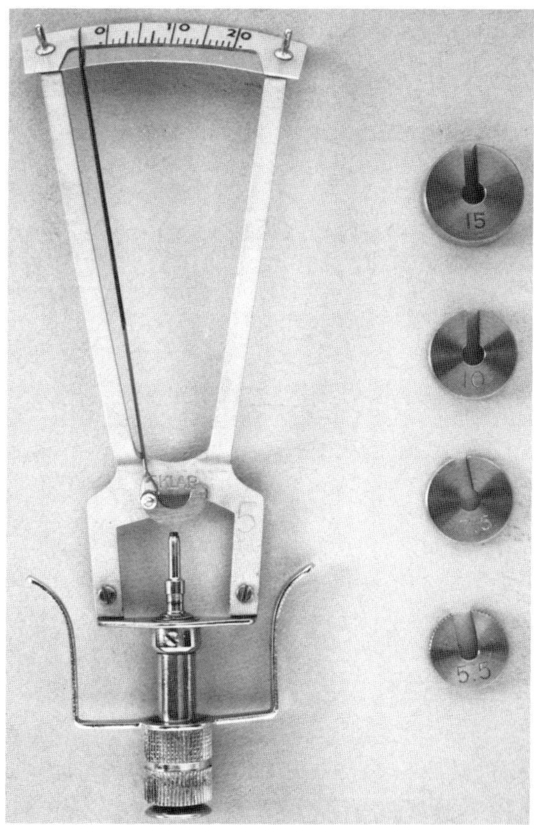

Fig. 2–19. Schiøtz tonometer (left) and weights (right).

to the ceiling. The physician separates the lids to keep them from touching the eyeball, taking care not to exert pressure on the globe with the fingers. Any pressure on the lids will falsely elevate the intraocular pressure. The instrument is then placed gently in a vertical position directly over the cornea and the plunger is allowed to exert its full weight. A reading between 5 and 7 with the 5.5-g weight indicates normal intraocular pressure. A reading less than 4 indicates elevated pressure (less indentation). Readings less than 3 are inaccurate with a 5.5-g weight, and a 7.5-g weight should be added and the testing repeated.

If an eye is very elastic with a low ocular rigidity (for example, in high myopia), it may undergo more than average expansion as the volume is displaced, giving a falsely low intraocular pressure. If the eye is very rigid with a high ocular rigidity (for example, in thyroid ocular disease), a falsely high measurement may be obtained. Applanation tonometery is more accurate in such cases.

Applanation tonometry for measuring intraocular pressure may be performed with an applanation tonometer mounted on a slit-lamp biomicroscope (*Goldmann*) (Fig. 2–17 *B*) or with a hand-held applanation tonometer (*Perkins*) (Fig. 2–20). Applanation tonometers flatten a small area of the cornea. Because the shape of deformation is constant, its relationship to the intraocular pressure can, in most cases, be derived from mathematical calculations. The applanation tonometer has two beam-splitting prisms within the applanating unit that optically convert the circular area of corneal contact into semicircles. The prisms are adjusted so that the margins of the semicircles overlap when 3.06 mm² of cornea is applanated.

The technique is the same for either the Goldmann or the Perkins tonometer. First, the tear film is stained with sodium fluorescein, and the cornea and biprism are illuminated with a cobalt blue light. The resulting fluorescence of the fluorescein stain facilitates visualization of the meniscus at the margin of contact between the cornea and biprism. On contact and with the cobalt blue light in place, two fluorescein semicircles are seen through the microscope, and the force against the

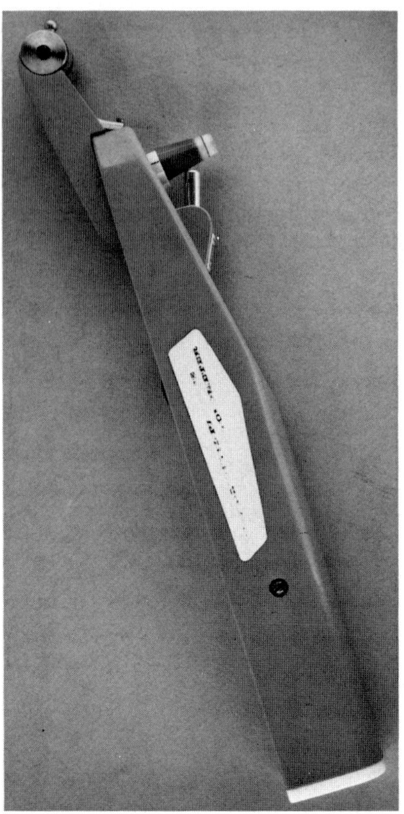

Fig. 2–20. Perkins applanation tonometer.

cornea is adjusted until the inner edges overlap (Fig. 2–21). The intraocular pressure is then read directly from a scale on the tonometer housing.

Common sources of error include 1) too much fluorescein, which creates a wider meniscus and thus results in falsely higher pressure estimates; 2) pressure on the eyelids or eye, which gives a falsely higher pressure estimate; 3) improper vertical alignment (one semicircle larger than the other), leading to falsely high intraocular pressure estimates; and 4) an irregular cornea distorting the semicircles and interfering with the accuracy of the intraocular pressure estimates.

The Perkins applanation tonometer uses the same biprism as the Goldmann applanation tonometer. The light source is powered by a battery instead of an electrical current. In both, the force is varied manually. In contrast to the Goldmann instrument, the Perkins

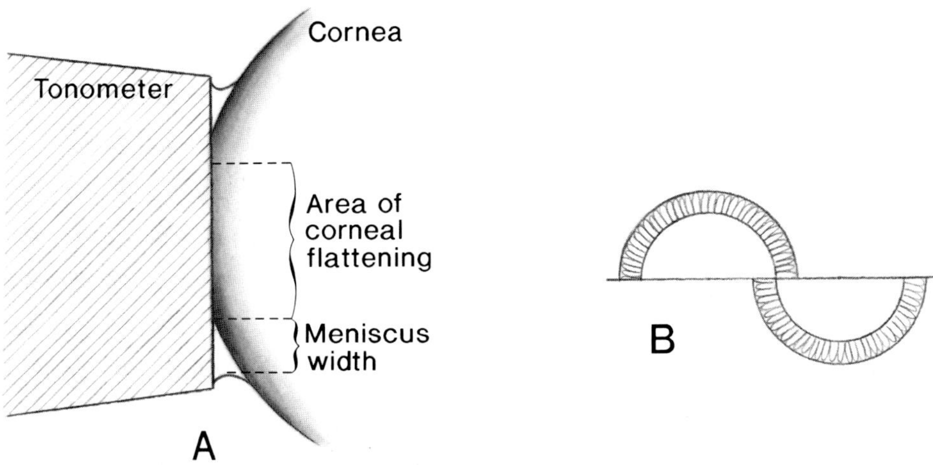

Fig. 2–21. *A*, The applanation tonometer measures the force necessary to flatten an area of the cornea that has a diameter of 3.06 mm². Fluorescein in the tear film is used to outline the area of flattening. *B*, An accurate intraocular pressure is determined when the inner edges of the semicircles, representing the fluorescein-filled tear meniscus, are aligned.

tonometer is a hand-held instrument with a counterbalance that makes it possible to use the instrument in either the vertical or the horizontal position. As a result, it is invaluable for bedside examinations.

With the *Mackay-Marg tonometer*, the measured force is that which is required to keep the flat plate of a plunger flush with a surrounding sleeve against the pressure of corneal deformation. The force required to keep the plate flush with the sleeve is electronically monitored and recorded on a paper strip. It has its greatest use in patients with corneal scarring or altered corneal shape such that conventional Schiøtz or applanation tonometers cannot be used with accuracy.

The advantage of an *"air-puff" tonometer* is that it does not touch the eye other than with a puff of air. A puff of room air creates a constant force, which momentarily deforms the cornea. The time from an internal reference point to the moment of presumed flattening is measured and converted to intraocular pressure on the basis of prior comparisons with readings from Goldmann applanation tonometers.

The patient sits with his or her head in a slit-lamp-like device, and a 3-msec puff of air (a blink takes 10 msec) is blown against the cornea. The indentation pattern is detected by the tonometer. The pressure is calculated from the amount of corneal flattening by the fixed air-puff pressure and displayed on a digital readout.

It is recommended that a minimum of three readings within 3 mm Hg be taken and averaged as the intraocular pressure. The noncontact tonometers are reliable within the normal intraocular pressure range, although the reliability is reduced in the higher-pressure ranges and is limited by an abnormal cornea or poor fixation. Applanation tonometry is by far the most commonly used technique in ophthalmic practice to measure intraocular pressure.

Direct ophthalmoscopy provides an enlarged, upright view of the retina (and more).

The basic principle of direct ophthalmoscopy is simple. If the patient's eye is emmetropic, light rays emanating from a point in the fundus emerge as a parallel beam. If this beam enters the pupil of an emmetropic observer, the rays are focused on the observer's retina and an image is formed. The direct ophthalmoscope uses this principle by utilizing a strong light that can be directed into the patient's eye by reflection from a small mirror. The light is then reflected from the fundus of the pa-

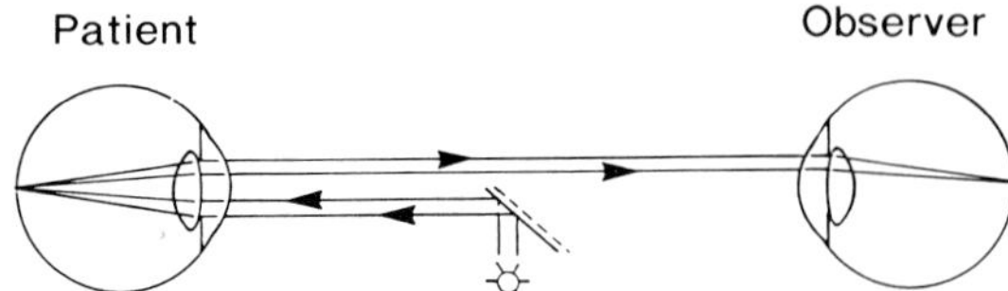

Fig. 2–22. Illumination method in direct ophthalmoscopy.

tient's eye back through a small aperture in the ophthalmoscope through the examiner's eye (Fig. 2–22). Therefore, the direct ophthalmoscope needs to have only an appropriate light source for illumination and lenses interposed between the patient and the observer to neutralize any refractive error of the observer or the patient plus any accommodation exerted by either. The lenses in the ophthalmoscope are black for plus or farsightedness and red for minus or nearsightedness.

The limiting factors in direct ophthalmoscopy are the degree of dilatation of the patient's pupil (increasing the angular size of the visible fundus) and the proximity of the observer to the patient (increasing the axial magnification of the image). The patient's pupil should, therefore, be widely dilated and the examiner positioned as close as possible to the patient.

The technique of ophthalmoscopy must be mastered.

The aperture of the direct ophthalmoscope is held as close as possible to the observer's eye and the subject's eye. The details of the fundus will then be in focus if both eyes are emmetropic. If either eye is ametropic, a graduated series of plus (convex) or minus (concave) lenses can be moved into the aperture by rotating the lens wheel with one finger. The examiner's right eye should be used to examine the patient's right eye, and the examiner's left eye should be used to examine the left eye. The patient should not be wearing glasses and should be fixating on a distant target while keeping his or her eyes as steady as possible.

The first step in ophthalmoscopy is to look for the red fundus reflection. The red reflex is due to parallel beams of light that are focused on a retinal point and reflected back in the same identical direction. To observe the red reflex, the examiner must be directly aligned with these parallel bundles of reflected light. The red reflex can be seen without magnification from a comfortable distance of 25 to 40 cm. The experienced examiner, when seeing a fundus reflection, can immediately rule out gross corneal lesions, dense opacities of the media, and total retinal detachments. If opacities are present, they will appear as black forms against the red background.

Once the examiner has visualized the red reflex, the ophthalmoscope should be moved as close to the patient's eye as possible. Black or positive lenses are then introduced into the aperture of the ophthalmoscope. Lens settings of +8 to +10 will focus the ophthalmoscope on the anterior segment to reveal corneal opacities or changes in the iris and lens.

As the examiner gradually rotates the lens wheel to bring lenses from +8 to +4 D into the aperture, the focus extends posteriorly into the vitreous. Vitreous opacities may occur as a result of inflammatory disease (uveitis), degenerative changes (asteroid hyalosis, posterior vitreous detachment), and hemorrhage.

A fundus examination includes inspection of the optic disc, macula, retinal vessels, and peripheral retina. If the patient has high myopia, the magnification of the image is increased; with high hyperopia, it is decreased. The retina can be examined with the direct ophthalmoscope as far anteriorly as the equator in patients with widely dilated pupils. The area from the equator to the ora serrata, however, can be examined adequately only with the binocular indirect ophthalmoscope or a three-mirror contact lens with the slit lamp.

The optic nerve head should be brought into focus and examined first (Fig. 2–23). The disc size, color, vascularity, and degree of cupping should be assessed. The optic nerve is generally round or oval and pink. The nasal edge is less distinct than the temporal edge. A white crescent may appear around the temporal edge, especially in myopic patients.

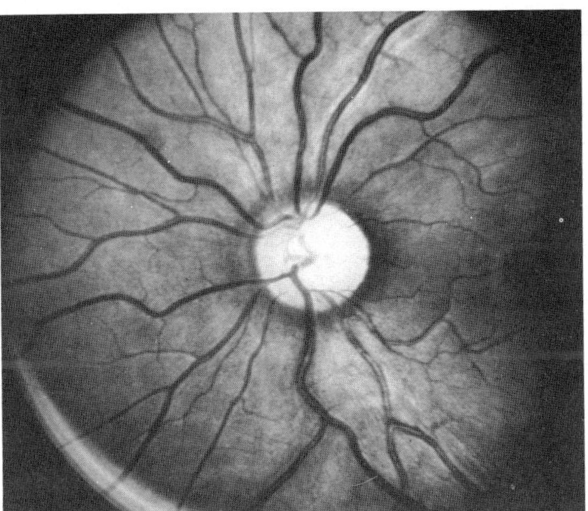

Fig. 2–23.   Normal optic nerve head.

This is formed by exposure of the sclera between the choroidal vasculature and the opening of the optic nerve. There may be excessive pigmentation in this area due to the presence of choroidal pigmentation.

The optic disc usually has a white central depression that is referred to as the physiologic cup. The bottom of this may be "dotted" (laminar dots) in appearance and represents the opening in the lamina cribrosa of the sclera. Normal cupping varies considerably in normal patients, but the average diameter is approximately one-third or less of the disc diameter. This is referred to as the cup/disc ratio and should be noted on the patient's record (for example, C/D = 0.3). In some patients, the optic nerve head may appear elevated. This condition may be pathologic (papilledema) or physiologic (hyperopia, optic nerve drusen) (Fig. 2–24). In either case, the height of disc swelling can be roughly approximated by knowing that each diopter corresponds to approximately ⅓ mm axial length. Therefore, 3 D of disc swelling would be approximately 1 mm in height.

The macula is an oval area located about 2 disc diameters temporal and slightly inferior to the optic nerve head (Fig. 2–25). It appears darker than the surrounding retina because of xanthophyll pigment. Centrally located is a small, yellow light reflex due to the slightly depressed center of the fovea (umbo). This foveal reflex dulls with age and with certain drug-induced retinal toxicities.

The periphery of the fundus may be examined by moving the ophthalmoscope in various directions and asking the patient to move his or her eye in various quadrants. Any fundus

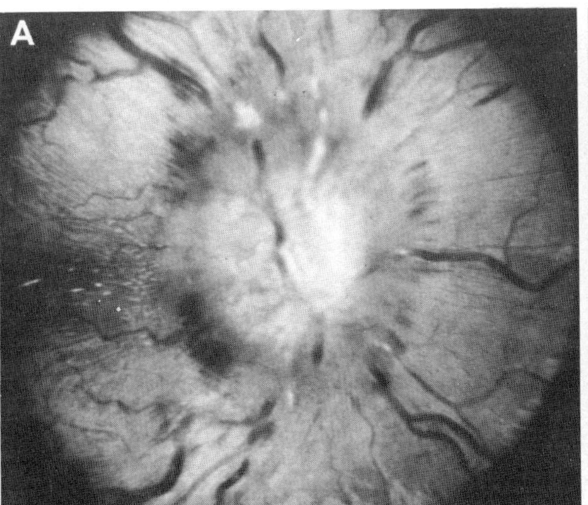
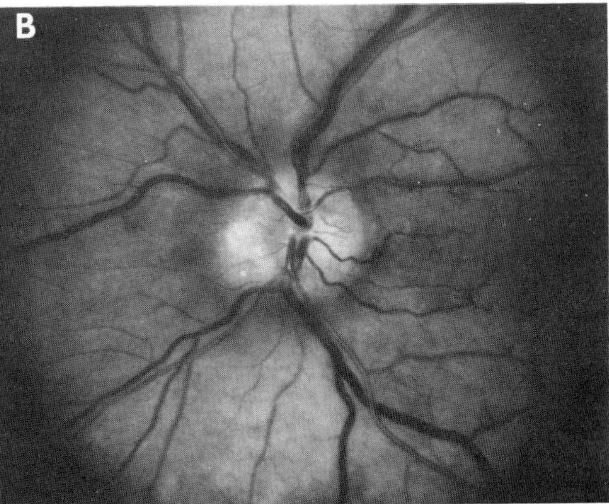

Fig. 2–24.   *A*, Papilledema. Disc margin blurred with obscuration of underlying vessels. Note associated nerve fiber layer hemorrhages and cotton-wool spots. *B*, Optic disc drusen. The nasal disc is full in appearance secondary to underlying disc drusen.

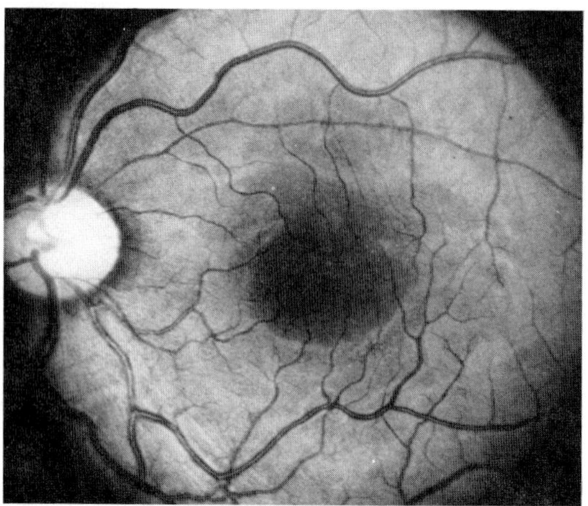

Fig. 2–25. Normal macula.

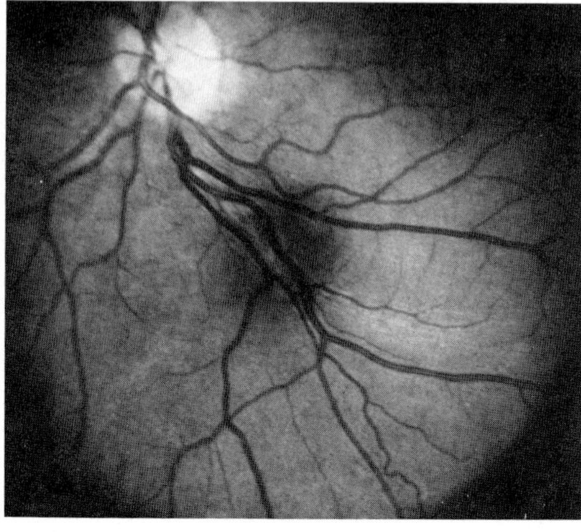

Fig. 2–26. Choroidal nevus. This nevus is adequately described as being 1 disc diameter in size and located 1 disc diameter inferotemporal to the optic nerve head.

lesion should be noted and described. Its size can be recorded using the diameter of the disc as a reference size (Fig. 2–26).

Retinal arteries and veins should be carefully examined. The arteries are redder and smaller in caliber than the veins in approximately a 4:5 ratio. Arteries and veins frequently cross each other. However, arteries never cross arteries and veins never cross veins. The examiner should evaluate such things as the transparency of the vessels, the presence of focal narrowing of the arterioles, the presence of tortuosity and widening of the venules, the presence of pressure effects such as arterial venous compression (nicking) where vessels cross each other, and hemorrhages or exudates around the vessels. Hemorrhages in the nerve fiber layer of the retina obscure the retinal vessels. Deeper intraretinal hemorrhages, in contrast, can be seen beneath the retinal vessels (Fig. 2–27).

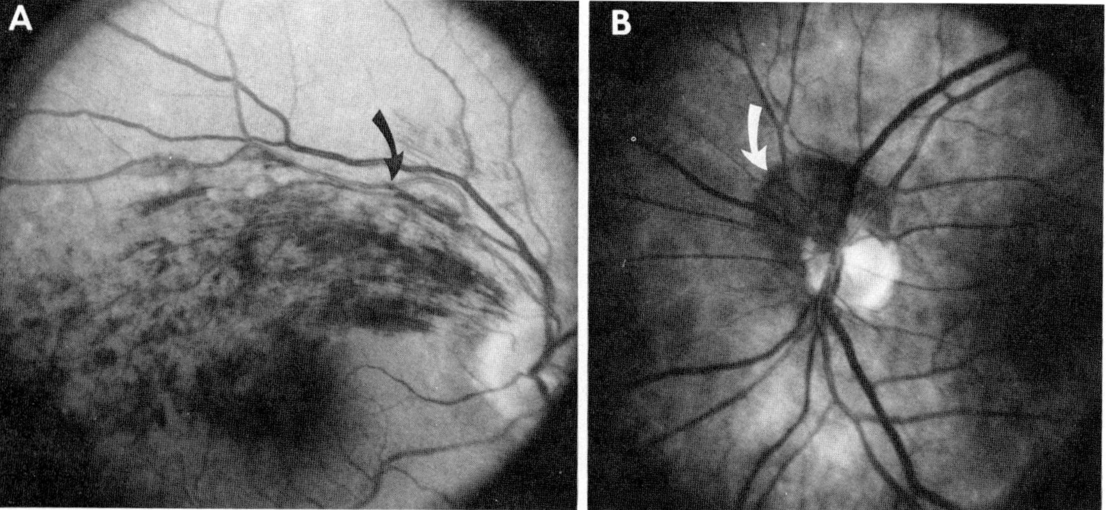

Fig. 2–27. *A*, Hemorrhage in the nerve fiber layer that obscures the underlying retinal vessels (*arrow*). *B*, Subretinal hemorrhage (*arrow*) is seen beneath the retinal vessels.

Indirect ophthalmoscopy provides a binocular, panoramic view of the retina.

Indirect ophthalmoscopy involves the use of a head-mounted, prism-directed light source coupled with the use of a hand-held condensing lens (usually +20 D) (Fig. 2–28).

For stereoscopic visualization, both eyes of the observer must receive light from the aerial image. For this to occur, two criteria must be met. First, the patient's pupil must be as widely dilated as possible. Cyclopentolate (Cyclogyl; 1%), tropicamide (Mydriacyl; 1%), and phenylephrine (Neo-Synephrine; 2.5%), or a combination eyedrop (Cyclomydril) of cyclopentolate and phenylephrine, is usually adequate. Second, the observer's interpupillary distance must be reduced. This interpupillary distance is reduced optically from 65 mm to 15 mm by the use of prisms in the headpiece.

Although most indirect ophthalmoscopes are designed for use through dilated pupils, some may be used through miotic or undilated pupils. These are especially useful in patients whose pupils cannot be dilated because of allergic reactions to topical drugs, risk of angle-closure glaucoma, or scarred miotic pupils.

The image seen with the indirect ophthalmoscope is stereoscopic with a large field of view (37°). Both are advantages over the direct ophthalmoscope. The image, however, is smaller than with the direct ophthalmoscope.

Every ophthalmologist must become proficient in the use of the binocular indirect ophthalmoscope. The advantages of this technique over direct ophthalmoscopy are a much larger field of view (approximately 10 times), a stereoscopic view, more illumination, and easy visualization of the peripheral retina. The only disadvantages are that the image is inverted, magnification is decreased, and the pupil should be widely dilated.

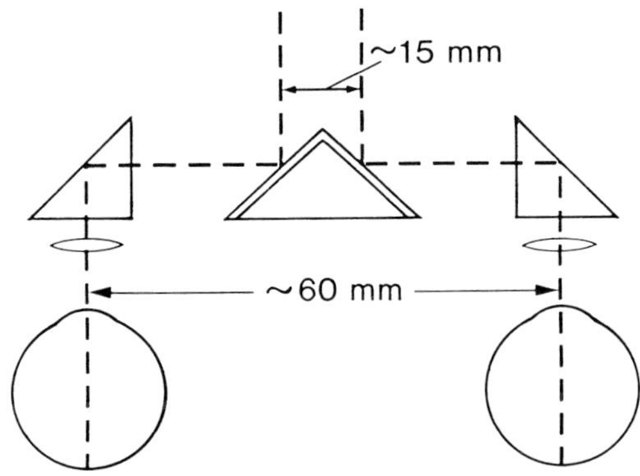

Fig. 2–28. Indirect ophthalmoscopic headpiece. The prism binocular optically narrows the observer's true pupillary distance to about 15 mm.

3

THE EYELIDS AND LACRIMAL DRAINAGE SYSTEM

George B. Bartley

The *anatomy* of the eyelids and lacrimal drainage system is intricate and worthy of detailed study to allow accurate diagnosis and proper treatment of local pathologic conditions. The skin of the eyelids is the thinnest on the body and lacks subcutaneous fat, factors that present both clinical advantages and challenges. For example, keloid formation on the eyelids is uncommon, and severe injuries can often be repaired with minimal or no permanent sequelae; few body tissues compare as favorably as a surgical fabric. Alternatively, the unusual distensibility of the eyelid skin may result in rapid, massive edema after slight trauma or an insect bite, and examination of the underlying globe is thus difficult or impossible.

The "backbone" of each eyelid is the *tarsal plate*, a firm, fibrous structure approximately 25 to 30 mm wide and 1 mm thick. Its height is about 10 mm in the upper eyelid and approximately half that in the lower eyelid. The tarsal plates are connected to the orbital rims by the *medial* and *lateral canthal tendons*; the medial tendon is anatomically more elaborate and prominent than its lateral counterpart, and its attachment to bone is considerably more secure.

The upper and lower eyelids have similar cross-sectional anatomy, and several distinct tissue planes can be identified from the anterior to the posterior aspect (Fig. 3–1). Immediately beneath the skin of each lid lies a layer of stri-ated muscle, the *orbicularis oculi*, that rings the eye in the frontal plane. The orbicularis is innervated by the facial nerve; loss of nerve function in Bell's palsy or after operation in the region of the parotid gland may result in a facial droop with lagophthalmos (inability to close the eyelids) of various degrees.

A horizontal incision through the fibers of the orbicularis several millimeters above the superior tarsal border reveals the *orbital septum*, a thin, glistening membrane that originates at the orbital rim and inserts into the retractors of each eyelid. Beneath the orbital septum lies an important surgical landmark, the *preaponeurotic fat*. The eyelid surgeon knows that immediately posterior to this fat pad in the upper lid is the *levator palpebrae superioris* muscle and aponeurosis, the principal elevating structure of the eyelid. The levator is a striated muscle and is innervated by the superior division of the oculomotor nerve. It originates at the orbital apex and embryologically should be considered an extraocular muscle.

The levator has five insertions that significantly define eyelid anatomy and function: 1) the subcutaneous tissue, forming the normal eyelid crease; 2) the anterior surface of the tarsal plate, allowing for eyelid elevation; 3) the medial canthal tendon (the "medial horn"); 4) the lateral orbital rim, dividing the lacrimal gland into orbital and palpebral lobes (the "lateral horn"); and 5) the conjunctiva of the superior fornix. Originating from and just

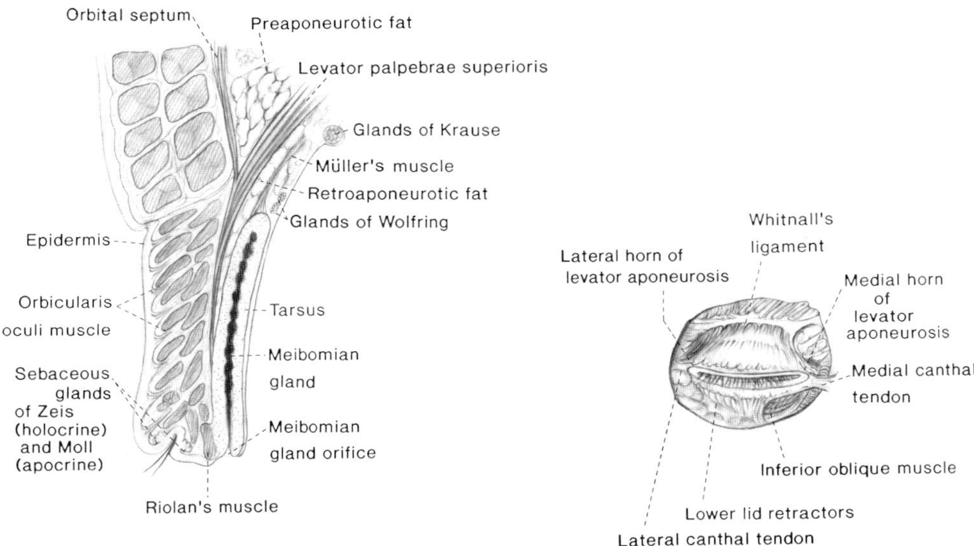

Fig. 3–1. Cross-sectional (*left*) and front (*right*) anatomy of the eyelids.

posterior to the levator is the smooth, sympathetically innervated, and richly vascularized *Müller's muscle*. Müller's muscle is intimately apposed to the most posterior tissue plane of the eyelid, the palpebral conjunctiva. In most eyelids a *"retroaponeurotic fat"* compartment may be identified between Müller's muscle and the overlying levator aponeurosis. The retracting structures in the lower eyelid that are analogous to the levator palpebrae superioris and Müller's muscle are the capsulopalpebral fascia and inferior tarsal muscle.

Several important anatomic landmarks are present in the margin of each eyelid. The eyelashes emerge from the anterior portion of the lid margin and are normally directed away from the globe. Associated with the eyelash follicles are *sebaceous glands (of Zeis)* and *sweat glands (of Moll)*. Immediately posterior to the eyelashes is a thin longitudinal stripe, the *gray line*. Although the gray line has often been described as the mucocutaneous junction between the keratinized skin anteriorly and the conjunctiva posteriorly, it has recently been shown to correspond with a strip of marginal orbicularis, also known as the *muscle of Riolan*. The *meibomian gland* orifices appear as small dots in the posterior half of the eyelid margin; the glands themselves are vertically oriented within the tarsus and can be identified as thin, parallel, yellowish lines when the eyelid is everted. The openings to the lacrimal drainage system, the

superior and inferior puncta, are found in the eyelid margin approximately 6 to 7 mm from the medial canthal angle.

Tears are produced by both the main and the accessory *lacrimal glands*. The main gland is superior and temporal to the eye and is divided by the lateral horn of the levator into an orbital lobe and a palpebral lobe, as mentioned above. Most of the *accessory lacrimal glands (of Krause and Wolfring)*, which provide the baseline minute-to-minute tears, are located in the conjunctiva of the upper eyelid and near the superior fornix, although glands are present in the lower lids as well. Tears course across the surface of the eye before exiting through the lacrimal drainage apparatus (Fig. 3–2). The open-

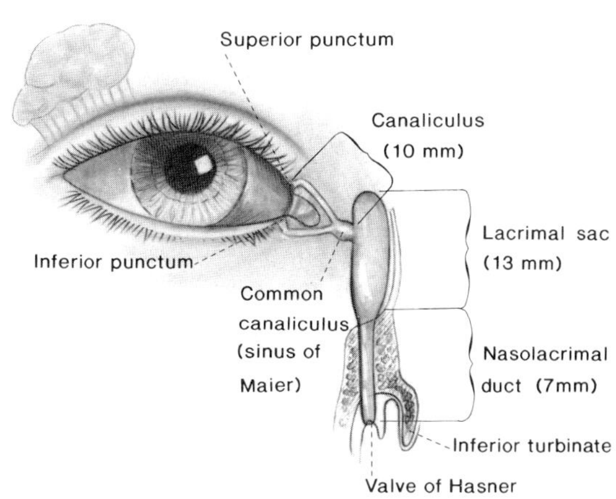

Fig. 3–2. Lacrimal drainage apparatus.

ings to the drainage system, the *puncta*, are oriented slightly posteriorly to allow tears to enter the canaliculi from the lacrimal lake, a small but identifiable ribbon of tears along the medial eyelid margin. The inferior punctum is slightly more temporal from the medial canthal angle than is the superior punctum. The *canaliculi* lie close to the lid margin and usually merge to form a common canaliculus before entering the *lacrimal sac*. The sac rests in its bony fossa just posterior to the medial canthal tendon. Tears pass from the sac into the inferior meatus of the nose via the *nasolacrimal duct*. The superficial location of the canaliculi in the eyelids and the transit of the nasolacrimal duct through its bony canal make the lacrimal excretory system vulnerable to trauma to the eyelids or midface and to disease originating in the nasal cavity or paranasal sinuses.

The eyelids may be involved by various inflammatory and infectious disorders.

Blepharitis and *dysfunction of the meibomian glands* are common and often related disorders. The patient complains of ocular and eyelid discomfort, itching, burning, blurred vision, and "granulated eyelids." Signs include eyelid erythema and edema, crusting of the eyelid margins, madarosis (loss of eyelashes), conjunctivitis, an oily tear film, hordeola and chalazia, and corneal scarring and vascularization in advanced cases.

Although two distinct types of blepharitis, staphylococcal and seborrheic, have often been described, most cases involve both components (Fig. 3–3). Excess oil secretion from the meibomian glands or the glands of Zeis produces favorable growth conditions for *Staphylococcus aureus* or *epidermidis*, and the lipid itself is irritating to the globe. Blepharitis commonly accompanies acne rosacea or acne vulgaris, and it is worsened by excess tea or alcohol consumption.

Because treatment requires good patient compliance, education about the cause and chronicity of the problem is important. Eyelid hygiene (warm compresses followed by gentle scrubbing of the eyelid margins with a cotton-tipped applicator soaked in dilute baby shampoo) is helpful for removing crusts from

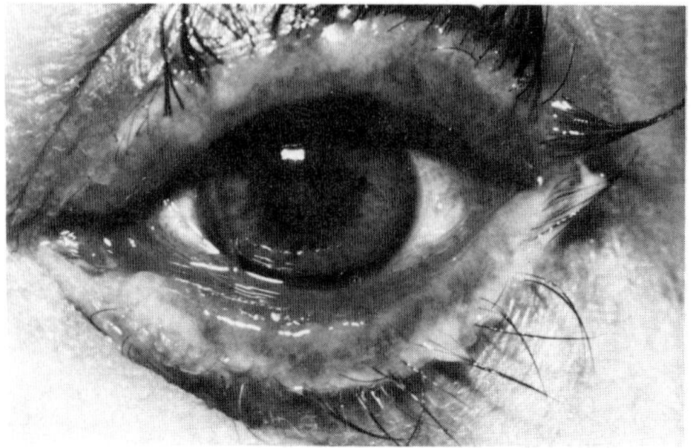

Fig. 3–3. Severe blepharoconjunctivitis with both infectious (bacterial) and inflammatory components.

the base of the eyelashes and restoring normal lid margin fauna. Excess oil can often be expressed from the meibomian glands, and an antibiotic-corticosteroid ointment may reduce the infectious and inflammatory components of the disorder. If local measures are unsuccessful, a course of oral tetracycline, 250 mg four times daily, may be useful.

A *hordeolum* (sty) is an acute infection of the glands of Zeis or Moll at the base of an eyelash follicle (external hordeolum) (Fig. 3–4) or of a meibomian gland within the tarsus (internal hordeolum) (Fig. 3–5); staphylococci are the usual offending microbes. The onset can be rapid, and discomfort is frequent. In some cases, the vision is distorted because of induced astigmatism from pressure on the globe by the mass. A hordeolum usually drains spontaneously, although its resolution can be hastened

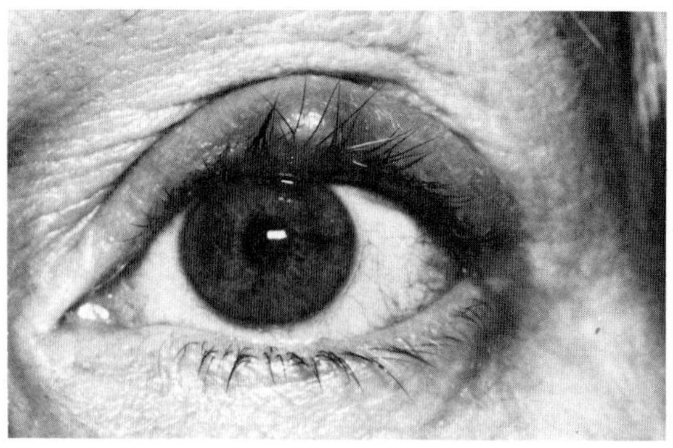

Fig. 3–4. Acute external hordeolum ("sty").

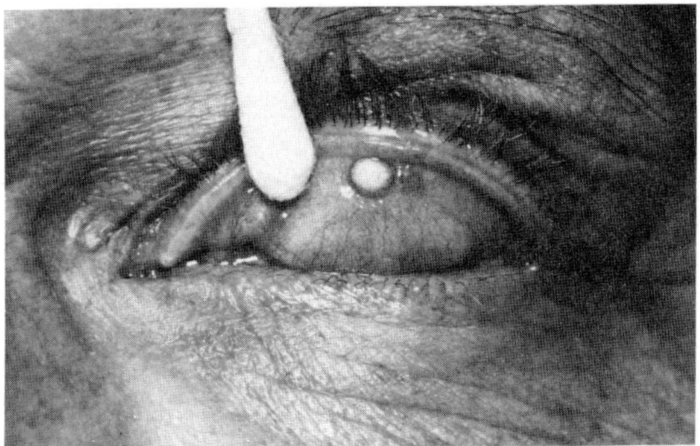

Fig. 3–5. Acute internal hordeolum.

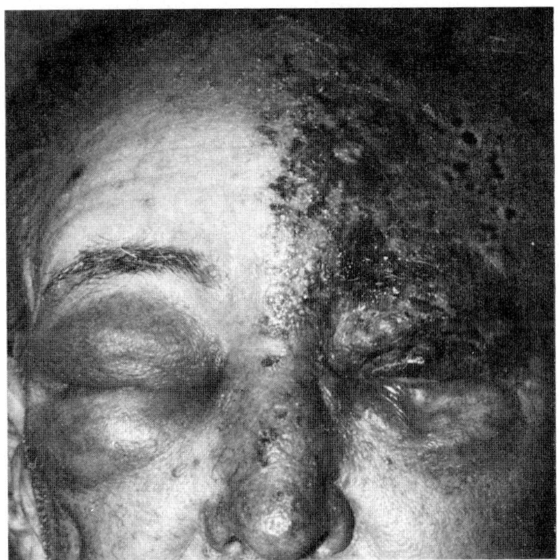

Fig. 3–7. Herpes zoster ophthalmicus. Although the virus involves the ophthalmic division of the left trigeminal nerve, the eyelid edema "spills over" to the right side as well.

by the application of warm compresses and antibiotic ointment four times a day.

A *chalazion* (Fig. 3–6) can be considered a chronic internal hordeolum with no active infection. Spontaneous resorption may occur over weeks to months, but a minor surgical procedure is often required once the inflammation has become encysted. If the tendency of the mass is to "point" posteriorly, a vertical conjunctival incision (with care taken to avoid the eyelid margin) is the preferred approach. A chalazion that is predominantly on the anterior surface of the tarsus is best excised through an incision parallel to the fibers of the orbicularis. The cyst wall of the chalazion should be removed, and the skin usually can be left to heal without sutures if the incision is small. One should suspect a sebaceous carci-

noma whenever a chalazion is unusually persistent or recurrent.

The signs and symptoms of *herpes zoster* (Fig. 3–7) often begin on the forehead or eyelids, and prompt diagnosis by the ophthalmologist may save the patient significant ocular and systemic morbidity. The globe is spared in many cases, but uveitis, retinal vasculitis, cataract, keratopathy, and eyelid scarring occur frequently. Hutchinson's sign (the appearance of vesicles on the tip of the nerve) indicates involvement of the dorsal nasal and nasociliary branch of the ophthalmic nerve and alerts the ophthalmologist to examine the patient carefully for the development of ocular inflammation. Postherpetic neuralgia and cerebrovascular insults are potential severe systemic sequelae of herpes zoster ophthalmicus.

The cutaneous vesicular eruption of herpes zoster characteristically has an erythematous base, whereas the skin beneath a simplex vesicle is typically uninflamed. The diagnosis can be confirmed by aspirating fluid with a 30-gauge needle from a vesicle for viral culture; the lesion can be unroofed if insufficient material is obtained. Postinfectious ocular sequelae of

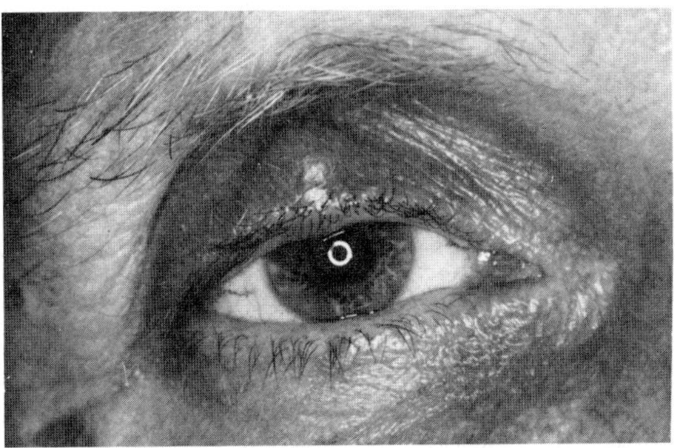

Fig. 3–6. Chalazion – chronic meibomian gland inflammation.

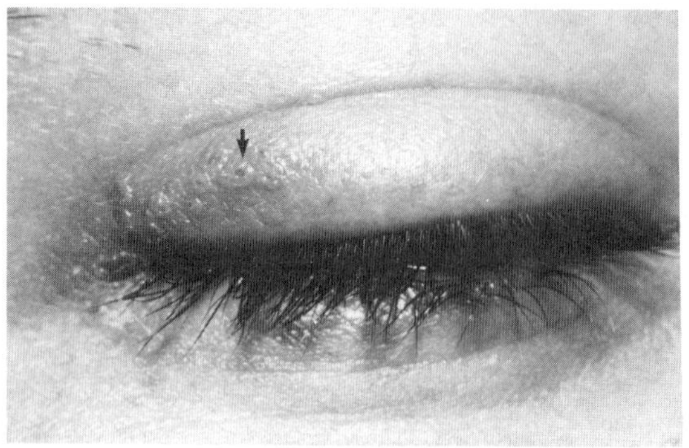

Fig. 3–8. Herpes simplex blepharitis. Eyelid vesicles (*arrow*) are not associated with the cutaneous inflammation seen in herpes zoster.

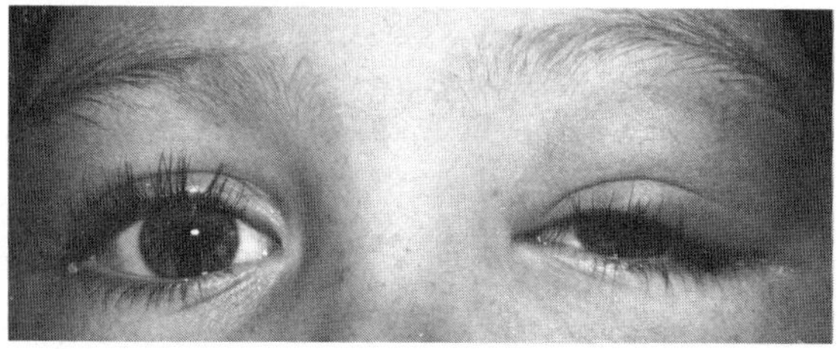

Fig. 3–9. Preseptal cellulitis: characteristic S-shaped lid, globe is quiet and white, and vision is normal.

herpes zoster ophthalmicus and the discomfort of the acute eruption can be reduced by the prompt institution of oral acyclovir, 600 mg five times a day for 10 days. The skin lesions may be treated with a topical antibiotic-corticosteroid ointment.

In contrast to herpes zoster, the cutaneous vesicles of *herpes simplex* (Fig. 3–8) tend to be confined to the epidermis, and the deep scarring that often occurs with herpes zoster is thus avoided. Local treatment is rarely necessary, although if the vesicles are present on the eyelid margin, seeding onto the globe may be reduced by the application of antiviral ointment such as vidarabine or idoxuridine.

Preseptal cellulitis of the eyelid may occur after minor or even occult trauma in which the surface flora, usually *Staphylococcus aureus*, is inoculated beneath the skin. The orbital septum is an important barrier to the spread of a superficial infection posteriorly into the orbit; in preseptal cellulitis the eyelid may be massively swollen and erythematous, but the globe is uninvolved and the vision and ocular motility are normal (Fig. 3–9). True orbital cellulitis may occur if the orbital septum has been breached; the eye is then at great risk, and significant systemic morbidity is possible. Orbital cellulitis is discussed in greater detail in Chapter 8.

Haemophilus influenzae should always be considered when preseptal cellulitis occurs in a young child with a coexistent upper respiratory infection. The eyelid has a characteristic, nearly pathognomonic, violaceous hue, and cultures from the conjunctiva may confirm the suspected diagnosis. Ampicillin should be administered promptly; close observation is necessary to monitor the possibility of antibiotic resistance and spread of the infection to the paranasal sinuses or orbit.

Degenerative changes take place in the lids with age, and some malpositions are related to disease states.

Entropion is a tendency for the eyelid margin to rotate posteriorly (Fig. 3–10). The eyelashes abrade the globe, resulting in corneal scarring and vascularization in severe cases. Entropion should be distinguished from *trichiasis* (see Fig. 3–15); in trichiasis, the eyelid margin is properly positioned but ocular irritation occurs from misdirected eyelashes.

Entropion is usually an involutional process, and several factors are contributory.

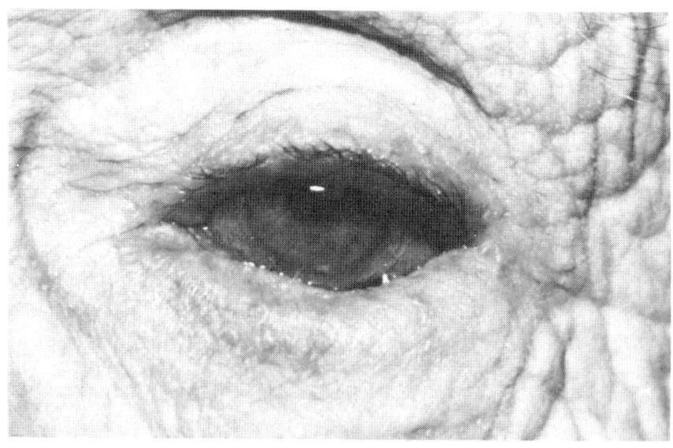

Fig. 3–10. Entropion with secondary keratoconjunctivitis.

Normal relationships between tissues are altered with age; for example, orbital fat atrophies, the eyelid becomes horizontally lax, and the lower lid retractors may disinsert from their attachment near the inferior tarsal border. The globe becomes relatively enophthalmic, particularly when the patient is supine and the eye moves posteriorly in the orbit, and the loose and unstable eyelid may rotate posteriorly against the globe. These factors help to explain why many patients with early or intermittent entropion have symptoms of ocular irritation and eyelid mattering on arising after sleep; entropion may not be present on examination in the office but can be induced by having the patient lie supine and blink forcibly.

The role of disinsertion of the lower eyelid retractors in involutional entropion has only recently been appreciated. The presentation and findings are similar to involutional myogenic ptosis of the upper eyelid, which is discussed below. The lower eyelid displays "inverse ptosis"; that is, it does not retract inferiorly as it should during downgaze and the globe appears as a "setting sun" behind the stationary lower lid. If the inferior fornix is inspected, a distinct reddish hue is often seen beneath the conjunctiva just inferior to the lower edge of the tarsal plate. This red tissue is the orbicularis of the lower eyelid, which becomes visible when the lower eyelid retractors, identifiable as a white band in the inferior fornix, disinsert and migrate away from the tarsal border.

Many satisfactory methods of treatment for involutional entropion have been described. Rotational sutures are sometimes useful for acute "spastic" cases in which entropion is the result of ocular irritation or for patients who are debilitated and cannot undergo a more involved operation. The technique is simple and can be performed at the bedside, although the result is usually only temporary. Another procedure for similar circumstances is cautery of the anterior lamella of the eyelid (skin and orbicularis); the intent is to elicit mild scarring that will evert the eyelid away from the globe.

Horizontal eyelid laxity may be addressed by various eyelid resection or suspension procedures, and disinsertion of the lower eyelid retractors may be repaired from either a conjunctival or a skin approach. Perhaps the most common operation in widespread use to treat involutional entropion is the modified Wies procedure: a full-thickness horizontal incision (blepharotomy) allows both advancement of the lower eyelid retractors and placement of rotational sutures. The Wies procedure can be combined with horizontal shortening of the eyelid if necessary.

In contrast to the involutional factors described above, acquired entropion may occasionally result from scarring of the conjunctival surface of the eyelid. Upper eyelid entropion is rare in the United States, but it is common in areas where trachoma is endemic. Both upper and lower eyelid scarring may occur with cicatricial pemphigoid, an uncommon but devastating autoimmune disorder.

Finally, entropion may occur as a rare congenital abnormality. Disinsertion of the lower eyelid retractors is the likely cause, and surgical repair must be accomplished promptly to prevent corneal scarring. Congenital entropion should not be confused with *epiblepharon* (Fig. 3–11), a common eyelid condition of children in which a redundant fold of pretarsal orbicularis and skin causes the eyelashes to turn toward the globe. Epiblepharon rarely leads to significant corneal irritation, and the fold of extra tissue usually disappears during normal midface and eyelid development.

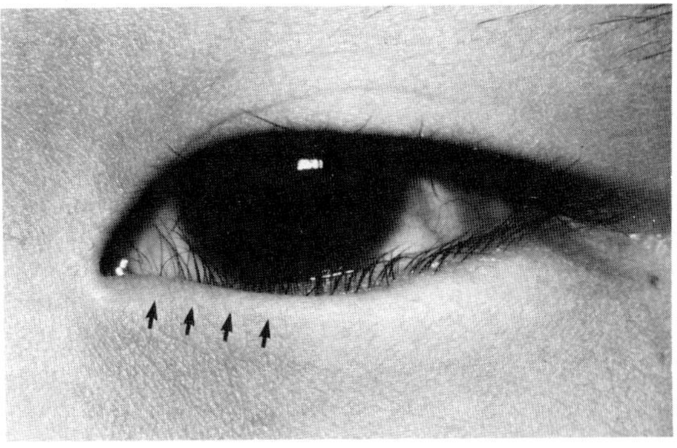

Fig. 3–11. Epiblepharon: a redundant fold of medial pretarsal skin and orbicularis (*arrows*) causes the eyelashes to turn toward the eye.

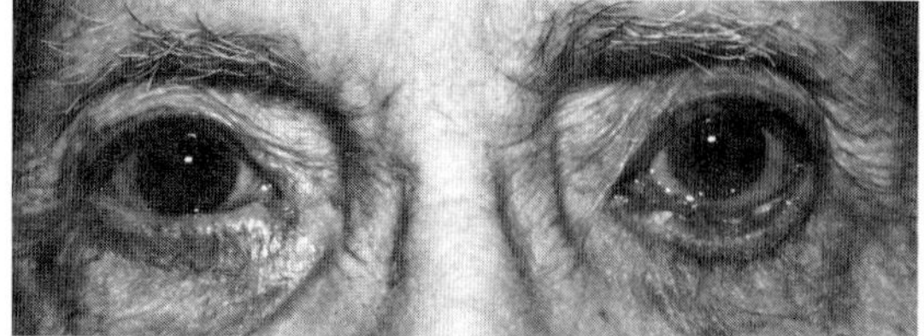

Fig. 3–12. Involutional ectropion of the left lower eyelid secondary to disinsertion of the lower eyelid retractors.

Ectropion is a tendency for the eyelid margin to rotate anteriorly, away from the globe (Fig. 3–12). Like entropion, ectropion is often associated with aging changes such as horizontal eyelid laxity and disinsertion of the lower eyelid retractors, yet the positional defect is opposite. This may be due in part to the common coexistent finding of vertical eyelid skin deficiency, which acts to pull the eyelid margin away from the globe instead of allowing it to rotate posteriorly, as seen in entropion. Patients with ectropion often are bothered by tearing that can occur because of various factors, including an isolated obstruction of the lacrimal drainage system, displacement of the inferior punctum away from the lacrimal lake (Fig. 3–13), or irritation of the globe by exposure. Frequent wiping of the tears may stretch the eyelid tissues further, worsening the ectropion and contributing to vertical eyelid shortening. It is often difficult to identify which causative factor occurred first, mild ectropion or mild tearing, but the result is a perpetuating cycle that can lead to complete eversion of the tarsal plates with keratinization of the palpebral conjunctiva. Operation is usually directed toward horizontally shortening the eyelid by tightening the lateral or medial canthal attachments, and skin grafting may be necessary if vertical eyelid scarring is prominent. As with entropion, repair of disinsertion of the lower eyelid retractors is often helpful.

Paralytic ectropion is a common complication of disorders affecting the facial nerve (Fig. 3–14). Nerve function may be compromised idiopathically (Bell's palsy), as a result of a neoplasm such as an acoustic neuroma in the cerebellopontine angle, or after parotid gland operation. An eyelid operation can be performed to minimize ocular exposure once it is apparent that spontaneous improvement in seventh nerve function is unlikely. In the meantime, it is imperative that the cornea be adequately moistened with artificial tears and lubricating ointments. A protective plastic shield is often useful to retain moisture around the eye while the patient is sleeping.

Ectropion is occasionally a complication of dermatologic conditions such as atopic dermatitis or discoid lupus erythematosus or of cicatricial situations such as trauma, burns, or surgical procedures to the face or eyelids; it may also be a mechanical result of large lesions on the eyelid margin. Treatment is directed toward the underlying cause.

Trichiasis (Fig. 3–15) refers to misdirected eyelashes; the eyelid margin is normally positioned, although coexistent entropion may occur. The abnormal eyelashes may be

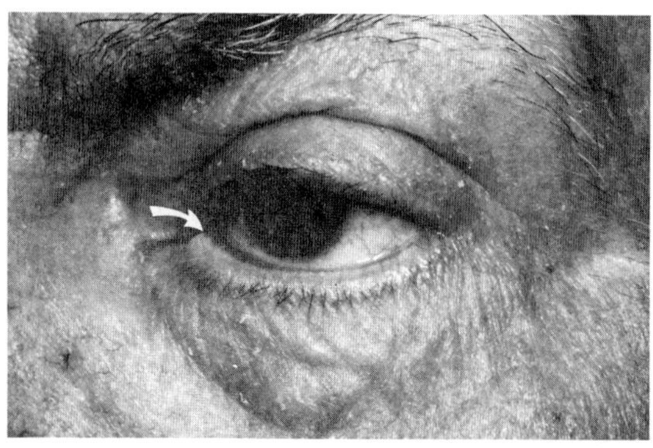

Fig. 3–13. Early ectropion involving primarily the medial portion of the lower eyelid ("punctal ectropion" or "medial ectropion"); punctum (*arrow*) is displaced anteriorly away from the lacrimal lake.

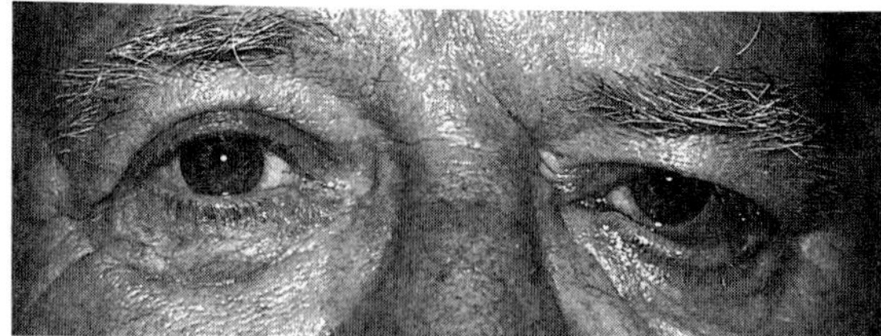

Fig. 3–14. Paralytic left lower eyelid ectropion and left brow ptosis after resection of carcinoma involving the left parotid gland and facial nerve.

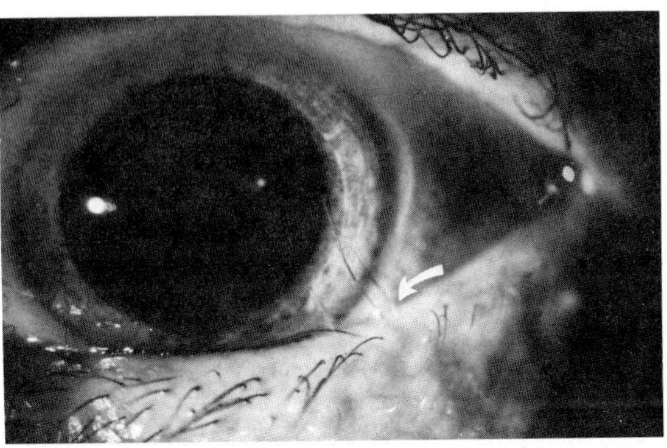

Fig. 3–15. Trichiasis: malpositioned eyelashes (*arrow*) point toward and abrade the eye; eyelid margin is normally positioned (in contrast to entropion).

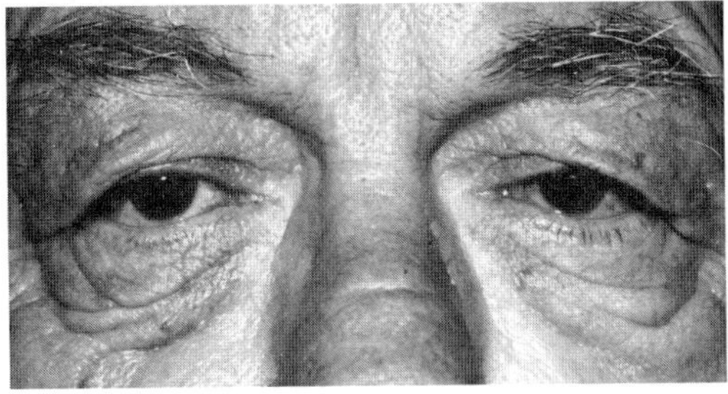

Fig. 3–17. Dermatochalasis: age-related, redundant eyelid skin.

removed by simple epilation ("plucking"), although relief is temporary because regrowth nearly always occurs. Cryotherapy is the preferred treatment for localized areas of multiple misdirected cilia, whereas argon laser therapy or electrolysis may be used to ablate isolated trichiatic lashes.

Distichiasis is a rare congenital abnormality in which abnormal eyelashes emerge from the meibomian gland orifices (Fig. 3–16). It may occur as an isolated finding or in association with other defects of development. Treatment is usually surgical.

Dermatochalasis and *blepharochalasis* are distinct entities, but unfortunately the terms often are used interchangeably to describe redundant eyelid tissue from any cause. *Der-*

matochalasis is common and refers to the stretched, redundant, baggy eyelid skin that occurs with age (Fig. 3–17). A frequent concomitant finding is anterior migration of orbital fat through a weakened orbital septum, producing prominent subcutaneous bulges in both the upper and the lower eyelids. In contrast, *blepharochalasis* describes an infrequent condition of thinned, stretched eyelid skin that results from multiple episodes of eyelid edema for which no cause is apparent (Fig. 3–18 *A*). Blepharochalasis usually has its onset while the patient is a teenager or young adult, and both

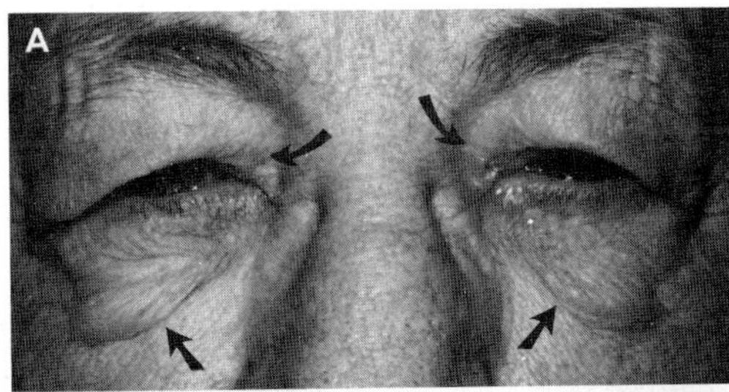

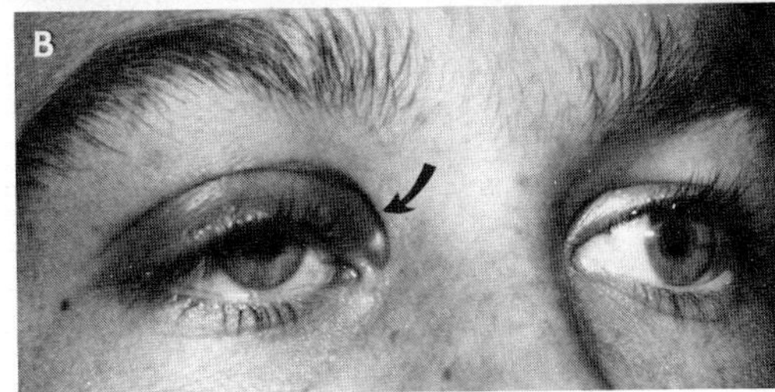

Fig. 3–18. Blepharochalasis. *A*, Thin, stretched eyelid skin after multiple episodes of idiopathic eyelid edema (*arrows*). *B*, The acquired epicanthal folds (more prominent on the right [*arrow*] than on the left) are the result of atrophy of the nasal eyelid fat pad and are characteristic of the blepharochalasis syndrome.

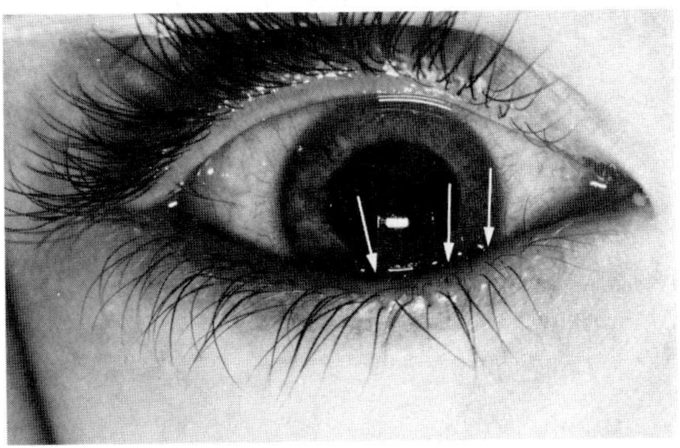

Fig. 3–16. Distichiasis: a congenital abnormality in which abnormal eyelashes (*arrows*) emerge from the meibomian gland orifices.

sexes are equally affected. Although not always present, a pathognomonic clinical feature of blepharochalasis is an acquired epicanthal fold from atrophy of the nasal fat pad following the recurrent eyelid swelling (Fig. 3–18 *B*). Surgical procedures for both dermatochalasis and blepharochalasis can be performed to remove excess eyelid tissue and to repair blepharoptosis if present.

Blepharoptosis (ptosis) is present when the position of the upper eyelid is abnormally low. Although individuals have considerable variation in lid position, in adults the upper eyelid usually rests 1.5 to 2.0 mm below the superior corneoscleral limbus (Fig. 3–19). The primary retractor or elevator of the eyelid is the levator muscle, whereas Müller's muscle contributes 1 to 2 mm of lift.

The diagnostic classification of patients with ptosis has encouraged much debate, but the most workable and widely accepted outline was proposed by Crowell Beard (*Ptosis*, Third Edition, C.V. Mosby Company, 1981). A droopy eyelid can be considered either "congenital" or "acquired." *Congenital ptosis* usually is the result of abnormal development of the levator muscle. Whereas a normally formed and functioning levator muscle allows the eyelid to follow the globe smoothly as the eye looks up and down, in congenital ptosis the eyelid excursion during upgaze and downgaze is greatly diminished. This lack of eyelid mobil-

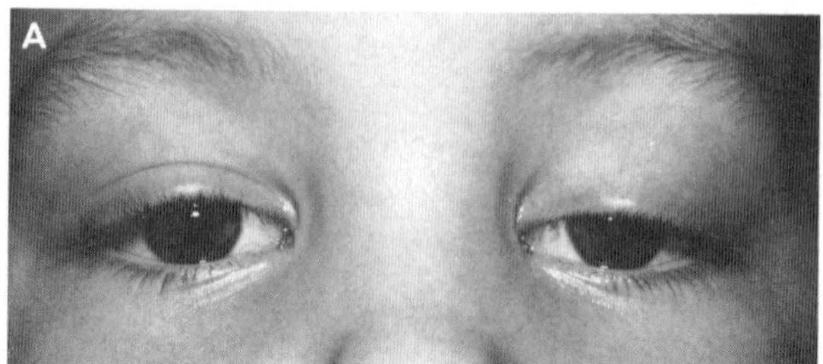

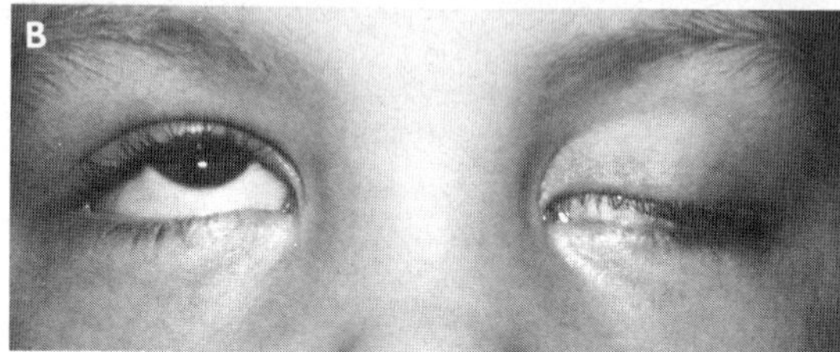

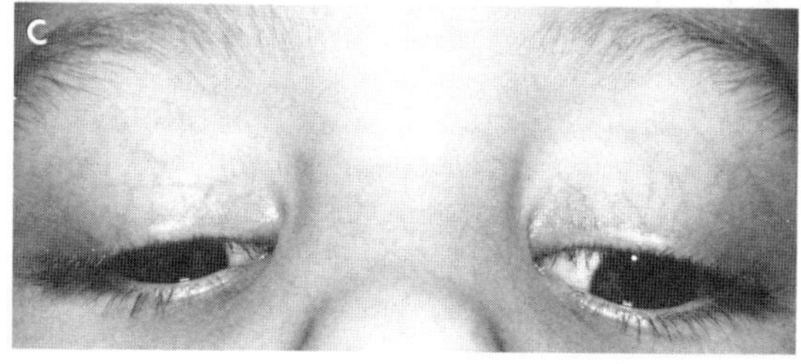

Fig. 3–20. *A*, Congenital ptosis, left upper eyelid. Note absence of the normal eyelid crease. *B*, In upgaze, poor function of the left levator muscle is apparent. *C*, In downgaze, the dystrophic left levator muscle fails to "relax" and the eyelid is higher than the normal right upper lid.

ity is an important clinical sign and results from the basic pathophysiology of congenital ptosis: the levator is dystrophic and fibrotic. Lid elevation in upgaze is poor because of lack of levator contraction, and the lid fails to follow the globe in downgaze because of inability of the muscle to relax (Fig. 3–20). The characteristic clinical features of congenital ptosis are outlined in Table 3–1.

Because the levator muscle and superior rectus muscle originate from a common embryologic tissue mass, it is not unusual for dysfunction of the superior rectus to accompany congenital ptosis. Amblyopia may be present in any patient with congenital ptosis, but the finding of coexistent strabismus makes a thorough search for poor vision even more imperative.

The surgical treatment of congenital ptosis is challenging. Some levator function may be

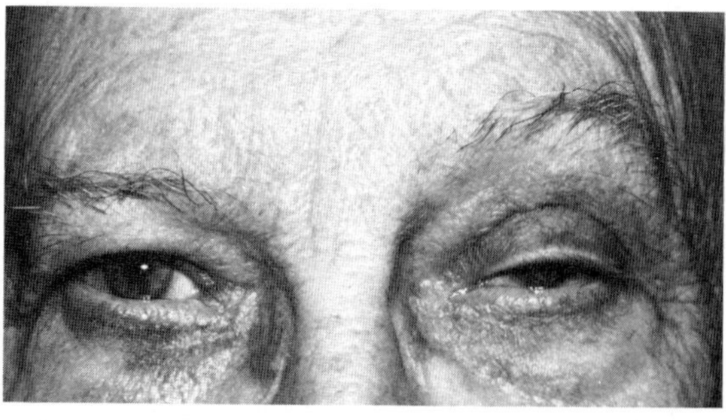

Fig. 3–19. Ptosis of the left upper eyelid after intraocular surgery; the right upper lid is in normal position, approximately 1.5 to 2.0 mm below the superior limbus. Note high left eyelid crease from levator disinsertion. The left frontalis muscle is contracted in an attempt to elevate the left brow and upper lid.

TABLE 3–1 Clinical Features of Congenital and Acquired Myogenic Ptosis

Feature	Congenital ptosis	Acquired myogenic ptosis
History	Present since birth	Usually gradual onset
		Patient may have had previous eyelid edema from insect bite, trauma, thyroid disease, blepharochalasis
Degree of ptosis	Mild to severe	Mild to severe
Levator function (excursion of eyelid from downgaze to upgaze)	Usually poor (5 mm or less)	Usually good (9 mm or more)
Position of eyelid crease	Often poorly developed	Usually higher than normal
Position of eyelid on downgaze	Usually "lags" and is higher than other upper lid if ptosis is unilateral	Follows globe down normally; lower than other upper lid if ptosis is unilateral
Other features	Weakness of superior rectus muscle may be coexistent	Iris may be seen through thin eyelid
		Tarsus may be laterally migrated

present if the muscle is not completely dystrophic; shortening the muscle by a resection procedure may help to "strengthen" its action. In severe cases with minimal or no eyelid excursion, the eyelid must be suspended in a "sling" procedure from structures in the superior orbit or in the region of the brow.

The levator muscle usually is normally developed in ptosis that develops later in life, in contrast to congenital ptosis. Beard described four broad and sometimes overlapping etiologic categories of *acquired ptosis*: myogenic, neurogenic, traumatic, and mechanical.

Most patients with droopy eyelids have acquired myogenic ptosis. In most cases, the pathophysiologic features are due to involutional changes involving the levator aponeurosis. The aponeurosis normally inserts onto the anterior surface of the tarsal plate. As the eyelid ages, the aponeurotic attachments may stretch and become thin. The position of the eyelid gradually drops, and severe ptosis of 5 mm or more may occur with complete disinsertion of the aponeurosis from the tarsus.

Unlike congenital ptosis, in which the dystrophic levator precludes normal eyelid excursion, the lid continues to move normally in upgaze and downgaze in aponeurotic disinsertion (Fig. 3–21). In addition to ptosis, the eyelid crease migrates superiorly because of the attachments of the levator to the subcutaneous tissues. The tarsus may migrate temporally, and the outline of the iris can frequently be observed through the diaphanous central eyelid tissues. Table 3–1 summarizes some of the important clinical findings of ptosis secondary to disinsertion of the levator aponeurosis. Surgical exploration of the eyelid to identify and advance the disinserted levator aponeurosis has a high rate of success.

Although disinsertion of the levator aponeurosis is the commonest cause of acquired myogenic ptosis, myasthenia gravis can be isolated to the muscles around the eye and should always be kept in mind. The edrophonium (Tensilon) test should be performed if myasthenia is suspected, especially if surgical correction of the ptosis is being contemplated

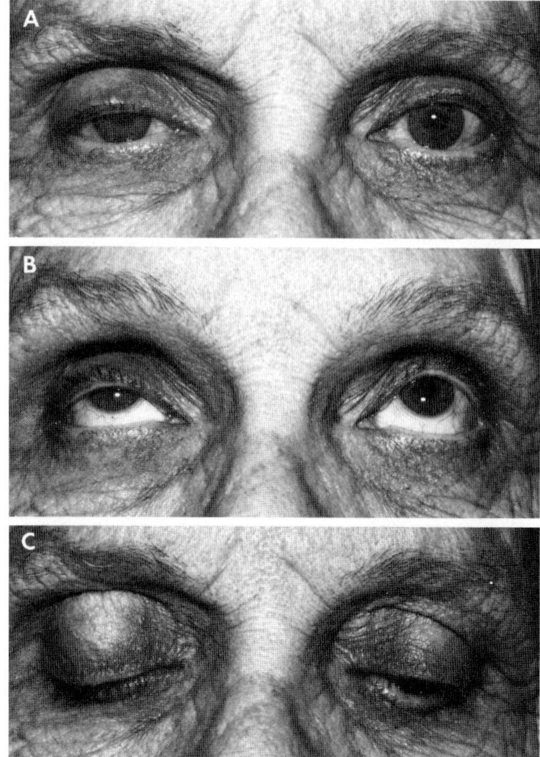

Fig. 3–21.   *A*, Acquired ptosis, right upper lid, from levator aponeurotic thinning. *B*, In upgaze, good levator function is demonstrated. *C*, In downgaze, the right upper lid is lower than the left upper lid (compare with Fig. 3–20 *C*).

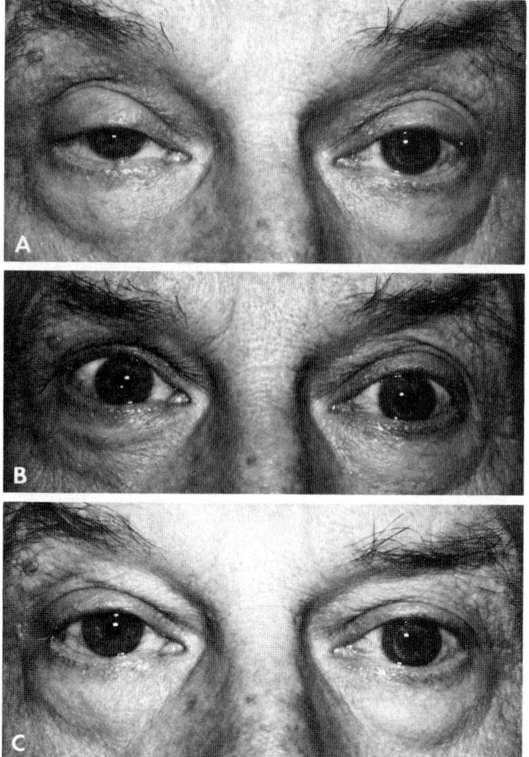

Fig. 3–22.   *A*, Acquired ptosis, right upper eyelid. *B*, Ptosis improved after intravenous injection of edrophonium (Tensilon). Patient needs medical evaluation and treatment for myasthenia gravis, not ptosis surgery. *C*, Resolution of ptosis with pyridostigmine therapy.

(Fig. 3–22). Testing for serum antibodies to acetylcholine receptors also can be helpful in diagnosing myasthenia. Other infrequent but systemically important causes of acquired myopathic ptosis include Kearns-Sayre syndrome, chronic progressive external ophthalmoplegia, and myotonic dystrophy.

Acquired neurogenic ptosis results from interruption of the oculomotor nerve to the levator or of the sympathetic innervation to Müller's muscle. When ptosis is the result of a third cranial nerve palsy, the globe usually is exotropic and hypotropic because of denervation of the ipsilateral medial and superior rectus muscles (the levator, medial rectus, and superior rectus are all supplied by the superior division of the third cranial nerve); the pupil may be dilated if the inferior division of the third cranial nerve is also involved. When it is apparent that all spontaneous improvement in third nerve function is complete, surgical procedures to straighten the eye and elevate the eyelid can be considered. A strabismus operation customarily precedes the ptosis operation. In Horner's syndrome, innervation of the sympathetic autonomic nervous system to the orbit is violated, and mild ptosis of 1 to 2 mm is accompanied by constriction of the ipsilateral pupil (Fig. 3–23). The differential diagnostic causes of Horner's syndrome are discussed in Chapter 7.

Finally, acquired ptosis may result from various traumatic mishaps or mechanical conditions. The levator muscle may be

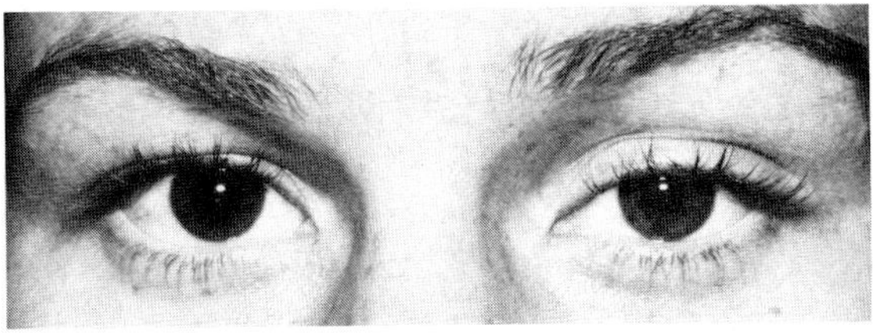

Fig. 3–23. Left Horner's syndrome: mild ptosis (from loss of function of Müller's muscle) and miosis (pupillary constriction).

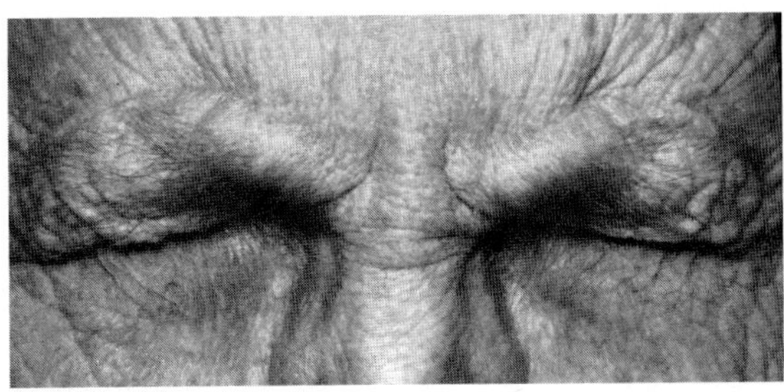

Fig. 3–25.   Essential blepharospasm: severe, involuntary eyelid closure.

damaged by lacerations of the eyelid, trauma to the orbit, or ocular or orbital operations of nearly any type. Mechanical causes of ptosis include tumors on the eyelid or in the orbit, and conjunctival or eyelid scarring from ocular inflammation or previous operation may result in an abnormally low eyelid position.

Eyelid retraction is the opposite of blepharoptosis—instead of being abnormally low, the resting position of the upper eyelid is at the superior limbus or higher. The lower lid may be retracted as well. Normally, the lower eyelid rests approximately at the inferior limbus; however, when it is retracted, the white sclera is seen between the eyelid margin and the limbus. Exceptions exist, but, in general, "scleral show," either superiorly or inferiorly, is abnormal (Fig. 3–24).

The most frequent cause of eyelid retraction is Graves' disease. When accompanied by proptosis, restriction of ocular motility, and clinical and laboratory evidence of thyroid dysfunction, the diagnosis is ensured. Occasionally, however, eyelid retraction may be the first and only subtle sign of Graves' ophthalmopathy. The ocular and orbital manifestations of Graves' disease are discussed further in Chapter 8.

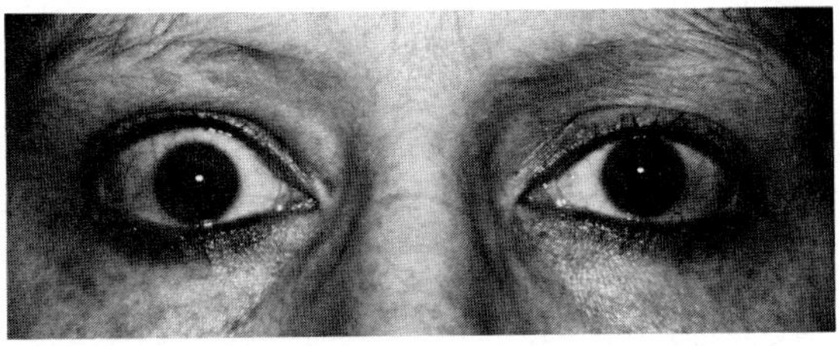

Involuntary, forceful blinking (*blepharospasm*) is a perplexing problem that has long been misunderstood by the medical community. Some patients with excessive blinking do so because of a local ocular cause such as blepharitis, dry eyes, a foreign body, trichiasis, or entropion. In many patients, however, no apparent contributing factor can be identified (essential blepharospasm). The severity of the spasms varies, but when they are severe the patient may be rendered functionally blind (Fig. 3–25). The exact cause remains a mystery, but the disorder is often associated with oromandibular dystonia, spastic dysphonia, or torticollis, and it may result from abnormal neurotransmission. Medical treatment with muscle relaxants is usually ineffective, but temporary relief can often be achieved by periorbital injections of botulinum toxin, which partially paralyzes the orbicularis oculi muscles. Severe cases may require surgical extirpation of the eyelid protractors (orbicularis oculi, corrugator supercilii, and procerus muscles).

Hemifacial spasm clinically resembles essential blepharospasm except that only one side of the face is involved (Fig. 3–26 *A*). A compressive stimulus to the facial nerve is the cause, and in many patients a dilated intracranial blood vessel can be identified (Fig. 3–26 *B*). The spasms can be treated with botulinum toxin or with operation.

Fig. 3–24.   Bilateral, asymmetric upper eyelid retraction secondary to Graves' disease.

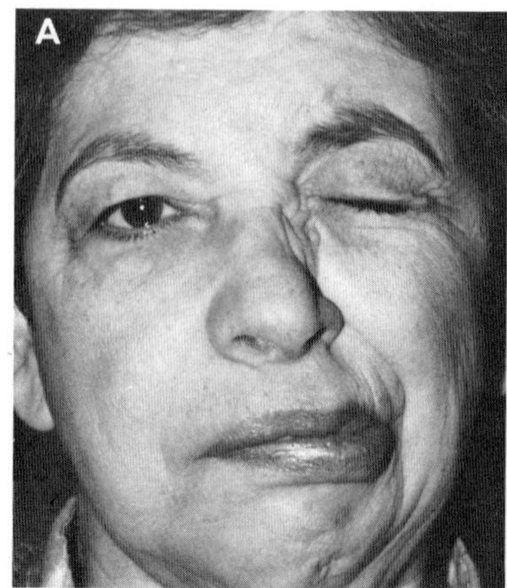
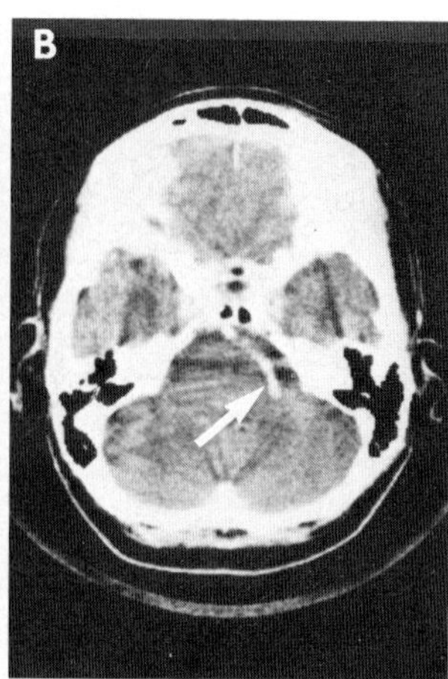

Fig. 3–26. Hemifacial spasm (*A*) caused by a dolichoectatic vertebral artery compressing the facial nerve (*arrow* on *B*, computed tomographic scan).

The most frequent benign growths on the eyelids are papillomas and nevi, whereas basal cell carcinoma is the commonest malignant tumor.

Many benign growths occur on the eyelids, and most can be removed easily if they are bothersome to the patient. Epithelial tumors such as *squamous papillomas* (Fig. 3–27), *seborrheic keratoses* (Fig. 3–28 and 3–29), and *cutaneous horns* (Fig. 3–30) are the most common. *Intradermal nevi*, which may or may not be pigmented, frequently arise along the eyelid margin. Clinical features of their benignancy include a smooth posterior surface from conformity to the shape of the globe and persistence rather than loss of eyelashes (Fig. 3–31). Sudoriferous cysts (hidrocystomas) (Fig. 3–32) and epithelial inclusion cysts (Fig. 3–33) are other frequent benign eyelid lesions.

Keratoacanthoma (Fig. 3–34) deserves particular mention because of its characteristic and

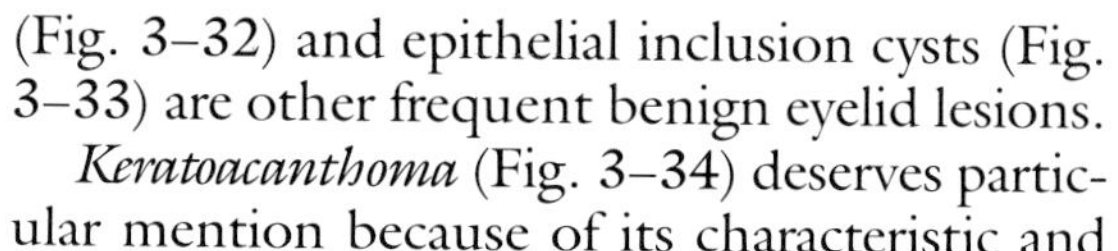

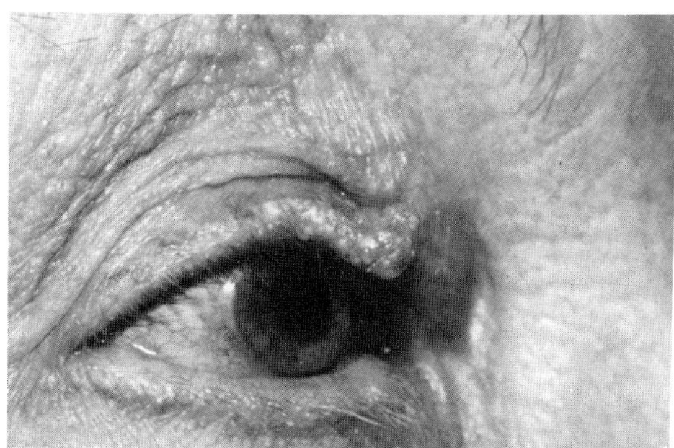

Fig. 3–28. Seborrheic keratosis; benign.

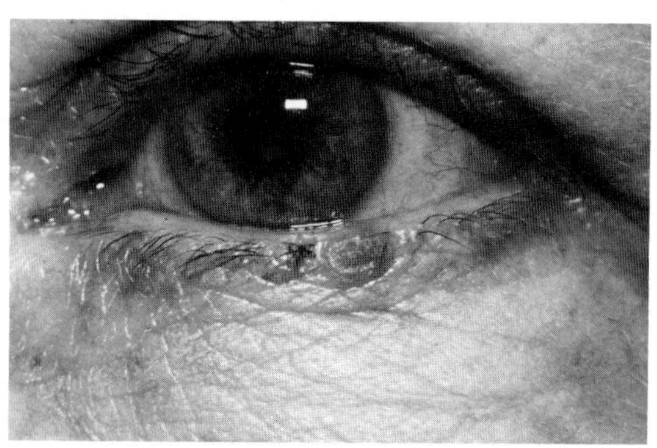

Fig. 3–27. Squamous papilloma: a benign lesion, but it may be confused with basal cell carcinoma.

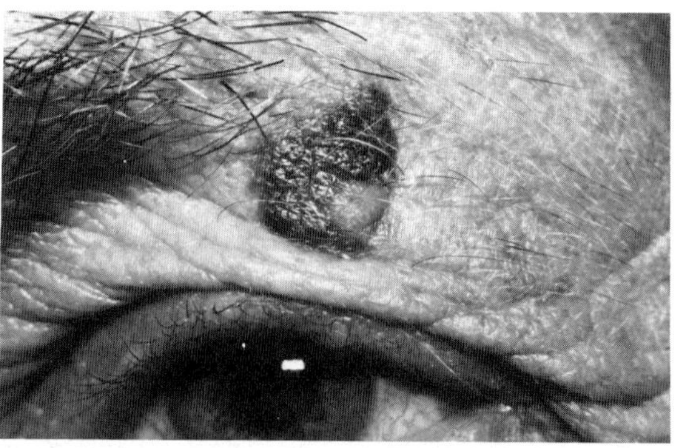

Fig. 3–29. Seborrheic keratosis. Pigmentation may raise the suspicion of melanoma, but the presence of hairs suggests benignancy.

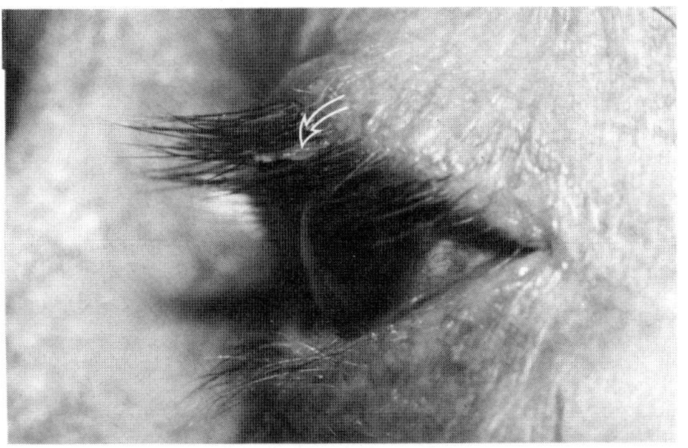

Fig. 3–30. Cutaneous horn (*arrow*) among upper eyelid lashes. These lesions are benign, but neoplastic changes occasionally occur in the base.

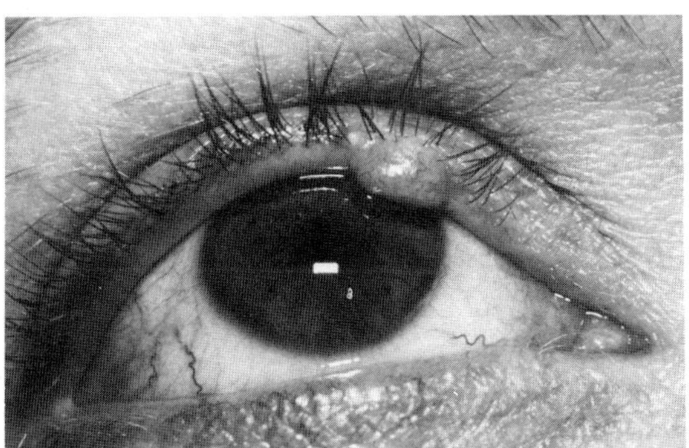

Fig. 3–31. Intradermal nevus, upper eyelid margin. Although these benign growths are often confused with basal cell carcinoma, intradermal nevi usually have a smooth surface that conforms to the shape of the globe, and madarosis (loss of eyelashes) near the lesion characteristically is not seen.

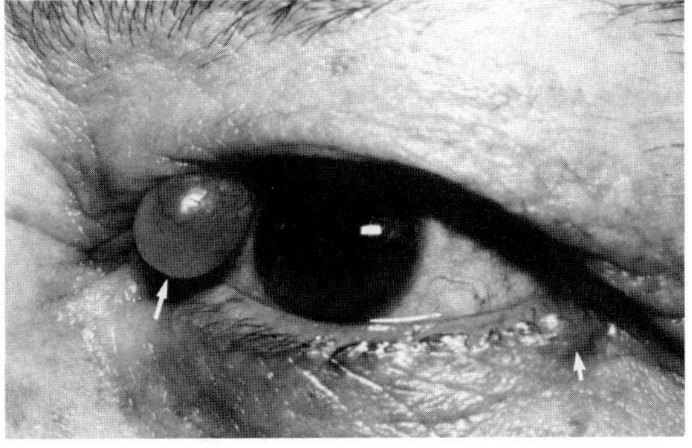

Fig. 3–32. Sudoriferous cysts (hidrocystomas) (*arrows*); benign.

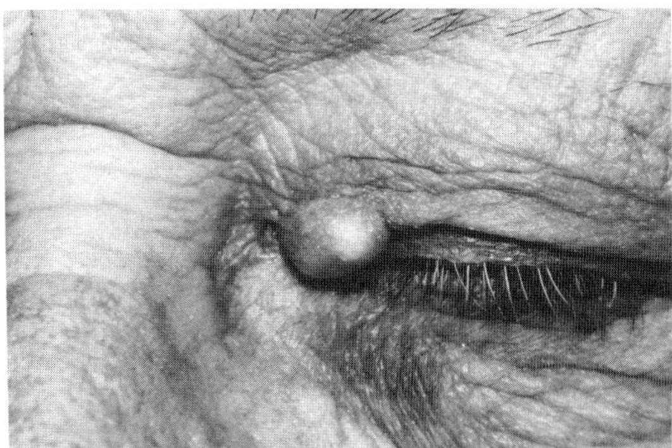

Fig. 3–33. Epithelial inclusion cyst; benign.

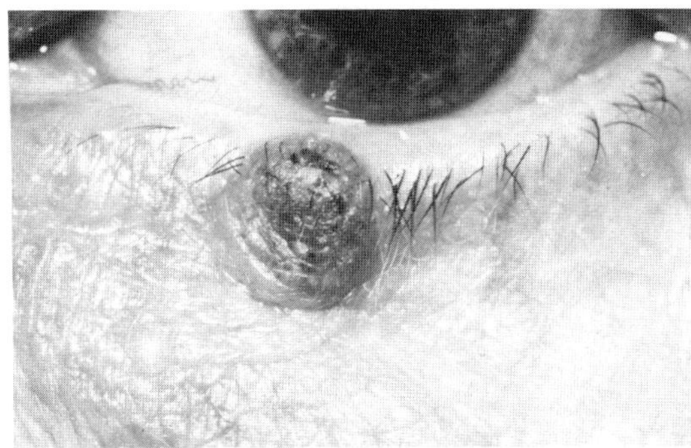

Fig. 3–34. Keratoacanthoma that appeared and grew to this size within 1 month. A biopsy is indicated.

often impressive clinical course. Although histologically benign, the lesion is often confused with basal cell carcinoma or squamous cell carcinoma and treated as such. A keratoacanthoma typically appears as a rapidly growing, elevated tumor with a central keratin-filled crater surrounded by rolled edges. A viral cause is suspected but unproved. Complete spontaneous regression can occur, but an excisional biopsy is reasonable to exclude the infrequent occurrence of true neoplastic differentiation in the base of the lesion.

Xanthelasmas (Fig. 3–35) are common lesions that characteristically localize on the nasal portions of both the upper and the lower eyelids. The growths are plaquelike, yellowish, slightly elevated, and soft to palpation. Microscopically, the lesions are composed of lipid-filled histiocytes, and approximately a third of

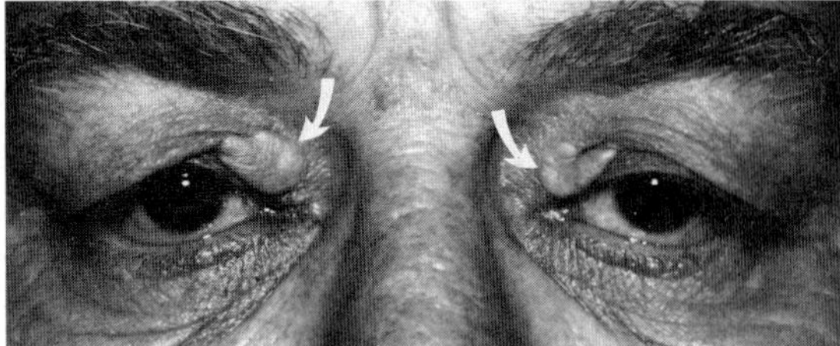

Fig. 3–35. Xanthelasmas. These benign lesions (*arrows*) may be associated with hyperlipidemia, as in this patient, whose serum cholesterol and triglyceride concentrations were elevated.

patients with eyelid xanthomas have an abnormality of serum lipid content. Surgical excision can be performed, although extensive lesions may require a skin graft or flap. The appearance of a typical eyelid xanthelasma may be mimicked by a rare but important entity, necrobiotic xanthogranuloma (Fig. 3–36). This eyelid lesion is more indurated than xanthelasma, and the process is often locally infiltrative. A systemic evaluation is mandatory in cases of necrobiotic xanthogranuloma because of the frequent association of a dysproteinemia such as multiple myeloma.

Basal cell carcinoma accounts for approximately 90% of malignant eyelid neoplasms. The tumor is most commonly located on the lower eyelid or in the medial canthus, although lesions on the upper eyelid or lateral canthus are not infrequent. Many clinical and histologic subtypes of basal cell carcinoma have been

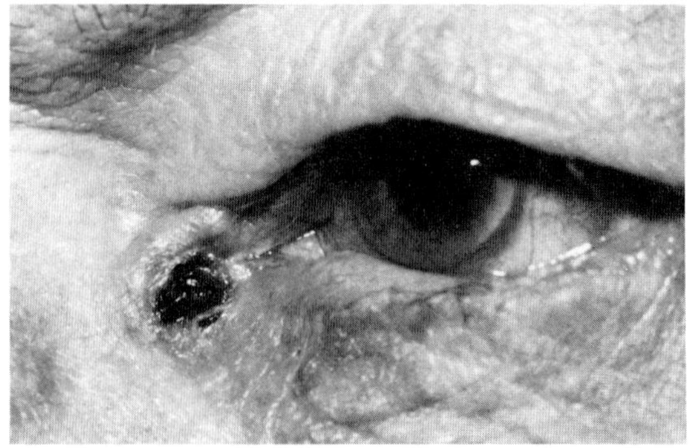

Fig. 3–37. Basal cell carcinoma with typical "rodent ulcer" appearance: raised, "pearly" edges and necrotic center. These neoplasms usually occur on the lower eyelid or in the medial canthus.

described, consistent with the myriad personalities of this common but often capricious invader. The "classic" basal cell tumor is shown in Figure 3–37: a circumscribed, elevated lesion with central necrosis and "pearly" rolled margins. Figures 3–38 through 3–40 demonstrate other common appearances.

The variable clinical pictures of basal cell carcinoma are matched by its wide range of malignant potential. Some lesions may be apparent to the patient for many years without demonstrating noticeable growth, and an incomplete incisional biopsy may sufficiently insult the tumor to lead to its demise. Unfortunately, the more typical course for basal cell carcinoma is to recur locally and invasively if

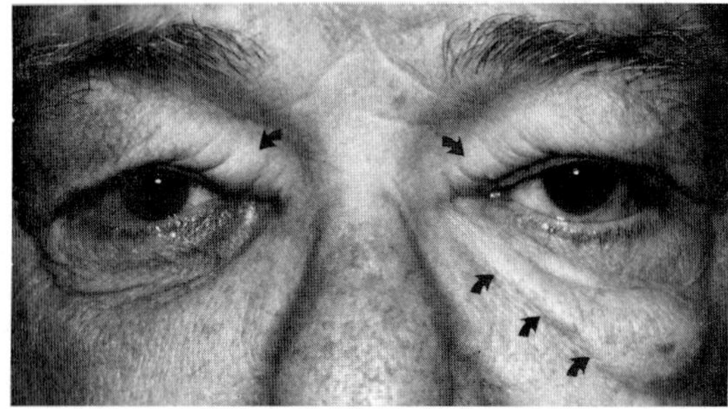

Fig. 3–36. Necrobiotic xanthogranuloma (*arrows*). This rare disease mimics xanthelasma, but it is important to recognize because of its frequent association with dysproteinemia.

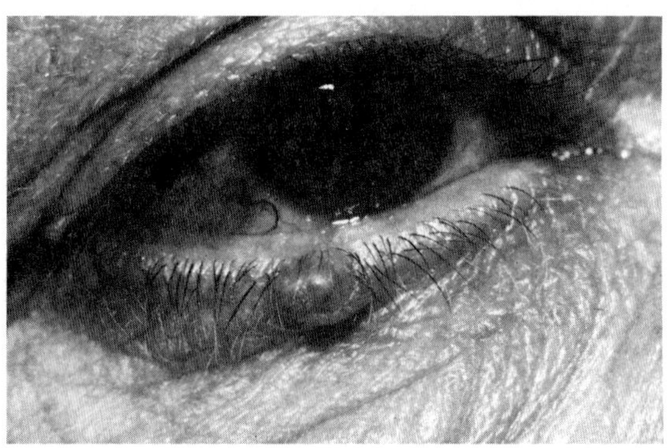

Fig. 3–38. Basal cell carcinoma that could be confused with a chalazion.

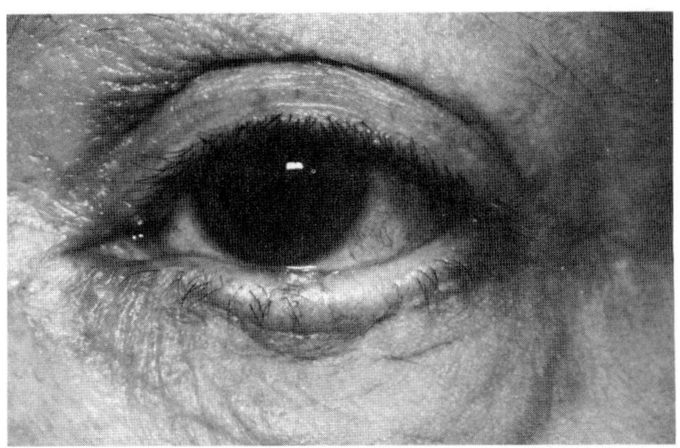

Fig. 3–39. Basal cell carcinoma that histopathologically was found to have spread horizontally to involve the entire lower eyelid margin. Note important feature of madarosis (loss of eyelashes).

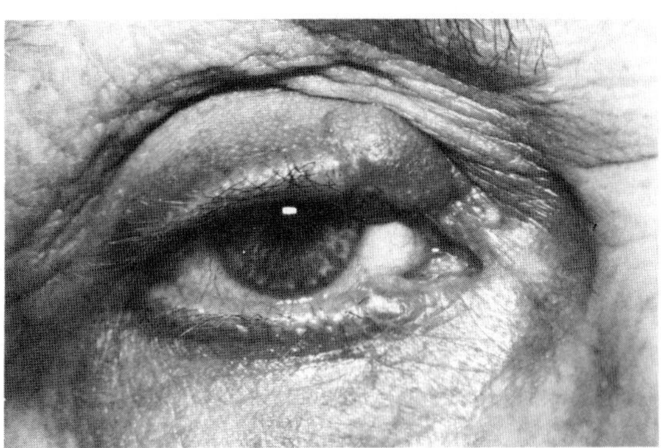

Fig. 3–41. Sebaceous carcinoma usually arises from the upper eyelid meibomian glands and should be suspected whenever a "chalazion" is unusually persistent or recurrent.

residual tumor is left behind, especially when the lesion arises in the medial canthus, where embryonic fusion planes may allow easy and unsuspected growth posteriorly into the orbit. The potential for clinically inapparent extension and local invasion should not be underestimated, and tumor-free surgical margins must be obtained by frozen-section analysis. Metastatic lesions are extremely rare but have been reported.

Sebaceous carcinomas arise from the oil-producing glands (primarily the meibomian glands) and are the second most common eyelid malignancy (Fig. 3–41). The upper lid is the usual site of origin, presumably because it has more meibomian glands than the lower lid; the neoplasm rarely arises elsewhere on the body. The tumor has significant malignant potential for both local invasion and metastasis. Sebaceous gland carcinoma can appear as a chalazion or a diffuse, unilateral blepharoconjunctivitis, demonstrating few characteristic clinical signs to reveal its identity, and it may elude diagnosis for many months. Adequate treatment is hampered not only by the common delay in diagnosis but also by the tendency for the neoplasm to arise multicentrically. Wide surgical excision is necessary because clinically normal tissue may harbor unsuspected extensions far from the primary tumor mass ("pagetoid spread"). *Any persistent or recurrent chalazion should be considered a sebaceous gland carcinoma until proved otherwise by biopsy.*

Squamous cell carcinoma commonly occurs on sun-exposed skin, and the eyelids are occasionally involved (Fig. 3–42). The frequency of squamous cell carcinoma is approximately equal to that of sebaceous gland carcinoma, but fortunately the malignant potential and mortality are much less. Both eyelids are equally affected and the clinical appearance can be variable, similar to the neoplasms described above. Surgical excision with microscopically tumor-free margins is the treatment of choice.

Other malignancies may affect the eyelids. Malignant melanoma is uncommon but important because of its poor prognosis.

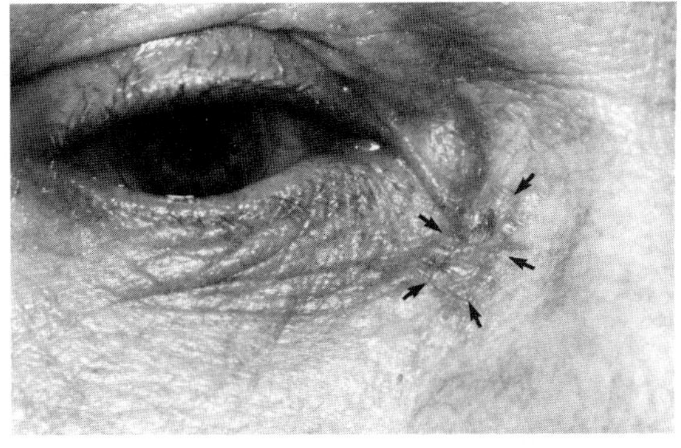

Fig. 3–40. Basal cell carcinoma, morpheaform type. Clinical margins of the tumor (*arrows*) are indistinct. Because the tumor often extends into apparently "normal" tissue, excision must be monitored carefully by frozen sections to minimize the risk of recurrence.

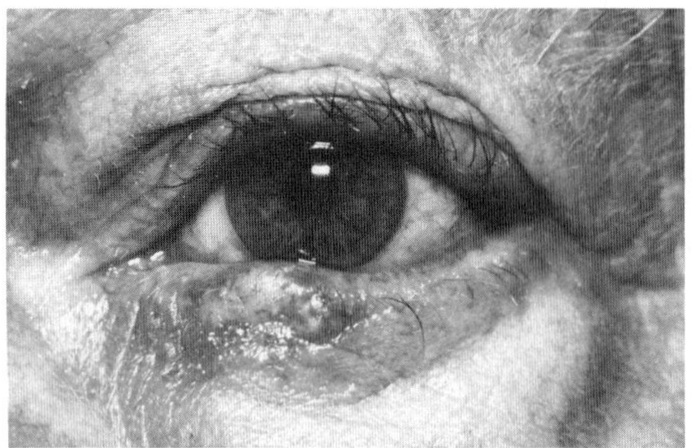

Fig. 3–42. Squamous cell carcinoma. Because of this tumor's medial location on the lower eyelid, the surgeon should be aware that excision most likely also will require lacrimal reconstruction.

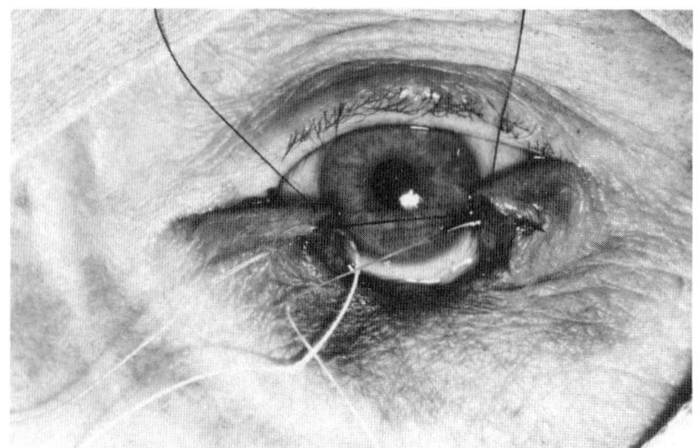

Fig. 3–43. Eyelid closure. The sutures to reapproximate the tarsus and orbicularis (white suture) give the repair its needed strength. The sutures that close the eyelid margin (black suture) are left long after tying and are draped away from the eye to prevent corneal irritation.

Although metastatic tumors rarely localize to the eyelids, the most common malignancy to do so is breast carcinoma.

Because of the intricate anatomy of the eyelid, seemingly minor trauma may cause significant functional and cosmetic problems.

A 1-cm laceration on many parts of the body may be relatively insignificant, and function and cosmesis can often be restored by simple closure. A traumatic insult of this size on an eyelid may result in severe complications that affect not only the eyelid but also, potentially, the lacrimal drainage system and the globe. When an eyelid laceration is evaluated in an emergency setting, the first priority must be to affirm that the eye itself is intact and unharmed. Unfortunately, in many cases, such as multiple life-threatening trauma, the ophthalmologist is often the last member of the medical team to be consulted. The delay during stabilization of the patient's general medical status may allow an eyelid with an originally small and manageable laceration to become massively edematous, precluding adequate visualization of the globe and making primary surgical repair of the eyelid difficult.

A *laceration through the eyelid margin* should be reapproximated carefully, with special attention to meticulous tarsal closure. A common mistake is to place several sutures in the eyelid margin while neglecting proper alignment of the tarsus; although both closures are important, it is the deep reapproximation that provides strength and security against notching or deformity of the eyelid. One should remember to leave the lid margin sutures long so that they may be draped away from the eye to prevent abrasions of the cornea (Fig. 3–43).

The lacrimal drainage structures must be evaluated carefully whenever a laceration involves the nasal portion of either the upper or the lower eyelid. *Canalicular lacerations* should be repaired promptly; postoperative anatomic and functional patency can be assisted by stenting the canal with silicone tubing (Fig. 3–44).

Horizontal lacerations superior to the tarsus in the upper eyelid may violate the levator aponeurosis, and primary repair is indicated to prevent ptosis. Care must be taken to avoid incorporating the orbital septum in the repair because postoperative scarring may lead to lagophthalmos. A ptotic eyelid may occasionally occur from blunt trauma to the periorbital region without laceration; gradual improvement usually can be expected over weeks to months. In a young child, amblyopia can result from occlusion of the eye by a traumatically ptotic eyelid, and temporary surgical elevation of the eyelid (with an alloplastic sling) may be necessary.

Avulsion of eyelid tissue may result in scars that are difficult to manage, particularly in a

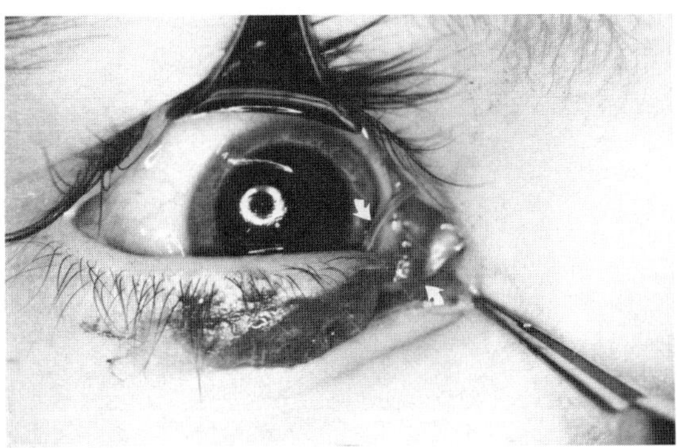

Fig. 3–44.   Eyelid and inferior canalicular lacerations from a dog bite. Crawford silicone lacrimal tubing (*arrows*) has been passed through the canaliculi to act as a stent during healing; the canalicular and eyelid lacerations are then repaired.

young person whose lids are not sufficiently lax to provide local flaps. Unnecessary debridement and wound freshening should be avoided whenever possible when repairing traumatic eyelid defects.

Excess tearing (epiphora) is a considerable inconvenience for the patient.

"My eye is always watering, and the tears run down my cheek" is a common complaint of patients. Tearing is a common concern; although the cause is rarely life-threatening, it can be a source of discomfort and considerable inconvenience for the patient. A thorough lacrimal examination includes a detailed history, careful inspection, probing and irrigation, and more sophisticated evaluations such as Jones' tests, dacryocystography, or dacryoscintigraphy if needed. Before *epiphora* (*tearing due to defective drainage*) can be diagnosed and treated, one must exclude *lacrimation* (*excessive tear formation*) as the origin of the problem.

Tearing in a child rarely may be a manifestation of congenital glaucoma, and associated signs such as buphthalmos (an enlarged globe) and corneal clouding should be sought. In adults, the most common cause of excessive lacrimation is, paradoxically, dry eyes. This phenomenon has been termed "pseudoepiphora of keratoconjunctivitis sicca." If the baseline minute-to-minute tear production is inadequate to keep the surface of the eye sufficiently moist, reflex tear secretion may be induced and tearing becomes manifest. The diagnosis can be confirmed by the findings of corneal and conjunctival rose bengal staining and low basal lacrimal secretion (Schirmer test after instillation of topical anesthesia). One should search for other local causes of ocular irritation such as trichiasis, foreign bodies, allergies, corneal abrasions, iritis, or dermatitis affecting the eyelids and face. Some eyedrops, such as betaxolol, can be irritating to the eye, whereas others with cholinergic properties, such as pilocarpine, may stimulate tear secretion. Lacrimation may at times be associated with systemic disorders such as acoustic neuromas, meningitis, subarachnoid hemorrhage, pseudobulbar palsy, and aberrant regeneration after facial nerve paralysis.

If excessive lacrimation has been excluded as the primary cause of tearing, defects in tear drainage should be sought. In many cases, the lacrimal apparatus is anatomically patent but local nonobstructive disorders prevent the proper transit of tears through the system. For example, the punctum may be displaced from the lacrimal lake in eyelid malpositions such as ectropion, that associated with Graves' ophthalmopathy, or that after operation or trauma to the eyelid. In some patients with seventh cranial nerve palsy, the puncta may be appropriately apposed to the globe, but laxity of the eyelids may preclude proper "pumping" of the tears into the system with blinking.

Most patients with tearing have blockage, either anatomic or functional, of the lacrimal drainage system. The evaluation of obstructive epiphora can be divided into three main components: 1) inspection, 2) probing and irrigation, and 3) tests for patency, if needed.

One should begin by inspecting the eyelids, medial canthal region, and the nose. The presence of upper and lower puncta should be confirmed, and any evidence of abnormal development such as a slit-shaped canaliculi or accessory puncta should be noted. Punctal stenosis may occur secondary to chronic topical glaucoma therapy, if potent antiviral drops or ointments such as idoxuridine have been used, or in association with systemic chemotherapy for cancer. Gentle digital pressure over the medial canthus is important; the lacrimal sac is normally not palpable, and if mucus or pus emerges from the puncta the presence of an obstructed nasolacrimal duct with dacryocystitis is confirmed. Finally, one should inspect the inferior turbinate for masses or other nasal abnormality that could impede the passage of tears through the terminal orifice, the valve of Hasner.

Next, the *anatomic patency of the nasolacrimal system* is evaluated by probing and irrigation. The inferior punctum is gently dilated with a thin, pointed dilator to allow insertion of a small (size 0 or 00) Bowman *probe* into the canaliculus. Placing mild lateral tension on the lower eyelid will put the canaliculus on stretch and facilitate easy passage of the probe. One must be careful not to "force" the probe; the lacrimal canals are delicate and iatrogenic trauma must be avoided. Any areas of resistance to the probe are noted, and insertion of 10 mm or more usually indicates that entry into the lacrimal sac has been achieved. The Bowman probe is removed and *irrigation* of the system is done with saline through a 23-gauge blunt-tipped cannula. Passage of irrigant to the nasopharynx confirms anatomic patency of the nasolacrimal duct. If an obstruction is present in the sac or duct, the saline will usually reflux through the superior canaliculus and punctum, often accompanied by mucus or pus. Blockage high in the sac or at the junction of the common canaliculus and the sac typically results in reflux of clear fluid through the superior canaliculus (Fig. 3–45), whereas reflux of saline through the cannulated inferior punctum points to canalicular obstruction that is preventing the irrigant from reaching the common canaliculus or sac. Irrigation through the superior punctum and canaliculus may be performed if any doubt exists concerning the site of blockage.

If a complete block in the lacrimal sac or nasolacrimal duct is confirmed by probing and irrigation, a bypass procedure is indicated and no further evaluation is typically necessary. Radiologic visualization of the system (*dacryocystography*) is useful in certain circum-

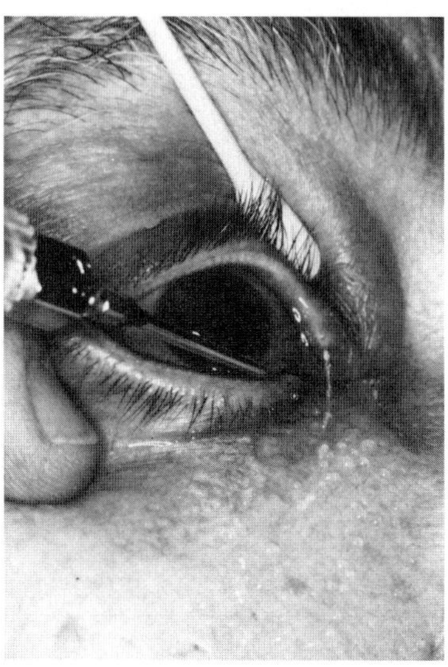

Fig. 3–45. Saline irrigated through the inferior canaliculus refluxes without mucus or pus through the superior canaliculus and punctum, indicating an obstruction at the common canaliculus or high in the lacrimal sac without acute dacryocystitis.

stances (for example, in cases of previous trauma, prior nasal or lacrimal operation, congenital anomalies, or a suspected obstructing dacryolith or tumor). Standard dacryocystography, consisting of a posteroanterior (Caldwell) skull film after irrigation of a radiopaque contrast material into the nasolacrimal system, may be helpful for confirming the site or cause of lacrimal obstruction (Fig. 3–46).

Some patients complain of persistent tearing despite the presence of anatomically patent puncta, canaliculi, lacrimal sac, and nasolacrimal duct. Several tests may help to identify whether the system is functioning properly.

The simplest evaluation is the *fluorescein dye disappearance test*: a drop of 2% fluorescein is instilled into each inferior cul-de-sac, and one observes whether the dye disappears normally from the tear film over a 5-minute period. The anatomic site of resistance within the nasolacrimal system is not identified by this test, and a malpositioned or stenotic punctum may prevent entry into an otherwise patent conduit.

The *Jones primary dye test* is similar to the dye disappearance test except that an attempt is made to identify whether fluorescein has passed through the lacrimal drainage system

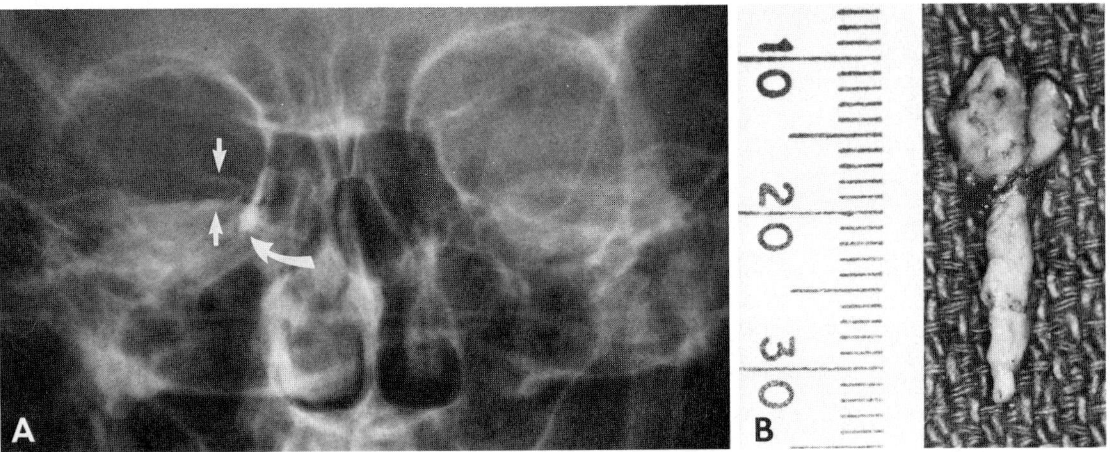

Fig. 3–46. *A*, Dacryocystography demonstrates obstruction of the nasolacrimal duct (*curved arrow*). The canaliculi (*small arrows*) can be identified. *B*, Nasolacrimal obstruction in this case was due to a dacryolith that formed a "cast" of the sac and duct.

into the nose. A cobalt light is used to examine beneath the inferior turbinate, or a cotton-tipped applicator is placed near the valve of Hasner; if fluorescence is identified or dye is recovered, the test is positive (that is, normal). If fluorescein has not passed into the nose, the *Jones secondary dye test* is performed: the dye is irrigated from the conjunctival fornix, and clear saline is then irrigated through the canaliculus. The patient leans forward to prevent the fluid from coursing posteriorly into the throat, and an emesis basin is placed next to the naris to collect the irrigant. Fluorescein in the recovered fluid indicates that some of the originally instilled dye passed into the system but was impeded from complete transit by a partial blockage—a positive Jones secondary dye test. If the fluid in the basin is completely clear, the secondary test is negative, consistent with a malfunctioning upper system that prevented entry of the dye.

The Jones dye tests are simple in concept and easy to perform, but many examiners are unfamiliar with nasal anatomy and uncertain of the sometimes ambiguous subjective results. In these circumstances, *dacryoscintigraphy* is an excellent objective evaluation of the functional status of the lacrimal drainage system. Eyedrops with radiolabeled technetium are instilled and passage through the system is followed scintigraphically. The radiation exposure

is minimal (approximately 1% of a standard skull radiograph), and the procedure is completely noninvasive. Incomplete or inadequate transit is identified by the pattern of radioactivity in the sac or duct (Fig. 3–47).

Dacryoscintigraphy is also useful in some cases of suspected "lacrimal pump failure" in which the eyelids are too lax or flaccid to propel

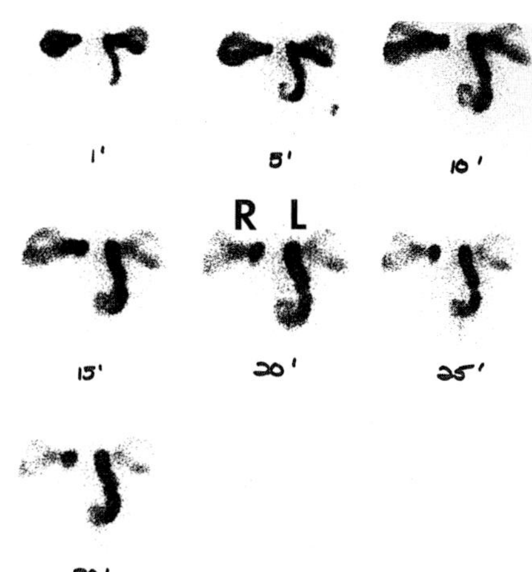

Fig. 3–47. Dacryoscintigraphy. This patient complained of tearing from the right eye. Lacrimal drainage systems were anatomically patent, as confirmed by irrigation, but dacryoscintigraphy demonstrates functional blockage of the right system.

the tears through the canaliculi to the sac. The possibility of false-negative results can be reduced if tests to evaluate the functional status of the nasolacrimal system are not performed immediately after the drainage apparatus has been probed or irrigated.

Table 3–2 summarizes the approach to a patient with tearing.

Lacrimal obstruction in children typically responds to probing, whereas in adults a bypass procedure is usually required.

Approximately 5% of all full-term newborns are born with an incompletely patent nasolacrimal system (*congenital dacryostenosis*); the obstruction is almost always due to a soft tissue membrane over the valve of Hasner. Rarely, a mass may be present at birth in the medial canthus from a swollen lacrimal sac (*congenital dacryocele*, lacrimal sac mucocele, or "amniotocele"), but in the typical case tearing is often not immediately apparent because reflex tear secretion from trigeminal stimulation does not commence until several weeks of age. A blocked tear drainage system soon becomes apparent to the parents as a watery eye, mattering on the eyelashes, and occasionally a swollen lacrimal sac. Most infants with congenital dacryostenosis are probably never seen by an ophthalmologist: in most cases the disorder resolves spontaneously, or first-line medical treatment, if required, is usually provided by the family physician or pediatrician. Gentle pressure in a downward direction may help to open the blockage at the valve of Hasner by increasing hydrostatic pressure within the lacrimal sac, and topical antibiotics such as sulfacetamide are typically prescribed. Persistent tearing and low-grade infection eventually bring the child to the ophthalmologist.

It is generally agreed that a congenital dacryocele noted at birth should be opened promptly by passing a probe through the system to reduce the possibility of facial or preseptal cellulitis. The treatment of "routine" congenital dacryostenosis, however, has been the topic of vigorous debate for many years. Some specialists have presented convincing evidence that one should wait for the obstruction to

---

TABLE 3–2 The Evaluation of Tearing

Is tearing due to lacrimation (excessive tear secretion) or epiphora (defective tear drainage) or both?

I. Lacrimation

    A. In a child, rule out congenital glaucoma

    B. Local causes of tearing
       1. Keratoconjunctivitis sicca
       2. Trichiasis
       3. Foreign bodies
       4. Allergies
       5. Corneal abrasions
       6. Iritis
       7. Dermatitis
       8. Eyedrops

    C. Systemic disorders associated with tearing
       1. Acoustic neuroma
       2. Meningitis
       3. Subarachnoid hemorrhage
       4. Pseudobulbar palsy
       5. Aberrant seventh cranial nerve regeneration

II. Epiphora

    A. Nonobstructive
       1. Eyelid malpositions
         a. Ectropion
         b. Graves' ophthalmopathy
         c. After trauma or operation
       2. Eyelid laxity (insufficient lacrimal pump function)
         a. Normal aging
         b. Seventh cranial nerve palsy

    B. Obstructive
       1. Complete anatomic blockage
         a. Site of obstruction may be anywhere in system (punctum, canaliculus, lacrimal sac, nasolacrimal duct, nose)
         b. Lacrimal sac may contain mucus and pus (dacryocystitis)
         c. Dacryocystography demonstrates complete block
         d. Jones primary and secondary tests both negative
       2. Incomplete anatomic blockage with functional obstruction
         a. Site of obstruction may be anywhere in system (punctum, canaliculus, lacrimal sac, nasolacrimal duct, nose)
         b. Dacryocystography usually normal
         c. Dacryoscintigraphy demonstrates delay in tear transit
         d. Jones primary test negative, Jones secondary test positive

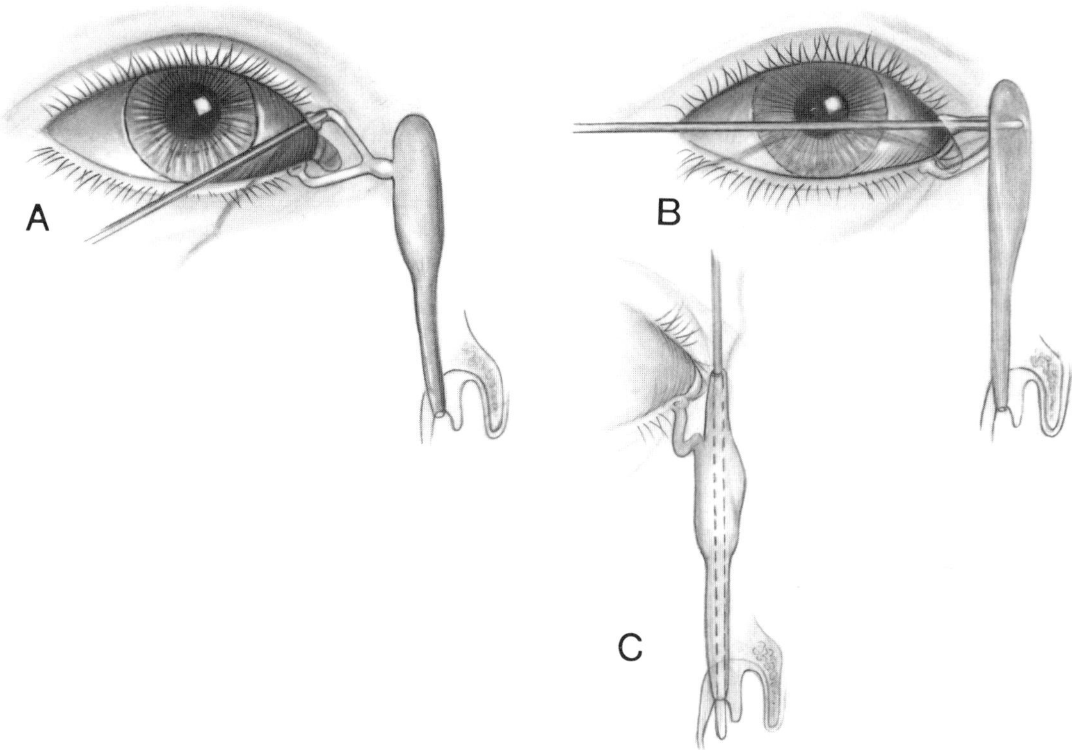

Fig. 3–48.   Nasolacrimal probing for congenital dacryostenosis; the obstruction typically is at the valve of Hasner, where the nasolacrimal duct opens into the inferior meatus.

open spontaneously until the child is a year old, at which time probing can be considered if needed (Fig. 3–48). Others have argued that the success of probing is greatly reduced if delayed and that earlier intervention is warranted. Our recommendations have been to use topical antibiotics and massage over the sac until the child is at least 6 months old; probing can then be performed if the parents wish. A single probing relieves the obstruction in more than 90% of cases. If the tearing and mattering persist, a second probing is performed; if significant obstruction is encountered, the nasolacrimal system is intubated with *silicone tubing*

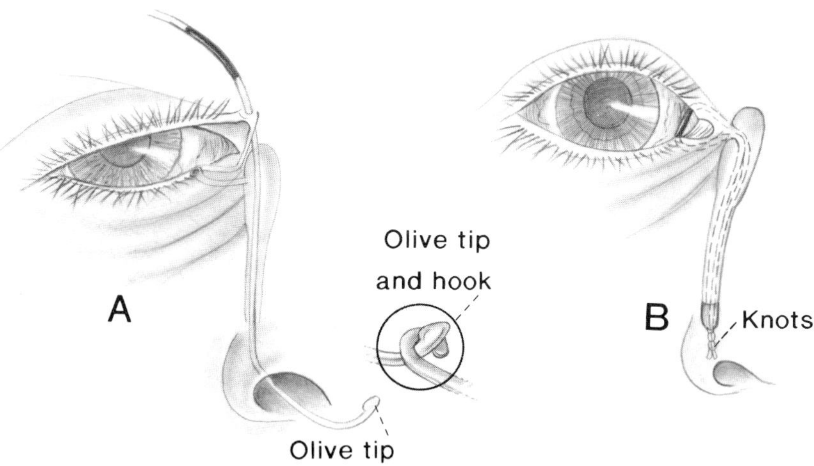

Fig. 3–49.   Crawford tubing for persistent congenital dacryostenosis; the tubes act as a stent to facilitate patency of the drainage system.

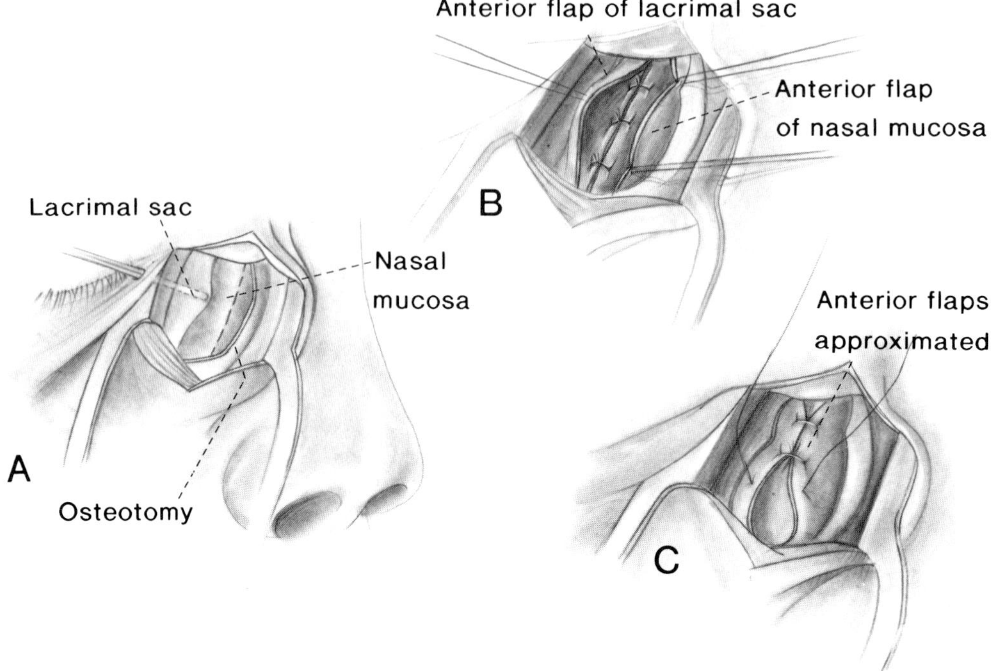

Fig. 3–50.   Dacryocystorhinostomy creates a new conduit for tear flow between the lacrimal sac and the nasal cavity.

that acts as a stent to decrease postoperative scarring and closure (Fig. 3–49). The tubes are removed after several months, and in almost all cases the tearing does not recur. If obstruction is persistent, a bypass can be performed by creating a mucosal anastomosis between the lacrimal sac and the middle meatus of the nose (a *dacryocystorhinostomy*) (Fig. 3–50).

Tearing due to nasolacrimal obstruction in adults is nearly always an acquired problem, and several factors are contributory. Chronic sinusitis can "spill over" and lead to scarring of the narrow nasolacrimal duct. Nasal operation may result in postoperative epiphora, and trauma to the mid-face often disrupts the lacrimal excretory system. Neoplasms in the sinuses, nose, or rarely the lacrimal sac itself can obstruct the transit of tears, and bloody epiphora should alert the clinician that an invasive process may be present. Occasionally a "stone" (dacryolith) can form in the lacrimal sac, and in other cases an infection can be localized to a single canaliculus (canaliculitis). In most patients, however, the etiologic sequence of nasolacrimal obstruction is not clear but

probably follows the course of a mild lacrimal sac infection, leading to scarring, which results in more infection and eventually complete blockage. A minority of patients have one or several bouts of fulminating *dacryocystitis* (Fig. 3–51). These infections usually respond well to broad-spectrum oral antibiotics, although occasionally intravenous therapy is necessary. Dacryocystorhinostomy is ideally delayed until the acute infection subsides.

In contrast to dacryostenosis in children, obstruction in adults rarely responds to simple

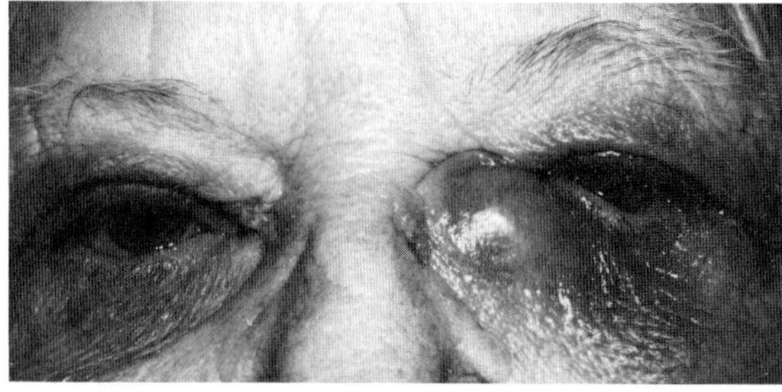

Fig. 3–51.   Acute dacryocystitis secondary to nasolacrimal duct obstruction.

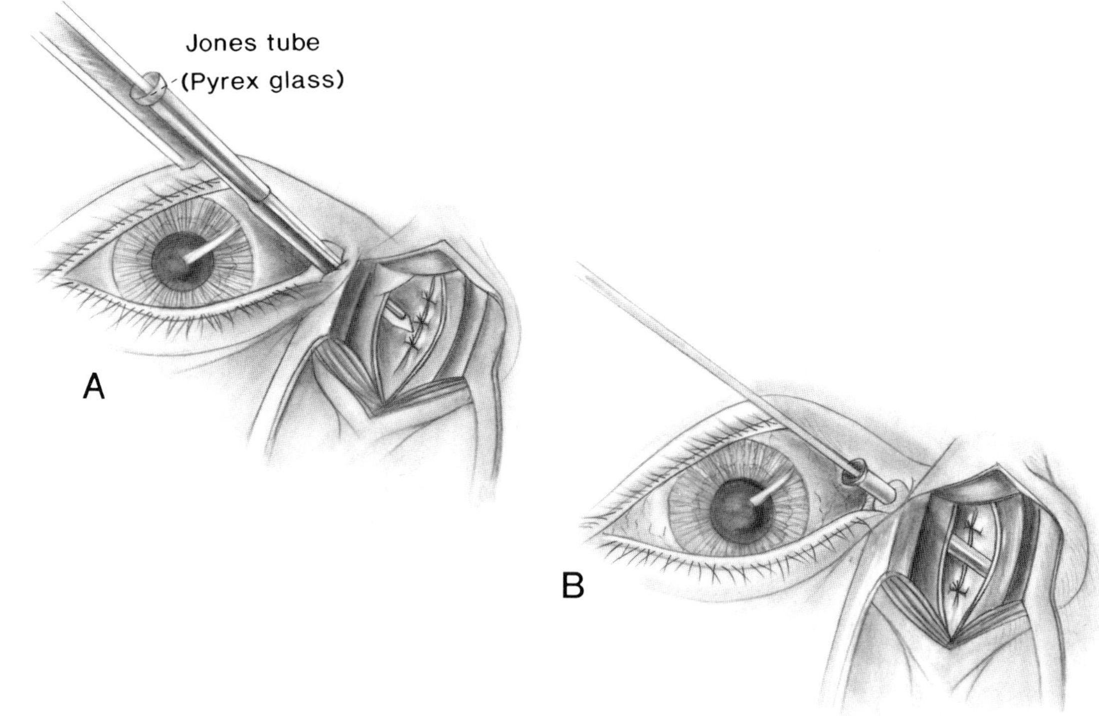

Fig. 3–52. Conjunctivodacryocystorhinostomy with Jones tube. When the tears cannot pass through the canaliculi, the entire nasolacrimal system is bypassed by a glass tube from the medial canthal angle to the nasal cavity.

probing through the lacrimal sac and duct, and a dacryocystorhinostomy is required. Silicone tubing can be placed through the system at the time of operation and is especially useful when common canalicular stenosis is present or if excessive postoperative scarring is expected (for example, in cases of trauma or prior operation or radiation). If the canaliculi are too diffusely scarred to allow tear passage or to permit placement of silicone tubing, a *Jones tube* made of Pyrex may be placed in conjunction with a dacryocystorhinostomy to allow tears to drain directly from the medial canthal angle to the nose (Fig. 3–52). Placement of Jones tubes is fraught with many potential problems, such as blockage, migration, and poor patient acceptance, and should be considered a procedure of last resort.

4

DISORDERS OF THE CORNEA, CONJUNCTIVA, AND LENS

Thomas J. Liesegang

CORNEA

The six layers of the cornea interact to provide a clear refracting surface for the eye.

The cornea is the major refracting surface of the eye related to its curvature and the index of refraction. The cornea is composed functionally of six layers: tear film, epithelium with its basement membrane, Bowman's layer, stroma, Descemet's membrane, and endothelium (Fig. 4–1). The *tear film* is intimately connected with the epithelial surface by microvilli. The *epithelium* is five to six layers of nonkeratinized epithelial cells attached to each other by desmosomes and to the basement membrane by hemidesmosomes. *Bowman's layer* is an acellular condensation of the anterior corneal stroma running parallel to the surface of the cornea. The *stroma* constitutes the major part of the cornea and is composed of lamellae of collagen running the full length of the cornea in a parallel arrangement and separated by a ground substance and keratocytes. *Descemet's membrane* is a thickened acellular structure that is a product of secretion of the endothelial cells. The *endothelium* is a single layer of flattened cuboidal cells lining the inner cornea. Several complex factors are involved in maintaining the transparency and the central corneal thickness at approximately 0.52 mm: the structural and func-

tional integrity of the endothelium and epithelium, the evaporation of the precorneal tear film, the intraocular pressure, and the uniform and regular arrangement of the lamellae of collagen.

The cornea is avascular, probably because of its compact lamellar structure. The special privilege of avascularity is very important for the success of corneal transplantation, but it may be altered by inflammation, infection, or edema. The cornea has a few characteristic ways to respond to insult: epithelial punctate keratitis and ulceration; stromal infiltration, edema, and neovascularization; and endothelial keratitic precipitates.

Some corneal degenerations may be physiologic or age-related.

Corneal degenerations are unilateral or bilateral changes in the cornea related to aging, corneal disease, or trauma. They may be central or peripheral and usually are asymptomatic. Occasionally, they may accompany systemic disease.

Many corneal degenerations occur with age. These *physiologic corneal degenerations* consist of thinning of the peripheral cornea, flattening of the vertical meridian (giving a plus refractive cylinder at 180°), an increased stromal relucency, and decreased transparency and luster. *Corneal arcus* is a common peripheral lipid

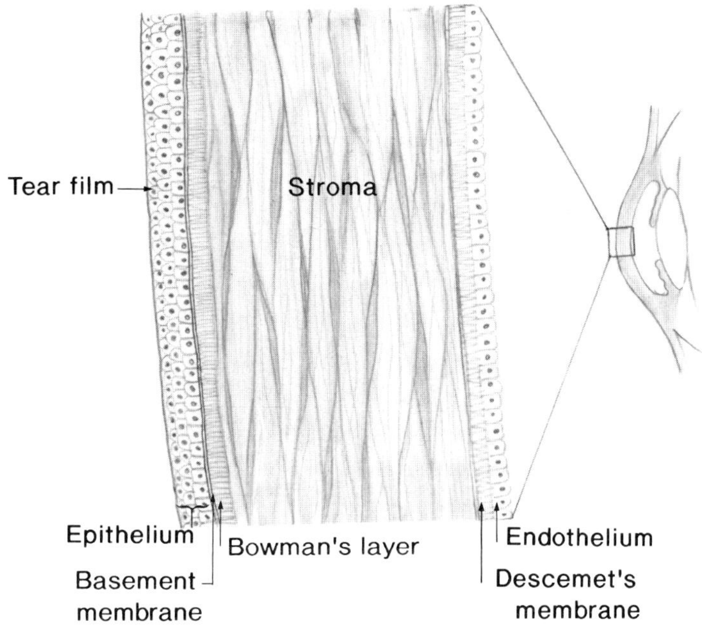

Fig. 4–1. The layers of the cornea include the tear film, epithelium with its basement membrane, Bowman's layer, stroma, Descemet's membrane, and endothelium.

deposit that begins in the inferior and superior cornea and eventually involves the whole corneal circumference (Fig. 4–2). There is usually a clear zone between the limbus and this deposit which consists of extracellular cholesterol, triglycerides, and phospholipids. Corneal arcus is related to age and is frequent in blacks. When it occurs in patients younger than 40 years, it may be associated with serum

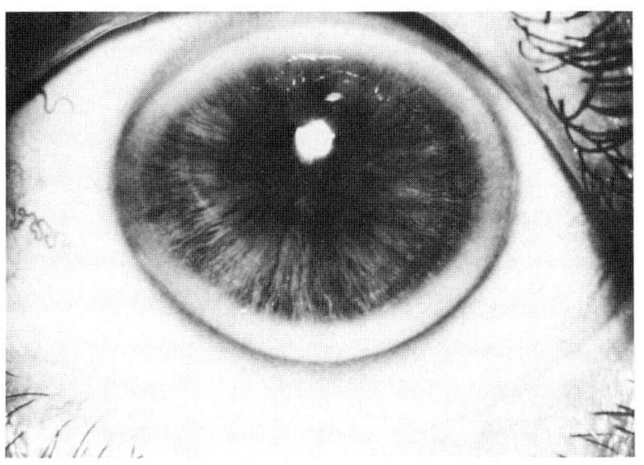

Fig. 4–2. Marked lipid deposit encircling the peripheral cornea, characteristic of corneal arcus.

lipid abnormalities. The *white limbal girdle of Vogt* is a common, white, irregular, chalky opacity in the limbal area, usually nasally and temporally. *Hassall-Henle bodies* are irregular nodular thickenings of Descemet's membrane in the peripheral cornea. They are pathologically similar to central cornea guttata. *Cornea farinata* are numerous tiny flecks in the deep corneal stroma and are best seen on retroillumination. *Anterior crocodile shagreen* refers to central gray-white polygonal opacities in the anterior stroma that consist of fibrous tissues in areas of interruption of Bowman's membrane; they are usually asymptomatic. *Posterior crocodile shagreen* refers to polygonal patches with dark clear lines in the deep corneal stroma that do not interfere with vision.

Some central corneal degenerations may cause significant visual disability.

Spheroidal degeneration refers to peripheral oily droplets beneath the epithelium and occasionally in the central cornea which appear in some individuals with age but may also be centrally associated with irradiation, chronic corneal disease, or certain regional climates. This is probably a form of elastotic and fibrillar degeneration of collagen. It is usually asymptomatic and requires no treatment. *Salzmann's nodular degeneration* consists of elevated white nodules usually arranged circularly in the middle of the cornea (Fig. 4–3). It is usually associated with previous chronic ocular disease and may be seen with spheroidal degeneration or map-dot corneal dystrophy. Salzmann's nodules consist of hyaline plaques between the epithelium and Bowman's membrane with an increase in basement membrane material and occasionally hypertrophy of the epithelium. Occasionally, superficial keratectomy is required, but the nodules have a tendency to recur.

Band keratopathy is a Swiss cheese or frosted-glass calcific turbidity at Bowman's level within the palpebral fissure (Fig. 4–4). It usually begins peripherally with a clear interval between the limbus (because it involves only Bowman's membrane). This deposition of hydroxyapatite calcium occurs with chronic ocular disease (uveitis), from several drugs, or from systemic diseases associated with hypercalcemia (Table 4–1). Band keratopathy usually evolves slowly but tends to develop quicker in cases of aqueous tear deficiency. With time, additional fibrosis may occur. The treatment of band keratopathy is to remove the epithelium and then to chelate the calcium with disodium EDTA.

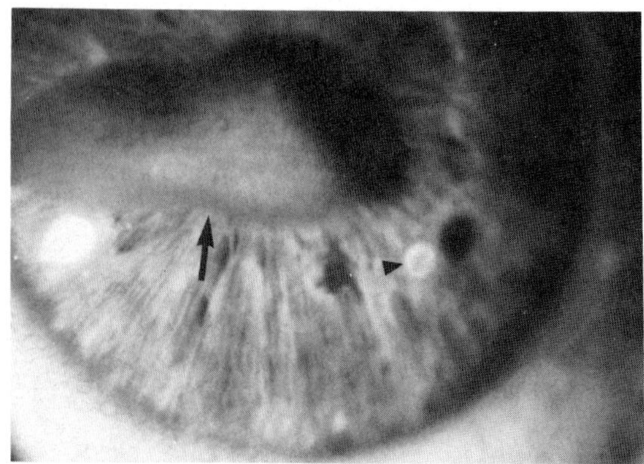

Fig. 4–4. Frosted-glass appearance of calcific band keratopathy (*arrow*) across the central anterior corneal surface in a patient with hypercalcemia. This cornea also has a Coats' white ring (*arrowhead*) in the peripheral cornea.

Sometimes, simple scraping can remove the calcium flecks. Band keratopathy tends to recur unless the inciting cause is eliminated.

Lipid degeneration of the cornea is a dense, yellow opacity in various areas of the cornea with cholesterol crystals and frequent corneal neovascularization (Fig. 4–5). The lipid is de-

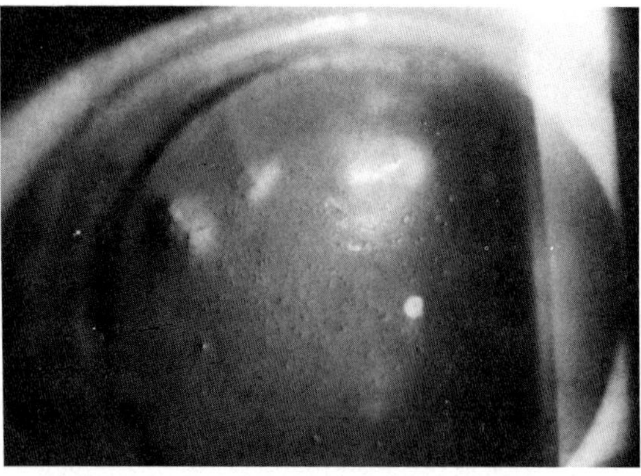

Fig. 4–3. Elevated white nodules of various sizes on the anterior surface of the cornea, characteristic of Salzmann's nodular degeneration.

TABLE 4–1 Causes of Band Keratopathy

Chronic ocular inflammatory disease (especially in rheumatoid arthritis, Still's disease, sarcoidosis)
  Keratitis
  Scleritis
  Iridocyclitis
Chronic ocular environmental disease
  Neurotrophic keratitis (especially herpes zoster)
  Exposure keratitis
  Long-standing glaucoma (especially miotic therapy)
  Spheroidal corneal degeneration
  Severe dry eye
  Chronic topical drugs (thimerosal, phenylmercuric nitrate)
Systemic disease
  Hypercalcemia, idiopathic
  Vitamin D intoxication
  Gout
  Fanconi's syndrome
  Milk-alkali syndrome
  Hypophosphatemia
  Myotonic dystrophy
Hereditary
  Dystrophic band keratopathy

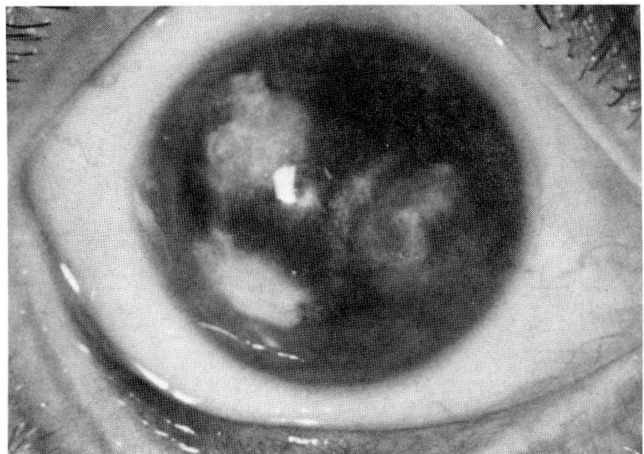

Fig. 4–5. Multiple corneal opacities of cholesterol and lipid throughout the cornea with some vascularization, characteristic of lipid degeneration of the cornea. Opacities in this disorder are yellowish white.

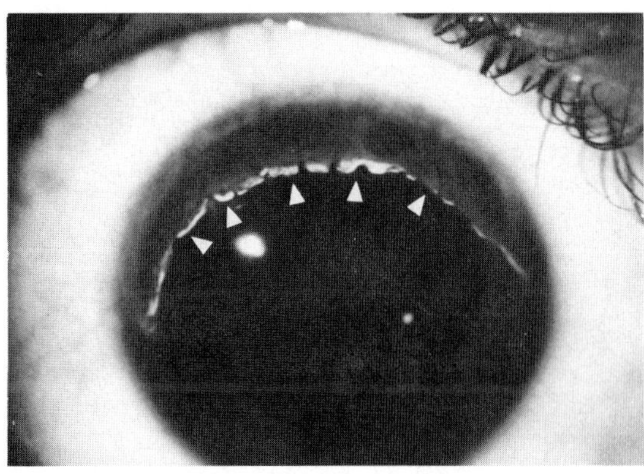

Fig. 4–6. Superior peripheral corneal thinning with the lipid deposit at the advancing edge (*arrowheads*) in an eye with Terrien's marginal degeneration. Deposits were yellowish.

posited around the blood vessels. Lipid keratopathy is secondary to chronic corneal disease but occasionally can be seen as a primary ocular disease without specific cause and may be related to systemic lipid abnormalities. *Coats' white ring* is a small, granular, white, oval ring that contains iron and is usually seen in the peripheral cornea (Fig. 4–4). It may be related to a prior foreign body.

Peripheral corneal degeneration may cause thinning and, rarely, perforation.

Terrien's marginal degeneration is a peripheral thinning of the cornea; it is associated with a mild opacification and superficial peripheral neovascularization. A lipid deposition occurs at the advancing edge of the thinning (Fig. 4–6). This tends to begin superiorly at the limbus with an intact epithelium and is bilateral, although asymmetric. It is asymptomatic except when a large corneal astigmatism develops. Terrien's degeneration tends to progress slowly and can rarely lead to a corneal perforation. It is probably related to lysosomal activity of histiocytic cells. In many instances, the condition itself subsides and the thinning is filled in with epithelium or a pseudopterygium. The patient should be warned to avoid trauma.

Senile marginal degeneration is an asymptomatic thinning of the peripheral cornea that occurs in elderly patients without conjunctival

injection, corneal neovascularization, or perforation. It begins superiorly and inferiorly and tends to be slowly progressive. *Pellucid marginal degeneration* is a thinning of the cornea concentric with the limbus and limited to the inferior cornea with a clear interval separating it from the limbus. It tends to occur in young men between the ages of 20 and 40 years and is bilateral without vascularization or lipid infiltration. It is slowly progressive with a plus refractive cylinder developed at 180°. Treatment consists of protective glasses, contact lenses for mild astigmatism, and occasionally penetrating keratoplasty or corneal wedge resection to reduce severe astigmatism.

The most common corneal dystrophies involving the epithelium and basement membrane are Meesmann's dystrophy, anterior membrane dystrophy, and Reis-Bücklers dystrophy.

The corneal dystrophies are bilateral, symmetric, central, avascular, hereditary (almost all are autosomal dominant), early in onset, slowly progressive, and without associated systemic disease. They commonly involve a single corneal layer and are typically grouped according to the corneal layer that is involved (Table 4–2).

The most common dystrophies involving the epithelium and basement membrane are

TABLE 4–2 Common Corneal Dystrophies

Type	Characteristics
Anterior corneal dystrophies	
Meesmann's epithelial dystrophy	Intraepithelial cysts of glycogen Later decrease in vision Begins in childhood
Anterior membrane dystrophy (Cogan's microcystic, map-dot-fingerprint)	Epithelial microcysts or aberrant thickening of basement membrane Bilateral, variable dots or lines Usually occurs in middle-aged women Eventually, recurrent erosions
Reis-Bücklers dystrophy	Defects of basement membrane and Bowman's layer Treadlike opacities with irregular corneal surface Significant visual loss Begins in childhood
Anterior crocodile shagreen (there is a senile form of this condition)	Granular deposits at Bowman's layer Polygonal, gray, central opacities Begins in childhood
Cornea verticillata (a component of Fabry's disease)	Intracellular vacuoles of glycolipids; bilateral, pigmented, vortex-shaped lines
Stromal dystrophies	
Granular dystrophy	Hyaline granules in superficial stroma; white "bread-crumb" appearance of granular superficial lesions Decreased vision Corneal erosions
Lattice dystrophy	Amyloid degeneration of collagen Lattice-like or round opacities Decreased vision and erosions
Macular dystrophy	Mucopolysaccharides in stroma Diffuse, confluent opacities in all layers of stroma Decreased vision and erosions
Central cloudy dystrophy of François	Diffuse, deep opacification with segmental areas of involvement that may extend to Bowman's layer No decrease in vision
Crystalline dystrophy of Schnyder	Cholesterol crystals in superficial stroma, usually oval or needle-shaped, polychromatic crystals Decrease in vision
Cornea farinata (pre-Descemet's dystrophy) (probably a senile degeneration)	Periodic acid–Schiff-positive deposits in deep stroma Punctate, gray-white opacities anterior to Descemet's membrane No symptoms
Endothelial dystrophies	
Posterior polymorphous dystrophy of Schlichting	Coalescent vesicles or bandlike figure on posterior corneal surface with thickening of Descemet's membrane Epithelial-like endothelium Minimal decrease in vision
Cornea guttata	Wartlike thickening of Descemet's membrane with thinning of the endothelium; "hammered" appearance of Descemet's membrane Affects middle-aged persons Minimal decrease in vision

(continued)

TABLE 4–2 (*continued*)

Type	Characteristics
Endothelial dystrophies (*continued*)	
Fuchs' corneal dystrophy	Cornea guttata plus stromal and epithelial edema; later, bullae and scarring Marked decrease in vision with photophobia
Ectatic corneal dystrophies (degenerations)	
Keratoconus	Thinning and conical protrusion of cornea, either central or inferior; striae of Descemet's membrane, breaks in Bowman's layer, or tears in Descemet's membrane Progression is highly variable and asymmetric Possible history of allergy
Keratoglobus	Globular configuration to cornea; cornea thin, especially peripherally, and occasionally larger in diameter; cornea may perforate with minimal trauma Occasional family history of keratoconus
Pellucid marginal degeneration	Bilateral, clear, inferior corneal thinning with high astigmatism Occasional perforation
Posterior keratoconus	Increased curvature of posterior corneal surface in either focal location or entire cornea; the anterior cornea is normal Nonprogressive Descemet's membrane and endothelium abnormal in area of concavity

Meesmann's dystrophy, anterior membrane dystrophy, and Reis-Bücklers dystrophy. *Meesmann's dystrophy* is a bilateral, symmetric, and autosomal dominant dystrophy involving the epithelial layer with epithelial vesicles visible on slit-lamp examination. There is occasional foreign body sensation associated with ruptured vesicles. Corneal sensation may be reduced, but vision is usually normal. The epithelial vesicles appear gray-white in direct illumination but appear clear on retroillumination. The disease is very frequently asymptomatic, although it may be gradually progressive. Superficial corneal scrapings are usually ineffective, although use of soft contact lenses may eliminate the epithelial cysts. Superficial lamellar keratoplasty may be indicated.

Anterior membrane dystrophy, also called map-dot-fingerprint dystrophy or Cogan's microcystic dystrophy, is a common bilateral disease of the corneal basement membrane. It is probably hereditary, although it is not usually detected until middle age. The three patterns of map, dot, and fingerprint lines can occur alone or in combination and can change with time on different examinations. The *fingerprint pattern* is the most common and consists of concentric contoured lines formed by reduplication and thickening of basement membrane material. The *map pattern* is a gray-white, irregular geographic design related to thickening of the basement membrane and proliferation of collagen material. The *dots* consist of gray-white round or irregularly shaped intraepithelial opacities that appear putty-like (Fig. 4–7).

Anterior membrane dystrophy is frequently asymptomatic, but occasionally it is associated with blurring of vision, irregular astigmatism, foreign body sensation, or corneal erosions. It appears to be aggravated by dry, hot climates or exposure of the corneas. Pathologic findings are a thick, abnormal basement membrane with the formation of microcysts in the epithelium. The treatment of recurrent erosions consists of pressure patching for acute episodes and prophylaxis involving the use of sodium chloride ointment and patching at bedtime along with artificial tears during the day. A soft con-

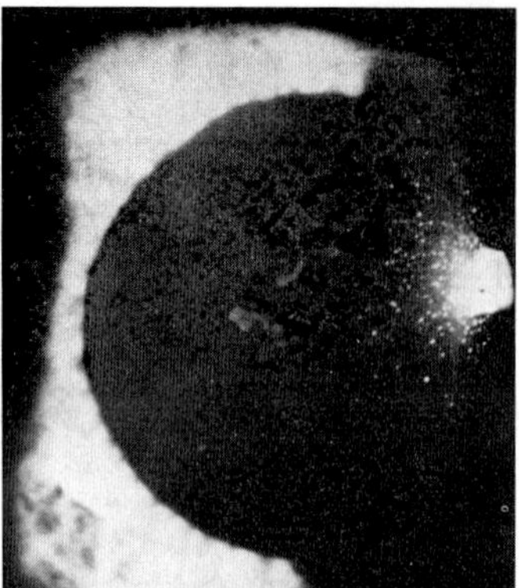

Fig. 4–7. The dot pattern of anterior membrane dystrophy with putty-like intraepithelial deposits that will vary in location over time.

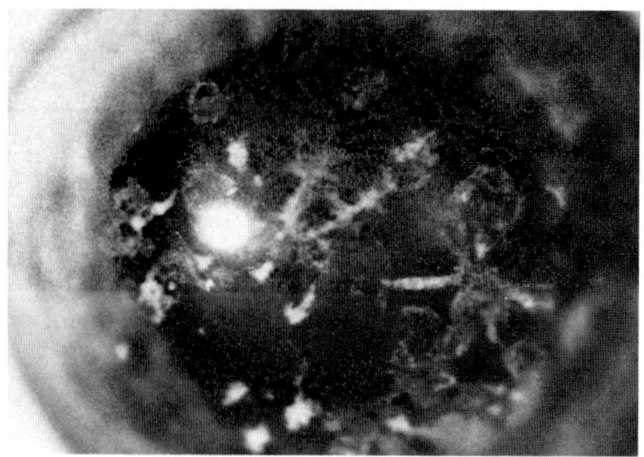

Fig. 4–8. Small, gray-white, sharply demarcated, crumblike opacities throughout the cornea in a patient with granular corneal dystrophy.

tact lens may be used as a "splint" for the healing cornea and may be necessary for several months. Occasionally, removal of the epithelium or basement membrane is indicated, and various techniques to scar the basement membrane have been attempted if recurrent erosions are recalcitrant to more conservative measures.

Reis-Bücklers corneal dystrophy is an autosomal dominant, bilateral, symmetric disease that usually becomes evident in childhood. There is diffuse ground-glass opacification (a blue haze) at the level of Bowman's layer. The corneal surface is irregular with astigmatism, and there are usually episodes of painful epithelial erosions. Over time the condition may become asymptomatic as the basement membrane is replaced by scar tissue. Occasionally, a superficial lamellar keratectomy or penetrating keratoplasty may be necessary.

The major dystrophies of the corneal stroma include granular dystrophy, lattice dystrophy, macular dystrophy, fleck dystrophy, central cloudy dystrophy, and central crystalline dystrophy.

Granular dystrophy is the most common of the classic stromal dystrophies. It is autosomal dominant, bilateral, and symmetric. Small, gray-white, sharply demarcated opacities that appear crumblike begin centrally and superficially and spread peripherally and deeply with time (Fig. 4–8). There is usually a clear inter-

vening stroma. Because the epithelium and endothelium may remain unaffected, the patient is frequently asymptomatic with normal vision. Pathologic examination shows hyaline deposits with phospholipids.

Lattice dystrophy is an autosomal dominant, bilateral disease that represents a primary localized form of amyloidosis. Initially, there are fine, irregular lines or dots or a central haze; with time, the lines become thicker and ropier in appearance and have a double-contoured, lattice-like structure. The disease is usually detected at a young age, and symptoms of recurrent erosions and irregular astigmatism are frequent. The pathologic finding is amyloid with all the specific staining characteristics.

Macular dystrophy is an autosomal recessive, bilateral condition that presents with poor vision at an early age. Initially, there are diffuse spots with fuzzy edges in the superficial central cornea. With time, there is diffuse cloudiness of the stroma between the opacities with irregularity of Descemet's membrane. There is irregular astigmatism as well as episodes of recurrent erosions. Macular dystrophy appears to be a disease of abnormal acid mucopolysaccharide metabolism and deposition.

Fleck dystrophy is an autosomal dominant, bilateral disease that occurs in early childhood. It is asymptomatic and does not progress to visual loss. The chief clinical feature is flattened, dandruff-like, small opacities within the corneal stroma that vary in size, shape, and depth. *Central cloudy dystrophy* is autosomal dominant,

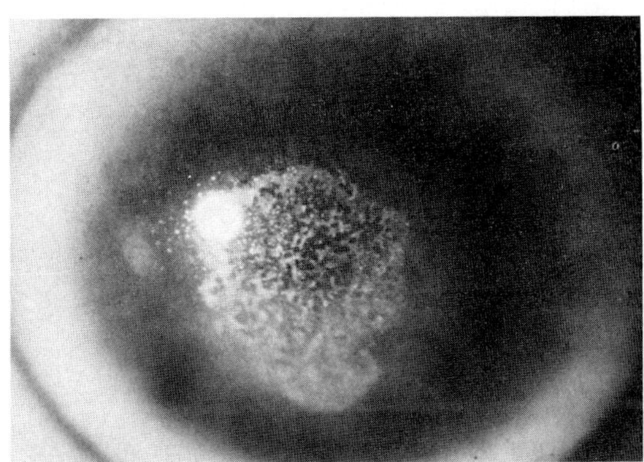

Fig. 4–9. Central, needle-shaped, crystalline, cholesterol deposits of the central cornea in a patient with central cystalline dystrophy of Schnyder.

nonprogressive, and asymptomatic. There is posterior stromal opacification that fades toward the periphery and may have a cracked-ice appearance; it is similar to posterior crocodile shagreen but is more extensive. *Central crystalline dystrophy of Schnyder* is an autosomal dominant, bilateral condition that is detected in childhood but is usually not progressive. There are fine polychromatic, needle-shaped cholesterol crystals with multiple different arrangements (usually ring-shaped) (Fig. 4–9). A diffuse corneal haze may be present. Schnyder's dystrophy is frequently associated with arcus senilis and hyperlipidemia.

Several conditions could be considered pre-Descemet's dystrophies.

There have been multiple descriptions of punctate lesions, filaments, or snowflakes in the deepest layers of the corneal stroma. These *pre-Descemet's dystrophies* may be associated with ichthyosis, keratoconus, or other ocular disease, but usually the corneal lesions are asymptomatic. Most cases are sporadic, although familial examples have been reported.

The major dystrophies of the corneal endothelium are posterior polymorphous dystrophy, cornea guttata, and Fuchs' corneal dystrophy.

Posterior polymorphous dystrophy is a bilateral, although often asymmetric, disease that may be either dominant or recessive. It may be congenital or may develop at an early age. It is recognized as grouped vesicles or a gray plaquelike lesion on the endothelium projecting into the anterior chamber. Occasionally, there are broad bands across the endothelium or thickened areas of Descemet's membrane. Usually this condition is asymptomatic, but occasionally it is progressive to the extent of requiring penetrating keratoplasty. Pathologically, endothelial cells have undergone metaplasia to an epithelial-like cell with abnormal Descemet's membrane.

Cornea guttata is a condition of wartlike excrescences on Descemet's membrane that are probably an abnormal product of endothelial cells. Cornea guttata is frequently autosomal dominant and is most commonly seen in middle-aged patients. The guttae are usually central and occasionally pigmented, and they may produce a beaten-metal appearance or additionally have a thickened Descemet's membrane. Numerous guttae can compromise endothelial function. Secondary cornea guttata may result from corneal degenerative or inflammatory diseases and may disappear with resolution of the underlying disorder.

Fuchs' corneal dystrophy is a bilateral, autosomal dominant trait characterized by progressive epithelial and stromal edema resulting from ineffective endothelial cells. It is an extreme form of cornea guttata. The earliest clinical signs may be a fine epithelial edema in association with cornea guttata that later may progress to stromal edema and epithelial bullae (Fig. 4–10). Late findings include fingerprint lines, subepithelial fibrosis, and vascularization. Symptoms are usually worse in the morning and better later in the day as evaporation helps to dry the cornea. Pathologic findings are decreased endothelial cell density and thinning over Descemet's warts with increased basement membrane–like material behind Descemet's membrane. Early in the course of the disease, sodium chloride ointment or drops may be effective for epithelial edema, as are other measures designed to dehydrate the stroma. Soft contact lenses may alleviate epithelial discomfort. Lowering the intraocular pressure sometimes will help the edema, but in advanced cases a penetrating keratoplasty is required.

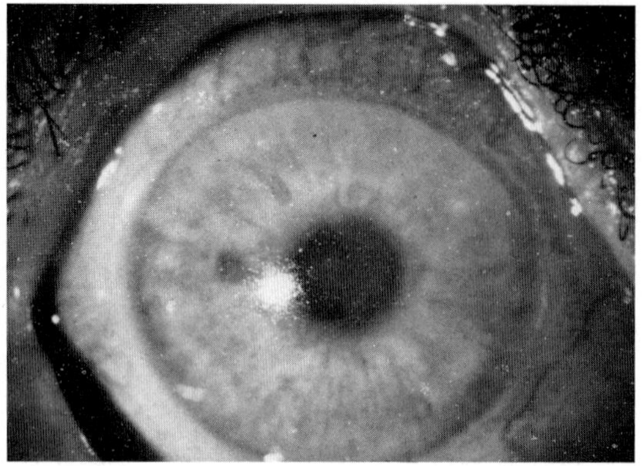

Fig. 4–10. A hazy cornea caused by epithelial and stromal edema in a patient with advanced endothelial cell loss from Fuchs' corneal dystrophy.

Keratoconus and related conditions are ectatic corneal dystrophies.

Keratoconus is a thinning and irregular protrusion and scarring of the corneal apex (Fig. 4–11). It begins in young patients as a bilateral process, but it is frequently asymmetric. Keratoconus takes several years to progress and then may become stable. It may occur in association with several ocular and systemic conditions. Clinical signs include thinning and scarring of the corneal apex, deep vertical stress lines that represent wrinkles in Descemet's membrane, increased visibility of corneal nerves, Fleischer's hemosiderin ring surrounding the cone, scars in Bowman's membrane, irregular

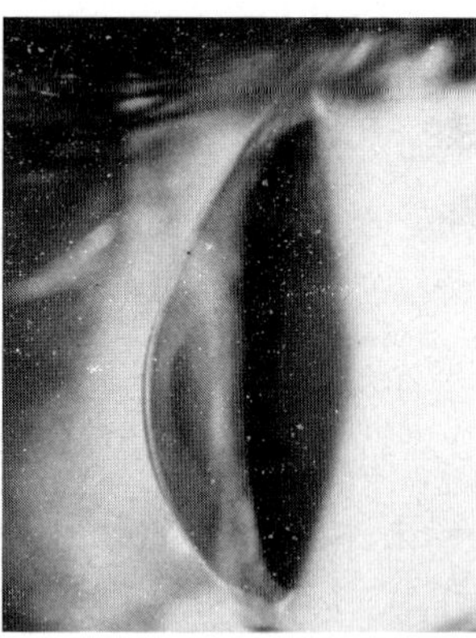

Fig. 4–11. A conical protrusion and thinning of the corneal apex in a patient with keratoconus.

high astigmatism, and occasional ruptures of Descemet's membrane with acute swelling of the cornea (hydrops). Rigid contact lenses are usually necessary to correct the irregular astigmatism. Penetrating keratoplasty in general has good results, although occasionally lamellar keratoplasty or epikeratophakia is preferred. Acute hydrops is treated conservatively because it usually resolves with time.

In *keratoglobus*, the diameter of the cornea is normal but there is total thinning of the cornea, especially peripherally. This bilateral condition may be familial. Ruptures in Descemet's membrane are frequent, and perforation may result from minor trauma.

Bacterial corneal infections may develop rapidly after trauma, in association with wearing of contact lenses, or in a compromised cornea.

Any bacteria can cause microbial keratitis in a host that is compromised by medications (such as corticosteroids) or by local or systemic disease. It most commonly occurs rapidly after trauma or in association with wearing of contact lenses. The most common organisms are *Staphylococcus* (*Staph. aureus*, *Staph. epidermidis*), *Streptococcus* (*Strep. pneumoniae*, viridans streptococci), *Pseudomonas* (*P. aeruginosa*), or other Enterobacteriaceae (*Proteus*, *Serratia*). Less commonly, bacterial infection is caused by *Neisseria*, *Moraxella*, or anaerobic bacteria.

The keratitis may be central or peripheral with epithelial ulceration, stromal abscess, mucopurulent exudate adherent to the ulcer surface, epithelial edema, and frequently a hypopyon. It may be difficult to distinguish an infection in an abnormal cornea with a pre-existing epithelial ulceration from, for example, herpes keratitis. Gram-positive cocci most commonly produce a well-defined epithelial ulceration and a deep stromal abscess (Fig. 4–12). *Pseudomonas* bacteria usually produce a liquefactive stromal necrosis with cellular infiltration of the surrounding cornea. The corneal destruction is caused by the invasion of organisms into the tissue as well as the release of exotoxins and endotoxins.

If an infection is suspected, adequate sam-

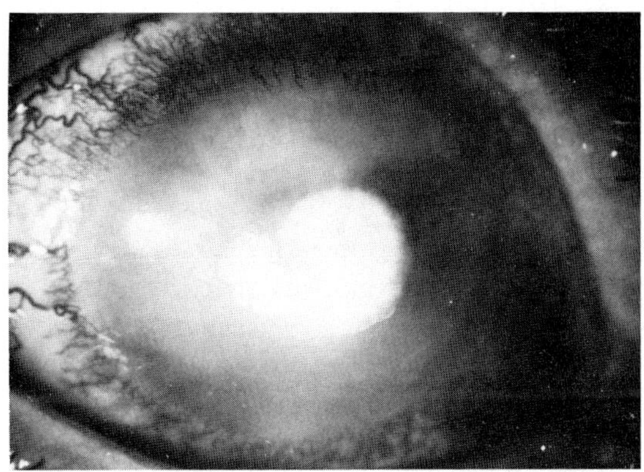

Fig. 4–12.   A white, deep corneal abscess and epithelial ulceration in a patient with corneal infection caused by *Staphylococcus aureus.*

ples should be obtained by corneal scraping for appropriate smears and cultures. Close communication with the microbiology laboratory is mandatory for the Gram stain and for the follow-up of culture reports. The decision about initial antibiotic coverage should be made on the basis of the Gram stain (Table 4–3). In severe cases or if the Gram stain is inconclusive, broad antibiotic coverage is indicated, usually with fortified topical antibiotics. In more severe cases, subconjunctival or intravenous administration may be needed. Later modification of the antibiotic therapy depends on the results of cultures, the clinical response, the patient's tolerance of medication, and the realization that the drugs may be toxic.

In addition to use of antibiotics, it is necessary to correct any lid abnormalities, tear film inadequacies, and elevated intraocular pressure. Nonhealing epithelial defects may require a soft contact lens. Topical corticosteroids should be used with great caution, but they may prevent tissue necrosis and structural alteration. Corneal perforation may occur, and a penetrating keratoplasty may be necessary (Fig. 4–13). Corneal ulcers heal slowly and should be examined frequently. Signs of improvement

TABLE 4–3   Organism Classification in Bacterial Keratitis, by Result of Gram Stain, Cell Shape, and Oxygen Requirements

		Oxygen requirements	
Result of Gram stain	*Cell shape*	*Aerobic or facultative*	*Anaerobic*
Positive	Cocci	*Micrococcus* *Staphylococcus* *Streptococcus*	*Peptococcus* *Peptostreptococcus*
	Rods	*Corynebacterium*	*Propionibacterium* *Actinomyces* *Arachnia* *Bifidobacterium* *Clostridium*
	Filaments	*Nocardia* *Streptomyces*	
Negative	Cocci	*Neisseria*	
	Coccobacillary	*Haemophilus* *Moraxella* *Acinetobacter*	
	Rods	*Pseudomonas* *Azotobacter* *Escherichia* *Citrobacter* *Klebsiella* *Enterobacter* *Serratia* *Proteus*	*Bacteroides* *Fusobacterium*

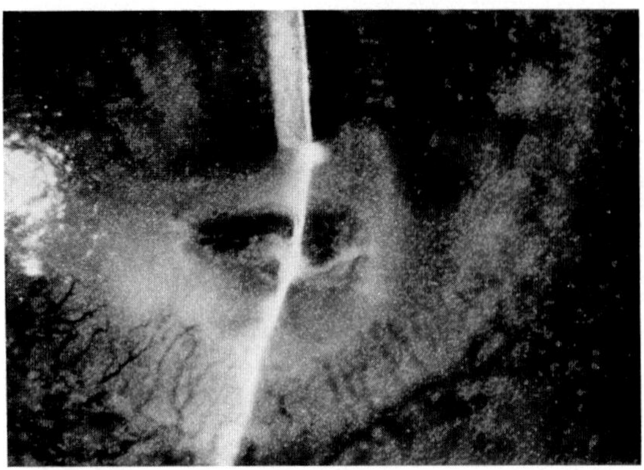

Fig. 4–13. A corneal perforation and flat anterior chamber in a patient with progressive corneal infection caused by *Staphylococcus aureus*.

TABLE 4–4 Equipment Needed for Obtaining and Testing Specimens of Corneal Ulcers

Topical anesthetic
Kimura spatula (preferably two)
Sterile cotton-tipped applicators (for lid and conjunctiva)
Glass microscope slides
Methyl alcohol fixative
Stains:
  Gram
  Giemsa
  Special
    Periodic acid-Schiff: for fungi
    Gomori methenamine-silver: for fungi
    Calcofluor white: for *Acanthamoeba* and fungi

include a reduction in the stromal abscess, rounding of the edges of the epithelial defect, a decrease in the amount of stromal edema, a decrease in the amount of anterior chamber inflammation, and progressive reepithelialization of the cornea.

The equipment necessary for appropriate staining and culturing of a corneal ulcer is listed in Table 4–4, and the appropriate culture media are listed in Table 4–5.

Fungal corneal infections may be caused by either filamentous fungi (multicellular fungi) or yeasts (unicellular fungi); these are found under different clinical settings.

Fungi are generally divided into filamentous fungi (multicellular fungi) and yeasts (unicellular fungi) (Table 4–6). Both of these classes are capable of causing corneal infection, but they are found under different settings.

Filamentous fungal keratitis commonly occurs in the southern United States in association with outdoor trauma, particularly with vegetable matter. Affected persons are healthy adults without preexisting ocular disease. *Fusarium* and *Aspergillus* are the most common organisms found. Fungal keratitis tends to present distinctive biomicroscopic features that suggest the diagnosis. Delicate, feathery, and hyphate

TABLE 4–5 Culture Media for Corneal Ulcers

Medium	*Purpose*	*Incubation temperature*
Routine		
Soybean casein digest broth (tryptic or trypticase soy broth)	Saturation of swabs	
Blood agar plate	Aerobic and facultatively anaerobic bacteria, fungi	35°C
Chocolate agar plate	Aerobic and facultatively anaerobic bacteria, *Neisseria*, *Haemophilus*	35°C
Thioglycollate broth	Aerobic and anaerobic bacteria	35°C
Sabouraud's dextrose agar plate with antibiotic	Fungi	Room temperature
Brain-heart infusion (BHI) broth with antibiotic	Fungi	Room temperature (rotary shaker)
Special		
Brucella blood agar plate	Anaerobic bacteria	35°C (anaerobic system)
Thayer-Martin agar plate	*Neisseria*	35°C
Middlebrook-Cohn agar start	*Mycobacterium*, *Nocardia*	35°C

TABLE 4-6 Fungi of Importance in Microbial Keratitis

Moniliaceae (nonpigmented filamentous fungi)
  Fusarium
  Aspergillus
  Acremonium
  Penicillium
  Petriellidium boydii
  Geotrichum candidum
  Myrathecum
  Volutella
  Cylindrocarpon
Dematiaceae (pigmented filamentous fungi)
  Curvularia
  Sphaeropsidales
  Melaanconiales
  Alternaria
  Drechslera
  Cladosporium
  Phialophora
Yeasts
  Candida

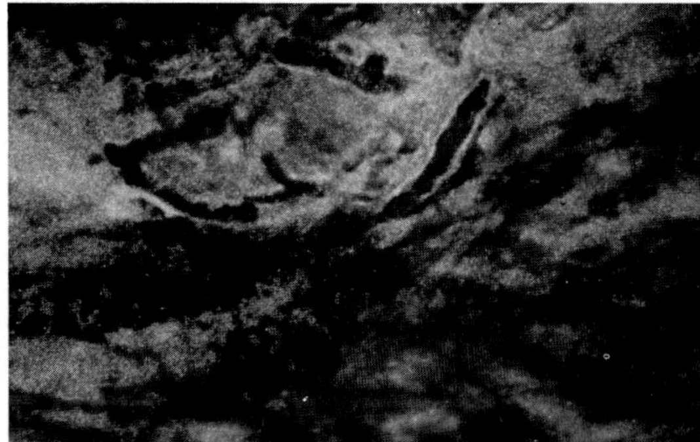

Fig. 4–15. Branching, septate, feathery hyphal elements in Gram-stained corneal scraping from a patient with *Aspergillus* corneal infection.

stromal infiltrates are seen either superficially or deep within the cornea and are associated with satellite lesions and a shaggy, gray, and elevated intact epithelium (Fig. 4–14). Frequently, endothelial rings or plaques are present on the back of the cornea with a hypopyon in the anterior chamber. Severely advanced disease may show total stromal abscess.

The Gram, Giemsa, Gomori methenamine-silver, or calcofluor stain may demonstrate the branching, septate hyphal elements that confirm the diagnosis (Fig. 4–15). A culture of mycelial colonies can be demonstrated on blood agar, Sabouraud's agar, or brain-heart infusion broth at 25°C (Fig. 4–16). Growth usually occurs within 48 hours. Therapy is initiated with topical natamycin 5%, which is available on request from Alcon Laboratories, Inc. Other antifungal agents are sometimes needed in this prolonged disease.

Yeast keratitis is most commonly caused by *Candida albicans*; it occurs throughout the world, usually in compromised hosts. It clinically presents with a dense, central stromal suppuration that may be yellow-white (Fig. 4–17). Budding yeast or pseudohyphae may be seen on Gram, Giemsa, or Gomori methenamine-silver stain. The growth in blood agar usually shows pasty white colonies.

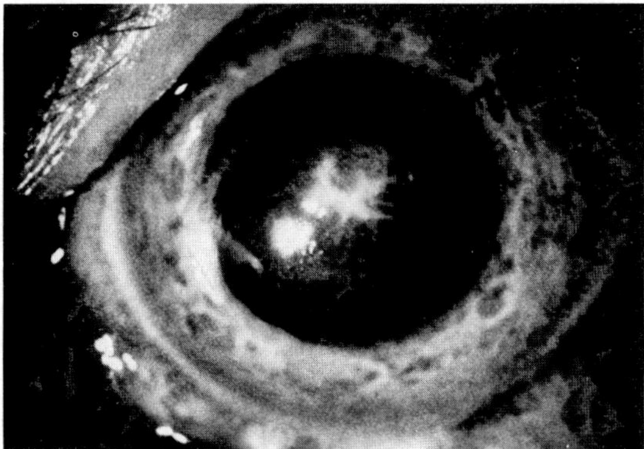

Fig. 4–14. A shaggy, feathery corneal infiltrate and raised intact epithelium in a patient with fungal corneal infection from *Alternaria*.

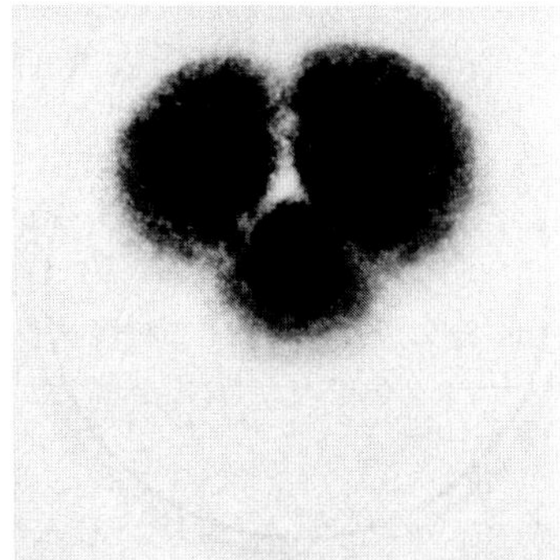

Fig. 4–16. Black, fluffy fungal colonies growing on Sabouraud's agar within 2 days in a patient with *Aspergillus* corneal infection.

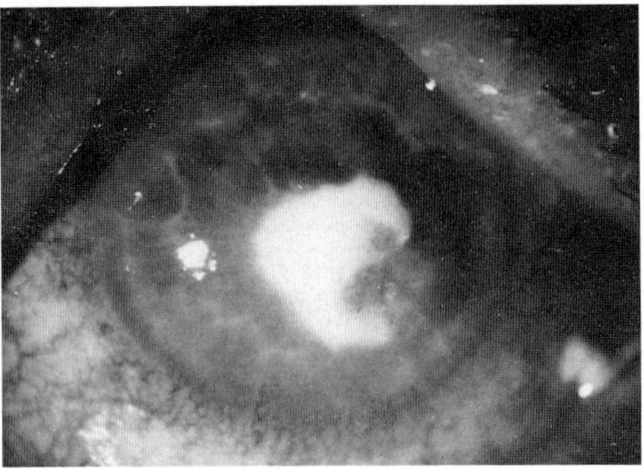

Fig. 4–17. A dense stromal abscess in an immuno-compromised patient with *Candida* corneal infection. Abscess was yellow-white.

Therapy is with topical amphotericin and natamycin. Occasionally, surgical therapy with a keratectomy, conjunctival flap, or lamellar or penetrating keratoplasty may be necessary. In general, corticosteroids are contraindicated in all types of fungal keratitis.

The protozoan Acanthamoeba *is implicated in an increasing number of corneal infections.*

The free-living protozoan *Acanthamoeba* has been identified in an increasing number of cases of keratitis. Most of the patients wear soft contact lenses and frequently have a history of relatively minor trauma. *Acanthamoeba* may present in various sections of the cornea without inciting biomicroscopically visible inflammation. Because of its multiple manifestations, it is frequently mistaken for corneal herpes simplex. Clinical features include recurrent epithelial defects, stromal infiltrates with a partial or complete ring configuration, a waxing and waning course, and relatively severe pain.

The diagnosis can be confirmed when amoebic cysts, which are double-walled and polygonal, are seen on routine smears. Optimal growth requires nonnutrient blood agar with an overlay of *Escherichia coli*. Occasionally, corneal biopsy may be indicated for deep corneal disease. *Acanthamoeba* keratitis is extremely resistant to most forms of therapy, although combinations of topical propamidine (Bro-

lene), neomycin, and miconazole and systemic ketoconazole have been useful. Therapeutic epithelial debridement may be indicated. Penetrating keratoplasty may be required for progressive stromal ulceration or for significant stromal scarring after a therapeutic response. The disease may recur at the host margin.

The herpes simplex virus establishes a "symbiosis" in the trigeminal ganglion and can cause frequent, recurrent ocular infection.

The herpes simplex virus is a large, intracellular DNA virus with humans as its only natural host. There are two subtypes based on the site of isolation. Type 1 is found in the oral, facial, ocular, and brain tissue. Type 2 is usually found in the genital area. The types can be differentiated by immunologic specificity, cell culture characteristics, and drug response. More than 90% of the U.S. population have antibodies to herpes simplex by adulthood, although this percentage varies with socioeconomic groups. The virus is spread by oral and sexual contact.

The initial encounter with type 1 herpes simplex virus is usually at an early age, and it is usually a mild disease with gingivostomatitis, rhinitis, fever, malaise, lymphadenopathy, and cutaneous vesicles that may not even be noticeable. Ocular involvement may occur during this primary infection and is frequently unilateral with a vesicular eruption, especially in the lower lid and the medial canthus. Occasionally, follicular conjunctivitis and corneal epithelial disease may be noted. Primary herpes simplex virus infection is usually self-limited.

Neonatal herpes is typically sequential to maternal herpetic cervicitis caused by type 2 herpes simplex virus. The onset usually occurs within the first week of birth; clinical manifestations include cutaneous lesions and ocular involvement with keratitis, chorioretinitis, or cataracts. The disease may progress to dissemination with a significant threat to life.

After the primary infection, the herpes virus develops a "symbiosis" with humans. The trigeminal ganglion is a reservoir for type 1 infections, and different stimuli can provoke viral shedding or overcome normal immunologic barriers. Recurrences may be frequent and tend to be highly localized to the various ocular structures. Certain herpes simplex viruses have a propensity to cause significant ocular disease; the initial herpes simplex virus that is encountered may determine the patient's future ocular course.

Ocular herpes simplex virus disease presents in multiple forms related to the active viral disease, host inflammatory response, or structural damage caused by the infection.

Herpes simplex virus is the "great masquerader" in the anterior segment and presents in multiple forms related to active viral disease as well as to the structural damage caused by the infection (Table 4–7).

Lid vesicles may occur on the upper and lower lids either in primary disease or with recurrent disease. No particular treatment for the skin disease has been found to be efficacious.

Follicular conjunctivitis with or without corneal involvement may occur in primary disease

TABLE 4–7 Classification of Ocular Disease Associated with Herpes Simplex Virus

Viral disease
  Blepharitis
  Conjunctivitis
  Epithelial disease
    Punctate
    Stellate
    Dendritic
    Geographic
  Stromal disease
    Disciform keratitis (central endotheliitis)
    Necrotizing keratitis (interstitial keratitis)
  Peripheral endotheliitis (trabeculitis)
  Uveitis
    Focal iritis
    Diffuse iritis
Nonviral disease (metaherpetic)
  Erosions
  Indolent ulceration
  Trophic ulceration
  Permanent altered corneal structure
  Permanent trabecular damage

or with recurrent herpes simplex virus. Antiviral therapy is applied to the conjunctiva, with surveillance for corneal involvement.

The cornea may be involved with either active epithelial viral disease or other nonviral epithelial disease. *Active corneal epithelial viral disease* may manifest as a punctate keratitis, a dendritic keratitis, or a geographic keratitis (Fig. 4–18). These patterns are different configurations of the raised clusters of opaque epithelial cells that stain brightly with rose bengal; they represent active viral infection of the epithelium. Geographic keratitis has been associated with corticosteroid use. Treatment of active herpes simplex virus keratitis requires topical antiviral medication with trifluorothymidine, idoxuridine, or vidarabine. Another alternative is simple mechanical debridement. Trifluorothymidine is preferable with geographic keratitis. Therapy is usually effective within 7 days, and lack of response suggests resistance or an incorrect diagnosis.

The herpes simplex virus can cause structural damage to the epithelium or its basement membrane and leave residual structural defects even though the virus is no longer present. An *indolent ulceration* is a sharply defined epithelial and stromal ulceration associated with inflammation in the stroma but without active epithelial herpes. This is probably a hypersensitivity stromal reaction. Indolent ulceration is usually treated with topical corticosteroids for the stromal keratitis, along with antiviral pro-

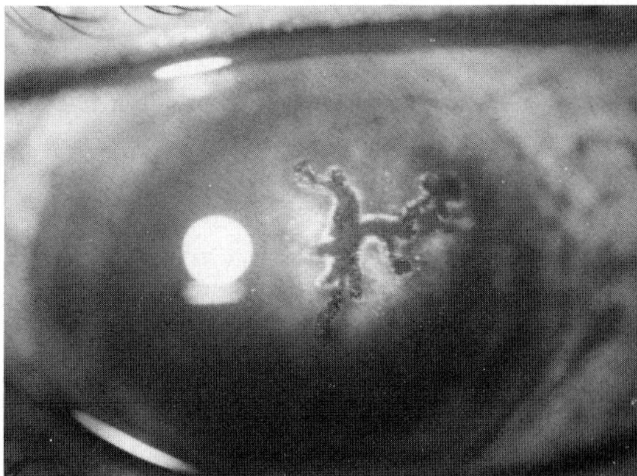

Fig. 4–18. A large fluorescein-stained corneal epithelial dendrite that has enlarged to a geographic keratitis. Herpes simplex virus was cultured from the lesion.

phylaxis. *Trophic ulceration* is an epithelial and stromal ulceration without active stromal inflammation; characteristics are stromal scarring, edema, and damage with poor healing of the epithelium over the ulcer. Therapy includes eliminating any toxic agents (such as antiviral therapy) and patching, lubrication, or soft contact lenses to promote epithelial healing. Punctate epithelial erosions and granularity may be a sign of resolving herpes or may be an indication of drug toxicity. In cases of drug toxicity, it is necessary to withdraw all medications to promote epithelial healing.

Three forms of stromal disease are caused by herpes simplex virus: necrotizing stromal keratitis, disciform keratitis, and permanent stromal structural alterations. *Necrotizing stromal keratitis* is a deep inflammation throughout the layers of the cornea; it can vary from a mild to a dense stromal abscess. It may be segmental or diffuse throughout the cornea. There is uveitis with smudgy keratitic precipitates, a coagulum, dilated iris vessels, and elevated intraocular pressure from the inflammation. There may be posterior synechiae within the anterior chamber. Occasionally, the stromal inflammation can progress to perforation or it may heal with scarring and vascularization. Necrotizing stromal keratitis usually follows multiple episodes of epithelial herpes, but the role of active virus in this specific disease is arguable. Viral particles have been identified, but the primary reaction is probably an immunologic event.

Therapy involves treatment of active epithelial disease if it is present. The stromal disease frequently may respond to cycloplegia alone. Topical corticosteroids are indicated to suppress the inflammation, which may cause stromal and intraocular scarring. Corticosteroids must be tapered slowly to avoid rebound keratitis. An antiviral prophylactic cover is needed until low-dose corticosteroids are used. With unresponsive, prolonged disease, systemic acyclovir should be considered. Topical acyclovir may be helpful in this condition, but it is not available in the United States.

Disciform keratitis is a distinctive central or eccentric disc of stromal edema that may be associated with a granular infiltrate and an intact

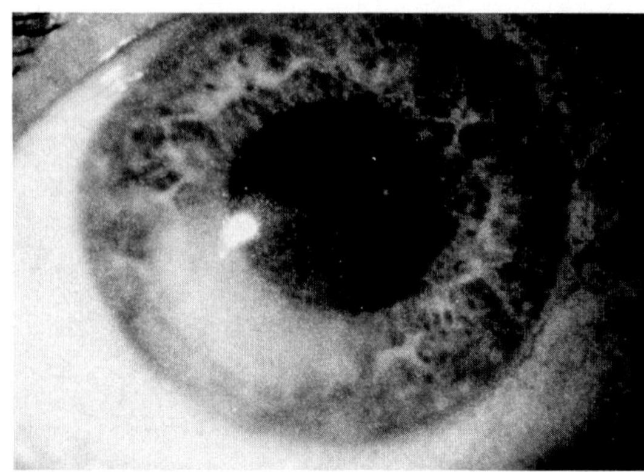

Fig. 4–19. An eccentric disc of corneal stromal edema with an intact epithelium in a patient with a previous episode of herpes simplex viral corneal infection. This represents herpes simplex viral disciform keratitis.

epithelium (Fig. 4–19). There may be an immune Wessely ring as well as mild wrinkles in Descemet's membrane (striae) and uveitis. This is probably a cell-mediated hypersensitivity response or, alternatively, may represent active viral disease of the corneal endothelium. Disciform keratitis usually responds to topical corticosteroids with an antiviral prophylactic cover.

After long or repeated bouts of recurrent stromal keratitis, there may be severe damage to the corneal endothelium with corneal edema, stromal vascularization, and scarring. *Permanent stromal structural alterations* will not respond to medical therapy. Depending on the symptoms and visual needs of the patient, consideration may be given to either a penetrating keratoplasty or a conjunctival flap when the disease is finally quiescent.

Inflammation within the eye (*uveitis* and *trabeculitis*) can occur with and without active corneal disease. There is inflammation as well as swelling of the tissues within the eye that can lead to a hypopyon or intractable glaucoma. Clinical signs include posterior synechiae, dilated iris vessels, anterior lens changes, and elevated intraocular pressure. Therapy is with cycloplegia and topical corticosteroids with a prophylactic antiviral cover. Elevated intraocular pressure should be treated as necessary. Systemic acyclovir may be indicated in severe cases.

The principles of drug use in herpes simplex virus relate primarily to the presence of active viral disease and to the attempt to reduce the inflammatory reaction.

Herpes simplex virus has multiple clinical manifestations and variable therapy during its clinical course. If the presence of active viral disease is equivocal, it is best to defer antiviral therapy. Rose bengal, rather than fluorescein, is better for evaluating the corneal epithelium. All of the presently available topical antiviral treatments are effective in epithelial disease, although trifluorothymidine and acyclovir are probably best in geographic disease, stromal disease, or uveitis. The epithelial disease should respond within a few days; in the absence of response, consideration should be given to drug resistance or other mechanisms of disease (such as drug toxicity or indolent or trophic ulceration). Most of the topical antiviral drugs can lead to significant epithelial toxicity if used on a prolonged basis.

If both active viral epithelial disease and stromal disease are present, it is best to begin therapy of the epithelial disease with a topical antiviral agent for a few days before instituting topical corticosteroids for the stromal disease. Optimally, the least amount of topical corticosteroid necessary should be used to suppress the stromal inflammatory reaction. A topical antiviral cover is usually used until the topical corticosteroid dose is extremely low. Topical corticosteroids should always be tapered and never be abruptly terminated. Corticosteroids should not be used in certain instances, such as in active epithelial disease, trophic ulcers, and nonresponsive stromal edema. Consideration should be given to the use of systemic acyclovir for deep stromal disease or uveitis, although at present it is not approved for this use in the United States.

Herpes zoster ophthalmicus is a reactivation of the varicella virus in the dorsal root ganglion of the trigeminal nerve.

Herpes zoster ophthalmicus is a reactivation of the latent varicella DNA virus in the dorsal root ganglion of the upper trigeminal nerve. Patients are usually older than 40 years, and there may be a prodrome of fever, malaise, headache, nausea, and preeruptive pain or hyperesthesia. Herpes zoster may occur after physical trauma or exposure to a patient with varicella and may be associated with acquired immunodeficiency syndrome (AIDS), malignancy, immunosuppressive therapy, or chronic illness. The clinical picture begins with skin eruption of erythematous papules and later vesicles in the ophthalmic division of the trigeminal nerve (Fig. 4–20). The dermis is affected with subsequent scarring that may cause entropion, trichiasis, ptosis, or exposure of the cornea. The severity of herpes zoster ophthalmicus varies tremendously. Postherpetic neuralgia with extreme and persistent pain in the distribution of the involved nerve is one of the more severe problems in patients older than 50 years.

Ocular findings of herpes zoster ophthalmicus include conjunctivitis with follicles, hyperemia, and vesicles. Episcleritis, scleritis, and uveitis are frequently found. Corneal epithelial changes may vary from a blotchy punctate epithelial keratitis to ulcerative keratitis or stromal corneal immune reactions with nummular infiltrates. If the corneal condition persists, it may lead to corneal scarring, vasculari-

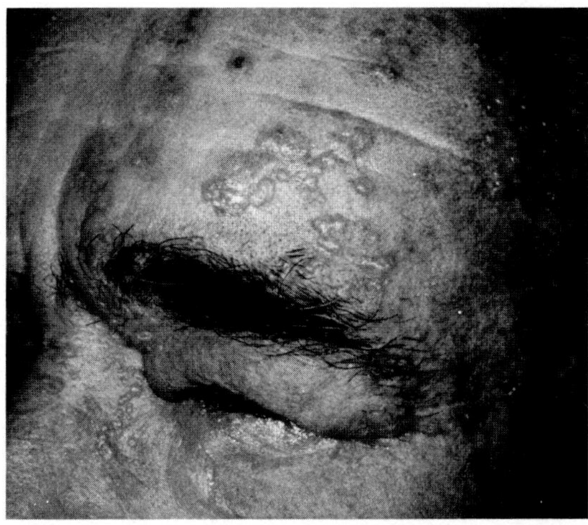

Fig. 4–20. Forehead and eyelid vesicles in the distribution of the ophthalmic division of the trigeminal nerve. Culture of the vesicle yielded the varicella zoster virus.

zation, lipid deposition, and neurotrophic keratitis. Other ocular involvement may include optic neuritis, chorioretinitis, and ocular motor paralysis. The acute retinal necrosis syndrome is a rare disorder that has been attributed to the varicella zoster virus.

The ocular findings in herpes zoster ophthalmicus are due to a combination of active viral replication, neural inflammation, and arteritis (Table 4–8). Persistent disease can lead to permanent structural damage and neuralgia. There may be severe central nervous system damage from the arteritis, including symptoms suggestive of a stroke.

If given early and in high doses, oral acyclovir has proved beneficial for all aspects of herpes zoster ophthalmicus, except for postherpetic neuralgia. In the early stages of the skin disease, various wet dressings have been useful under the direction of a dermatologist. Surveillance is necessary for secondary bacterial infection. A corticosteroid antibiotic ointment to the skin may be beneficial. Most of the inflammatory signs of herpes zoster in the cornea and sclera may respond to cycloplegia and topical corticosteroids. Neurotrophic keratitis is frequently resistant to therapy and may require patching,

TABLE 4–8 Manifestations of Herpes Zoster Ophthalmicus

Cutaneous eruption
Scarring of lids with entropion, trichiasis
Postherpetic neuralgia
Corneal disease
   Epithelial dendrites, plaques, or erosions
   Focal stromal keratitis, interstitial keratitis
   Endothelial damage
   Scarring with lipid deposition, band keratopathy
   Peripheral thinning or melt
Neurotrophic keratitis
Keratoconjunctivitis sicca
Scleritis/episcleritis
Secondary inflammatory glaucoma
Secondary cataract
Ischemic vasculitis of iris, anterior segment, retinal
   vessels, or optic nerve
Cranial nerve palsy with arteritis
Central nervous system arteritis with diffuse
   neurologic signs

lubrication, or soft contact lens therapy. Closure of the eyelids with a tarsorrhaphy is occasionally necessary. The most persistent problem with herpes zoster ophthalmicus is the postherpetic neuralgia, which may be lessened if systemic corticosteroids are used within the first 2 weeks of therapy. Corticosteroids should be used with caution in immunosuppressed patients. Capsaicin topical cream is occasionally helpful for postherpetic neuralgia. Oral antidepressants or surgical ablation of the trigeminal nerve is occasionally used.

The superficial cornea may manifest a nonspecific inflammatory response.

There are multiple causes of an inflammatory process of the epithelium or superficial corneal stroma (Table 4–9). A specific cause can sometimes be determined from associated findings of the lid, conjunctiva, cornea, or skin and from the location of the keratitis. There are four specific reactions of the corneal epithelium: punctate epithelial erosions, punctate epithelial keratitis, punctate infiltrates, and filamentary keratitis. *Punctate epithelial erosions* are clear, fine pits in the epithelium that stain brightly with fluorescein. Lesions of *punctate epithelial keratitis* are opaque, gray spots elevated on the epithelium that stain variably with fluorescein. *Punctate infiltrates* are clusters of opaque inflammation that are just beneath Bowman's membrane and very frequently are in the peripheral cornea. *Filamentary keratitis* consists of elongated, desquamated epithelium and mucus that remain attached to the epithelium by a small pedicle. The specific type of keratitis usually suggests more limited diagnostic possibilities.

There are many corneal inflammatory conditions with specific clinical findings.

Superficial punctate keratitis of Thygeson is a bilateral disease with elevated, discrete, coarse, punctate epithelial keratitis. The conjunctiva is normal and the eye otherwise appears to be quiet and white. The disorder tends to run a chronic course with exacerbations and remis-

TABLE 4–9 Etiologic Agents in Epithelial Keratitis

Infections
  Herpes simplex virus
  Herpes zoster virus
  Molluscum contagiosum
  Measles
  Mumps
  Adenoviral disease
  Infectious mononucleosis
  Chlamydia inclusion
  Trachoma
  Staphylococcal blepharitis
Mechanical
  Exposure, poor blink
  Keratitis sicca
  Trichiasis
  Entropion
  Occlusion
  Spray keratitis (aerosols)
  Posttraumatic erosion
  Overuse of contact lenses
Toxic
  Medication (neomycin, gentamicin, timolol,
    topical anesthetics)
  Radiation
  Chemicals or toxins
  Ultraviolet light
  Arc welding
  Acne rosacea
Others
  Neurotrophic
  Anterior membrane dystrophy
  Recurrent erosions
Unknown cause
  Superficial punctate keratitis of Thygeson
  Superior limbic keratitis of Theodore

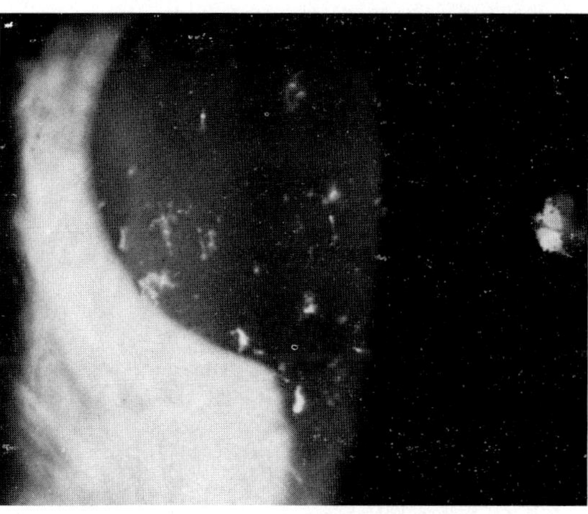

Fig. 4–21. Multiple corneal filaments in a patient with keratitis sicca and a filamentary keratitis.

eye. The patient notes a foreign body sensation, and single or multiple strands of epithelial cells and mucus attached to a corneal receptor site are the prominent clinical findings (Fig. 4–21). Filamentary keratitis tends to be chronic and recurrent. Multiple forms of therapy have been tried to help remove or eliminate the filaments.

Recurrent erosions cause a typical syndrome of acute onset of pain and tearing that is worse on awakening. There is usually a history of a previous corneal abrasion in the area where the epithelial defect is found (Fig. 4–22). Recurrent erosions also may be associated with other corneal conditions, such as anterior membrane dystrophy and some of the other corneal dystrophies. If the patient is seen immediately, there is usually an epithelial defect with adjacent edematous epithelium. Usually, however, by the time the patient is seen the epithelium has healed but is somewhat thickened or may contain gray deposits. This defect is probably caused by a faulty hemidesmosomal attachment of the epithelium to a damaged basement membrane. The treatment for the acute episodes consists of patching, but the main therapy is prophylactic to help prevent the erosions from recurring. Lubrication, hypertonic ointments, and patching at bedtime are the initial suggested therapies. Soft contact lens therapy, scraping of the cornea, or microdiathermy are other techniques in recalcitrant patients.

sions over years. Patients notice a foreign body sensation, tearing, and photophobia. The number of lesions on the cornea varies, and each lesion is composed of fine granules or microcysts arranged in a discrete oval pattern, usually in the central cornea and confined to the epithelium. Superficial punctate keratitis is thought to be of viral cause. Trifluorothymidine, topical corticosteroids, or soft contact lens therapy all have been successful in some patients.

Filamentary keratitis has multiple causes but is most common in keratitis sicca, in the recurrent erosion syndrome, after anterior segment surgery, and in association with patching of the

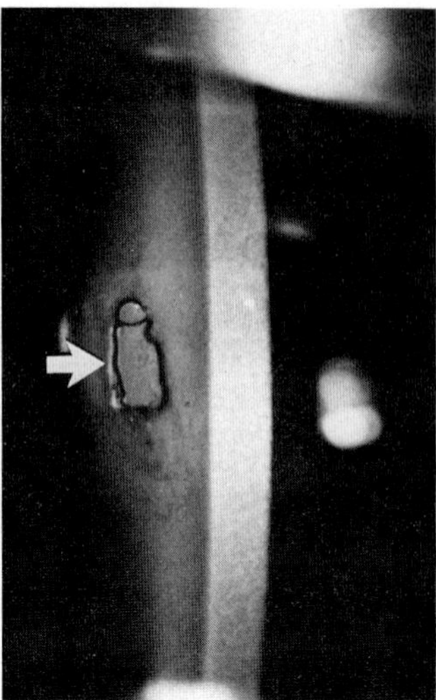

Fig. 4–22.   A large, recurrent corneal epithelial defect (*arrow*) in a region of the cornea that previously had suffered a large corneal abrasion.

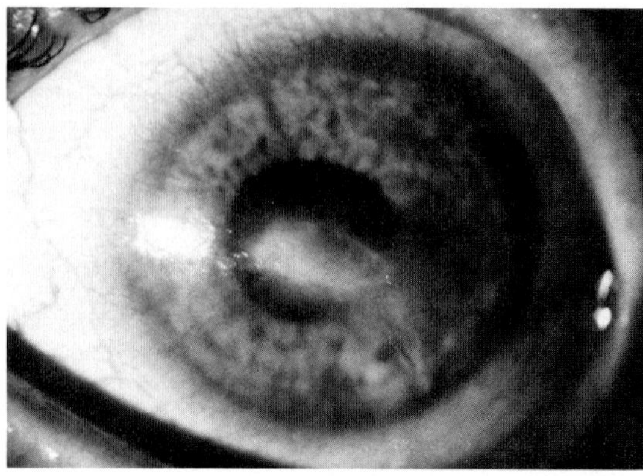

Fig. 4–23.   A horizontal, central, neurotrophic corneal ulcer in a patient who had resection of the fifth cranial nerve for tic douloureux. There was no corneal sensation.

Exposure keratitis may occur whenever there are abnormalities in the blink reflex, or it may occur in the presence of lid defects or exophthalmos that interferes with normal closure and protection of the cornea. Clinically, it is seen as a lack of the normal corneal luster and there is desiccation in a horizontal band across the lower portion of the cornea. Many elderly patients probably sleep with their lids partially opened (nocturnal lagophthalmos). Once the condition is recognized, therapy consists of frequent lubrication, taping the lids nightly, and treating the underlying problem (such as lid malposition or exophthalmos).

Neurotrophic keratitis results from corneal and conjunctival denervation, as seen in diabetes, herpes simplex, or herpes zoster, or from surgical lesions of the fifth cranial nerve. Clinically, there is a corneal haze with punctate epithelial erosions, ulcerations (Fig. 4–23), and, rarely, stromal melting with perforation. This disease is probably related to an abnormal cell turnover and lack of neurotrophic factors. Treatment consists of lubrication and patching, and usually a tarsorrhaphy is necessary until the underlying condition resolves.

Radiation keratitis is a superficial burn to the surface of the cornea with a clinical picture that varies from punctate epithelial erosions to punctate epithelial keratitis to a stromal melt. It may occur several weeks to months after radiation therapy for various types of lid, orbital, or retinal tumors. With healing, later changes include scar formation and vascularization of the cornea.

Toxic keratitis consists of a coarse punctate epithelial keratitis or swirls of heaped-up opaque epithelium that stains with fluorescein. Multiple topical drugs or their preservatives can cause this toxic reaction. It is necessary that this condition be recognized so that the offending agent can be withdrawn.

Interstitial keratitis is a deep inflammation of the corneal stroma associated with infectious organisms or an immune reaction.

Interstitial keratitis is a deep inflammation of the corneal stroma that has multiple causes (Table 4–10), but it is most commonly associated with syphilis, tuberculosis, or the vasculitis associated with Cogan's syndrome (Fig. 4–24). Luetic keratitis is a bilateral inflammation usually caused by congenital syphilis, but it is occasionally seen in acquired syphilis. Congenital ocular syphilis usually presents in the first or second decade of life with photophobia associated with deep inflammation, infiltration, and vascularization of the cornea. Usually the second eye becomes involved within 1 year. Acquired

TABLE 4–10 Diseases Associated with Interstitial Keratitis

Viral disease
  Herpes simplex
  Herpes zoster
  Infectious mononucleosis
  Rubeola (measles)
  Mumps
  Rubella
  Influenza
  Variola and vaccinia
Bacterial disease
  Congenital or acquired syphilis
  Tuberculosis
  Leprosy
  Lymphogranuloma venereum
Parasitic disease
  Onchocerciasis
  Cysticercosis
  Leishmaniasis
  Trypanosomiasis
  Malaria
Unknown cause
  Cogan's syndrome
  Sarcoidosis
  Mycosis fungoides

ocular syphilis usually occurs 10 years after the primary infection; it is typically unilateral and may involve only a portion of the cornea. Interstitial keratitis is probably an immune reaction against treponemal antigens remaining in the stroma because the organism itself is rarely recovered. The prolonged inflammation clears but it usually leaves a thin cornea with deep ghost vessels and anterior chamber synechiae.

Cogan's syndrome is a bilateral interstitial keratitis that occurs in adults in association with pain and photophobia but no findings of syphilis. There are usually vestibuloauditory symptoms of vertigo, tinnitus, eighth nerve deafness, and nystagmus as well as a systemic vasculitis with serologic findings. In the early stages, the characteristic corneal finding is a bilateral, subepithelial, peripheral keratitis. The disease has an acute phase lasting several months and then it may move on to a chronic phase.

There are multiple untoward corneal responses to soft contact lenses, including toxic, allergic, and infectious reactions.

There is an increasing recognition of the multiple side effects associated with use of soft contact lenses. Some of the preservatives in the contact lens solution can cause a toxic keratitis with erosions of the corneal epithelium. Allergic reactions to contact lens solutions may cause conjunctival hyperemia, anterior stromal infiltrates, a corneal pannus, or a mixed follicular and papillary conjunctival reaction (Fig. 4–25). *Giant papillary conjunctivitis* is an inflammation of the upper lid that is probably an allergic reaction to soft contact lenses or to deposits on soft contact lenses. Use of soft contact lenses can be as-

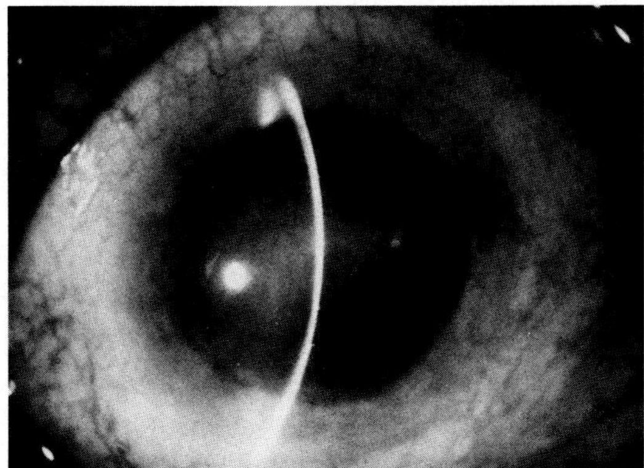

Fig. 4–24. A mild, diffuse corneal haze with corneal thinning and ghost vessels in a patient with interstitial keratitis in both eyes. The result of the fluorescent treponemal antibody absorption test was positive.

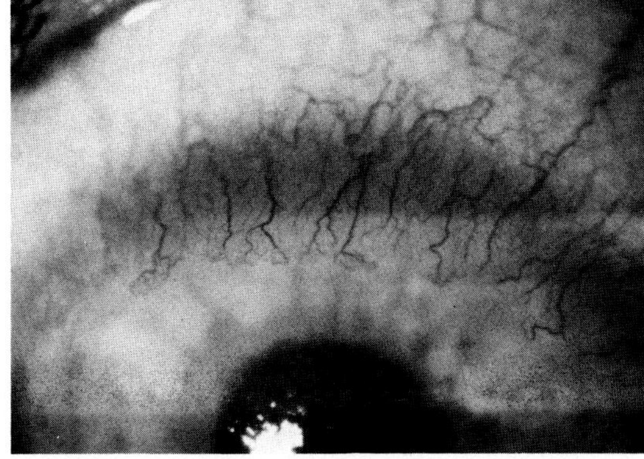

Fig. 4–25. A superior vascular corneal pannus and a punctate epithelial keratitis in a patient using "daily-wear" soft contact lenses. The patient had gradually increasing intolerance of the soft contact lenses.

sociated with irritation and decreased vision in the presence of excessive deposits of protein, lipid, or calcium on the lenses as well as with corneal edema resulting from hypoxia or tight-fitting lenses. There is increasing evidence that there are morphologic and functional changes in the corneal endothelium with long-term use of hard or soft contact lenses, but whether these changes are reversible is unclear. Microbial keratitis from bacteria, fungi, or *Acanthamoeba* is much more common in the presence of soft contact lenses, especially extended-wear lenses.

Persons who wear contact lenses should be instructed carefully on the appropriate care of these devices. Patients who develop a red eye while wearing their contact lenses should immediately remove them and seek ophthalmic care if the condition does not resolve quickly.

Marginal keratitis is a spectrum of diseases resulting from several potential stimuli producing an infiltrative, ulcerative, or vascular lesion at the limbus.

Marginal keratitis is an infiltrative, ulcerative, or vascular lesion at the limbus resulting from several potential stimuli. Causes include microorganisms (or their toxins), antigens, exogenous toxins, or reactions of the perilimbal vasculature. Immune mechanisms of disease (immediate or delayed), vascular obstruction, and the release of proteolytic enzymes (protease, proteoglycanase, and collagenase) are all potential mechanisms of disease. Many local ocular diseases may be associated with marginal keratitis, including blepharitis, conjunctival infections, or various conjunctival allergies. Marginal keratitis can also occur as a corneal immune reaction from herpes simplex, herpes zoster, or an extension of scleritis. Various systemic disorders, especially the collagen vascular diseases, can be associated with a marginal keratitis (Fig. 4–26).

Mooren's ulcer is a chronic, slowly progressive, unilateral or bilateral, peripheral, deep ulceration of the cornea with overhanging redundant edges. The eye is usually red and painful as the necrosis spreads circumferentially and toward the central portion of the cornea (Fig.

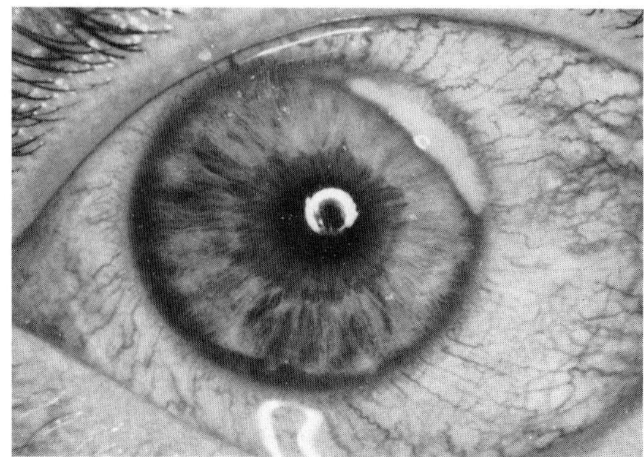

Fig. 4–26. A dense peripheral corneal infiltrate and corneal necrosis in a patient with Wegener's granulomatosis.

4–27). This results in either a very thin vascularized cornea or a perforation. There may be evidence of systemic or local immunologic derangements, and this disease may respond to systemic immunosuppressive therapy.

The multiple forms of therapy for marginal keratitis depend on the specific ocular or systemic disease that has caused the condition. Aggressive systemic medical therapy or a surgical procedure is occasionally necessary.

Corneal edema has multiple causes that may act either alone or in combination.

Corneal edema usually results from any disease process that damages the corneal endothelium because the endothelial layer is primarily responsible for pumping fluid out of the cornea (Table 4–11). The endothelium can be damaged in certain corneal dystrophies (such as Fuchs' corneal dystrophy) or in association with operation, trauma, or vitreous touching the cornea. The endothelium may also be damaged by elevated intraocular pressure, as in acute glaucoma. Several stromal inflammatory conditions can damage the endothelium secondarily, such as herpes simplex, herpes zoster, anterior segment ischemia, or toxic keratopathy. The corneal endothelium can be attacked primarily by lymphocytes as a form of graft rejection after penetrating keratoplasty. Corneal edema is usually manifest first in the

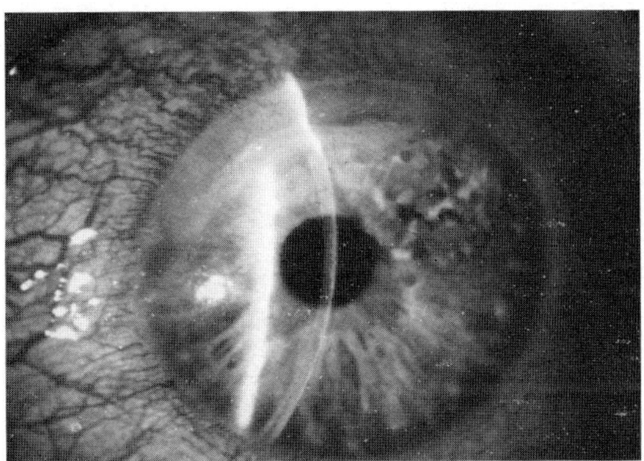

Fig. 4–27. A painful, peripheral corneal gutter that is spreading circumferentially around the eye in a patient with Mooren's corneal ulcer. The other eye perforated from the same condition.

epithelium with a corneal haze (bedewing). Later, stromal edema, epithelial blisters, and then corneal scarring and vascularization occur.

Endothelial damage should be avoided during intraocular operations. If corneal edema occurs, measures to help improve the condition include lowering the intraocular pressure, controlling stromal and intraocular inflamma-

TABLE 4–11 Clinical Disorders Associated with Corneal Edema

Primary disorders
  Cornea guttata
  Fuchs' endothelial dystrophy
  Posterior polymorphous dystrophy
  Proliferative endotheliopathies
    Iridocorneal endothelial syndrome
    Associated with trauma, interstitial keratitis
Secondary disorders
  Associated with increased intraocular pressure
  Trauma (surgical and nonsurgical)
  Iridocyclitis
  Radiation
  Vitreous adhesion syndrome
  Ocular hypoxia (contact lens, anterior segment ischemia)
  Diabetes mellitus
  Immune-related corneal graft rejection
  Later stage of several corneal dystrophies
  Later stage of corneal inflammation (herpes simplex, herpes zoster, interstitial keratitis)

tion with topical corticosteroids and cycloplegia, reducing epithelial edema with hypertonic agents, and using soft contact lenses for comfort. Definitive treatment usually necessitates a penetrating keratoplasty.

Keratorefractive procedures are designed to alter the shape of the cornea.

The anterior corneal surface is the most powerful refracting interface of the eye. Altering the curvature of the cornea has a profound effect on the refraction of the eye. Recently introduced surgical techniques use these principles to change the refraction of the eye to a more emmetropic state. These procedures can be grouped under the term *"keratorefractive surgery"* and have generated increased knowledge and instrumentation for studying the physiology, optics, biocompatibility, and topography of the cornea. In general, the procedures are designed to flatten the anterior surface of the cornea to reduce myopia, to steepen the anterior surface of the cornea to reduce hyperopia, or to flatten certain sectors of the cornea to reduce astigmatism. Because they are frequently performed on eyes that otherwise are healthy, the risk-benefit ratio is an important concern. In contrast, *lamellar keratoplasty* (partial-thickness corneal replacement) and *penetrating keratoplasty* (full-thickness corneal replacement) are generally used to treat significant corneal disease, corneal thinning, or corneal scarring.

Keratorefractive procedures may be effected by local heat or laser, surgical incisions, corneal lathing techniques, or the introduction of inserts into or onto the corneal surface. The safety, efficacy, and predictability of keratorefractive procedures are still a matter of debate. This section defines the procedures in current practice.

External procedures that alter the shape of the cornea include orthokeratology, thermokeratoplasty, and excimer laser sculpturing.

Orthokeratology attempts to reduce refractive errors by the use of contact lenses that change the shape of the cornea. The contact lenses are fit extremely flat or steep in order to produce a desired effect on the cornea. The change in corneal topography frequently takes months, and the cornea tends to resume its normal shape when the contact lens is withdrawn. Ophthalmologists rarely use this technique.

Thermokeratoplasty is the application of heat to shrink the anterior corneal surface and cause corneal flattening. It has been used in keratoconus for years but has also been used for refractive purposes. The heat can be applied by cautery or by a more controlled radiofrequency probe.

The *excimer laser* is currently being evaluated for direct sculpting of the anterior surface of the cornea. This technique of photorefractive keratectomy removes tissue from the anterior stromal surface in a sculpturing fashion and shapes the cornea to a smooth surface either steeper or flatter to obtain the desired refractive power. It can additionally remove superficial corneal scars or abnormal corneal elevations.

Corneal incisions that alter the corneal shape include radial keratotomy, corneal relaxing incisions, corneal wedge resection, and astigmatic keratotomy procedures.

Radial keratotomy ("cutting the cornea") is a procedure in which radial, nearly full-thickness, peripheral corneal incisions (from 4 to 32) are used to flatten the cornea and reduce myopia. The central 3 mm of the cornea is spared (Fig. 4–28). The incisions are made with a diamond blade after careful measurements; the excimer laser can make similar incisions. Fyodorov of the U.S.S.R. popularized this technique, and it has undergone considerable scrutiny by U.S. ophthalmologists. Radial keratotomy is effective, but its safety and predictability remain long-term concerns.

Corneal relaxing incisions and *corneal wedge resection* are generally used to correct astigmatism resulting from an abnormal curvature of the anterior surface of the cornea. The proce-

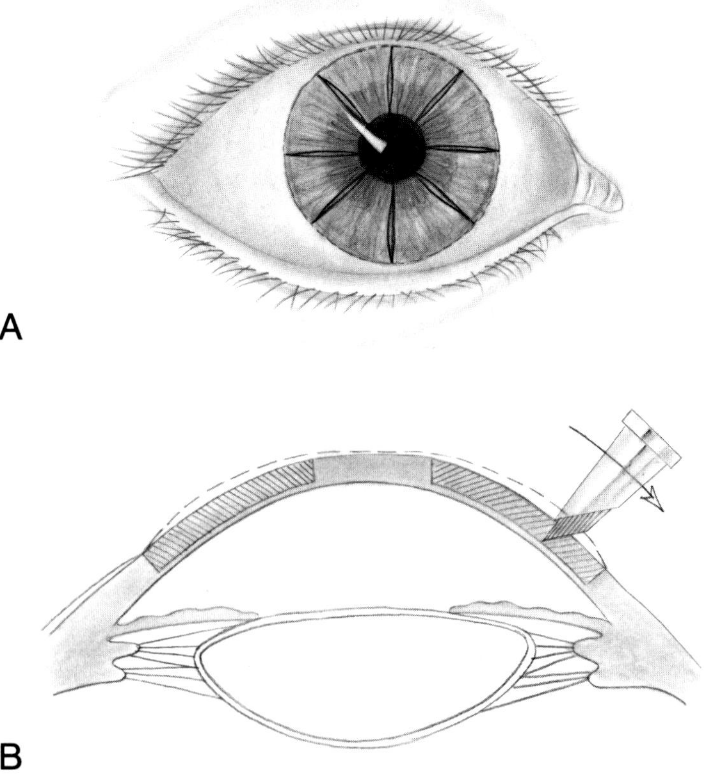

Fig. 4–28. Radial keratotomy for myopia. Nearly full-thickness incisions of the cornea are made with a calibrated diamond blade in a radial fashion with sparing of the central cornea. *A*, Frontal view. *B*, Axial view.

dures are most commonly used after corneal transplantation when the degree of astigmatism may be extremely high. Deep corneal relaxing incisions can be made with topical anesthesia at the slit lamp along the interface between the donor corneal button and the host recipient cornea, usually for three clock hours on either side of the cornea at the steepest corneal astigmatic area (Fig. 4–29). These result in a flattening of the cornea along this meridian and a decrease in the astigmatism. The corneal wedge resection is done in the operating room; approximately 0.5 to 1.0 mm of corneal tissue is removed in a deep ellipse in the interface between the donor and the recipient cornea in the meridian of the flattest corneal curvature (Fig. 4–30). The wound is then sutured tightly to steepen the corneal curvature in this meridian.

In *astigmatic keratotomy procedures*, a pattern of incisions is made in the steepest corneal meridian and a clear, unoperated optical zone remains. The incisions are circumferential or tangent with the optical zone. No one pattern has emerged with satisfactory predictability.

Corneal lathing techniques are forms of lamellar keratoplasty that change the shape of the cornea by carving the tissue or by inserting lenticules.

Keratomileusis ("carving the cornea") is a form of a lamellar keratoplasty in which a portion of the patient's own anterior cornea is removed with a surgical microkeratome in the operating room, is altered in shape by a computer-guided cryo-

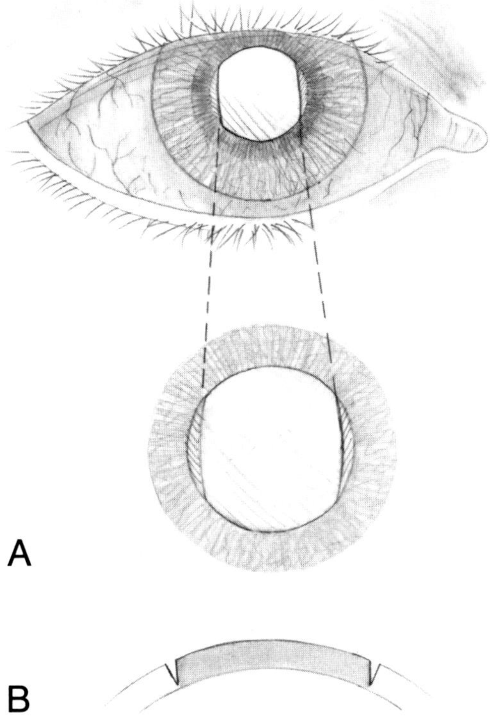

Fig. 4–29. Relaxing corneal incisions to reduce astigmatism in a patient after corneal transplantation. Incisions are made for three clock hours in both sides of the corneal transplant in the axis of the steepest corneal curvature in an attempt to flatten the cornea in this axis. *A*, Frontal view. *B*, Axial view.

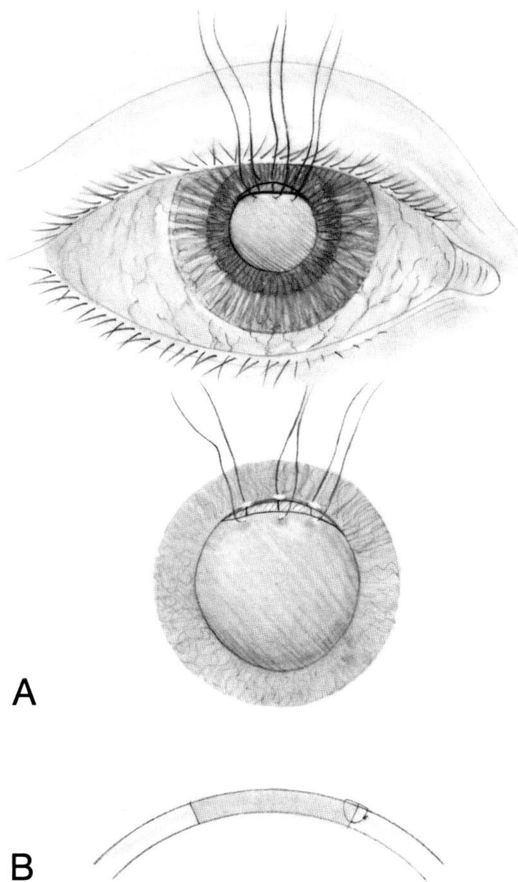

Fig. 4–30. Corneal wedge resection to reduce astigmatism in a patient after corneal transplantation. A crescentic piece of corneal tissue is removed from the corneal transplant in the axis of the flattest corneal curvature, and tight sutures are placed in an attempt to steepen the cornea in this axis. *A*, Frontal view. *B*, Axial view.

lathe, and then is resutured back onto the cornea. Myopic or hyperopic refractive errors can be corrected. In hyperopic keratomileusis, the anterior corneal surface is steepened by removing corneal tissue from the peripheral portion of the removed lamellar disc (Fig. 4–31 *A*). In myopic keratomileusis, the anterior corneal surface is flattened by removing corneal tissue from the central portion of the removed lamellar disc (Fig. 4–31 *B*).

Keratophakia is a lathing technique that uses donor corneal tissue to correct aphakic refrac-

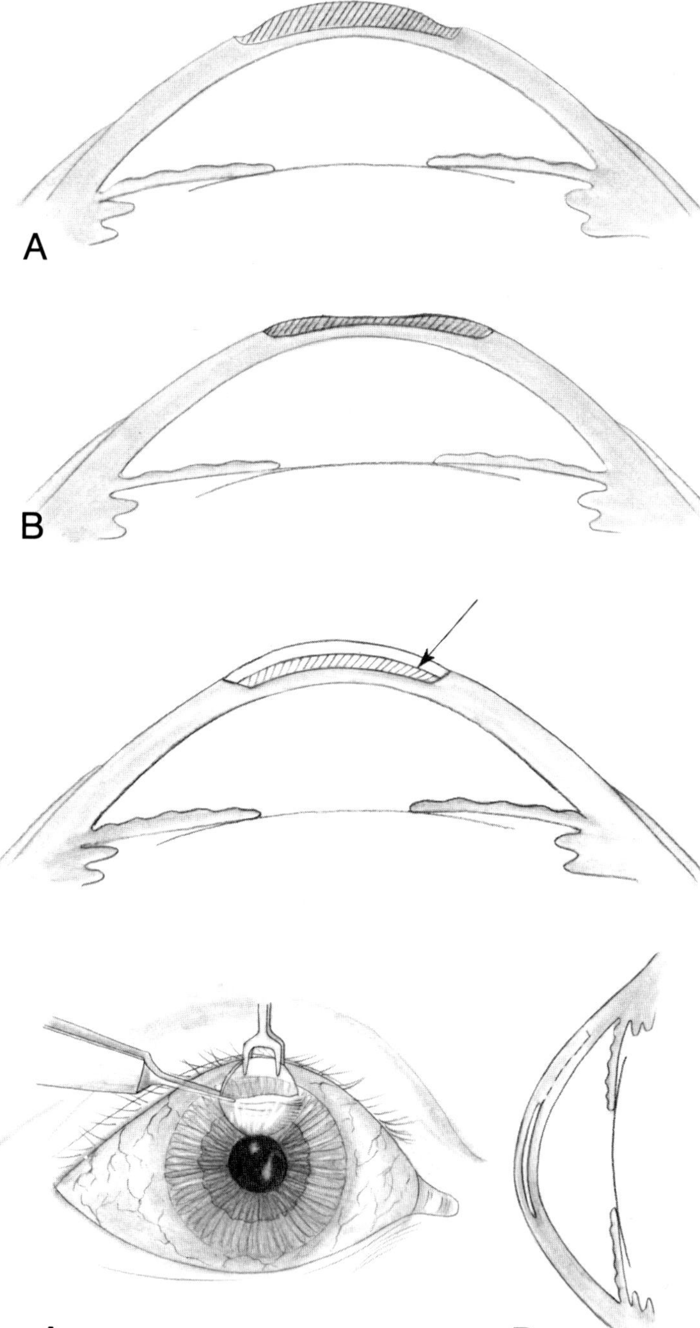

Fig. 4–31. Keratomileusis. A lamella of corneal tissue is removed, frozen and reshaped on a cryolathe, and returned to the normal bed. In hyperopia, the peripheral corneal tissue is thinned to result in a steeper central cornea (*A*); in myopia, the central corneal tissue is thinned (*B*).

Fig. 4–32. Keratophakia for hyperopia. A lamella of corneal tissue is removed and additional donor corneal tissue (*arrow*) is placed as a sandwich between the stromal bed and the corneal lamella, which is then sutured back in place.

Fig. 4–33. Intracorneal implantation. A pocket is created within the corneal stroma, and a hydrogel lens of high refractive index is placed centrally within the cornea. *A*, Frontal view. *B*, Axial view.

tive errors. The curvature of the cornea is steepened by placing a lenticule in the cornea between the anterior lamellar disc and the underlying corneal stromal bed (Fig. 4–32). In addition to the use of lathed donor corneal tissue as an intrastromal implant, several other materials—such as glass, Plexiglas, silicone, polysulfone, polymethyl methacrylate, and hydrogel lenses—have also been used to increase the refractive power of the cornea. A further modification of this technique is the simple creation of an intrastromal pocket in which to insert the alloplastic material (intracorneal implants) (Fig. 4–33).

In epikeratoplasty, a refractive lenticule is sewn on the surface of the eye.

In the *epikeratoplasty* technique, a "living contact lens" of donor cornea is sutured onto the surface of the eye. The lenticule is lathed from cryopreserved corneal tissue or from fresh tissue. The shape of the corneal lenticule is determined by mathematical formulas after determination of the axial length of the eye and the curvature of the recipient cornea. This procedure was conceived for aphakic eyes that require a central lenticule that is thicker than the periphery of the disc (Fig. 4–34 *A*). In addition, it has been modified for hyperopia, which also requires a thicker central lenticule, and for myopia, which requires a thinner central lenticule (Fig. 4–34 *B*). It has been used in keratoconus eyes with no power, in order to provide additional thickness to the cornea or to compress the conical protrusion of the cornea (Fig. 4–34 *C*). Some of the most encouraging work has been done in pediatric patients with aphakia who are unable to tolerate contact lenses; these patients will develop amblyopia unless the refractive error is corrected during their critical early years.

The sclera is an inert, avascular coat that is covered by three layers of blood vessels.

The sclera is an inert, avascular coat of the eye made up of collagen and elastic tissue in an interlacing fashion. Up until age 3 years, it is

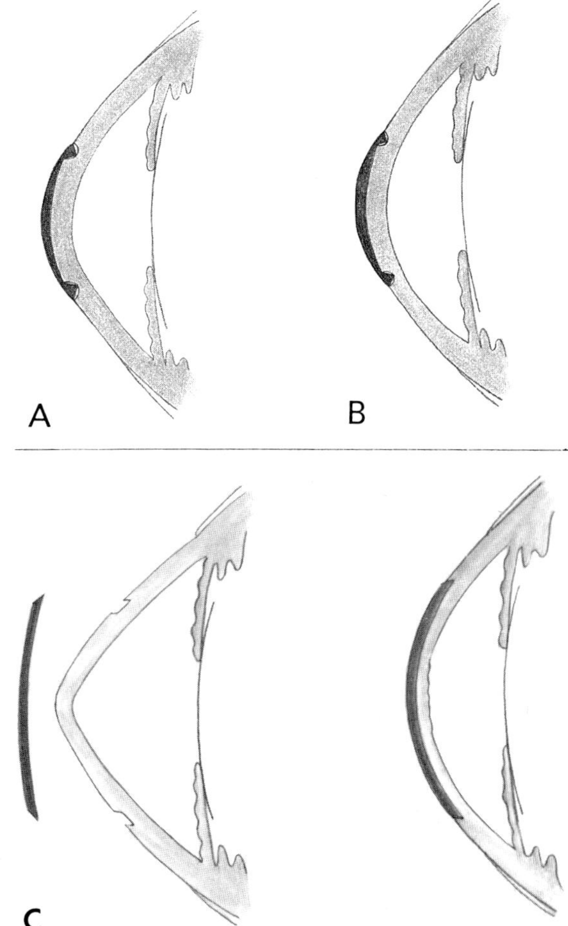

Fig. 4–34. Epikeratoplasty techniques. The central corneal epithelium is removed and a donor lenticule is sutured onto the surface of the cornea within a circular groove. In epikeratoplasty for hyperopia or after cataract operation, the central corneal thickness is more than that of the periphery (*A*). In epikeratoplasty for myopia, the central corneal thickness is less than that of the periphery (*B*). In epikeratoplasty for keratoconus, the central and the peripheral corneal thickness are equal but the whole corneal surface is flatter because of compression of the central conical cornea (*C*).

resilient and stretches in response to intraocular pressure. Many blood vessels and nerves are transmitted through the sclera. The episclera is a thin, vascular membrane that surrounds and provides nutrition to the sclera. Three layers of blood vessels cover the sclera; they become most evident when the eye is inflamed. The *deep episcleral plexus* is a syncytium of vessels that becomes dilated in scleritis. The *superficial episcleral vessels* are usually radially arranged and become evident in episcleritis. The *conjunctival plexus* is derived from the anterior ciliary arteries and is freely movable and blanches with phenylephrine (Neo-Synephrine). Scleral inflammation is best diagnosed under natural lighting conditions (rather than fluorescent or halogen lights) because the purplish hue of scleritis and the salmon-pink hue of episcleritis are evident. The red-free light of the slit lamp (green light) allows the best visualization of the blood vessels to determine which layer is inflamed.

Episcleritis is usually a benign, recurrent inflammation of the superficial layers of the sclera.

Episcleritis is a benign, recurrent inflammation of the fascial coat of the eye; it is more of a nuisance than a serious problem. Episcleritis is of acute onset and frequently bilateral. There is mild discomfort, and the disease itself is self-limited. Episcleritis is nontender compared with scleritis, in which the eye characteristically is painful. The maximal congestion is in the area of the radially oriented superficial episcleral vessels. Episcleritis may be associated with systemic disease such as collagen disease, herpes zoster, gout, or syphilis. Complications of episcleritis are rare.

There are two forms of episcleritis: simple and nodular episcleritis (Table 4–12). *Simple episcleritis* is more common and consists of a diffuse edema and redness of the episclera. These episodes usually last 1 to 2 weeks. *Nodular episcleritis* consists of a single red nodule or multiple red nodules of the episclera that may

be mobile and occasionally slightly tender and have surrounding congestion. Nodular episcleritis has a more prolonged course than does simple episcleritis. Both types of episcleritis are usually self-limited, but they resolve quicker with topical corticosteroids.

Scleritis is a potentially destructive inflammatory disease that is characterized by pain and scleral inflammation of either the anterior or the posterior sclera.

Scleritis is a potentially destructive disease that tends to involve the anterior exposed sclera more frequently than the posterior sclera. The prominent clinical feature is a radiating or boring pain. It typically has a gradual onset and a protracted course and may be bilateral. Scleritis is recognized by a purplish hue, indicating scleral edema and inflammation. It may be associated with systemic disorders such as collagen vascular disease, ulcerative colitis, Behçet's disease, sarcoidosis, or herpes zoster. Up to 30% of patients may die from a vascular disease within 8 years of an episode of scleritis.

Anterior scleritis is classified as diffuse scleritis, nodular scleritis, or necrotizing scleritis (Table 4–12). *Diffuse scleritis* is the most benign; it has an insidious onset and involves a large segment of the sclera (Fig. 4–35). *Nodular scleritis* is more painful, more protracted, and

TABLE 4–12 Morphologic Classification of Episcleritis and Scleritis

Episcleritis
  Simple
  Nodular
Anterior scleritis
  Diffuse
  Nodular
  Necrotizing
    With inflammation
    Without inflammation (scleromalacia perforans)
Posterior scleritis

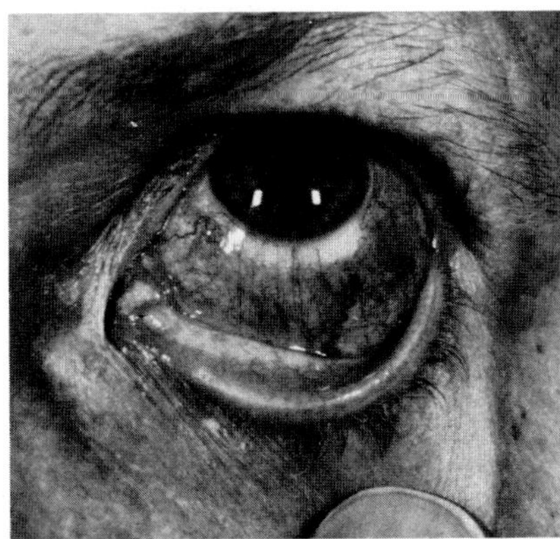

Fig. 4–35. Sclera in a patient with diffuse scleritis associated with a collagen vascular disease; entire sclera had a diffuse reddish-purplish hue.

more frequently recurrent. *Necrotizing scleritis* is of two types: with adjacent inflammation or without adjacent inflammation. *Necrotizing scleritis with adjacent inflammation* presents with acute pain and localized patches of avascular sclera (Fig. 4–36). This disease tends to be bilateral, progressive, and chronic with a high complication rate and a high mortality rate due to an underlying systemic disease. *Necrotizing scleritis without adjacent inflammation* (scleromalacia perforans) is most common in females in association with rheumatoid arthritis. This condition may be asymptomatic and quiet as the sclera becomes necrotic and sloughs over several months (Fig. 4–37). Sometimes the patient is unaware of this progressive condition. As the upper lid is lifted the superior sclera may reveal a porcelain appearance with uvea easily seen through the patches of thinned or absent sclera.

Posterior scleritis may begin posteriorly or may be an extension from anterior scleritis. There is swelling of the sclera that may be difficult to detect clinically but that can be confirmed by ultrasonography. Posterior scleritis may be associated with an exudative retinal detachment, choroidal detachments, retinal hemorrhages, disc edema, angle closure, or proptosis and may follow a prolonged course.

Therapy for scleritis involves identifying an underlying disease and initiating specific treatment if possible. Topical corticosteroids are used in most cases to increase comfort, but usually systemic therapy is necessary to quiet

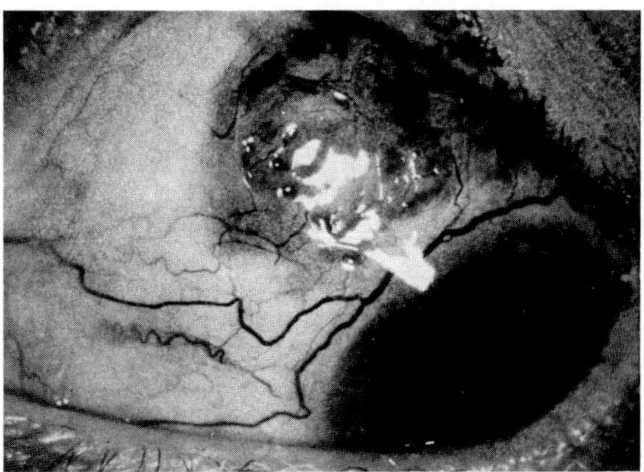

Fig. 4–37.   A painless, porcelain-white sclera with a large patch of avascular necrotic sclera revealing the underlying uvea in a patient with necrotizing scleritis without adjacent inflammation; patient had rheumatoid arthritis.

the inflammatory conditions. Systemic corticosteroids or various nonsteroidal anti-inflammatory agents are usually the initial agents tried, and immunosuppressive agents are warranted in severe situations. Surgical therapy is occasionally indicated.

CONJUNCTIVA

The conjunctival response to insult may be either nonspecific (hyperemia, edema, hemorrhage) or specific (papillae, follicles).

The conjunctiva is a mucous membrane of stratified columnar epithelial cells with three distinct regions: palpebral, forniceal, and bulbar (Fig. 4–38). The *palpebral conjunctiva* begins at the mucocutaneous junction within the keratinized epithelium of the skin and changes to nonkeratinized epithelium; it is adherent to the tarsus. The *forniceal conjunctiva* has numerous folds with attachments to the eyelid retractors (levator palpebrae superioris in the upper eyelid and capsulopalpebral fascia in the lower eyelid). The *bulbar conjunctiva* is loosely adherent to subconjunctival tissue called Tenon's capsule; it fuses with Tenon's capsule at the limbus where the conjunctival epithelium converts to the squamous epithelium covering the cornea.

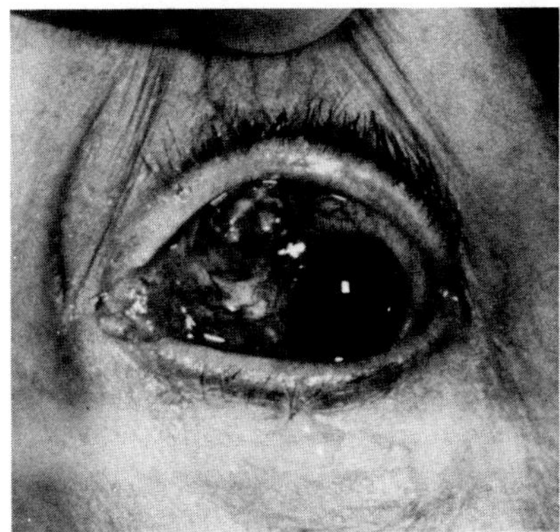

Fig. 4–36.   An extremely painful necrotizing scleritis with thinning and exposure of uveal tissue in a patient with Wegener's granulomatosis.

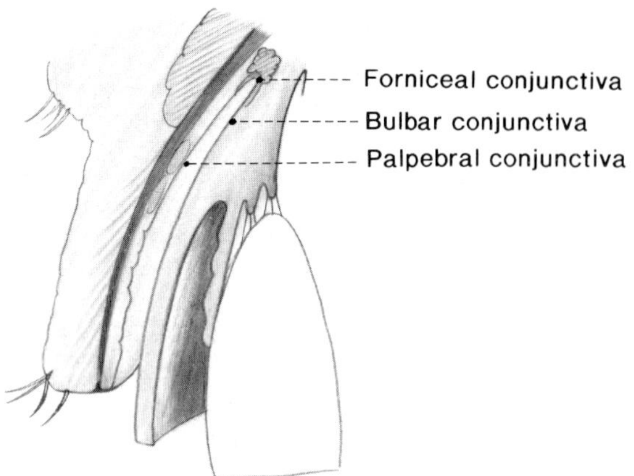

Fig. 4–38. A cross section of the lid and anterior surface of the eye, showing the adherence of the conjunctiva to the lid (palpebral conjunctiva), to the globe (bulbar conjunctiva), and the loose conjunctiva in the fornix (forniceal conjunctiva). Numerous glands throughout the conjunctiva help secrete lubricating tears.

Specialized structures within the conjunctiva include the *semilunar fold* (plica), which is a smooth, soft, movable membrane at the inner canthus, and the *caruncle*, which is an elevation of tissue between the plica and the inner canthus consisting of mucous membrane, sebaceous glands, and cutaneous elements. Both mucus-secreting goblet cells and accessory lacrimal glands are present throughout the conjunctiva and supply components of the tear film.

Symptoms suggestive of conjunctival disease include burning, discomfort, discharge, itching, and mild pain. The commonest conjunctival response to most insults consists of hyperemia, edema, and hemorrhage. More specific responses such as papillae, follicles, membranes, ulcerations, and scarring have a more limited differential diagnosis. A *papilla* varies in size and is usually on the palpebral conjunctiva. It is a perivascular inflammatory infiltration; its configuration depends on the fibrous attachments to the underlying tissue (Fig. 4–39 *A*). Small papillae cause the surface to have a slightly irregular appearance, and large, polygonal, flat-topped papillae are termed "pave stone" or "giant" papillae. The large papillae have a more specific clinical significance, whereas the smaller papillae are seen in

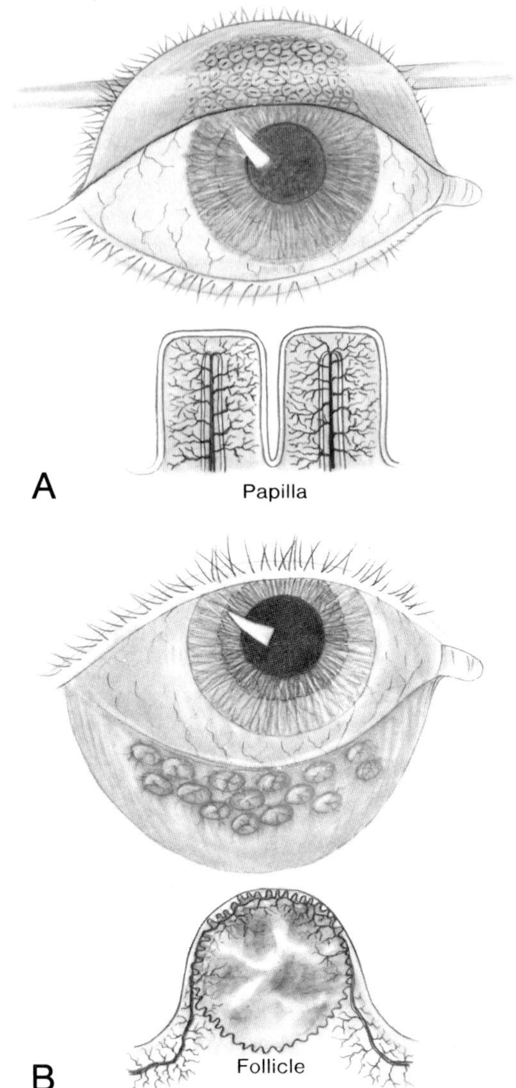

Fig. 4–39. The clinical and gross pathologic features of conjunctival papillae (*A*) and conjunctival follicles (*B*). A papilla is a central vessel core surrounded by chronic inflammatory cells. A follicle is a collection of lymphocytes in the conjunctiva, typically surrounded by blood vessels.

many conditions. *Follicles* are composed of discrete aggregates of lymphoid tissue within the superficial stroma. Small follicles have a slightly irregular, velvety appearance. Follicles are avascular, although small conjunctival vessels encircle them (Fig. 4–39 *B*). They are common in the fornix and have a diagnostic significance when they occur on the bulbar or palpebral conjunctiva. In addition to the clinical features

TABLE 4–13 Cytologic Features of Giemsa-Stained Conjunctival Scrapings

Cytologic features	Diagnostic considerations
Polymorphonuclear response	Bacterial or fungal conjunctivitis Neonatal chlamydial conjunctivitis Any conjunctivitis with inflammatory membranes or necrosis Erythema multiforme Acute toxic drug response Early ocular pemphigoid
Mononuclear response	Adenoviral conjunctivitis Herpes simplex Acute hemorrhagic conjunctivitis Chronic toxic conjunctivitis (molluscum, from drugs)
Polymorphonuclear and mononuclear response	Chlamydial conjunctivitis Trachoma Any chronic conjunctivitis Chemical burns
Eosinophilic response	Vernal conjunctivitis Atopic conjunctivitis Hay fever conjunctivitis Ocular pemphigoid Erythema multiforme Drug allergy
Other cell changes	
Intracytoplasmic inclusions	*Chlamydia*
Multinucleated giant cells	Herpes, trachoma, *Chlamydia*, neoplasia
Keratinization	Dry eyes, xerophthalmia
Increased goblet cells	Dry eyes, chronic conjunctivitis

described in the following pages, examination of Giemsa-stained conjunctival scrapings often confirms a diagnosis or suggests further specific laboratory tests (Table 4–13).

Pingueculae and pterygia are conjunctival degenerations probably associated with excess ultraviolet radiation.

A *pinguecula* is a yellow-white, elevated mass near the nasal limbus in the palpebral fissure. It is bilateral and consists of hyaline degeneration of collagen and elastin. It may be inflamed, and excision is occasionally done for cosmetic reasons. A *pterygium* is a triangular fold of bulbar conjunctiva with the apex extending onto the cornea (Fig. 4–40). It is usually loosely adherent to the cornea except at the apex. Pterygia are usually nasal, but they may occur at the temporal limbus. They are more common in regions of excess sun, wind, and dust and consist of a degenerative hyperplastic process. In most cases a pterygium follows a benign course,

but some can be aggressive. A surgical procedure is indicated because of corneal astigmatism or for cosmetic reasons. Young patients in tropical regions tend to have recurrences. Simple excision is done for primary cases, whereas recurrences are usually treated with excision and a conjunctival autograft. Beta

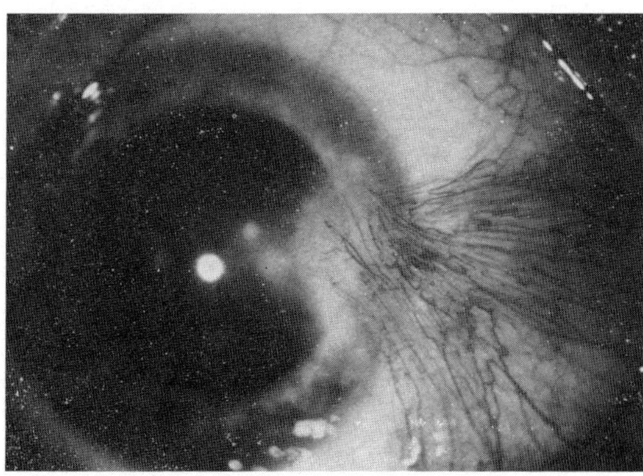

Fig. 4–40. A pterygium that is inflamed and progressive.

radiation or topical antimetabolites, such as mitomycin or thiotepa, are also used to help prevent recurrences. Lamellar keratoplasty may be necessary because multiple operations are usually associated with corneal thinning.

Acute bacterial conjunctivitis may be caused by a multitude of potential pathogens.

Multiple organisms are capable of producing conjunctivitis, although only a few produce severe, purulent, hyperacute conjunctivitis in the normal host (Table 4–14). The more common organisms in catarrhal conjunctivitis ("pinkeye") are *Staphylococcus aureus*, *Streptococcus pneumoniae*, and *Haemophilus aegyptius*, whereas the organisms responsible for severe, purulent, hyperacute conjunctivitis are usually *Streptococcus*, *Corynebacterium diphtheriae*, *Neisseria*, and *Haemophilus influenzae*. There are multiple routes of infection, including airborne, genitourinary transmission, spread from adjacent tissue, and occasionally endogenous spread.

The typical signs of acute bacterial conjunctivitis are conjunctival hyperemia, edema, and papillae, sticky lids, and a seromucoid or purulent discharge. Marked lid edema is characteristic of *Haemophilus influenzae* and *Corynebacterium diphtheriae*, whereas membranes are associated with *Streptococcus* and *Corynebacterium*. Petechial hemorrhages on the tarsal conjunctiva are especially common with *Streptococcus pneumoniae* and *Haemophilus influenzae*. There is usually no preauricular lymphadenopathy or skin involvement with bacterial conjunctivitis. The cornea is usually clear in bacterial conjunctivitis, although severe keratitis may result from infections with *Corynebacterium diphtheriae*, *Neisseria*, and *Haemophilus aegyptius*. Other complications include sepsis (especially with *Corynebacterium diphtheriae*, *Neisseria*, *Haemophilus*, and *Pseudomonas*), dacryocystitis, and conjunctival scar formation.

Treatment is based on the severity of the conjunctivitis. Mild conjunctivitis may be treated with a single antibiotic such as erythromycin, whereas severe conjunctivitis (lid edema, copious discharge, membranes, keratitis) requires evaluation with Gram and Giemsa stains and cultures from direct inoculation on blood and chocolate agar. The initial therapy is based on the results of the Gram stain. Fortified (high-concentration) topical antibiotics are occasionally used and are specially prepared by the pharmacy. Frequent cleansing of the eye and cycloplegia to reduce ciliary spasm and increase comfort may be indicated.

Gonococcal and Haemophilus influenzae conjunctivitis require prompt diagnosis and therapy.

The aerobic, gram-negative diplococcus *Neisseria gonorrhoeae* has a special affinity for mucous membranes and the genital tract. It grows best under increased CO_2 tension with chocolate agar or the Thayer-Martin medium. For epidemiologic reasons, it is important to distinguish *Neisseria gonorrhoeae* from *Neisseria meningitidis*. In adults, *Neisseria gonorrhoeae* conjunctivitis usually occurs from self-contamination and is characterized by an acute onset with marked purulence; it may progress to a severe keratitis (with perforation) or to sepsis, arthritis, or dacryoadenitis. Gonococcal conjunctivitis in newborns usually occurs within the first week after placental membranes have ruptured and shows a profuse purulent discharge with swollen eyelids. The Credé prophylaxis of 1% silver nitrate is usually effective. It is not always possible to distinguish *Gonococcus* from

TABLE 4–14 Bacteria and the Clinical Spectrum of Conjunctivitis

Acute conjunctivitis
  Staphylococcus aureus
  Streptococcus pneumoniae
  Haemophilus aegyptius
Hyperacute conjunctivitis
  Neisseria gonorrhoeae
  Neisseria meningitidis
  Corynebacterium diphtheriae
  Haemophilus influenzae
  β *Streptococcus*
Chronic conjunctivitis
  Staphylococcus aureus
  Moraxella lacunata
  β *Streptococcus*
  Branhamella catarrhalis
  Proteus, Klebsiella, Serratia

Chlamydia infection by clinical examination alone in a neonate.

The treatment of gonococcal conjunctivitis should include inoculation of secretions on chocolate agar or Thayer-Martin medium. The patient should be hospitalized and isolated, and the eyes should be irrigated often with sterile saline solution. Parenteral penicillin, ceftriaxone, or spectinomycin along with topical erythromycin is indicated. Sexual contacts should be treated, and consideration should be given to culture and treatment of concomitant *Chlamydia* infection in adults or neonates.

In young children, there is a specific form of severe conjunctivitis with chemosis, exudate, and preseptal cellulitis. This is related to lack of antibody titer against *Haemophilus influenzae* type B, and this infection typically occurs in the winter. Affected patients may have an upper respiratory infection, fever, and a purplish discoloration of the lid. This infection has a propensity to progress to orbital cellulitis. Treatment consists of systemic ampicillin (beware of resistance and consider systemic chloramphenicol if indicated), topical chloramphenicol, and frequent lavage.

Acute follicular conjunctivitis has a limited differential diagnosis with either a viral or a chlamydial cause.

The development of subconjunctival lymphoid follicles of acute onset has a limited differential diagnosis (Table 4–15). By noting the type of discharge, the presence of skin lesions, associated upper respiratory infection, and the presence of keratitis and preauricular lymph nodes, one can confirm a more specific diagnosis. The differential diagnosis includes pharyngoconjunctival fever, epidemic keratoconjunctivitis, herpes simplex conjunctivitis, adult inclusion conjunctivitis, Newcastle's disease, and epidemic acute hemorrhagic conjunctivitis.

The triad of fever, upper respiratory infection, and watery conjunctivitis of acute onset usually indicates *pharyngoconjunctival fever* caused by adenovirus type 3, 4, or 7 (Fig. 4–41).

Epidemic keratoconjunctivitis is an acute conjunctivitis with signs similar to those of pharyngoconjunctival fever, although there are

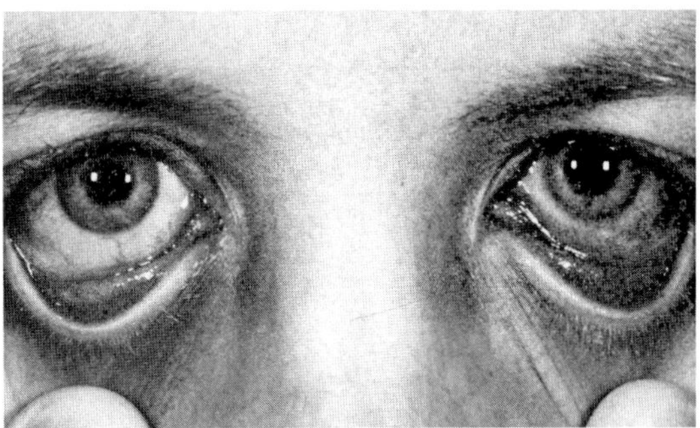

Fig. 4–41. Acute pharyngoconjunctival fever involving first the left eye and later the right eye in a patient with fever and sore throat.

normally no systemic symptoms. Epidemic keratoconjunctivitis is caused by adenovirus type 8 or 19 and is characterized by an explosive onset with watery discharge, acute follicular conjunctivitis (especially in the lower conjunctiva), periorbital pain, and marked foreign body sensation. The plica, caruncle, and upper lid are acutely inflamed, and occasionally there is hemorrhagic conjunctivitis. The preauricular lymph nodes are usually tender, and there may be an associated membranous conjunctivitis in about a third of the cases (Fig. 4–42). The incubation period is 8 to 9 days, and the patient is infectious for 14 days. This particular virus is very frequently seen in epidemics spread by health-care workers who examine these patients (especially the ophthalmologist). The disease initially involves one eye, and the second eye is infected to a lesser degree a few days later.

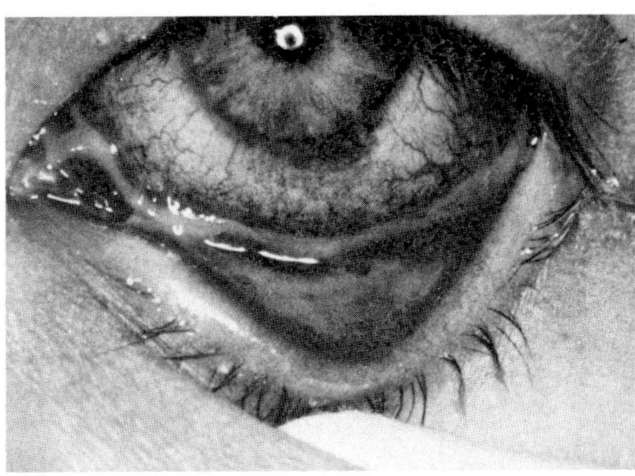

Fig. 4–42. Epidemic keratoconjunctivitis with a pseudomembranous conjunctivitis and a conjunctival follicular reaction.

TABLE 4–15 Diagnostic Features of Acute Follicular Conjunctivitis

Disease	*Characteristics*
Pharyngoconjunctival fever (adenovirus type 3, 4, 7)	Watery discharge, conjunctival hyperemia Acute systemic symptoms, 7 to 14 days Preauricular lymph node Fine epithelial keratitis, briefly Mononuclear conjunctival response Confirmed by culture, antigen detection, serologic testing No sequelae
Epidemic keratoconjunctivitis (adenovirus type 8, 19)	Watery discharge, conjunctival hyperemia Epidemics; infectious for up to 14 days Transmission from hand to eye Hyperacute onset, tender and enlarged preauricular lymph node Pseudomembranes in 1/3; occasional subconjunctival hemorrhage Stages of superficial corneal involvement (fine or focal keratitis, subepithelial opacities, subepithelial infiltrates that may last months) Mononuclear conjunctival response; neutrophils in pseudomembrane Confirmed by culture, antigen detection, serologic testing
Herpes simplex conjunctivitis (mainly herpes simplex type 1)	Watery discharge Usually children or young adults May be primary or recurrent herpes simplex virus Usually unilateral with frequent lid or corneal herpes (may be subtle) Pseudomembranes, occasionally Small preauricular lymph nodes May proceed to corneal stromal disease Mononuclear conjunctival response with multinucleated giant cells Confirmed by culture or antigen detection
Inclusion conjunctivitis (*Chlamydia* oculogenitalis)	Mild mucopurulent discharge Conjunctival redness, chemosis, and bulbar and palpebral follicles Enlarged preauricular lymph node Venereal hand-to-eye transmission Persistent infection until treated Corneal punctate or subepithelial infiltrates Superior corneal micropannus Polymorphonuclear conjunctival response with epithelial intracytoplasmic inclusions Confirmed by culture or fluorescent antibody stain
Hemorrhagic conjunctivitis (picornavirus)	Serous to mucoid discharge Chemosis and later bilateral subconjunctival hemorrhages Follicles not prominent Hand-to-eye transmission Massive epidemics reported Small preauricular lymph node Occasionally neurologic problems Occasionally epithelial or subepithelial keratitis Mononuclear conjunctival response
Neonatal inclusion conjunctivitis	Seen under certain conditions
Acute trachoma	Seen under certain conditions

The corneal lesions occur in many patients and run a characteristic course, beginning as a diffuse epithelial keratitis and evolving to punctate focal epithelial opacities, which are followed by stromal opacities and later subepithelial opacities. Approximately 25% of patients develop marked subepithelial opacities that may interfere with vision (Fig. 4–43). They usually resolve, but they may take months or occasionally years. These chronic opacities are probably an immune response that can be suppressed with topical corticosteroids, but they will return when the treatment is withdrawn. Topical corticosteroids are considered in cases of membrane formation and subepithelial infiltrates. Epidemic keratoconjunctivitis is self-limited, and treatment is only supportive. Because the physician is a primary vehicle of transmission, it is important that frequent handwashing and limited direct contact with these patients be the rule.

Both type 1 (oral strain) and type 2 (genital strain) *herpes simplex virus* can cause a primary or recurrent follicular conjunctivitis with sparing of the cornea. The primary disease usually occurs in children younger than 5 years and may be associated with a mild systemic illness with gingivostomatitis, lymphadenitis, and fever. The conjunctiva is red with a follicular conjunctivitis, a watery discharge, and small preauricular lymph nodes. This is usually a unilateral condition, and careful examination may show vesicular skin lesions on the lid. The diagnosis is confirmed by viral culture, immunofluorescent antibody techniques, or a rising serologic titer (in primary infection only). Therapy for the ocular condition consists of topical antiviral agents, mainly as a prophylaxis against corneal lesions. Topical corticosteroids should be avoided, and the patient should be followed closely for the development of corneal disease.

Chlamydia is an obligate intracellular parasite that contains both DNA and RNA. There are several serotypes, and types D-K generally are associated with genital, ocular, and systemic disease. Chlamydial conjunctivitis occurs in sexually active adults, and the genital tract is the reservoir in both males and females. The conjunctival infection is characterized by a mucopurulent discharge with a follicular conjunctivitis (Fig. 4–44). It is usually bilateral but asymmetric. There is some edema of the bulbar conjunctiva along with enlarged preauricular lymph nodes, but conjunctival membranes are usually not present. Many patients are inappropriately treated with topical corticosteroids and have some minimal relief. Later in the course, corneal findings include a peripheral keratitis with epithelial lesions and infiltrates, limbal swelling, micropannus, corneal neovascularization, and conjunctival scarring. The diagnosis is confirmed with a Giemsa stain (which shows polymorphonuclear cells and a

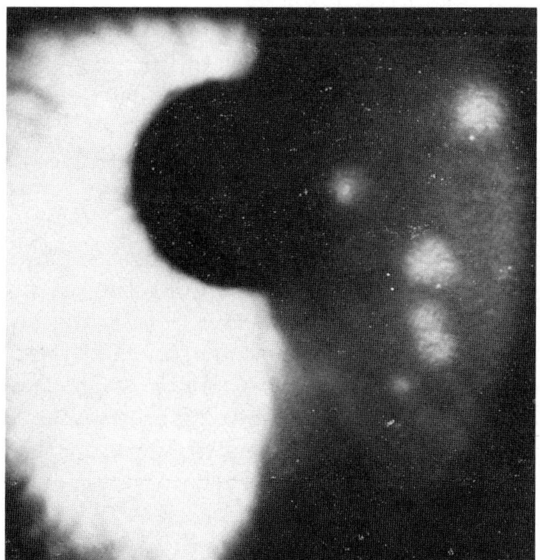

Fig. 4–43. Subepithelial opacities characteristic of late corneal involvement from epidemic keratoconjunctivitis.

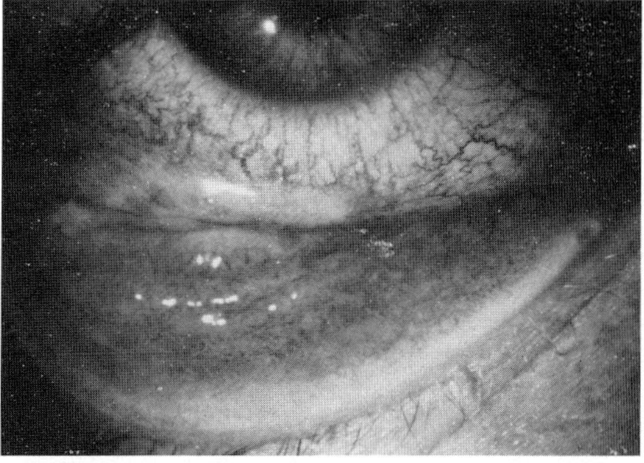

Fig. 4–44. Acute follicular conjunctival response with mucopurulent discharge characteristic of chlamydial conjunctivitis.

lymphocytic reaction with inclusion bodies), with a chlamydial culture, or with a fluorescent monoclonal antibody test (Microtrak). Treatment is with tetracycline for 3 to 4 weeks (substitutes include erythromycin or rifampin). It is necessary to treat any sexual contacts at the same time, and in most states this communicable disease must be reported to the state health board.

Enterovirus group 70 (picornavirus) has been associated with major epidemics of *acute hemorrhagic conjunctivitis* in the Orient as well as the United States. This disease has a short incubation period and is self-limited but has a very characteristic explosive onset. There is usually an upper respiratory infection, subconjunctival hemorrhages diffusely in the upper bulbar conjunctiva, small preauricular lymph nodes, a fine epithelial keratitis, periorbital pain, and anterior uveitis. Systemic symptoms include generalized myalgia and rarely a motor paralysis of the lower extremities.

Chronic follicular conjunctivitis is most commonly seen in association with chlamydial infection or as a toxic reaction to topical drugs.

Follicular conjunctivitis persisting for several weeks is called subacute or chronic (Fig. 4–45). The differential diagnosis is different from that of acute follicular conjunctivitis (Table 4–16). It may begin as an acute follicular conjunctivitis and may persist or insidiously progress unless it is treated.

Chlamydial infections with serotypes A–C cause *trachoma*, the leading cause of preventable blindness in the world. It is seen in the United States among Mexican-Americans, Chinese-Americans, American Indians, and Filipinos and in a "trachoma belt" in the Ozark Mountains. It is thought that a combination of bacterial pathogens (especially *Haemophilus aegyptius*) makes the disease more severe in trachoma regions than do the strains of oculogenital acute inclusion conjunctivitis. The presentation is with a chronic follicular conjunctivitis. The cornea is involved with peripheral inflammatory infiltrates, pannus formation, limbal follicles, and Herbert pits (cicatricial depressions of the peripheral cornea). Later,

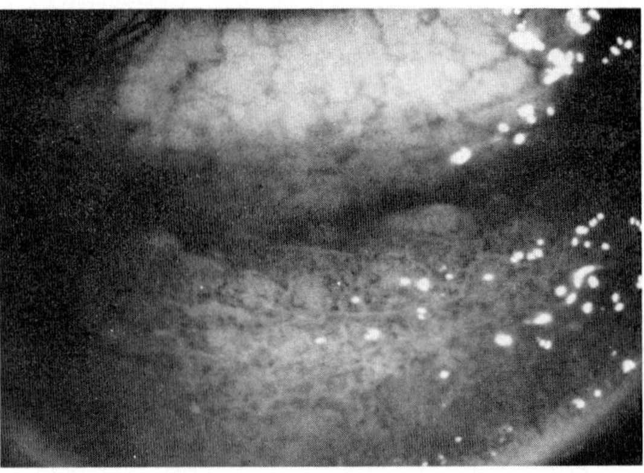

Fig. 4–45. Subacute follicular conjunctivitis in a patient with a reaction to dipivefrin (Propine), used to treat glaucoma.

there is scarring of the upper palpebral conjunctiva with linear lines (Arlt lines). Because of the conjunctival scarring, tear deficiency, dacryostenosis, entropion, trichiasis, corneal scarring, and Salzmann's nodules are frequent.

There are four stages of the disease, and the classification is based on conjunctival findings. In stage I there are immature follicles, and in stage II, mature follicles. Stage III shows scarring of the conjunctiva along with follicles, and stage IV, extensive scarring of the conjunctiva.

The diagnosis of trachoma is generally confirmed by a Giemsa stain (showing inclusion bodies in the earlier stages of the disease) or with fluorescent antibody staining, serologic testing, or special tissue culture techniques. Treatment of patients with active disease is with a 3-week course of either systemic tetracycline or erythromycin. Mass treatment of endemic areas has been successful with topical tetracycline.

Chronic conjunctival irritation from drug use (especially idoxuridine, dipivefrin, or atropine), constant cosmetic use, or irritation from a virus such as molluscum contagiosum can lead to a chronic *toxic follicular conjunctivitis*. The follicles are probably a toxic reaction to the degradation products from various compounds. This can have the appearance of trachoma with follicles, papillary hypertrophy, conjunctival scarring, keratitis, and pannus. Therapy involves recognizing the condition and withdrawing the offending agent before excessive conjunctival scarring occurs.

TABLE 4–16 Differential Diagnoses of Chronic Follicular Conjunctivitis

Disease	Comments
Chronic inclusion conjunctivitis (*Chlamydia* oculogenitalis)	Large bulbar and palpebral conjunctival follicles Redness to conjunctiva with mucoid discharge Associated genital infection Cornea changes progress with chronicity
Chronic blepharitis (especially *Moraxella lacunata*)	Usually in adolescents with angular blepharitis Subacute conjunctivitis with mucoid discharge Tarsal follicles No lymph node enlargement May be associated lacrimal drainage infection Polymorphonuclear conjunctival response with gram-negative diplobacilli
Molluscum contagiosum (molluscum contagiosum virus)	Lid molluscum evident Usually in young adults Usually self-limited Occasional conjunctival scarring Fine epithelial keratitis with pannus Mononuclear conjunctival reaction Eosinophilic cytoplasmic inclusions in lid nodule Probable toxic reaction to viral antigen
Trachoma (*Chlamydia trachomatis*)	Endemic in certain geographic areas Follicles on tarsus Linear and stellate tarsal scars Vascular pannus develops Lymphocytes and polymorphonuclear conjunctival response
Oculoglandular syndrome (multiple agents, including cat-scratch disease)	Focal granulomatous conjunctivitis with surrounding follicles Preauricular lymph node, ± fever Mononuclear and polymorphonuclear conjunctival reaction
Drug-induced follicular conjunctivitis (multiple agents, including antivirals, neosporin, gentamicin, glaucoma medications, preservatives)	Rarely preauricular lymphadenopathy Occasional epithelial keratitis May proceed to pannus, keratinization A "toxic" reaction
Eye makeup-induced conjunctivitis (especially mascara)	No lymph nodes Pigment (mascara) in conjunctival cysts that may appear like follicles Usually asymptomatic
Folliculoses of childhood (lymphoid hyperplasia)	Part of generalized lymphoid hyperplasia occasionally seen in children No inflammation Follicles most prominent in fornix

Chronic conjunctivitis is not a specific diagnosis; rather, it is a term used to categorize many conditions causing protracted conjunctival discomfort.

Chronic conjunctivitis is not a specific diagnosis; rather, it is a term used to categorize many conditions that cause protracted conjunctival discomfort (with or without ocular signs). This condition may be either unilateral or bilateral, and a careful history and examination may elucidate the cause. The major causes are listed in Table 4–17. Most of these conditions are discussed at length in various other areas throughout this chapter.

TABLE 4–17 Differential Diagnoses of Chronic Conjunctivitis

Infections
  Staphylococcal blepharoconjunctivitis
  Moraxella blepharoconjunctivitis
  Chlamydial inclusion disease
  Trachoma
  Parasitic (pediculosis) blepharitis
  Molluscum contagiosum
  Parinaud's oculoglandular syndrome
  Viral papilloma
Oculodermal disease
  Seborrheic blepharoconjunctivitis
  Acne rosacea
  Pemphigoid
  Psoriasis
Adnexal disease
  Meibomian gland dysfunction
  Keratitis sicca
  Superior limbic conjunctivitis
  Nasolacrimal obstruction, canaliculitis
  Lacrimal ductal stones
Allergic disease
  Atopic conjunctivitis
  Vernal conjunctivitis
  Contact dermatoconjunctivitis
  Phlyctenular keratoconjunctivitis
Toxic irritants
  Topical drugs
  Foreign bodies, pollution, chlorine
  Cosmetics
  Chemical irritants
Neoplasms
  Squamous cell carcinoma, meibomian gland
    carcinoma
  Pinguecula (inflamed)
  Pterygium (inflamed)
Structural lid disease
  Lid malposition
  Exposure
  Trichiasis

The cause of ophthalmia neonatorum cannot be distinguished by clinical examination alone and requires a systematic approach.

Any conjunctivitis that occurs in the first month of life is called ophthalmia neonatorum (Fig. 4–46). The specific cause of the conjunctivitis cannot be distinguished by clinical examination alone. The differential diagnosis of

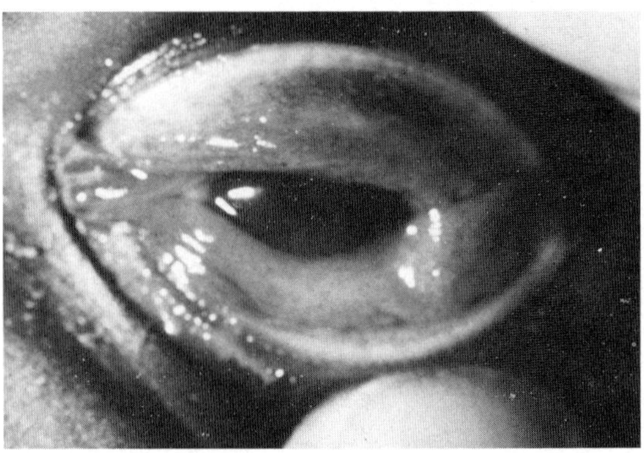

Fig. 4–46. Ophthalmia neonatorum in a 4-week-old infant caused by *Chlamydia*.

ophthalmia neonatorum is outlined in Table 4–18.

Chemical conjunctivitis occurs from silver nitrate prophylaxis. This conjunctivitis is minimal and transient; the Giemsa stain shows nonspecific inflammation. *Staphylococcal conjunctivitis* is acquired from the mother or from handling within the nursery. This is a mild conjunctivitis with hyperemia and mucoid discharge. The Gram stain should reveal the organisms, and treatment is with topical antibiotics.

Inclusion conjunctivitis is acquired from the mother during delivery. It may be a systemic disease with both genital tract and lung infection in a newborn. The eyelids and conjunctiva are swollen, but the conjunctiva does not show follicles. A micropannus or pseudomembranes may occur. The disease, if untreated, may become chronic. The Giemsa stain is positive in about 95% of cases (Fig. 4–47). Treatment is with topical tetracycline or erythromycin; if systemic symptoms or findings are present, systemic erythromycin is administered. *Neisseria gonorrhoeae* is acquired from the mother at birth. This presents with a very purulent discharge, and treatment is with topical erythromycin and parenteral penicillin. It is necessary to treat the mother and all sexual contacts. *Nasolacrimal duct obstruction* is evident with mucus in the nasal corner of one eye, especially each morning. This is common and resolves on its own; occasionally, nasolacrimal duct probing is necessary. *Herpes simplex virus* can be ac-

TABLE 4–18 **Differential Diagnoses of Ophthalmia Neonatorum**

Agents/disease	Post-partum day of onset	Clinical features	Laboratory findings
Silver nitrate irritation (Credé)	1	Injection Rarely purulent Rarely pseudomembranes	Polymorphonuclear cells
Inclusion conjunctivitis (*Chlamydia*)	5–10	Purulent conjunctivitis Occasional scars Pseudomembranes Micropannus	Polymorphonuclear cells Cytoplasmic inclusions Fluorescent antigen tests, chlamydial culture (+)
Neisseria gonorrhoeae conjunctivitis	3–5	Mucopurulent conjunctivitis Occasional corneal ulcer or ring abscess	Polymorphonuclear cells Gram (-) diplococci in epithelial cells
Bacterial conjunctivitis, especially *Staphylococcus aureus, Haemphilus, Streptococcus pneumoniae*	5–10	Catarrhal to purulent conjunctivitis Epithelial keratitis	Polymorphonuclear cells Organism seen occasionally in or around polymorphonuclear cells or in epithelial cells
Primary herpes simplex	3–10	Watery conjunctivitis Other ocular herpes	Multinucleated giant cells Fluorescent antigen, herpes simplex virus culture (+)
Nasolacrimal duct obstruction	2–5	Unilateral mucoid discharge	Variable organism in culture

quired from the mother during passage through the genital tract. This is type 2 herpes simplex virus and can progress to corneal dendrites, skin vesicles, chorioretinitis, and vitritis. The Giemsa stain shows multinucleated giant cells. Therapy is with topical and possibly systemic antiviral agents.

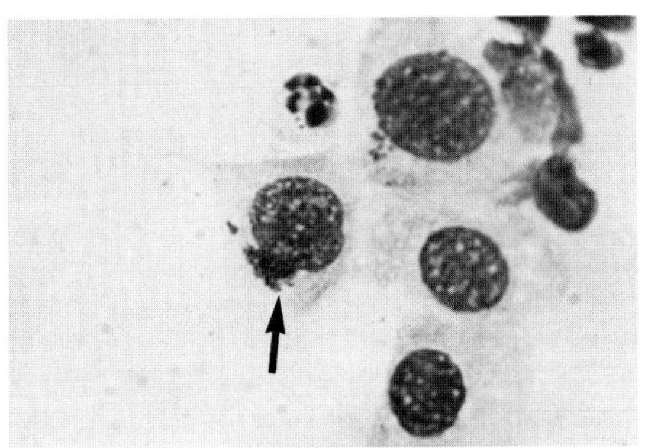

Fig. 4–47. Giemsa staining of conjunctival scraping demonstrating basophilic intracytoplasmic inclusion bodies (*arrow*) within conjunctival epithelial cells, characteristic of *Chlamydia*.

Because of the multiple causes of ophthalmia neonatorum, a systemic approach is necessary. Gram and Giemsa staining of conjunctival scrapings (after the purulent material has been wiped away) should be performed. Inoculation should be done directly onto blood agar and chocolate agar (or Thayer-Martin medium). More specific tests such as the Microtrak fluorescent monoclonal antibody test for *Chlamydia* or herpes simplex antibody testing depend on laboratory availability. Treatment is based on the results of the scraping and the cultures.

Inflammatory membranes of the conjunctiva may indicate a specific cause.

The diseases that can cause inflammatory membranes of the conjunctiva are limited (Table 4–19). It is important to differentiate true membranes from pseudomembranes. With *true membranes*, an inflammatory exudate is firmly adherent to the underlying conjunctiva; when grasped with a forceps, the epithe-

**TABLE 4–19 Differential Diagnoses
of Inflammatory Membranes
of the Conjunctiva**

True membranes
  Neisseria gonorrhoeae conjunctivitis
  Diphtheria conjunctivitis
  β-Hemolytic streptococcal conjunctivitis
  Stevens-Johnson syndrome
Pseudomembranes
  Bacterial conjunctivitis (especially *Streptococcus
    pneumoniae, Staphylococcus, Pseudomonas, Neisseria
    meningitidis*)
  Viral conjunctivitis (especially adenovirus 3 and 8,
    herpes simplex)
  Ocular pemphigoid
  Chemical burns
  Ligneous conjunctivitis

lium is torn away with the membrane, and bleeding results. *Pseudomembranes* have less adherence to underlying epithelium, and a hemorrhage does not occur when they are removed.

There are multiple manifestations of ocular allergy.

Because of the eye's prominent location, the ocular mucous membrane component, and prior exposure to topical drugs or atmospheric antigens, allergic ocular disease is common. The clinical presentation of anterior segment allergic diseases depends on the immunologic mechanisms involved (immediate versus delayed hypersensitivity) and the specific ocular tissue affected. Table 4–20 lists allergic diseases of the lids, conjunctiva, cornea, and sclera and the type of immunologic mechanism that has been implicated, at least in part.

Hay fever conjuctivitis is a classic example of an immediate humoral antibody response to airborne allergens.

Hay fever conjunctivitis is an immediate humoral antibody response to airborne allergens. The antigens react with IgE in the conjunctiva and lead to symptoms of puffy lids with edema, tearing, itching, red eyes, sneezing, runny nose, and a flushed feeling. The conjunctiva shows a pale, boggy edema that can evolve to a papillary reaction. Affected patients usually have a history of atopy, and the disease is typically seasonal and related to either grass or weeds. The diagnosis can be confirmed by Giemsa staining, which shows polymorphonuclear cells with eosinophils or eosinophilic granules. The disorder is usually self-limited after the allergen is eliminated. Cold compresses, astringents, and oral antihistamines may help. Desensitization has limited value. Topical cromolyn or low-dose topical corticosteroids are occasionally necessary in a "burst" dose to get the disease under control. Long-term use of topical corticosteroids is discouraged.

Drug sensitivity and contact conjunctivitis require a period of sensitization before expression.

Ocular allergic symptoms may occur after a period of sensitization to multiple topical drugs, including atropine, phenylephrine, anesthetics, antibiotics, and multiple vehicles that are incorporated in drugs. The amount of lid and skin involvement with *drug hypersensitivity* varies. The conjunctiva usually shows papillary hyperemia, which is most severe in the inferior tarsal conjunctiva. Giemsa stain reveals eosinophils. Treatment includes elimination of the compound and a "burst" dose of topical corticosteroids to the conjunctiva or steroid cream to the lids. Severe reactions may require oral or intramuscular corticosteroids. Dermatologic aids (wet dressings) may be helpful. Antihistamines and desensitization are usually of no value.

Contact conjunctivitis is a cell-mediated delayed hypersensitivity reaction that includes an initial sensitization period and then a delay period for expression. It appears unrelated to atopy. The most common offenders are the miotics, phenylephrine, aminoglycosides, idoxuridine, and drug vehicles (especially thimerosal). Hyperemia occurs initially, and edema of the conjunctiva is noted later. Follicles and corneal involvement with punctate epithelial erosions, macroepithelial erosions, and thickening of the

TABLE 4–20 Allergic Diseases of the Lids, Conjunctiva, Cornea, and Sclera and Their Proposed Immunologic Mechanism

Type I (anaphylactoid)	Type II (cytotoxic)	Type III (immune complex)	Type IV (cell mediated)
Hay fever Vernal keratoconjunctivitis Atopic keratoconjunctivitis Giant papillary conjunctivitis Angioedema of lids Corneal edema (bee sting) Urticaria	Drug-related conjunctivitis Mooren's ulcer Long-standing corneal allograft reaction	Catarrhal marginal keratitis Marginal keratitis in immune disease (such as rheumatoid arthritis) Scleritis/episcleritis Ocular pemphigoid Membranous conjunctivitis Ligneous conjunctivitis Parinaud's conjunctivitis Herpes simplex stromal keratitis Keratitis of mumps, infectious mononucleosis, adenoviral disease, and *Chlamydia* Stevens-Johnson syndrome Sjögren's syndrome	Phlyctenulosis Corneal allograft reaction Contact dermatoconjunctivitis Interstitial keratitis of lues, tuberculosis, leprosy
No complement involved	Complement involved	Complement involved	No complement involved

epithelium may occur. There may be later associated skin involvement (an eczematoid reaction) but little or no pruritus. There are usually no eosinophils on Giemsa stain. The therapy is the same as that for drug-induced hypersensitivity.

Vernal and atopic conjunctivitis are ocular manifestations of an "atopic state."

Vernal conjunctivitis is an ocular manifestation of the "atopic state." It is a chronic, recurrent, and bilateral disease that usually occurs in males before the age of 10 years and lasts for approximately 10 years. It is usually exacerbated with a seasonal pattern in temperate zones. There is typical evolution of itching, conjunctival hyperemia, mucoid discharge, papillary hypertrophy, and later giant papillae with vari-

ous degrees of corneal involvement. There are two basic forms, which occasionally occur together. The palpebral form is characterized by papillary hypertrophy of the upper tarsal conjunctiva with flat, cobblestone vegetations (Fig. 4–48). The lower tarsal conjunctiva has edema and hyperemia, and corneal involvement is more severe than in the limbal form. Eosinophils are abundant on Giemsa-stained scrapings of the conjunctiva. The limbal form is more frequent in blacks and consists of a papillary hypertrophy in the limbal zone superiorly which may enlarge to hyperplastic gelatinous tissue (Fig. 4–49). At the limbus there are Trantas' dots, which consist of degenerated epithelial cells or eosinophils in the deep epithelium. Pannus formation is common, and only a few eosinophils are seen on the Giemsa stain.

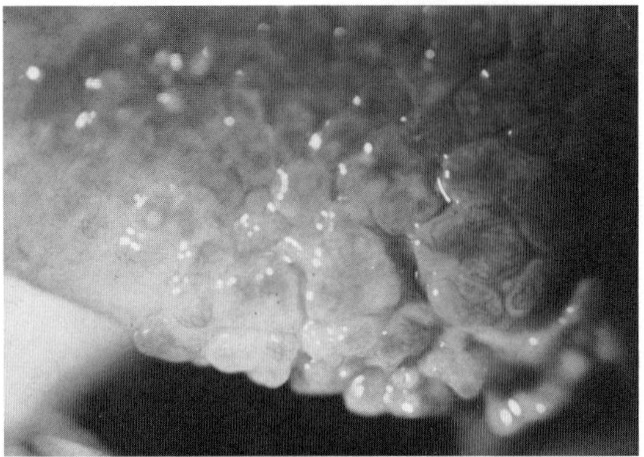

Fig. 4–48. Papillary form of vernal conjunctivitis with large, flat, cobblestone papillary conjunctival reaction of the upper lid.

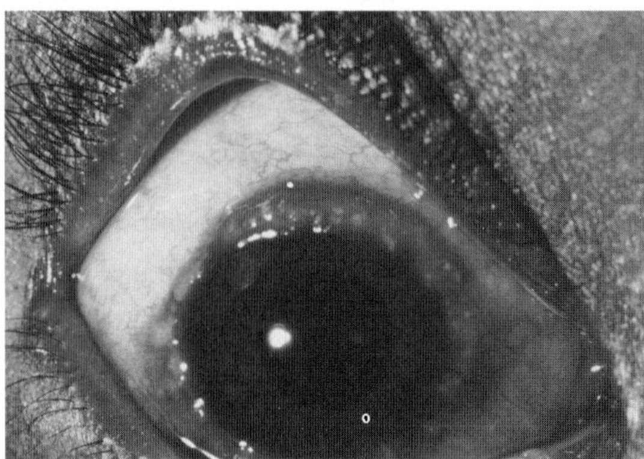

Fig. 4–49. Limbal form of vernal conjunctivitis with gelatinous, papillary hypertrophy in the limbal zone.

Corneal involvement is usually more severe in the palpebral form and consists of punctate epithelial erosions, punctate epithelial keratitis, macroepithelial ulcerations (shallow, gray, oval, and in the upper third of the cornea), plaque formation, stromal keratitis, and pannus formation.

An important part of the therapy for this condition is patient education regarding the seasonal nature of the disease, the long-term consequences, and the side effects of corticosteroid use. It is usually not possible to eliminate the allergen or to accomplish desensitization. Measures are directed at controlling the allergic conjunctival response with mucolytic agents (for filaments or copious mucous discharge), topical vasoconstrictors, and finally topical corticosteroids. Steroid solutions such as medrysone (HMS) that generally do not penetrate into the eye are probably the safest to use. Prompt control of acute symptoms may be possible with "burst" dosage and rapid reduction and continued surveillance of the patient. Topical cromolyn may help to reduce the need for corticosteroids and occasionally can be used alone. Topical cyclosporine is of possible benefit. Other nonsteroidal antiinflammatory agents seem to be of little value. Surgical excision of giant papillae or superficial keratectomy for plaques is occasionally necessary. Mucous membrane grafting and cryotherapy are other alternatives for advanced cases. Soft contact lenses can occasionally be helpful in the management of persistent keratitis.

Atopic conjunctivitis (or dermatoconjunctivitis) is an allergic disease of the skin and conjunctiva mediated by IgE. There is a frequent history of other atopy, and the condition may be exacerbated by certain stimuli. Early skin changes include roughening, cracking, and redness; later in the course, chronic inflammation with thickening, scaling, lichenification, and hypopigmentation may occur. The most common skin sites are the eyelids, face, neck, axilla, and antecubital and popliteal spaces. Ocular symptoms consist of itching and hyperemia, and signs include thickening of the bulbar and palpebral conjunctiva, epithelial keratitis and vascularization of the peripheral cornea, and occasionally giant papillary hypertrophy (cobblestones). There is a frequent association with keratoconus, retinal detachment, and a typical shieldlike atopic cataract. Affected patients are especially vulnerable to viral infections with herpes simplex. Treatment is aimed at removing any obvious trigger or irritant as well as cleansing, cold compresses, and cold creams to the skin. The judicious use of a topical corticosteroid for the skin or eye is frequently necessary. Cromolyn sodium 4% has been effective as a topical drop, and plasmapheresis is of value in some refractory patients.

Erythema multiforme may occur in a minor form (with predominant skin involvement) or a major form called Stevens-Johnson syndrome (with severe mucous membrane and ocular involvement).

There are two forms of *erythema multiforme*: the minor type involves primarily the skin, and the major type involves mucous membranes and the conjunctiva. This latter type is called *Stevens-Johnson syndrome*; it is probably a vasculitis with many reported associations (such as microbial organisms, collagen disease, malignancy, and multiple drugs). Circulating immune complexes have been reported. Stevens-Johnson syndrome occurs generally in young patients with a prodrome of 1 to 14 days. Features are fever, myalgia, coryza, and the rapid evolution of a polymorphic skin and mucous membrane eruption.

The skin lesions are macular or vesiculobullous and generally symmetric on distal extremities. The mucous membrane lesions may involve the mouth, nose, and genitalia and usually parallel the skin lesions, although they may be isolated. Early ocular lesions consist of vesicular eruptions of the lids and conjunctiva with possible conjunctival pseudomembranes, mucoid discharge, epithelial and stromal corneal ulceration, and uveitis (Fig. 4–50). Later ocular complications include entropion, trichiasis, symblepharon, dry eye, corneal scarring, and pannus formation. Serious systemic complications include sepsis, dehydration, and renal failure. Even with modern therapy this disease may still carry a mortality of up to 10%. A rare subset of patients may suffer recurrent attacks.

Treatment generally requires hospitalization with isolation, hydration, and surveillance for bacterial infection. Therapeutic considerations include systemic corticosteroids, immunosuppressives, or cyclosporine. Early therapy of the ocular condition requires topical corticosteroids and lysis of conjunctival adhesions to help prevent symblepharon. Therapy for the later ocular complications includes lubrication for dry eyes, management of lid malposition and tri-

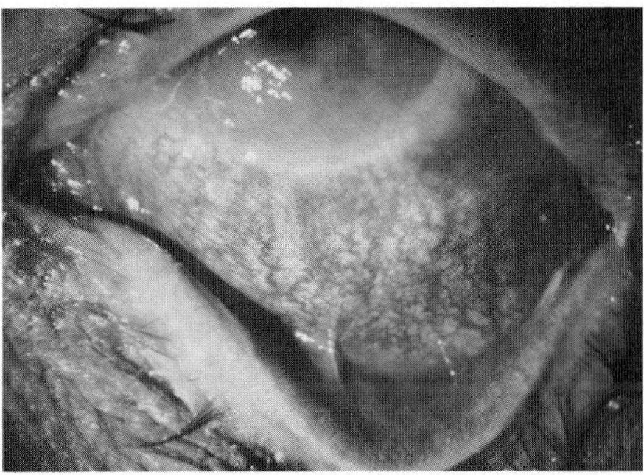

Fig. 4–50. Acute Stevens-Johnson syndrome in a young man with mucoid discharge and a pseudomembrane across the corneal surface.

chiasis, mucous membrane grafting, and the use of therapeutic soft contact lenses.

Ocular pemphigoid (cicatricial pemphigoid) is an autoimmune disease affecting the basement membrane of skin and mucous membrane.

Ocular pemphigoid is an autoimmune disease with immunoglobulins deposited at the basement membrane of skin and mucous membranes. Circulating antibasement membrane antibodies are also found. The long-term use of certain ocular medications (such as echothiophate or, rarely, timolol) may produce a similar picture. Ocular pemphigoid is seen predominantly in women older than 60 years without previous antecedent disease. The disorder runs a course of activity over many years during which either advancement or remission is possible. Ocular pemphigoid and bullous pemphigoid are probably variants of the same disease process.

Mucous membrane lesions consist of subepithelial blisters; there is generally a painless gingivitis or vesiculobullous eruption of the oral mucosa, pharynx, esophagus, and genitalia. The skin lesions are a vesiculobullous lesion or localized plaques. Early eye involvement consists of conjunctival hyperemia, thickening, and ulceration. There may be seromucoid discharge, shortening of the conjunctival fornix,

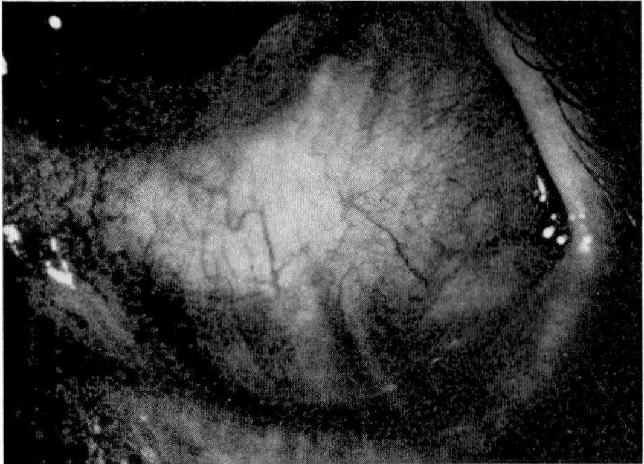

Fig. 4–51.   Foreshortening of the inferior conjunctival fornix and bandlike subconjunctival scarring, characteristic of ocular pemphigoid, in an elderly woman.

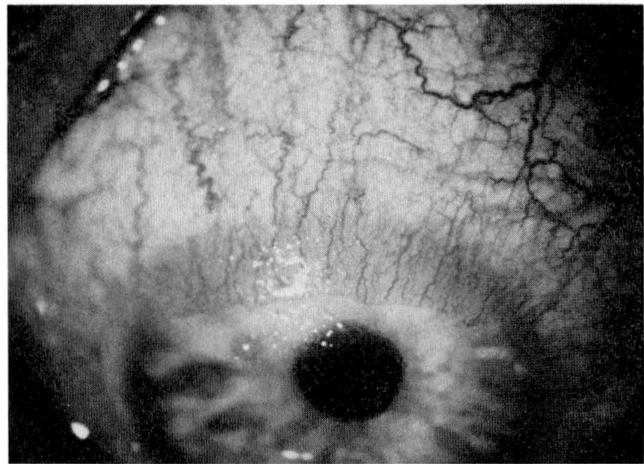

Fig. 4–52.   Redundant, edematous, hyperemic, bulbar conjunctiva at the superior limbus in superior limbic keratoconjunctivitis.

corneal ulceration, and pannus formation (Fig. 4–51). Late ocular complications include lid malpositions with trichiasis, extensive symblepharon and dry eye with corneal scarring, vascularization, and epidermalization.

Pemphigoid is an autoimmune disease that requires systemic therapy with dapsone, corticosteroids, or immunosuppressives, and co-treatment by a dermatologist or internist to monitor the medications and the systemic disease is mandatory. Topical corticosteroids seem to be of no benefit. Lubrication and the surgical treatment of lid malposition and trichiasis are important. In severe cases when the disease becomes quiescent, mucous membrane grafting or superficial keratectomy may be indicated. In severe bilateral cases a keratoprosthesis through the lid may be the only option for vision.

Superior limbic keratoconjunctivitis is an inflammatory condition; it is frequent in females and is associated with thyroid disease.

Superior limbic keratoconjunctivitis is of unknown cause, although frequently it occurs in association with thyroid disease. The vast majority of patients are women who are 20 to 70 years old. It is usually bilateral and has a tendency for remissions and exacerbations. Symptoms include tearing, burning, and hyperemia. Signs include edema of the superior bulbar

conjunctiva with a redundant conjunctiva, papillary, velvety hyperemia of the superior tarsal conjunctiva, and punctate epithelial erosions of the superior cornea (Fig. 4–52). Upper corneal filaments occur in about 50% of patients.

Many therapeutic regimens—including lubricating agents, cromolyn, acetylcysteine (Mucomyst), topical vitamin A therapy, soft contact lenses, 1% silver nitrate, cryotherapy, and thermocautery—have been tried. Success has probably been best obtained with a resection of the superior bulbar conjunctiva. Affected patients should be evaluated for a dysthyroid state.

Phlyctenulosis is a nodular keratoconjunctivitis that is probably a manifestation of allergy to a bacterial antigen.

This nodular keratoconjunctivitis is probably a manifestation of hypersensitivity in the conjunctiva or cornea to some allergen (especially tuberculosis or *Staphylococcus aureus*). *Phlyctenulosis* usually occurs in children living in crowded conditions. The phlyctenule consists of a small, pinkish-white nodule in the center of a hyperemic area in the conjunctiva (Fig. 4–53). The central microabscess becomes necrotic and sloughs as the lesion clears. The lesion can occur on the cornea (usually at the limbus) with a white mound and a triangular

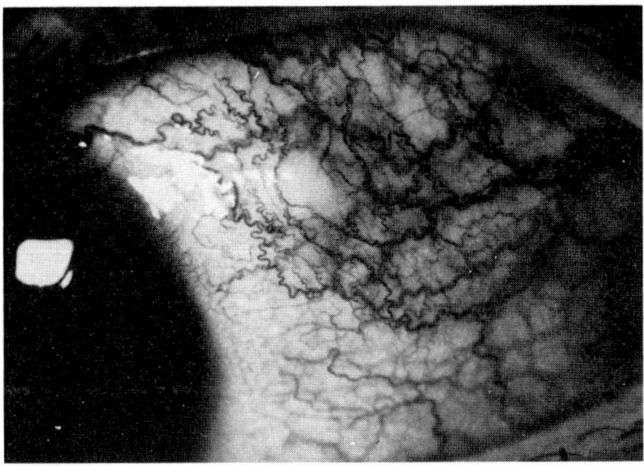

Fig. 4–53. Phlyctenule of the bulbar conjunctiva in an adolescent with staphylococcal blepharitis.

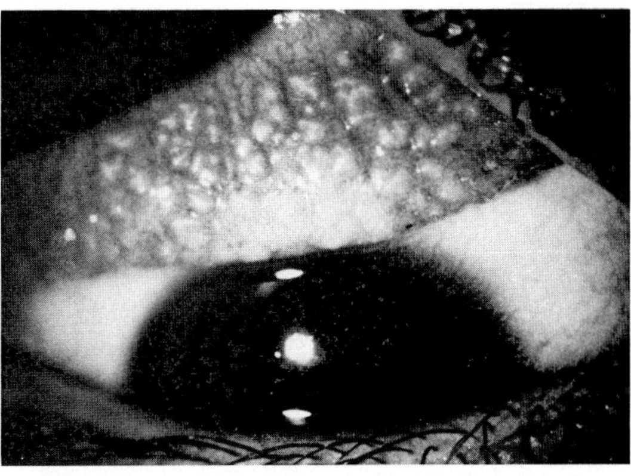

Fig. 4–54. Chronic giant papillary conjunctivitis of the upper tarsal conjunctiva associated with long-term use of soft contact lenses.

fan of blood vessels. The mound usually ulcerates and heals with a corneal scar. Phlyctenulosis is a self-limited disease, usually lasting 2 weeks. It may be recurrent if associated with either tuberculosis or *Staphylococcus aureus*. More severe cases involve the central cornea.

The patient should be evaluated for tuberculosis and chronic staphylococcal blepharitis and be treated appropriately. For cases in which a cause is not evident, the condition usually responds to topical corticosteroids, and occasional cycloplegia is necessary.

Giant papillary conjunctivitis is an immunologic response to antigen deposited on the surface of soft contact lenses.

Giant papillary conjunctivitis usually occurs on the upper tarsal conjunctiva in persons who wear soft or hard contact lenses or an ocular prosthesis, and occasionally it is a reaction to nylon suture after cataract or corneal transplantation. It resembles vernal conjunctivitis in appearance and may develop months or years after successful use of contact lenses (Fig. 4–54). Giant papillary conjunctivitis probably is an immunologic reaction to an antigen deposited on the contact lens surface. Symptoms include increased mucus, mild itching, and decreased tolerance to contact lenses.

Therapy includes a different method of sterilization, use of unpreserved saline, or a differ-

ent contact lens. Occasionally the use of contact lenses has to be discontinued permanently. Cromolyn or topical corticosteroids are occasionally helpful on either a short- or long-term basis. Long-term use of topical corticosteroids is discouraged.

The preocular tear film has three components: mucin, aqueous, and lipid.

The preocular tear film is a three-component structure. *Mucin* is derived from conjunctival goblet cells and spreads uniformly over the cornea and conjunctiva to reduce the surface tension. The *aqueous* layer is produced by the main and accessory lacrimal glands and additionally supplies inorganic salts, lysozyme, immunoglobulins, and oxygen. The *lipid* surface layer is produced by the meibomian glands and helps in lubricating, retarding evaporation, and stabilizing the surface (Fig. 4–55).

Disorders of any of the three components result in a tear film dysfunction (Table 4–21). Decreased aqueous production is characteristic of keratoconjunctivitis sicca; abnormal mucous secretion occurs with vitamin A deficiency or conjunctival scarring conditions such as pemphigoid; and abnormal lipid production is characteristic of meibomian gland dysfunction of the lids. Because the different layers are intimately related, abnormalities in

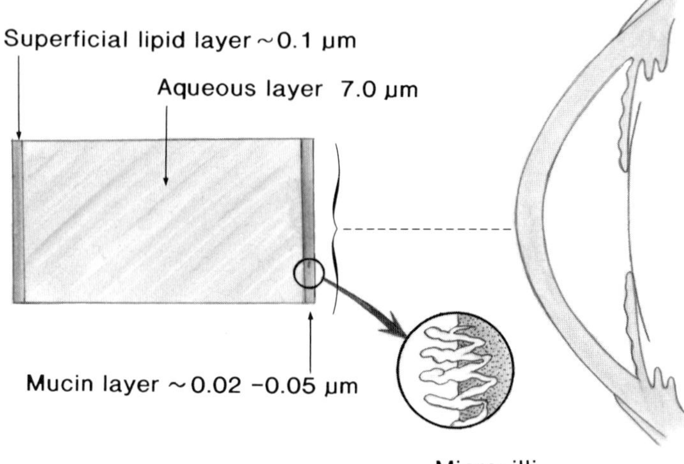

Fig. 4–55. The layers of the tear film and its relationship to the anterior corneal surface.

one layer will affect the other layers with similar resultant symptoms and clinical findings.

The symptoms of tear dysfunction may be vague and the clinical findings protean.

The symptoms of tear dysfunction may be vague and include symptoms of foreign body sensation (sandiness, scratchiness), fatigue, or dryness. There may be blurred or variable vision related to the loss of the smooth refractive surface of the tear film. Symptoms tend to be worse late in the day with prolonged use of the eyes (such as reading) or with exposure to environmental conditions (such as wind, heat, or low humidity). Pain may occur with filaments or with erosions.

Clinical signs of tear film dysfunction are multiple and include abnormalities detected on examination of the lids, conjunctiva, tear film, or cornea (Table 4–22). Incomplete blinking and various forms of blepharitis (such as seborrheic, staphylococcal, or meibomian gland dysfunction) are common accompanying disorders that exacerbate the ocular symptoms. Examination of the conjunctiva may reveal conjunctival foreshortening (in pemphigoid) or diffuse bulbar conjunctival injection or redundancy of the inferior temporal bulbar conjunctiva. The tear film may contain in-

TABLE 4–21 Disorders Associated with Tear Dysfunction

Abnormal tear film
  Aqueous deficiency
    Congenital
    Acquired
      Systemic diseases (Sjögren's syndrome, collagen vascular disease, sarcoidosis)
      Neurogenic (fifth nerve or seventh nerve paralysis)
      Associated with systemic medications (tranquilizers, psychotropic drugs)
  Mucous deficiency
    Goblet cell loss (vitamin A deficiency, chemical burns)
    Conjunctival scars (pemphigoid, Stevens-Johnson syndrome, radiation)
  Lipid dysfunction
    Meibomian gland dysfunction
Inadequate tear movement across cornea
  Poor blinking
  Lagophthalmos
  Irregular surface of globe (from tumor, mass)

TABLE 4–22 Signs of Tear Film Dysfunction

Incomplete blinking
Conjunctival injection
Redundant conjunctiva
Tear film debris
Decreased tear film meniscus
Irregular corneal surface reflex
Punctate epithelial keratitis
Mucous plaques or filaments
Corneal thinning or perforation

creased debris, and the height of the tear film meniscus at the lid margin may be low. Examination of the cornea may reveal an irregular corneal surface reflex, punctate epithelial keratitis, or corneal filaments and mucous plaques (Fig. 4–56). These findings result from damaged epithelial cells that have become keratinized or that have developed breaks in their membranes, with mucous adherent to the degenerated cells. Blinking may cause pain in the presence of filaments that are attached to the corneal epithelium. Corneal thinning and even perforation may occur, especially in rheumatoid arthritis, probably related to immune complex vascular disease.

Simple office tests can confirm tear dysfunction.

The use of *rose bengal* or *fluorescein* applied topically can facilitate the diagnosis of dry spots or damage to the corneal epithelium. In keratoconjunctivitis sicca, rose bengal reveals a strip of punctate staining across the globe within the palpebral fissure. Rose bengal may also stain filaments, mucous threads, mucous particles in the tear film, and abnormal conjunctival keratinization (Fig. 4–56). Fluorescein is especially useful for examining the corneal tear film. With fluorescein instillation and examination with a cobalt-blue filter light at the slit lamp, the patient is asked to blink completely, and then an estimate is made of the length of time the tear film remains stable and intact until a random corneal dry spot develops (normal tear breakup time is usually more than 10 seconds).

The *Schirmer test* is a quantitative measurement of tear production. A folded 5-mm end of a standard Whatman 41 filter paper strip is placed over the lower lid between its middle and lower third in a dimly lit room. The patient looks straight ahead and blinks normally. After 5 minutes, the amount of wetting of the filter paper is measured. The test can be performed with or without topical anesthesia, and this may correlate with the baseline secretion (with anesthesia) versus reflex secretion (without anesthesia). The test is not precise and has many variabilities; however, it is simple and inexpensive and can frequently provide good

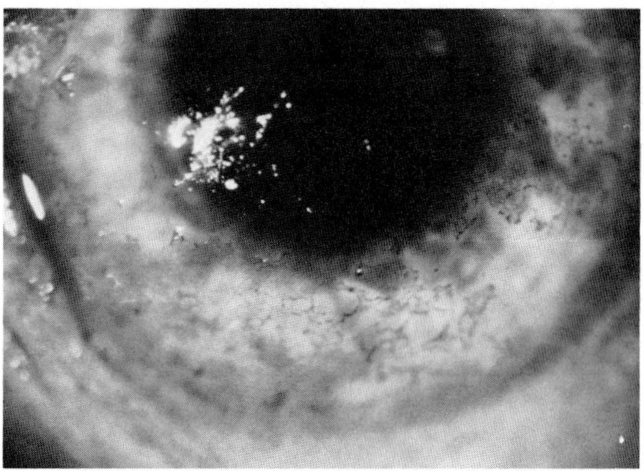

Fig. 4–56. Severe keratitis sicca, demonstrating rose-bengal-stained conjunctiva and corneal filaments, punctate epithelial keratitis, and an irregular corneal surface.

clinical information. Measurements of tear lysozyme levels, tear osmolarity, and tear disappearance are research tools at the present time.

Sjögren's syndrome (primary or secondary) requires evaluation by an internist.

Sjögren's syndrome consists of keratoconjunctivitis sicca, xerostomia, and arthritis. A concept is emerging that the disease may have different manifestations, that is, aqueous tear deficiency alone (keratitis sicca), in association with dry mouth (primary Sjögren's syndrome), or as a manifestation of systemic connective tissue disease (secondary Sjögren's syndrome). This concept is supported by the fact that clinical, laboratory, genetic, and immunologic characteristics of primary and secondary Sjögren's syndrome are different. The essential histopathologic feature of Sjögren's syndrome is lymphocytic destruction of the exocrine glands. As the disease progresses, the normal lacrimal gland architecture is replaced by both B and T lymphocytes.

The incidence of Sjögren's syndrome is unknown and difficult to judge in view of the natural decrease in tear flow that occurs with age. The diagnosis of Sjögren's syndrome is important because of a high incidence of associated systemic diseases such as lymphoma or thyroid dysfunction. The ophthalmologist should attempt in the review of systems to identify patients with complaints of dry eye who may have primary or secondary Sjögren's syndrome and to obtain proper consultation.

Management of tear deficiency involves several approaches.

Several classes of systemic medications can decrease tear flow and should be eliminated if possible. Associated local ocular diseases, especially blepharitis, should be treated. The mainstay of therapy is with *artificial tear substitutes*, which are derivatives of cellulose, polyvinyl alcohol, povidone, or other soluble polymers. Solutions or ointments free of preservatives (thimerosal, benzalkonium chloride, chlorobutanol, EDTA) are available for selected patients. The patients should avoid factors that increase evaporation of the tear film (such as wind and heat), and protective glasses may be helpful. Punctal occlusion reduces tear drainage and prolongs the tear film and may be indicated in severe cases. Systemic medications that increase tear production are not of proven benefit.

A conjunctival papilloma may be viral or irritative in origin (in young patients) or may be a squamous cell carcinoma (in older patients).

A *papilloma* is a sessile or pedunculated graypink lesion with fronds of fibrovascular tissue covered with epithelium. In young patients it tends to be viral or irritative in origin, whereas in older patients it tends to be larger and more vascular and may develop into a squamous cell carcinoma. Viral papillomas usually disappear spontaneously, although surgical excision, cryotherapy, CO_2 vaporization, and immunotherapy are alternative methods of treatment.

Conjunctival intraepithelial neoplasia is a precancerous dysplasia of the conjunctiva usually adjacent to the limbus which occurs in older men.

Conjunctival dysplasia is a disease of older men and appears as a leukoplakic lesion or as a vascular, gelatinous, or granulomatous tumor adjacent to the limbus. It may extend onto the corneal epithelium and present a frosted-glass appearance. The normal cellular polarity from basal layer to the surface may be maintained, but atypical and dyskeratotic cells are seen in the deeper layers of the epithelium. Conjunctival dysplasia should be surgically excised, and corneal dysplasia can usually be softened with cocaine and then wiped off. Recurrences are common unless the surgical margins are free of tumor.

A conjunctival squamous cell carcinoma occurs when the malignant epithelial cells invade through the basement membrane.

When a conjunctival intraepithelial neoplasia extends through the basement membrane it represents *squamous cell carcinoma*. This malignant epithelial tumor may invade locally as well as metastasize. The lesions are usually solitary, although occasionally multiple gelatinous, elevated, reddish gray demarcated tumors that grow exophytically are seen at the interpalpebral limbus. Treatment of the conjunctival lesion consists of excision with a 2-mm border until free margins are obtained. Tumor on the cornea can usually be loosened with cocaine and then wiped off or surgically removed. Supplementary cryotherapy reduces recurrences, but occasionally enucleation or exenteration is necessary for large recurrences.

Lymphoid conjunctival lesions may be a benign lymphoproliferative disorder or evolve to a localized or systemic lymphoma.

Conjunctival lymphoid tumors usually present in middle-aged patients as "salmon patches" with a predilection for the fornices. There is usually a painless fullness in the cul-de-sac, and the lesions may be either unilateral or bilateral (Fig. 4–57). This may evolve from a *benign lymphoproliferative disorder* or may be part of a localized or systemic *lymphoma*. Biopsy is necessary to confirm the diagnosis. Fresh tissue should be evaluated immunologically and

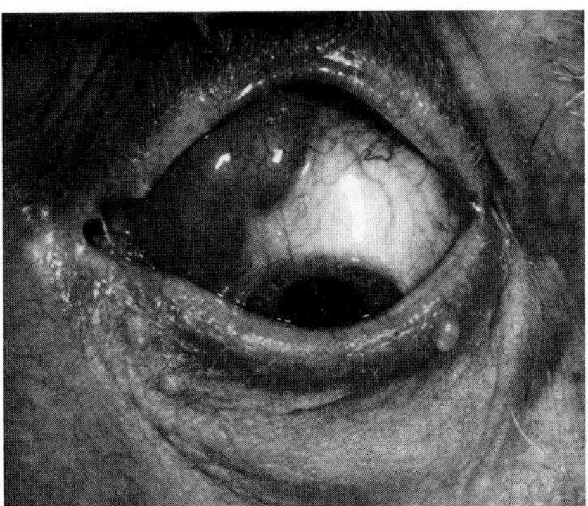

Fig. 4–57. Large, salmon-colored, smooth tumor in the superior nasal fornix, characteristic of a conjunctival lymphoma.

histochemically for the ratio of B and T lymphocytes because this has prognostic significance. Patients with lymphoma should undergo medical evaluation for systemic disease. Treatment may consist of local radiation or systemic chemotherapy depending on the grade of lymphoma and the presence of disease elsewhere.

Benign melanotic conjunctival lesions are usually congenital.

Melanotic lesions of the conjunctiva must be differentiated from other causes of nonmelanotic ocular pigmentations such as thinned sclera (from a staphyloma), metabolic disorders (ochronosis), and pigment deposits (epinephrine, argyrosis, mascara, hemosiderin) (Table 4–23). Most of the melanotic lesions in the conjunctiva are congenital.

Benign epithelial melanosis is a common patchy, flat, brownish pigmentation of the conjunctiva that occurs especially in blacks. It is found in the limbal area and is usually stationary, although it may spread onto the cornea or caruncle. Melanosis is similar to a skin freckle; it has no malignant potential.

Benign episcleral spots are common slate-colored, pigmented spots characteristically seen several millimeters back from the limbus. They represent uveal melanocytes associated with perforating anterior ciliary vessels or with

TABLE 4–23 Differential Diagnoses of Conjunctival Pigmented Lesions

Pigmentations not related to melanin
  Ochronosis
  Pigment deposits (epinephrine, mascara, argyrosis)
  Senile hyaline plaque
  Foreign body (usually iron)
  Staphyloma with thinned sclera
Melanocytic pigmentations
  Congenital pigmentations
    Benign epithelial melanosis
    Ocular melanosis
    Oculodermal melanosis (nevus of Ota)
    Axenfeld nerve loop
  Acquired melanosis
    Primary acquired melanosis (unilateral)
    Secondary pigmentations (radiation, hormones, chronic conjunctival disorders)
  Pigmented nevi
  Malignant melanoma
    Primary arising from nevi, acquired melanosis, or congenital melanosis or arising de novo
    Secondary melanoma from metastases or an extension of intraocular melanoma

an intrascleral (Axenfeld) nerve loop. They have no malignant potential.

Melanosis oculi is unilateral, slate-blue, mottled, episcleral pigmentation. There is usually a unilateral increase in all ocular pigment, especially in the conjunctiva, uveal tract, and less commonly in the sclera. It is more frequent in blacks, but when it occurs in whites it rarely may be associated with a uveal melanoma. Melanosis oculi is usually congenital but may become obvious only at puberty.

The *nevus of Ota* is unilateral melanosis oculi with the addition of skin pigmentation (Fig. 4–58). This has an affinity for Orientals and blacks, and when it occurs in whites, vigilance for choroidal melanoma and rarely conjunctival melanoma is warranted.

Nevi are by far the most common pigmented lesions in the conjunctiva and are probably congenital; 90% appear by age 30 years. The amount of pigmentation varies, and approximately 30% are actually nonpigmented. Nevi are usually well circumscribed with an abrupt demarcation from normal conjunctiva (Fig. 4–59). Most occur on the bulbar conjunctiva,

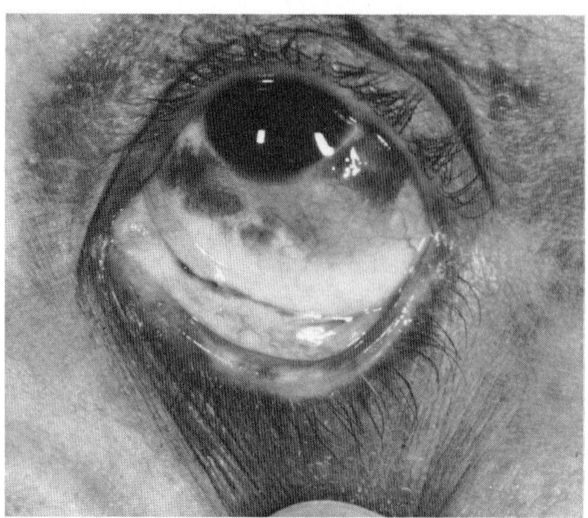

Fig. 4–58. Slate-gray pigmentation of sclera and episclera associated with gray pigmentation of the eyelids in a patient with the nevus of Ota.

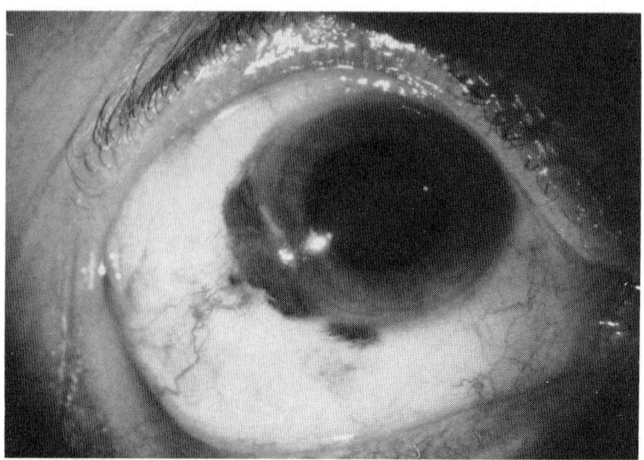

Fig. 4–60. Unilateral acquired melanosis of the conjunctiva that originally was flat and now has an elevated nodular appearance consistent with a conjunctival melanoma.

although some rarely occur on the fornix or on the caruncle. Most show a cystic appearance, which helps to confirm the diagnosis. They are less frequent than skin nevi but have a more frequent conversion to malignancy.

Acquired melanosis is a unilateral, diffuse, brown pigmentation of the conjunctiva or cornea that usually develops in exposed areas in middle-aged patients (Fig. 4–60). This runs a variable course and may be stationary or protracted. The pigmentation may spread extensively in a horizontal pattern before becoming elevated. Elevation is a sign of conversion to malignancy and may occur in multifocal areas. Acquired melanosis on the palpebral conjunctiva or in the fornices has a high probability of being malignant.

Secondary acquired melanosis is a benign stimulation of the basal layer melanocytes of the conjunctiva associated with several diseases or irritants to the conjunctiva. This condition is usually bilateral with flat pigmentation and generally has no malignant potential. It is associated with radiation therapy, chemicals (arsenic, thorazine), hormones (Addison's disease and pregnancy), and chronic conjunctival disorders (trachoma, vernal conjunctivitis, xeroderma pigmentosum).

Malignant melanoma of the conjunctiva may arise from congenital melanosis, acquired melanosis, or nevi or may arise de novo.

Most *conjunctival melanomas* arise from acquired melanosis or de novo; perhaps the worst prognosis is for those that arise from acquired melanosis. Less commonly they arise from nevi or congenital melanosis. Conjunctival melanomas may also arise secondarily from local spread of uveal melanoma or from metastatic origin.

Malignant melanomas are usually located in the fornix or the caruncle. Cell type does not seem to have the significance it does with uveal melanoma, although the presence of increased mitotic figures is associated with the worst prognosis. All suspicious lesions or areas of elevation in patients with primary acquired melanosis need to be biopsied. Melanomas should

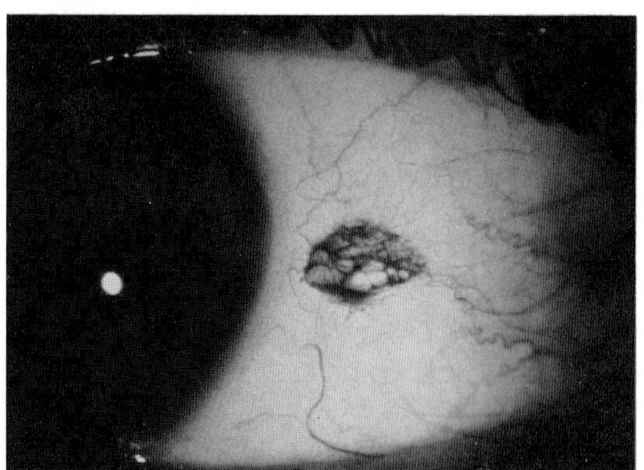

Fig. 4–59. A circumscribed conjunctival nevus; the presence of cysts commonly indicates benignancy.

generally be excised with a margin of several millimeters, and then cryotherapy is applied to the base, margins, and surrounding pigmentation. Superficial sclerectomy is occasionally needed. With deep ocular or fornix involvement, exenteration may be necessary. A metastatic evaluation and computed tomography scanning should precede an aggressive surgical procedure.

LENS

The lens continues to increase in size with age.

The lens is a biconvex disc, flatter on the anterior surface than on the posterior surface. It is surrounded by a *capsule*, which has been secreted as a basement membrane by the lens *epithelium* (Fig. 4–61). Beneath the capsule anteriorly is a monolayer of cells that differentiate into the long, thin *lens fibers* that constitute the bulk of the lens. As new cortical lens fibers grow concentrically, the central older fibers become more densely packed and form the lens nucleus. The lens is attached to the ciliary processes by *zonules*; the ciliary muscle contracts when the eye is focusing on a near object, and the contraction allows the zonules to relax and the lens to become thicker. This ability to *accommodate* is gradually lost during middle age as the lens increases in size and becomes more rigid. The lens is the least hydrated tissue in the body, with the main bulk composed of protein.

The lens is best examined through a dilated pupil and with different forms of biomicroscopic illumination.

The lens is best examined through a fully *dilated pupil* in a darkened room. *Diffuse light* is best for examining the anterior and posterior lens capsule. *Retroillumination* is optimal for viewing anterior or posterior subcapsular opacities. *Direct focal slit illumination* is best for demonstrating the different zones of the lens and localizing opacities to the capsule, subcapsule, cortex, adult nucleus, infantile nucleus, fetal nucleus, or embryonic nucleus (Fig. 4–61). These different zones of involvement, along with other features, suggest the cause for the cataract.

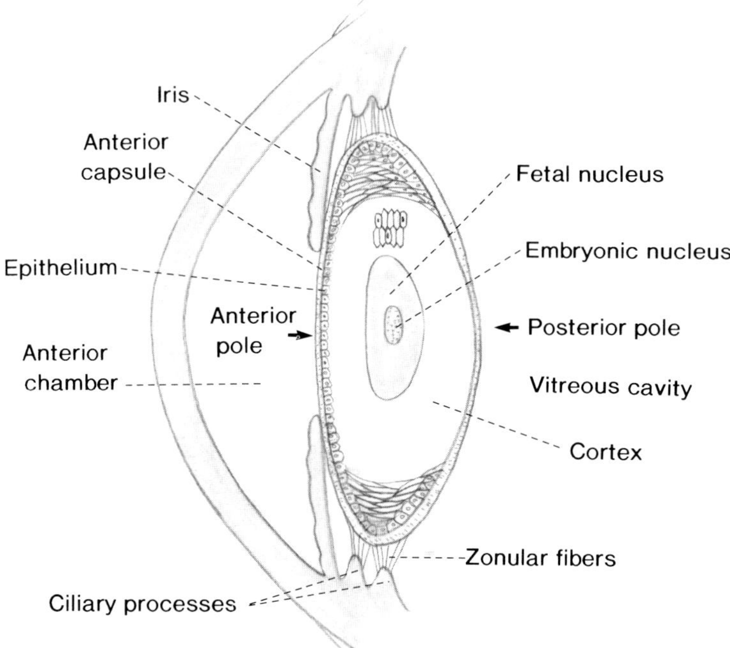

Fig. 4–61. The components of the adult lens and its attachments to the ciliary processes by zonular fibers.

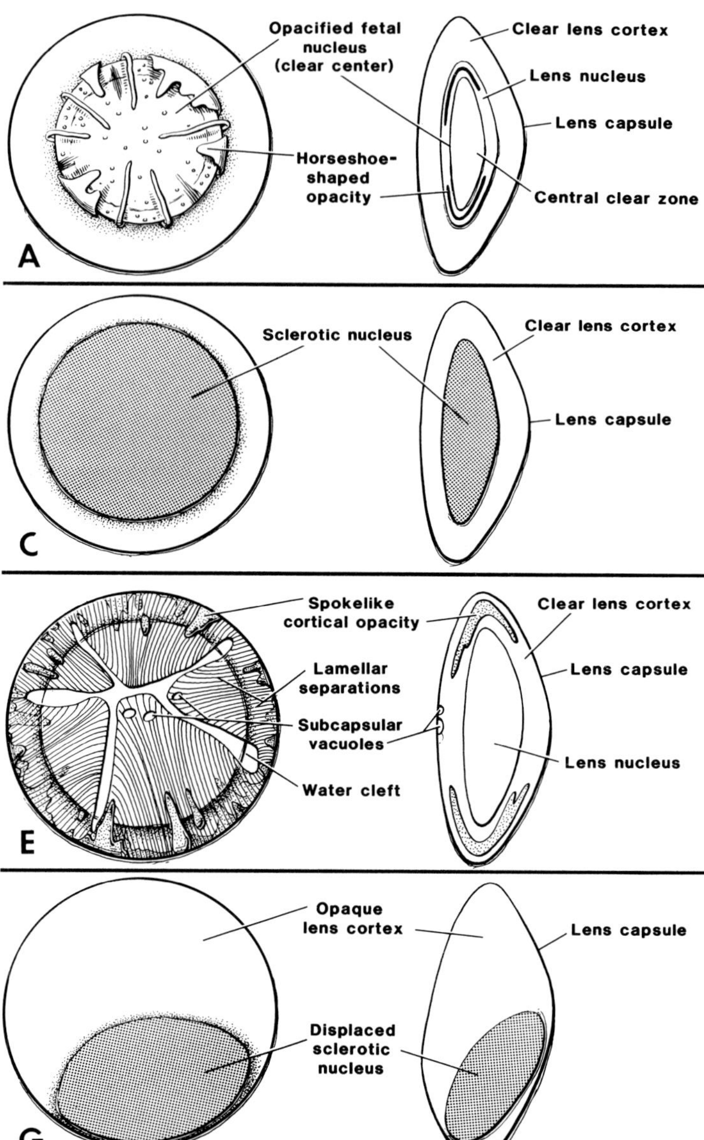

Fig. 4–62. Types and locations of some of the cataract forms. *A*, Congenital zonular cataract in various layers of the lens nucleus. *B*, Congenital coronary cataract in cortex of the lens. *C*, Common nuclear sclerotic cataract of aging. *D*, Posterior subcapsular cataract. *E*, Immature cortical cataract with beginning hydration of the lens. *F*, Total white opacification of the cortex with mature or "ripe" cataract. *G*, Morgagnian cataract with totally liquified cortex and a floating nucleus. *H*, Hypermature cataract with wrinkled capsule and loss of cortical fluid. (From T.J. Liesegang: Cataracts and cataract operations. Mayo Clin Proc 59:556–567, 1984. By permission of Mayo Foundation.)

There are many possible causes of cataract, which is defined as any opacification of the crystalline lens.

A cataract is any *opacification* in the crystalline lens. Not all cataracts are visually significant. They may be classified on the basis of *morphology, cause,* or *time of occurrence.* There are some basic mechanisms of cataract formation. Opacification of the lens fibers may occur from increased water content of the lens after injury to the lens's cation pump as a result of formation of opaque epithelial fibers from various causes, from the deposition of various materials within the lens, or from aging of the lens protein, which results in a deep amber brunescent cataract. A classification of cataracts is presented in Table 4–24. The major cataract types are shown in Figure 4–62 and are described in greater detail below.

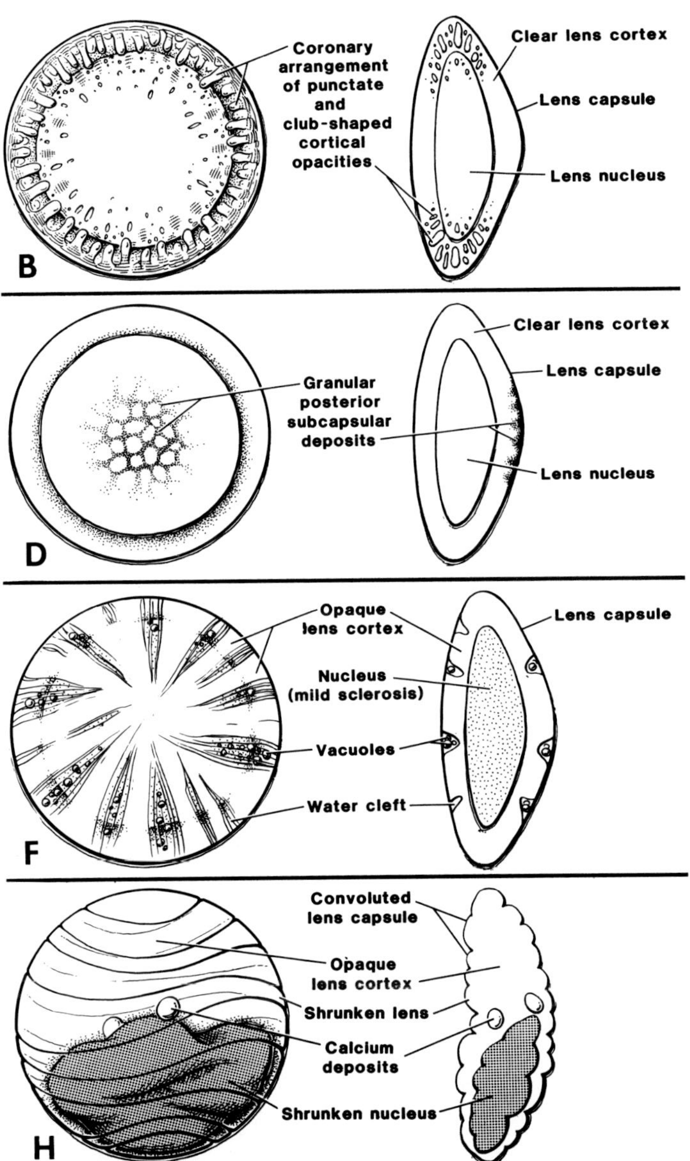

The main symptoms of cataracts are blurred vision, glare, distortion, and altered color perception.

The major indications for removal of a cataract are disabling visual symptoms. *Blurred vision* is the most common symptom, frequently being most prominent at night or with demanding visual tasks. *Glare* is due to the diffusion of light by the cataract, especially posterior subcapsular cataracts. *Distortion* is related to image duplication and occurs especially with nuclear-type cataracts. *Decreased color perception* correlates with a change in nuclear color and transparency with an aging nuclear cataract. Behavioral changes may occur in either children or older adults who may not be able to verbalize or notice a gradual decrease in their

TABLE 4–24 Classification of Cataracts

Congenital cataracts
  Hereditary
  Associated with ocular disease
  Associated with systemic disease
Developmental defects and abnormalities
  Lens colobomas
  Ectopia lentis
  Lenticonus
  Lentiglobus
  Microspherophakia
Age-related cataracts
  Coronary
  Nuclear
  Cortical
  Subcapsular
Metabolic and toxic cataracts
  Associated with systemic disease
  Associated with drugs, toxins, radiation
Traumatic cataracts
  Blunt or penetrating trauma
  Associated with intraocular foreign body
Complicated cataracts
  Associated with intraocular inflammation or
    disease

vision related to cataracts. Cataract surgery is, for the most part, elective except under some unusual circumstances cited below.

Congenital cataracts are occasionally hereditary, related to ocular disease, or associated with systemic disease.

Congenital cataracts are frequently associated with low birth weight and other central nervous system abnormalities such as mental retardation, convulsions, or cerebral palsy. Others may be related to ocular abnormalities such as persistent primary hyperplastic vitreous, anterior chamber cleavage syndrome, or aniridia. Cataracts that develop in the first year of life (infantile cataracts) are frequently associated with metabolic or systemic disease. Another type is hereditary, but a large portion of congenital cataracts are of unknown cause.

Congenital cataracts may be described by the portion of the lens that is involved. *Anterior polar cataracts* (Fig. 4–63) may occur with other anterior segment anomalies. A *posterior polar cataract* often occurs in association with a

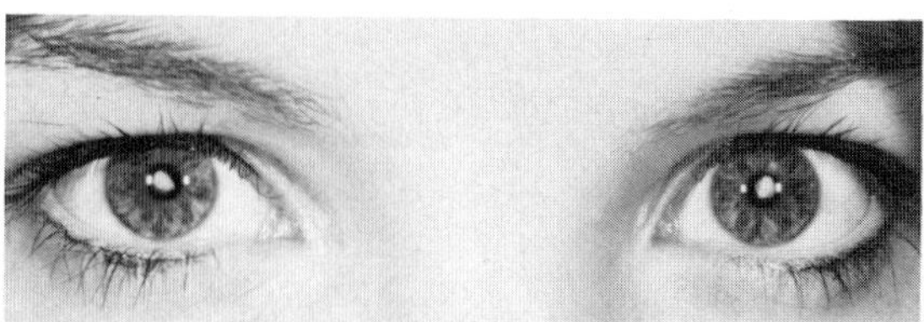

Fig. 4–63. Bilateral congenital anterior polar cataract filling the pupillary space in an 18-year-old girl. The patient had 20/80 vision when the pupils were dilated and 20/800 when the pupils were constricted.

persistent hyaloid artery remnant. An opacity in the *embryonal nucleus* in the center of the lens is frequently of autosomal dominant inheritance and may not affect vision. *Lamellar cataracts* are opacities at various levels of the fetal nucleus and are the most common congenital cataracts; they are usually hereditary but can also be associated with hypocalcemia, hypoglycemia, and galactosemia (Fig. 4–64).

A total congenital cataract is a dense, white, nuclear opacity that may resorb over time and leave only capsular remnants (called a membranous cataract). Congenital rubella is the most common cause of this cataract, although other maternal infections or metabolic disorders may be implicated.

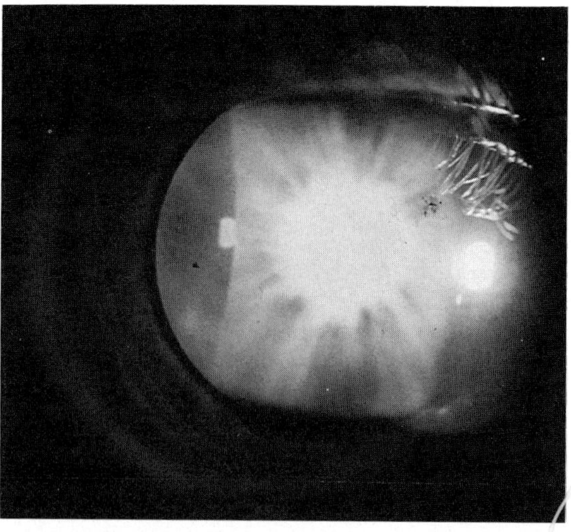

Fig. 4–64. A lamellar (zonular) cataract involving the central nucleus with spokes (or riders) surrounding the nucleus in an adolescent.

Small lens opacities of no visual significance often occur.

Small opacities are common in the periphery of the cortex, encircling the central axis, or even in the nucleus of the lens. They may be blue, white, or brown. These probably develop during life for unknown reasons and are never visually significant.

Involutional cataracts may be related to chronic exposure to ultraviolet light.

The most common type of cataract is associated with aging and possibly with chronic ultraviolet exposure from sunlight. Most patients older than 50 years have some form of a cataract; visually significant cataracts are very common in elderly persons. The predominant locations for these involutional lens changes are cortical, nuclear, and then subcapsular.

Cortical cataracts appear as vacuoles, water clefts, or radial separations of the lens fibers, representing aggregation of lens protein (Fig. 4–62 *E* and *F* and 4–65). A *nuclear cataract* (Fig. 4–62 *C*) may manifest with a hydrated nucleus, giving a more whitish appearance to the nucleus with marked distortion of the visual image, but it is more likely to be a dehydrated nucleus with marked compaction of the lens fibers, an increase in protein concentration, and the accumulation of a brown pigment, urochrome (Fig. 4–66). Hue discrimination is affected by nuclear cataracts, which

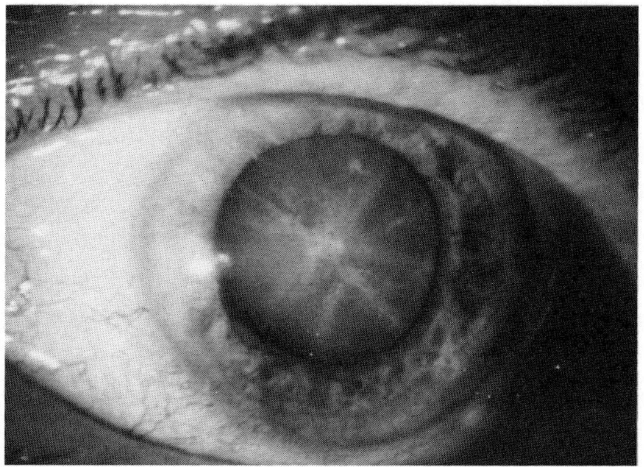

Fig. 4–65. A white, swollen, mature cataract with cortical opacities and water clefts.

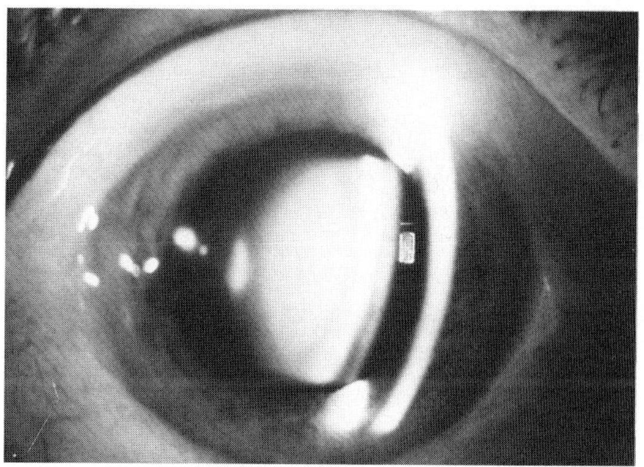

Fig. 4–66. A dense nuclear sclerotic cataract in an elderly man; cataract was yellowish brown.

may even progress to a dark-black nucleus. A *subcapsular cataract* (Fig. 4–62 *D*) consists of granules or cysts just inside the posterior capsule. Subcapsular cataracts may be seen alone in middle-aged men, but they are usually associated with nuclear cataracts.

Several metabolic disorders are associated with specific types of cataracts.

Uncontrolled *diabetes mellitus* may be associated with marked shifts in the fluid content of the normal lens. These fluid shifts may result in myopia or in the rapid formation of subcapsular granular (snowstorm) cataracts. These changes probably relate to the accumulation of *sorbitol* inside the diabetic lens. Some of these acute changes may be reversible. Chronic diabetes causes the common involutional lens changes to occur at a much earlier age.

Galactosemia caused by the absence of a specific enzyme may cause a cataract in infants with a characteristic "droplet" opacity in the anterior and posterior subcapsular areas which may progress to maturity within a few months unless galactose is restricted in the diet. A milder form caused by galactokinase deficiency may yield a nonspecific infantile cataract.

Many other metabolic conditions can be associated with infantile cataracts; blood and urine screening tests may detect the majority of potential associations.

Several drugs or therapies have been implicated in cataract formation.

Prolonged topical or systemic *corticosteroids* may cause posterior subcapsular cataracts. In children, these may regress after withdrawal of the corticosteroid. Miotic agents, especially *echothiophate iodide* (used for glaucoma), are a recognized cause of anterior subcapsular cataracts after prolonged use. Several other systemic drugs have been reported to cause cataracts, but most of these are no longer available. Lovastatin (Mevacor) was initially reported to cause cataracts, but the data are inconsistent. *Ionizing radiation* has an effect on the germinal epithelium at the lens equator; it causes more damage in younger lenses. *Infrared radiation* and *laser radiation* can cause posterior subcapsular or localized lens opacities. Recently, *near ultraviolet light* from the sun has been implicated in the formation of lens opacification.

Blunt or penetrating trauma may result in cataract.

Significant blunt ocular trauma may result in a specific star-shaped or *rosette cataract* of either the anterior or the posterior subcapsular zone of the lens (Fig. 4–67). Penetrating injury to the lens may seal if small enough, but large tears usually result in a rapidly maturing, white, swollen cataract. Electric shock and lightening cause specific cataract changes. Metallic intraocular foreign bodies result in incorporation of metal particles in the lens capsule and epithelium over a long period. A *sunflower cataract* is seen with a copper foreign body or with Wilson's disease. Iron deposited in the lens causes an orange flower-petal cataract.

Specific cataracts may be associated with some dermatologic or systemic diseases.

Lens opacities associated with dermatologic disease are usually bilateral and symmetric and occur at a relatively young age. *Atopic dermatitis* is associated with an anterior or posterior subcapsular shield-like cataract. Rothmund syndrome, Werner syndrome, and a few other der-

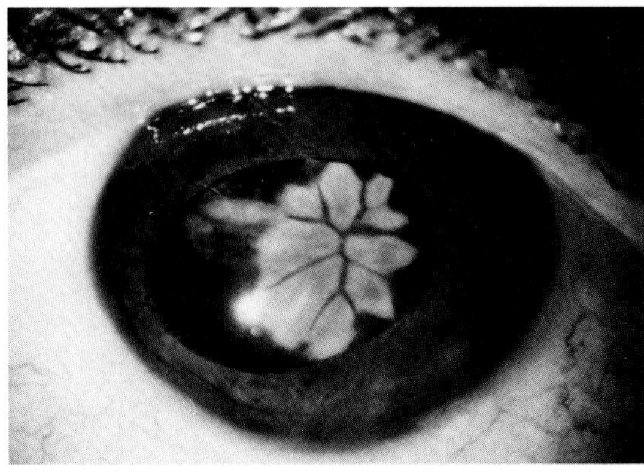

Fig. 4–67. A rosette-type cataract under the anterior surface of the lens, characteristic of a cataract from severe blunt trauma. The pupil was also irregular from the trauma.

matologic conditions have specific cataract types. *Down's syndrome* is associated with scattered punctate or flakelike opacities in the cortex with prominent suture lines. *Myotonic dystrophy* has characteristic multicolored punctate particles in the subcapsular area; these may be the presenting feature of the disease. Cataracts are also frequently involved in various skeletal syndromes, neuroectodermal syndromes, chromosome disorders, or oculorenal syndromes.

Chronic ocular inflammation and various ocular diseases are associated with cataract formation.

Chronic uveitis, especially as seen in Fuchs' heterochromic uveitis and juvenile rheumatoid arthritis, is associated with a high incidence of cataract. The cataracts usually begin as posterior subcapsular opacities but have a marked tendency to proceed to a mature (totally white) cataract. These are called *"complicated"* cataracts in that they are the result of interference with normal lens metabolism. Similar cataracts can also result from ocular ischemia or anterior segment necrosis from various causes that compromise the ocular circulation. Acute attacks of glaucoma may damage the lens epithelium, and anterior subcapsular opacities are left in the aftermath (*Glaukomflecken*).

Cataract extraction is usually elective during the immature stages; it becomes necessary in a few situations.

Small lens opacities are termed "immature" or "incipient." Over time, the opacities spread to produce swelling of the entire lens, called a "mature" cataract. With further progression, the lens may develop a milky liquid cortex with a floating nucleus within it, called a *hypermature or morgagnian cataract* (Fig. 4–62 *G* and *H* and 4–68). The capsule may undergo dystrophic calcification. The capsule may become permeable with protein diffusing into the aqueous humor. The entire cataract may resorb and only the capsule remains (membranous cataract).

Phacolytic glaucoma is a complication of a mature cataract in which the lens protein leaks from the lens and incites a macrophagic response; the inflammatory material then obstructs the flow of aqueous through the trabecular meshwork (Fig. 4–69). Lens extraction is necessary.

Phacomorphic glaucoma is a swollen lens brought on either by senescent changes or by a rupture in the lens capsule. The anterior chamber depth decreases and the angle may close (Fig. 4–70). Lens extraction is necessary.

Phacoantigenic uveitis is a granulomatous inflammation that occasionally is initiated by lens protein released through a ruptured lens capsule. The lens had previously been sequestered and not recognized as "self" by the immune

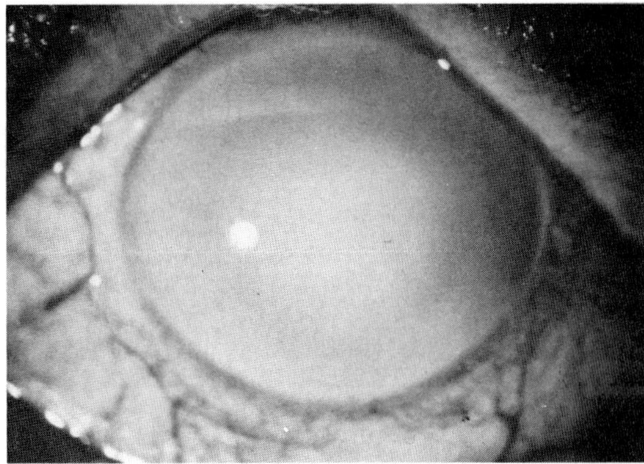

Fig. 4–69. The anterior chamber is filled with a white, milky fluid that represents cortical material that has leaked through the lens capsule in a patient with a hypermature cataract. The intraocular pressure was elevated and removal of the cataract was required.

system. The unpredictability of this event is difficult to explain.

Other significant changes in the crystalline lens may warrant lens removal.

Microspherophakia is a bilateral, abnormal weakness in the lens zonules resulting in a spherical lens with small diameter. The lens may dislocate or block the pupil. Areas of extreme thinning of the capsule may be present on the anterior or posterior capsule (*lenticonus*). This may cause a localized opacity or may

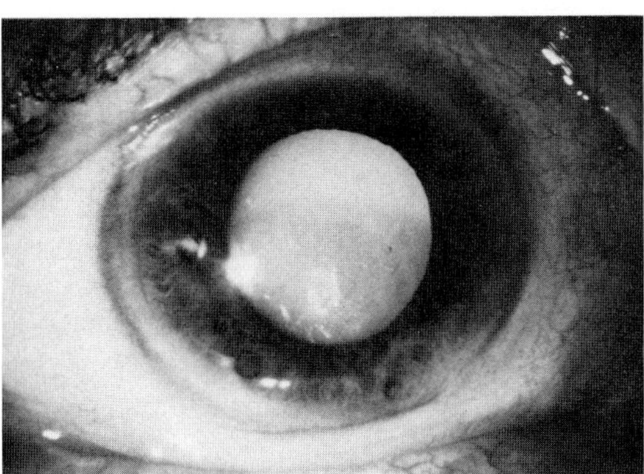

Fig. 4–68. A hypermature (morgagnian) cataract with a dense nucleus floating in a white liquid contained within the lens capsule; nucleus was yellow.

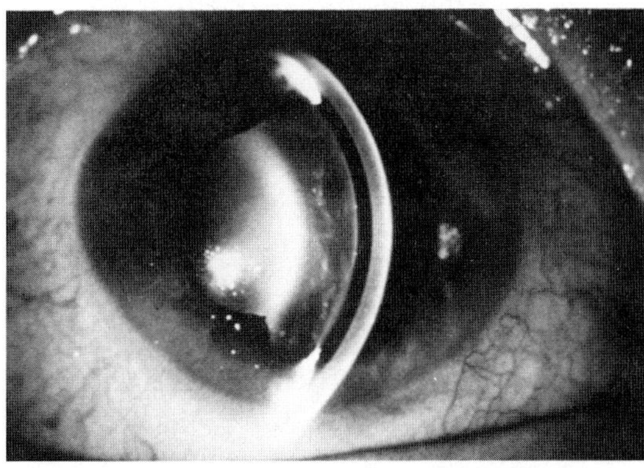

Fig. 4–70. A swollen nuclear and cortical cataract that has caused shallowing of the anterior chamber and elevated intraocular pressure, characteristic of phacomorphic glaucoma.

progress to capsule rupture and significant cataract. A coloboma of the lens may be associated with a local absence of lens zonules. *Ectopia lentis* is a more extreme form of zonular absence. A partial dislocation of the lens is a subluxation, and the absence of all zonular attachments is called a luxation, a dislocation, or an ectopia lentis (Fig. 4–71). Ectopia lentis is most frequently associated with blunt trauma or certain inherited diseases (Marfan's syndrome, Weill-Marchesani syndrome, homocystinuria) or related to various inflammatory disorders (syphilis). Hypermature cataracts may also develop weakened lens zonules.

Subtle forms of *subluxation* may manifest as increasing myopia or astigmatism, monocular diplopia, iridodonesis (abnormal tremulousness of the iris), phacodonesis (abnormal movement of lens), deep anterior chamber depth, or vitreous herniation into the anterior chamber. Complete dislocation of the lens results in significant visual changes and may result in pupillary block glaucoma or eventuate in phacolytic glaucoma (Fig. 4–72).

True *exfoliation* of the lens capsule is a rare condition in which the superficial layers of the capsule split off in a scroll. Infrared radiation (which affects glassblowers) is the most common cause, although it may be seen in trauma or in elderly persons. *Pseudoexfoliation* of the lens is a common condition in which gray,

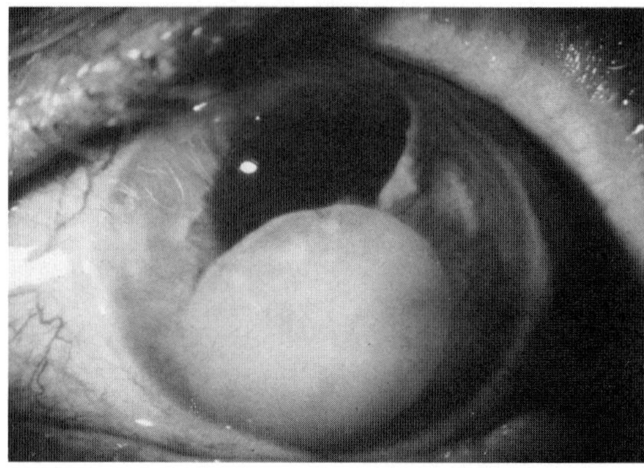

Fig. 4–72. A cataractous lens dislocated into the anterior chamber in a patient with previous severe blunt trauma that caused pupillary damage and dehiscence of all the lens zonules.

amorphous material is layered on the pupil, lens capsule, or back of the cornea (Fig. 4–73). It has also been seen on the iris, on the ciliary body, and in the trabecular meshwork. Although pseudoexfoliation often is identified in one eye, the disorder is considered to be bilateral and signs are usually seen in both eyes. The origin is unknown but probably represents a systemic basement membrane disease. Recognition is important because affected patients have a high risk of developing glaucoma, and they may have weak lens zonules that may rupture during an extracapsular cataract operation.

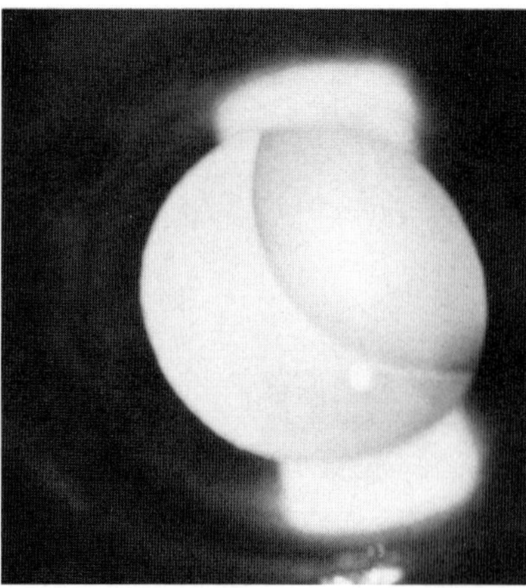

Fig. 4–71. A dislocation of the crystalline lens in the superior nasal direction from dehiscence of the lens zonules in a patient with Marfan's syndrome.

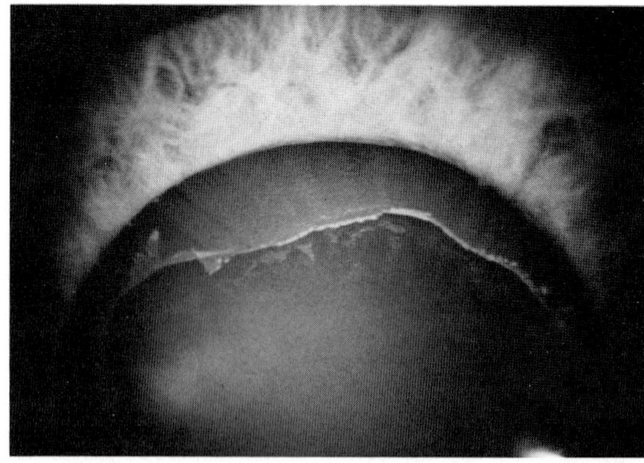

Fig. 4–73. White, gray, amorphous, flaking material on the anterior lens capsule, characteristic of pseudoexfoliation of the lens.

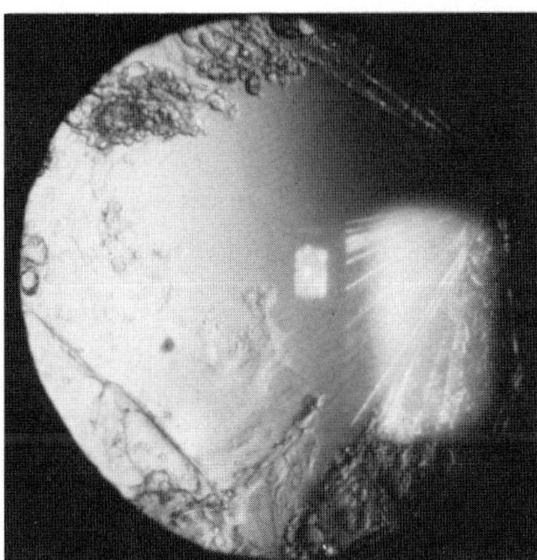

Fig. 4–74. A retroillumination view of the posterior capsule of the lens after extracapsular cataract operation, showing some wrinkling and proliferation of lens fibers causing "pearl formation." The central axis is still clear but may opacify over time.

A secondary cataract refers to capsular clouding that may occur after partial removal of the cataract.

The most common type of cataract surgery now performed is an extracapsular cataract operation in which the contents of the lens are removed and the posterior capsule of the lens and the zonular attachments to the ciliary body are left. An intraocular lens is usually placed within this capsular remnant. The *posterior capsule* may become hazy related to scarring, wrinkling, or the persistent proliferation of lens fibers, which cause small cysts on the posterior capsule (Fig. 4–74). If opacification of the posterior capsule occurs, the patient notices a decrease in vision similar to that with the original cataract. This membrane is thin and can be opened with a YAG laser as an office procedure if necessary.

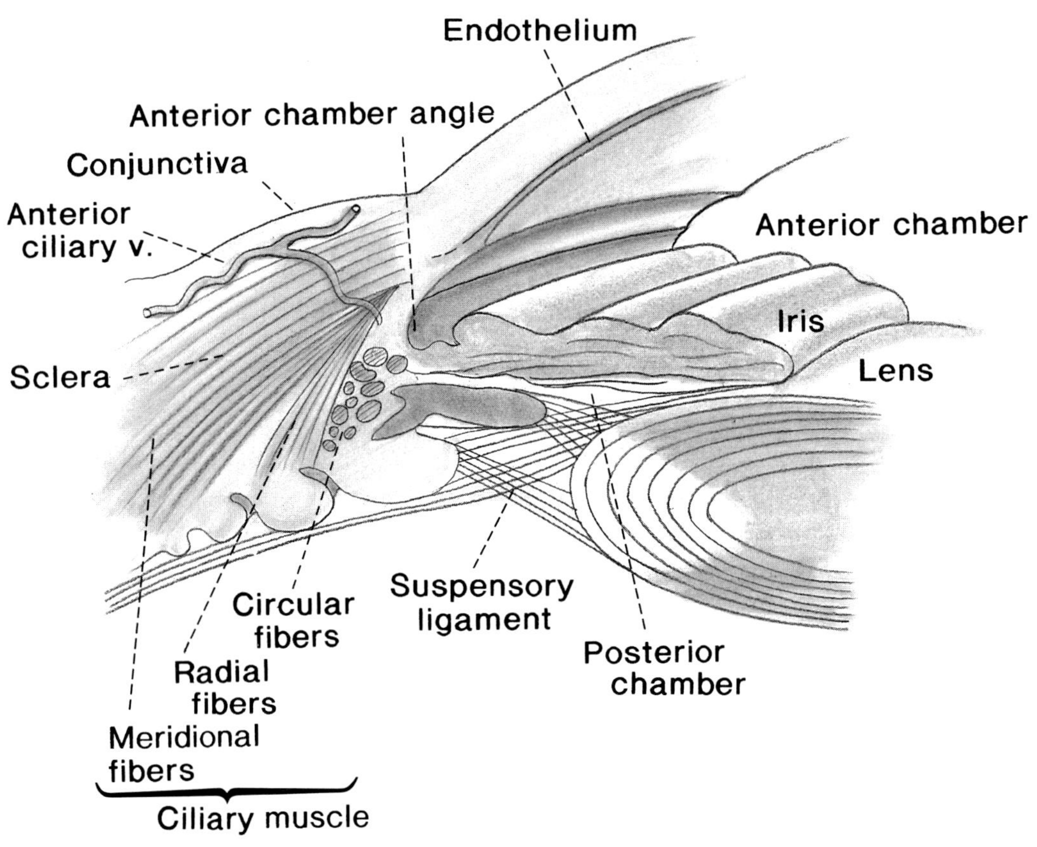

Endothelium
Anterior chamber angle
Conjunctiva
Anterior ciliary v.
Anterior chamber
Sclera
Iris
Lens
Circular fibers
Radial fibers
Meridional fibers
Suspensory ligament
Posterior chamber
Ciliary muscle

5

GLAUCOMA

Douglas H. Johnson
Richard F. Brubaker

Glaucoma is the leading cause of blindness in the United States and a leading cause of blindness in the world. It affects more than 2 million Americans of all ages, from newborns to the elderly. It is most common with age, involving some 3% of people older than 65 years. The term "glaucoma" (*glaukos*, bluish green) dates from ancient Greek times and referred to blindness from multiple causes, later coming to mean blindness with elevated intraocular pressure. Although the basic concepts and treatments of glaucoma have been known for nearly a century, new discoveries in the pathogenesis and treatment make the field ever changing.

Glaucoma is characterized by optic nerve damage in association with elevated intraocular pressure.

Glaucoma is actually a group of diseases of the eye, having a common feature of progressive *optic nerve damage* usually caused by *elevated intraocular pressure*. As optic nerve damage occurs, characteristic *visual field defects* develop, which can lead to blindness if the disease remains unchecked. Two types of glaucoma exist: *open angle*, in which aqueous drainage is impeded by a nonporous trabecular meshwork, and *closed angle*, in which aqueous cannot reach the meshwork because it is occluded by the iris (Fig. 5–1). The *angle* is the anatomic space between the anterior surface of the iris and the posterior surface of the cornea. At the apex of the angle lie the *trabecular meshwork* and *Schlemm's canal*, the drainage pathways for aqueous humor. Various subtypes of open-angle and angle-closure glaucoma exist.

Four essential facts are needed to understand the basic concepts of glaucoma.

1. *Pupillary block occurs in all eyes to some extent.*

The normal flow of aqueous is from the posterior chamber to the anterior chamber through the pupil (Fig. 5–1). Aqueous must squeeze between the lens and iris to enter the pupil and, hence, the anterior chamber. Normally, a slight resistance to this flow is encountered at the lens-iris interface, termed *pupillary block*. Because of this slight resistance, aqueous builds up in the posterior chamber, behind the iris, until its pressure overcomes the lens-iris apposition at the pupil, and a "puff" of aqueous enters the anterior chamber through the pupil. In the normal eye, this resistance is very slight, less than 1 mm Hg of pressure. However, if the resistance to flow through this lens-iris interface is increased, the build-up of aqueous behind the iris causes the iris to balloon forward like a sail in the wind, giving the iris a convex appearance when viewed with the slit lamp.

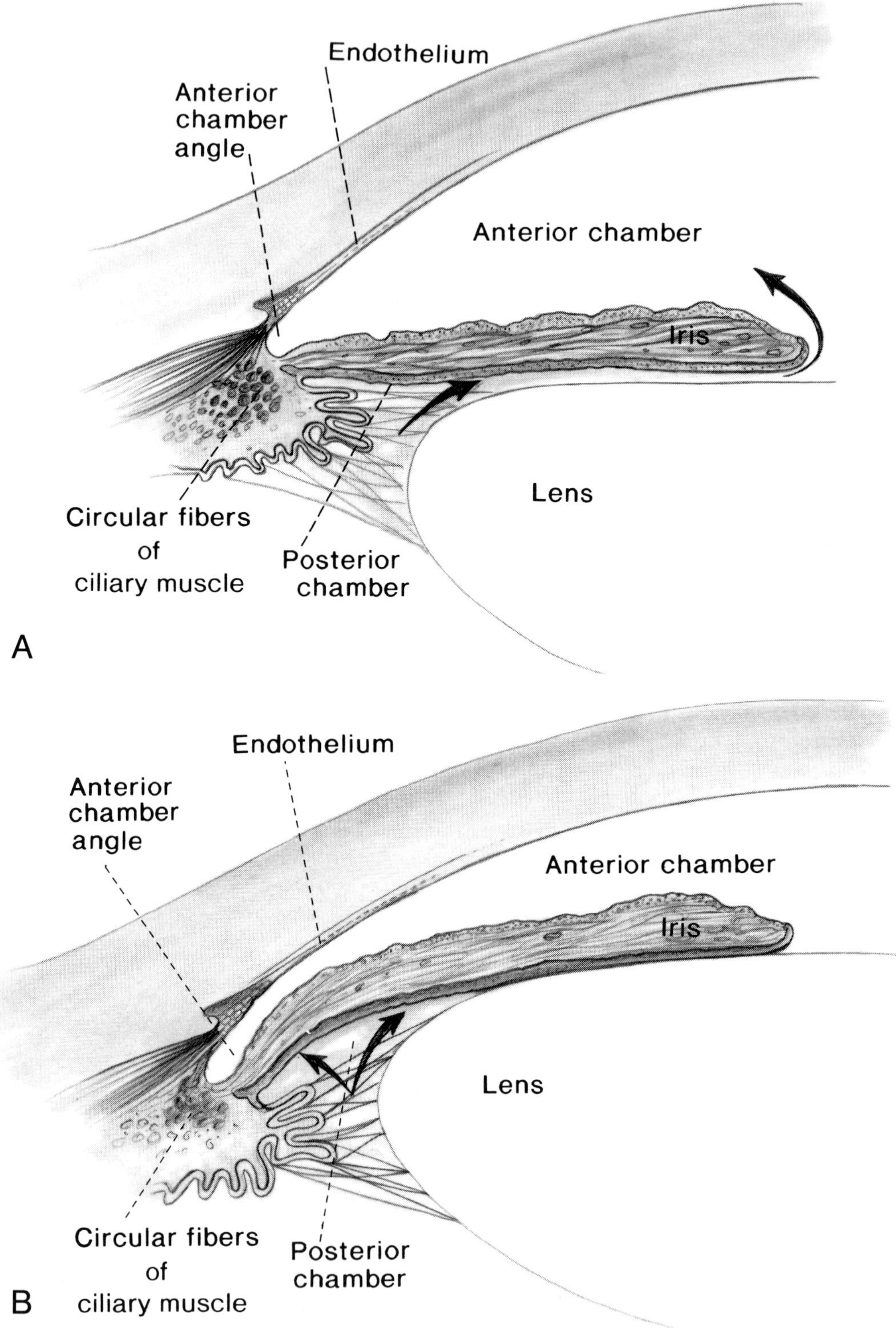

Fig. 5–1. Pupillary block of aqueous flow. Most eyes have minimal resistance to aqueous flow between the iris and the anterior surface of lens (*A*). Eyes with shallow chambers and narrow angles have lens physically closer to cornea, creating tighter contact between lens and iris. This positioning traps aqueous humor in the posterior chamber behind the iris (*B*).

2. The shape of field defects is determined by the anatomy of the retinal nerve fiber layer.

The typical *arcuate scotoma* of glaucomatous optic nerve damage results from the pattern of the retinal nerve fiber layer. The retinal nerve fiber layer consists of axons from the ganglion cells located throughout the retina (Fig. 5–2). As they course toward the optic nerve from the temporal retina, they arch around the macula, with fibers from the superior retina arching above the macula, and fibers from the inferior retina arching below it. This pattern prevents the fibers from directly crossing the macular area, thus allowing central macular photoreceptors to be undisturbed by overlying nerve fibers. Nerve fibers entering the optic nerve from the nasal retina run in a fairly straight line, without an arcuate pattern. The fibers enter the optic nerve in specific areas, with the arcuate fibers entering the superior and inferior poles of the optic nerve head. This anatomic organization at the optic nerve head results in bundles of related axons being simultaneously subject to damage from glaucoma, and this damage results in the characteristic visual field changes of glaucoma.

3. Visual field loss usually follows certain patterns.

The earliest field defects in glaucoma classically include the *paracentral scotoma* and the *nasal step* (Fig. 5–3 B). As glaucomatous damage increases, the paracentral scotomas enlarge, become denser (that is, require brighter or larger target stimuli to be seen in the scotomatous area), and finally coalesce to form an arcuate scotoma (Fig. 5–3 C). About 60% of the scotomas begin superiorly, whereas the remainder begin inferiorly. With further damage, scotomas begin in the inferior field as well (or in the superior field if the initial damage was inferior). Finally, the arcuate scotomas encircle the macula, creating a *"central island"* of vision (Fig. 5–3 D), usually also with a remaining *temporal crescent* of vision. By this time the patient usually is handicapped by these large scotomas and may be legally blind because of the field loss, despite retaining 20/20 central acuity. Ultimately, the central island of vision can be lost, leaving the patient with only "hand motion" vision from the remaining temporal field (Fig. 5–3 E).

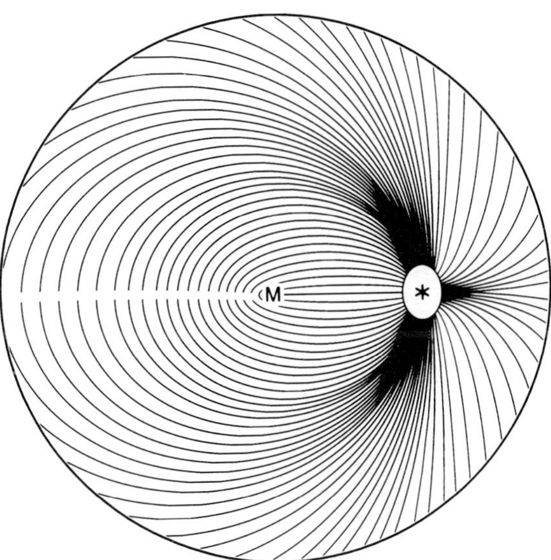

Fig. 5–2. Retinal nerve fiber layer, right eye. Note characteristic arching pattern of temporal fibers. This prevents fibers from covering the macula (M) and interfering with visual acuity. Nasal fibers run directly to optic disc (indicated by an asterisk), without arcuate pattern.

4. Progressive damage to the optic nerve produces cupping of the optic disc.

Damage to the optic nerve, with resultant visual loss, is the common sequela of all types of glaucoma. The damage, which occurs because of axonal loss at the optic disc, can occur both diffusely and in localized areas. Clinically, this damage is seen as a general enlargement of the optic cup, which may also become vertically elongated (Fig. 5–4). As more axons (the nerve fibers from the retinal ganglion cells, which form the nerve fiber layer) are lost, the cup continues to enlarge. In addition, the lamina cribrosa becomes more prominent, as seen with the ophthalmoscope. With further damage, the lamina begins to bow posteriorly, and the cup becomes deeper. At some sites around the perimeter of the disc, usually the superior or inferior pole, the cup can reach the rim of the scleral opening. Further damage results in total loss of all optic disc tissue, leaving only a large, deep cup with prominent laminar markings. Because of the marked posterior and lateral displacement of the lamina cribrosa at this stage of total cupping, the disc acquires the

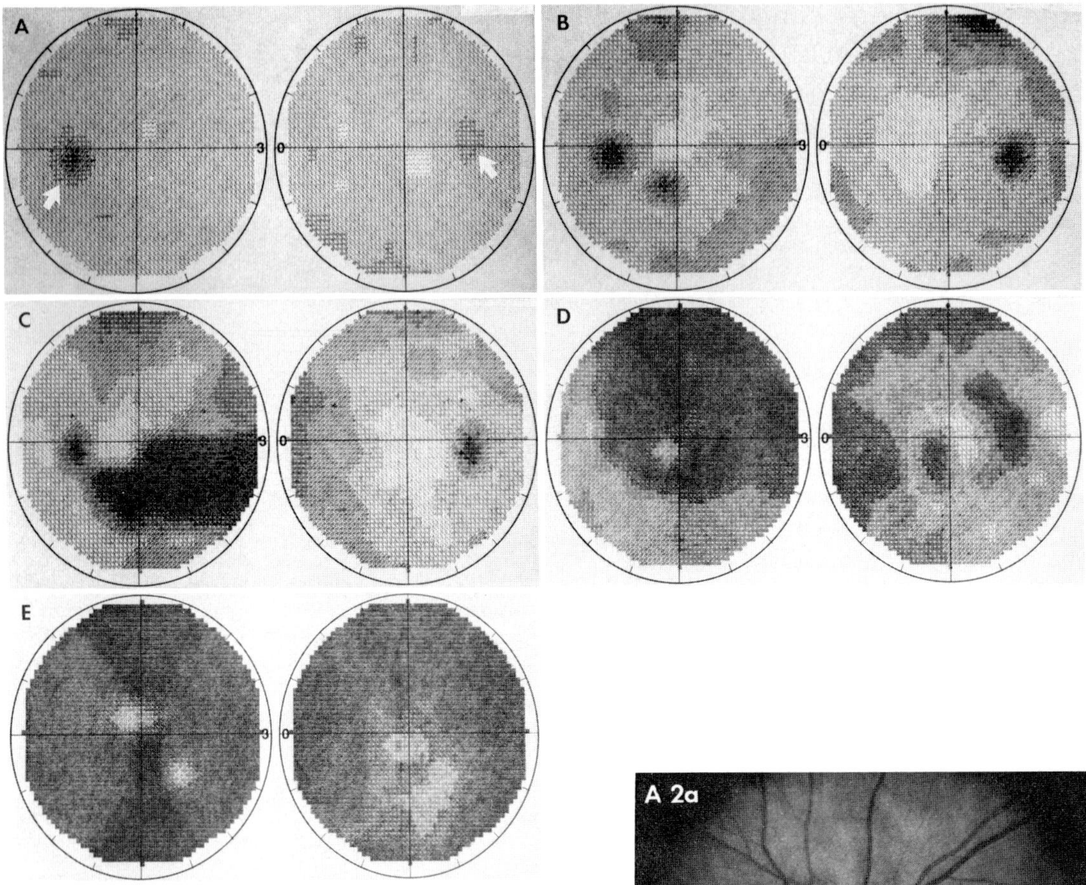

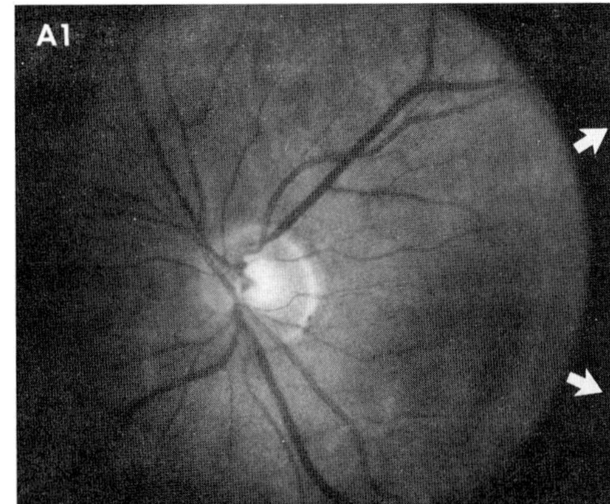

Fig. 5–3.

Fig. 5–4 *A*.

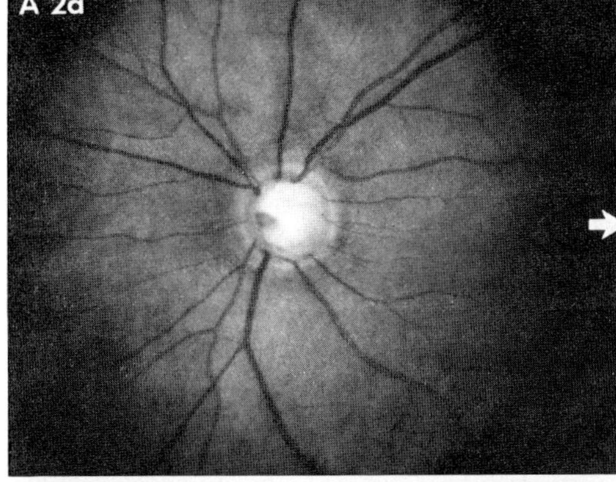

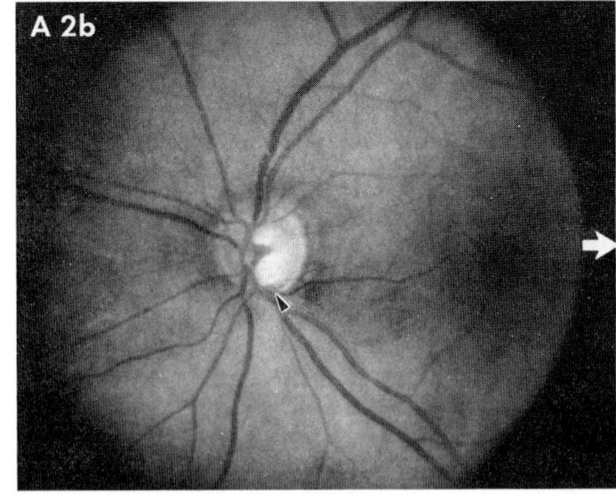

Fig. 5–3. Characteristic visual field loss in glaucoma. *A*, Normal fields, central 30°. Unlike most other pictures or representations in ophthalmology, visual fields are always displayed "as the patient sees them"; that is, the field on the left side indicates the patient's left eye, and the right field indicates the patient's right eye. The normal blind spots (which correspond to the optic nerve heads, which have no photoreceptors) are indicated by *arrows*. Most visual field defects begin in, or include portions of, the central 30°, especially in glaucoma. Thus, testing of the central 30° is the most fruitful for diagnosing and following glaucoma. *B*, Early visual field defects in glaucoma. Left eye has inferior paracentral scotoma and less dense inferior nasal step. *C*, Moderate degree of visual field loss in glaucoma. Left eye has developed dense inferior arcuate scotoma. *D*, Advanced glaucomatous field loss. Left eye has central island of vision, surrounded by extensive superior field loss and inferior arcuate scotoma. Right eye has earlier stages of loss. *E*, End-stage glaucomatous field loss. In each eye only a central island of vision remains. Testing of the more peripheral field usually demonstrates some preservation of the temporal field as well (the "temporal crescent").

shape of a bean pot, and this total cupping is often referred to as *"bean pot cupping."*

The superior and inferior poles of the disc are more susceptible to these changes. The anatomy of the lamina cribrosa, which is the collagen framework of the optic nerve head, may explain this preferential cupping. The lamina consists of a series of 10 collagen sheets layered one upon the other, through which run holes for passage of the axons of the optic nerve. The superior and inferior poles of the lamina contain the largest axonal holes and the thinnest collagen framework. It is thought that these areas are anatomically weaker and the

Fig. 5–4. *A*, The optic disc in glaucoma. *A 1*, Normal disc. *A 2*, Moderate cupping. Cupping may occur in two fashions: general enlargement of entire cup (*2a*) or vertical elongation with loss of neural rim tissue at superior or inferior pole (*2b*) (this figure shows inferior loss, *arrowhead*). *A 3*, Advanced cupping. *3a*, Generalized loss of neural rim has continued, extending nearly to edge of disc in all areas. *3b*, Alternatively, cupping may worsen by continued vertical elongation, to superior and inferior poles (*arrowheads*). *A 4*, Total glaucomatous cup. Whether by a continued generalized enlargement of cup (as in *2a* and *3a*) or vertical elongation with eventual loss of entire disc substance (as in *2b* and *3b*), the final result is loss of all of the neural rim of the disc. Vessels appear to emerge from edge of disc rather than from center of disc as in *A 1*.

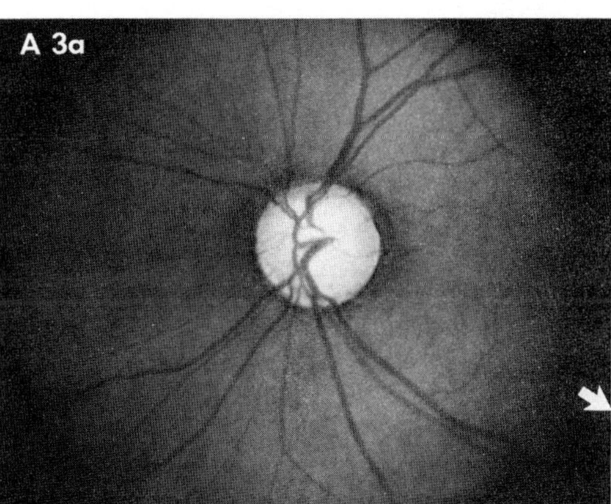

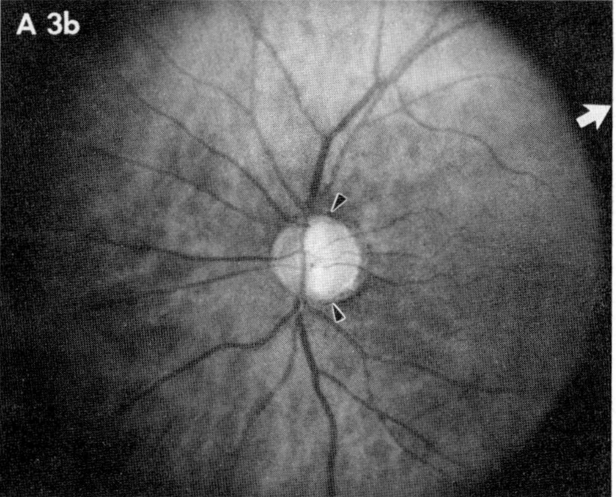

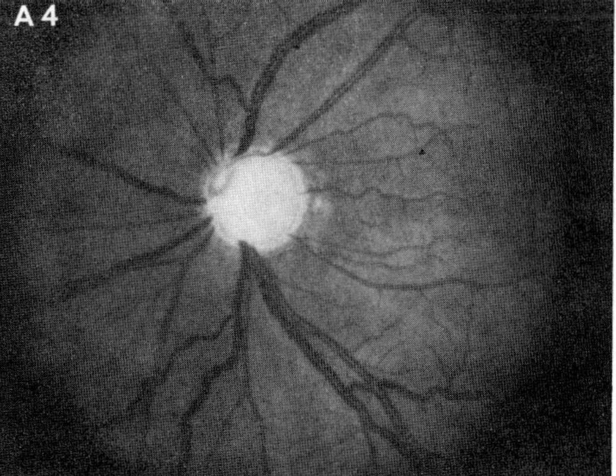

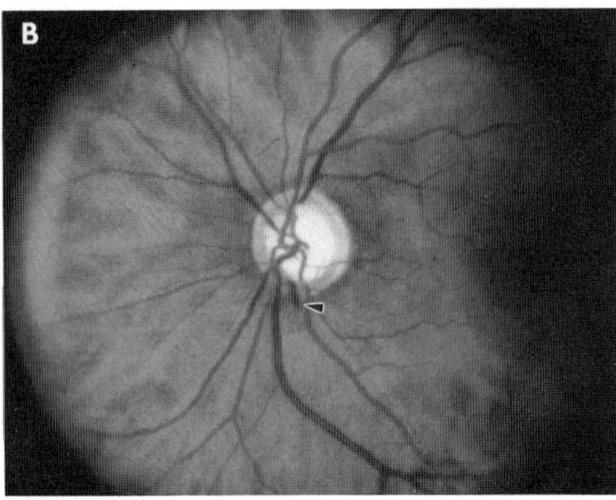

Fig. 5–4 (cont). *B*, Splinter hemorrhage at disc margin (*arrowhead*). Such hemorrhages appear characteristically at the inferior or superior pole of the disc and may cross the disc rim, as pictured here, or begin at the edge of the rim and extend onto adjacent retina.

lamina more prone to stretching and backward displacement by intraocular pressure in those areas. This proposed mechanism of optic nerve damage, the *mechanical theory*, states that the distortion and displacement of the lamina cause a misalignment of the axonal holes in the successive layers of the lamina. The misaligned holes are thought to compress and shear the axons, resulting in blockade of axonal transport and ultimately in axonal death. An alternative theory of optic nerve damage, the *vascular theory*, presupposes that ischemia or a decreased perfusion pressure of the vessels supplying the optic nerve initiates the pathologic nerve changes. This vascular-caused loss of axons, or their supporting tissue, would then cause the characteristic optic nerve cupping. These two theories of optic nerve damage, the mechanical

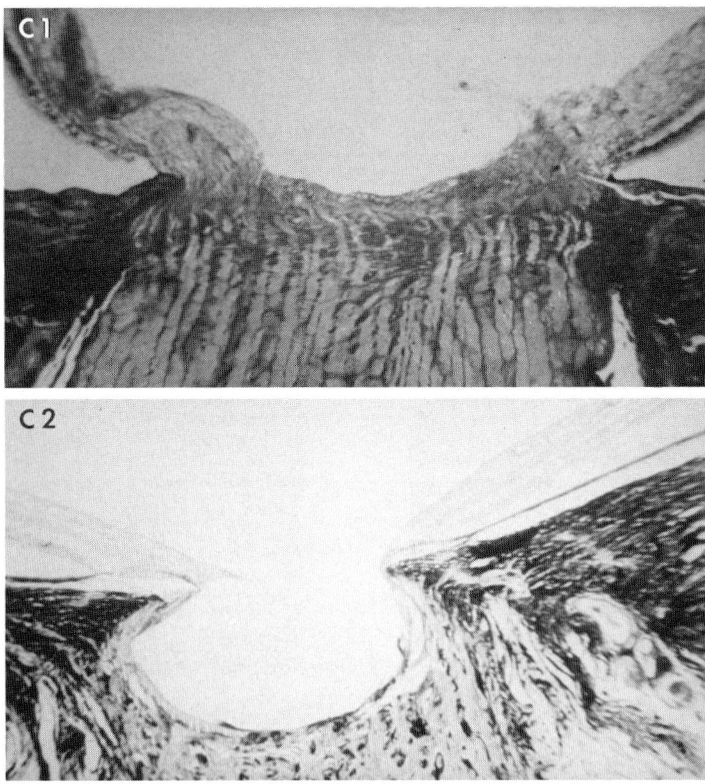

Fig. 5–4 (cont).   *C*, The optic disc, cross-sectional microscopic view. *C 1*, Normal optic disc, minimal optic cup. *C 2*, Advanced glaucomatous cupping. Loss of all rim tissue, posterior displacement and compression of lamina cribrosa, and extensive undermining of disc margins give "bean pot" appearance.

theory and the vascular theory, are not mutually exclusive, although the mechanical theory currently is considered the more plausible mechanism of glaucomatous optic nerve damage.

The clinical features of one type of glaucoma may be remarkably different from those of another type.

The diagnosis of glaucoma refers to the triad of elevated intraocular pressure, visual field loss, and optic disc damage. In addition, the term is often applied to an eye with pressure high enough to risk optic nerve damage if untreated. Various ocular conditions can cause the elevated intraocular pressure, and hence the term "glaucoma" is relatively nonspecific. The best treatment often hinges on the specific cause of elevated pressure, and an understanding of the mechanisms creating the problem is necessary before proper treatment can begin. Although angle-closure glaucoma is much less common than open-angle glaucoma, it will be discussed first. The underlying causative mechanism is better understood and it often requires emergency treatment.

Most angle-closure glaucomas occur rapidly and require immediate treatment.

Primary angle-closure glaucoma is triggered by pupillary block.

As discussed above, the normal flow of aqueous is from the posterior chamber to the anterior chamber through the pupil (Fig. 5–1). Pupillary block may cause the iris to balloon forward (*iris bombé*). If the peripheral iris touches the cornea, the trabecular meshwork can become occluded (Fig. 5–5). If it becomes occluded through all 360° of the angle, aqueous humor drainage from the eye stops. The intraocular pressure rapidly rises to very high levels, and headache, eye pain, and redness of the eye result. In addition, nausea and vomiting may occur, caused by the extreme ocular pain. The high intraocular pressure, which can be 50 to 90 mm Hg, can cause the cornea to appear steamy (edematous) (Fig.

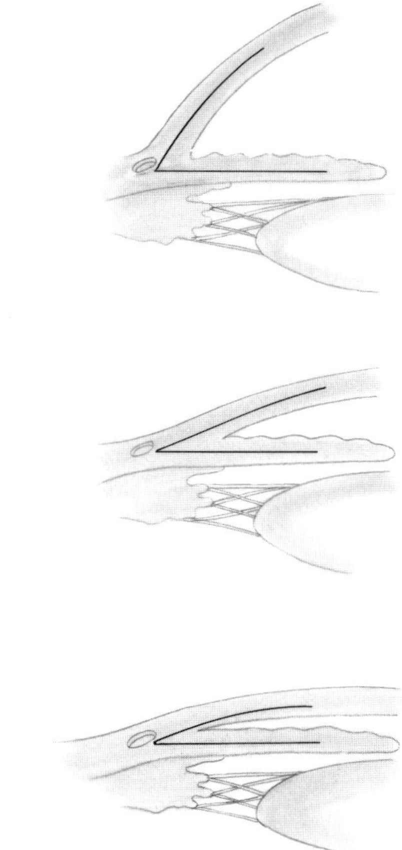

Fig. 5–5. Wide and narrow angles. Angle is formed by intersection of cornea and iris. Most angles are wide, approximating 45°. Note that eyes with narrow angles have shallower axial depth (distance from lens to cornea).

5–6), and this condition results in halos around lights and blurry or smokey vision. The pupil appears mid-dilated (5 to 6 mm) and does not react to light. Because circulation of blood to the eye is compromised at such high pressures, permanent visual loss can occur within hours. The diagnosis is made by observing the angle with *gonioscopy*.

Primary angle closure is more common in farsighted eyes.

Angle-closure glaucoma is more common in relatively small, hyperopic eyes. These eyes often appear to have a "crowded" anterior segment, with narrow angles and a relatively shal-

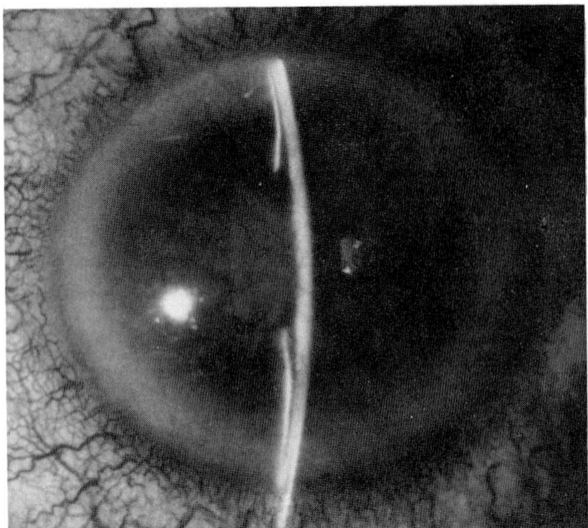

Fig. 5–6. Angle-closure glaucoma. Eye appears injected, with prominent, dilated vessels. Shallow chamber is evidenced by proximity of iris to cornea, as seen in slit-lamp beam. Corneal edema, seen as gray wrinkles and more generally as obscured clarity of iris details, is also present.

low axial depth (distance from the cornea to the lens as viewed with the slit lamp) (Fig. 5–5 and 5–7). This particular anatomic configuration makes pupillary block worse than in normal eyes and gives the iris a convex contour. Older patients are at an increased risk of angle closure, for as eyes age the lens becomes larger, has greater contact with the iris, and slowly increases the amount of pupillary block. Angle-closure glaucoma is much less common than

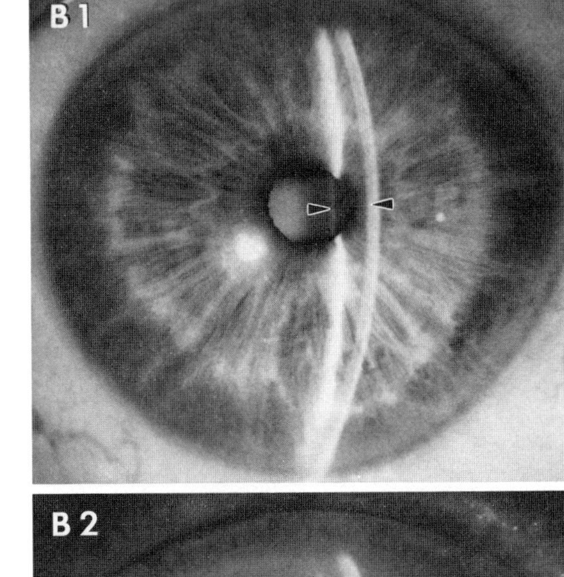

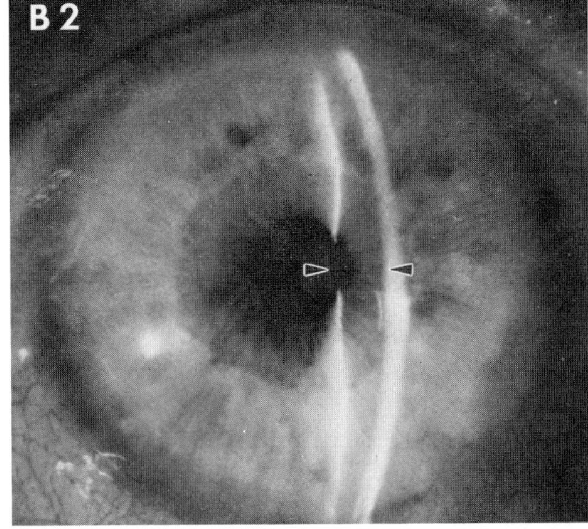

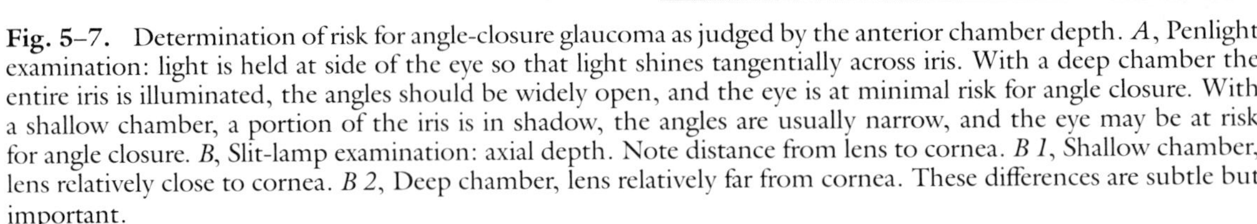

Fig. 5–7. Determination of risk for angle-closure glaucoma as judged by the anterior chamber depth. *A,* Penlight examination: light is held at side of the eye so that light shines tangentially across iris. With a deep chamber the entire iris is illuminated, the angles should be widely open, and the eye is at minimal risk for angle closure. With a shallow chamber, a portion of the iris is in shadow, the angles are usually narrow, and the eye may be at risk for angle closure. *B,* Slit-lamp examination: axial depth. Note distance from lens to cornea. *B 1,* Shallow chamber, lens relatively close to cornea. *B 2,* Deep chamber, lens relatively far from cornea. These differences are subtle but important.

open-angle glaucoma. At all ages, the most significant risk factor in precipitating an attack is a mid-dilated pupil (5 mm in diameter). This pupil position causes the greatest amount of pupillary block. In eyes with deep chambers and wide angles, a mid-dilated or widely dilated pupil does not increase pupillary block enough to cause problems. In narrow-angled, shallow-chambered eyes, this amount of pupillary dilation may be enough to close the angle.

A pupil may dilate to the mid-position by several mechanisms, including stress, excitement, response to the dark, or instillation of dilating eyedrops. Some eyes that receive pupil-dilating eyedrops may not experience angle closure until several hours after the patient leaves the physician's office. This can occur because a widely dilated pupil may actually cause less pupillary block than a mid-dilated pupil, and the angle will remain open temporarily. As the dilating

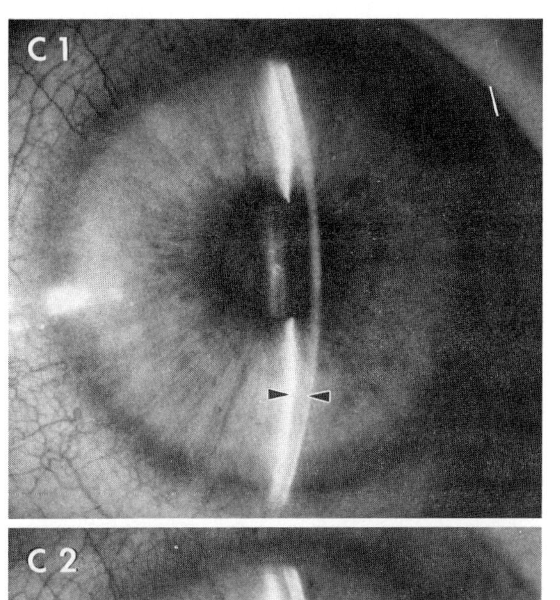

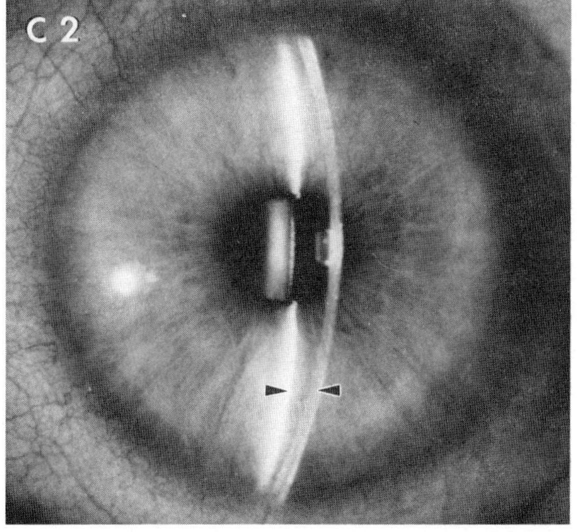

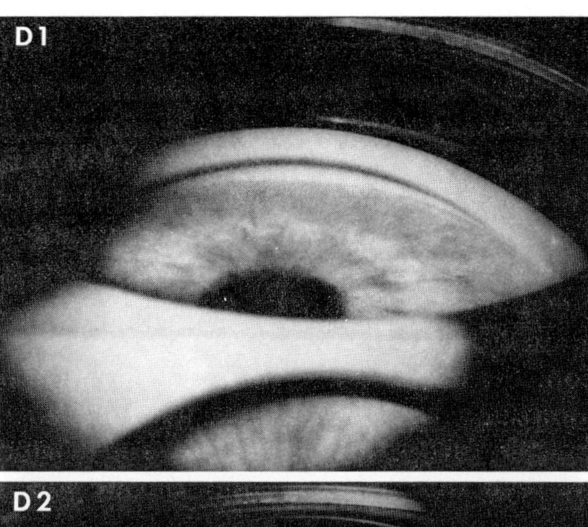

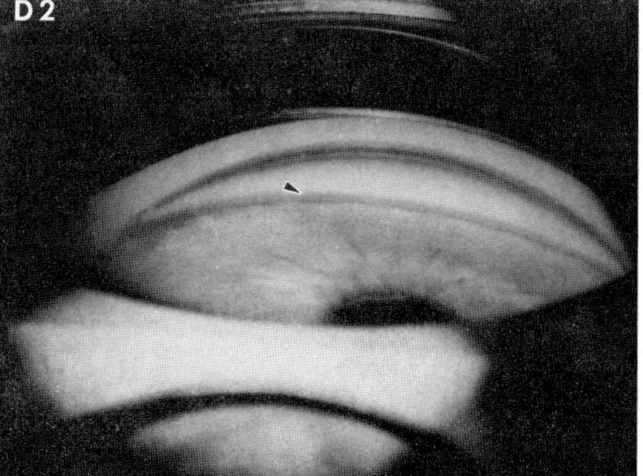

Fig. 5–7 (cont). *C,* Slit-lamp examination: peripheral depth. Note distance from iris to cornea. *C 1,* Eye that had a previous attack of angle-closure glaucoma, shown before treatment with laser iridotomy. Note proximity of iris to cornea in mid-periphery, with apposition of iris to cornea at extreme periphery. *C 2,* Same eye after laser iridotomy. Iris is farther from cornea. Note that axial depth (lens to cornea) distance was unchanged by iridotomy. *D,* Gonioscopy: closed and open angles. *D 1,* Angle closed; no view of angle structures seen. *D 2,* Angle open, dark line of pigmented trabecular meshwork (*arrowhead*) visible above white line of scleral spur. The dark line of the ciliary body band is below these structures and is seen just anterior to iris insertion.

eyedrop wears off, the pupil gradually constricts, going through the stage of mid-dilation, which may precipitate an attack of angle closure.

The treatment of primary angle-closure glaucoma is surgical.

The treatment of primary angle-closure glaucoma requires relieving the pupillary block. This is best accomplished by creation of a hole in the peripheral iris, allowing aqueous to bypass the pupil and enter the anterior chamber by a new route. Laser can be used to create this hole, making a full-thickness *iridotomy*. An intraocular surgical procedure also may be performed if laser therapy is unsuccessful. This entails creation of a *peripheral iridectomy*, the removal of a small, full-thickness piece of iris. The creation of a hole in the iris, either with laser or operation, permanently relieves pupillary block and is curative for primary angle-closure glaucoma.

Medical treatment is used initially to break the attack of angle-closure glaucoma (Table 5–1). Although laser therapy can be attempted early in the course of treatment of angle closure, it often is difficult or impossible to apply through a cloudy, edematous cornea. In addition, the inflamed and thickened iris that accompanies an attack makes laser treatment difficult. An operative procedure on an inflamed eye with an elevated pressure can be equally hazardous, although in some cases it may be the only therapeutic option to break the attack of angle closure.

The fellow eye of an acute angle-closure glaucomatous eye should be treated prophylactically.

The fellow eye of an eye with spontaneous angle closure is at great risk of having an attack. Some studies indicate that the fellow eye has a 50% chance of an attack within 5 years, despite prophylactic daily pilocarpine treatment to constrict the pupil and prevent pupillary block. Because of this risk, the fellow eye should also have an iridotomy, even if the eye has been asymptomatic. Although it is wise to avoid laser therapy or a surgical procedure on both eyes of a patient on the same day, the fellow eye should be treated within a reasonable period.

Subacute and chronic angle-closure glaucomas cause few or no symptoms.

Certain cases of narrow angles with pupillary block may not undergo precipitous closure of the entire drainage angle but may develop a more insidious form of angle closure. *Subacute angle closure* is characterized by symptoms similar to but less severe than those of an acute attack. Often the symptoms are mild enough

---

TABLE 5–1 Treatment of Primary Angle Closure

I. Confirm the diagnosis: gonioscopy

II. Lower the pressure
 1. Topical β-adrenergic blocker (timolol, bunolol, or betaxolol): 1 drop
 2. Pilocarpine 2%: 1 drop every 10 minutes, three times
 3. Systemic methazolamide or acetazolamide:
  either methazolamide (Neptazane; 100 mg orally)
  or acetazolamide (Diamox; 500 mg orally)
  NOTE: may be given parenterally if needed
 4. Systemic osmotic agent (if no medical contraindications):
  isosorbide (Ismotic):
  or glycerin (Osmoglyn): } 1 to 1.5 g/kg body weight
  or intravenous mannitol, 20% sol:

III. Perform iridotomy/iridectomy
 1. YAG or argon laser iridotomy
 2. Surgical iridectomy if laser unsuccessful

IV. Treat fellow eye prophylactically with laser iridotomy

that the patient does not seek help or attributes the problem to something else, such as "recurrent headaches." An episode with elevated pressure may last several hours before it spontaneously ends. Recurrent subacute attacks may cause optic nerve damage, producing field loss. They may also damage the trabecular meshwork and create a form of open-angle glaucoma superimposed on the intermittent attacks of angle closure.

Chronic angle-closure glaucoma is the silent killer of the trabecular meshwork. With prolonged iris-meshwork contact, adhesions (*peripheral anterior synechiae*) can form. Because the entire angle does not close simultaneously, intraocular pressure does not elevate dramatically during the initial stages of the disease. Instead, as the angle progressively narrows with time, synechiae between iris and meshwork form, permanently closing more and more of the drainage angle. Finally, enough angle becomes scarred by iris that the remaining open angle cannot adequately drain the aqueous humor and the intraocular pressure begins to rise.

Peripheral iridotomy or iridectomy is the treatment for both subacute and chronic angle-closure glaucoma. If more than 50% of the angle has been scarred shut by chronic angle closure, the intraocular pressure is usually elevated and more extensive medical or surgical treatment is required.

Factors other than pupillary block can cause secondary angle closure.

Unlike primary angle closure, *secondary angle closure* is not caused by pupillary block. Several distinct syndromes that cause secondary angle closure are known, and they can be grouped into those causing permanent closure by iris adhesions and those causing temporary closure by reversible iris contact.

Several syndromes can cause permanent closure.

1. *Neovascular glaucoma results from vasoproliferation in the angle.*
The stimulus for neovascularization probably comes from an ischemic retina (Table 5–2).

TABLE 5-2 Common Causes of Neovascular Glaucoma

1. Diabetes mellitus
2. Central retinal vein occlusion
3. Branch retinal vein occlusion
4. Central retinal artery occlusion
5. Ischemia from carotid disease
6. Intraocular tumor
7. Retinal detachment, long-standing
8. Chronic uveitis

Neovascularization in the anterior segment usually arises at the pupillary margin of the iris and also in the trabecular meshwork, consistent with an aqueous-borne factor. As new vessels arise, they are accompanied by fibrous tissue that causes permanent synechiae of the drainage angle, often in a period of only days or weeks. Once the angle is closed in this fashion it is impossible to reopen, and a downhill course invariably begins. Unless the stimulus for neovascularization is arrested, the problem will continue and doom any surgical intervention to failure, because continued fibrovascular proliferation will occlude surgical attempts to relieve the elevated pressure.

The treatment of neovascular glaucoma is *panretinal photocoagulation*, done in time to prevent further fibrovascular angle synechiae. This treatment often is effective in arresting and causing regression of neovascularization in the angle. If the angle is already entirely closed, laser treatment should still be performed to prevent further fibrovascular proliferation. Four to six weeks after panretinal photocoagulation, filtration surgery may be attempted. Standard medical therapy (eyedrops and systemic carbonic anhydrase inhibitors) may control the pressure during this interim period. If corneal edema or other media opacities prevent adequate visualization of the fundus despite medical therapy to lower the intraocular pressure, panretinal photocoagulation cannot be performed and surgical treatments must be used. A cyclodestructive procedure such as *cyclocryotherapy*, which decreases the formation of aqueous humor, is effective in permanently lowering intraocular pressure in these cases.

Other procedures include the surgical implantation of a *seton* or silicone drainage tube, designed to drain aqueous humor to the orbital space.

2. Iritis can cause synechial angle closure.

Peripheral anterior synechiae are adhesions between the peripheral iris and the trabecular meshwork. They can be caused by various factors, including iritis, a shallow or flat anterior chamber after intraocular surgery, and several syndromes, such as iridocorneal endothelial syndrome and aniridia. As described above, chronic angle closure may also produce peripheral anterior synechiae, although by a different mechanism. If more than half of the angle is scarred due to any cause, intraocular pressure often becomes elevated.

Ideally, treatment is directed at the offending cause: eliminating iritis, early re-formation of flat chambers postoperatively, and finding a cure for the pathogenesis of the syndromes that cause the angle closure. Surgical techniques to break adherence have been described, although peripheral anterior synechiae are usually considered permanent and the ophthalmologist is happy enough to prevent further formation of synechiae. Any resultant elevated intraocular pressure arising from angle closure is treated with the usual medical and surgical therapies.

Several conditions cause angle closure that can be reversed.

Some types of angle closure are caused by treatable conditions that can be diagnosed only by a thorough understanding of the causes of angle closure coupled with astute observation of the eye. Establishing a specific diagnosis is important and can make the difference between a "tough case" in which the patient does not do well and an "interesting case" in which the patient is cured with the proper therapy.

1. *Inadequate iridectomy* is a common factor in cases of persistent or recurring acute, subacute, or chronic angle closure. The clinician may erroneously assume that pupillary block has been relieved, because of a laser or surgical procedure, but the opening in the iris may be inadequate. It may be inadequate immediately after the procedure because laser iridotomies may not be as large as desired or because the surgical iridectomy may not be full thickness through the iris (this *can* happen). In addition, laser iridotomies can spontaneously close over several weeks. The adequacy and continued patency of these openings must be confirmed until it is certain that they are functional and stable.

2. *A plateau iris configuration* is a condition in which the central portion of the anterior chamber is normal or of near normal depth but the peripheral portion of the anterior chamber is very shallow. In this condition the shape of the iris and its insertion into the angle play a major role in the juxtaposition of the iris with the cornea. This abnormal configuration can lead to significant angle closure, differing in mechanisms from primary angle-closure glaucoma, in which pupillary block plays the major role. In most cases of plateau iris, however, pupillary block is also present and contributes to the plateau configuration to some extent. In cases worrisome in regard to angle closure, a peripheral iridotomy must be performed, and the angle then reassessed by gonioscopy. Often the iridotomy will relieve the plateau configuration, and this result indicates that pupillary block was playing a greater role than suspected. For cases in which the plateau iris configuration persists, a miotic drug should be added temporarily. If miotics open the angle significantly but the iridotomy did not, a true plateau iris is present. Rarely, such an eye may experience angle closure after dilation of the pupil despite a patent and functional peripheral iridectomy and an adequate depth to the central anterior chamber. This condition is termed *plateau iris syndrome* and should be treated with long-term miotic therapy.

3. *Malignant glaucoma* describes the association of a shallow anterior chamber, a closed angle, and elevated intraocular pressure in the face of a patent iridectomy. This condition generally is observed after surgical iridectomy for angle closure or after filtration surgery for glaucoma. More than one anatomic relationship may be responsible for this condition, but most observers believe it is due to *ciliolenticular block*. In these eyes, the crystalline lens is large

relative to the size of the eye and the placement of the ciliary processes. The ciliary processes rotate forward and contact the crystalline lens, preventing the aqueous humor from easily passing between them and the lens and entering the posterior chamber. Some portion of newly formed aqueous humor may be misdirected into the vitreous cavity, increasing the pressure in the vitreous cavity and forcing the lens and iris against the cornea. Medical treatment consists of cycloplegics, such as atropine, which pull the ciliary processes away from the lens. If successful, this treatment must be continued indefinitely. Surgical treatment can be carried out either by removing the anterior vitreous or by removing both the crystalline lens and the anterior vitreous face. These procedures allow aqueous humor to enter the posterior chamber rather than the vitreous, relieving the pressure that tends to close the angle.

4. A *dislocated lens* may cause unilateral shallowing of the anterior chamber and angle closure. The lens may move forward, causing the iris to move forward and temporarily close the angle. These changes often occur when the patient is upright and may be relieved by lying supine. In some circumstances the lens can move forward enough to get entrapped in the pupil and cause pupillary block. A dislocated lens usually occurs because of trauma, which breaks the zonular fibers, or a congenital condition such as Marfan's syndrome, in which the fibers are abnormally lax. Examination of patients with dislocated lenses demonstrates that the axial depth (cornea to lens distance) of the chamber is considerably less than the normal 3 mm and that asymmetry between the two eyes will exist. This condition differs from primary angle closure, in which the axial depths between eyes are usually similar. Another sign may be *phacodonesis*, in which the crystalline lens is observed to shake with eye movement, because of its loose tether.

5. *Choroidal effusions*, due to various causes, can produce a shallow anterior chamber with or without angle closure and with or without elevated intraocular pressure. These effusions may follow extensive laser procedures of the retina or may result from retinal detachment operation in which a tight encircling band displaces the posterior portion of the eye and alters the position of the ciliary body. It is important to recognize angle closure after a retinal operation, even if the pressure is not elevated, because permanent synechiae can form and intraocular pressure may rise at a later time.

Open-angle glaucomas are characterized by an asymptomatic and gradual onset, by progressive cupping of the optic disc, and often by elevated intraocular pressure.

Although glaucoma is classically associated with an elevated pressure, the evaluation of the optic disc is of equal importance. A diagnosis of "normal examination, no glaucoma" cannot be made without a disc examination. In addition, the observation of an optic disc with significant cupping may alert the clinician to glaucoma in a patient even before the intraocular pressure is known.

The average normal intraocular pressure is 16 mm Hg.

This average increases slightly with age, and the average normal intraocular pressure range for all ages extends from 10 to 22 mm Hg. Patients with glaucoma often have pressures of 30 mm Hg or higher, although others may undergo optic nerve damage at pressures in the 20s. A particular subset of people with *low-tension glaucoma* may experience optic nerve damage at normal pressures and will be considered later in the chapter. In general, if pressures from 23 to 29 mm Hg are observed, a patient with normal discs and fields is considered to have a higher risk of developing glaucoma in the future and must be reexamined; these patients are considered *"glaucoma suspects."* If the optic disc is suspicious for glaucoma, or if other significant risk factors are involved, even lower pressures may be of concern.

Once glaucoma has been diagnosed, treatment is usually aimed at lowering the intraocular pressure. The amount of pressure lowering needed to prevent further glaucomatous damage is a matter of judgment. Most ophthalmologists establish a *"target pressure,"* or goal, for each eye to help guide them in therapy. Although guidelines for these target pressures have been suggested, exact algorithms do not exist, and therapy must take into account the amount of glaucomatous damage, the intraocular pressure, and the presence of risk factors such as family history of glaucoma, myopia, diabetes, and age. In general, an eye with significant damage from glaucoma has less resistance to future damage than a normal eye, and a proportionately lower pressure is required (Table 5–3). If additional glaucomatous damage is noted despite treatment, the intraocular pressure must be lowered further, usually another 4 or 5 mm Hg, thus establishing a new target pressure. Because all techniques to lower pressure are accompanied by side effects and risks, the therapist must weigh any potential benefit against these risks.

Primary open-angle glaucoma has no other associated ocular abnormalities.

Primary open-angle glaucoma is the most common type of glaucoma, accounting for at least 50% of all cases. Because of the insidious nature of open-angle glaucoma, with its gradual and painless loss of vision, it does not produce symptoms that would bring a patient to seek help until relatively late in its course. Eyes are characteristically normal-appearing, with no specific findings on examination, aside from the elevated intraocular pressure and optic disc cupping.

The cause of primary open-angle glaucoma

TABLE 5–3 Guidelines for Desirable Intraocular Pressures*

Visual field	Pressure
Abnormal disc, normal field	Glaucomatous loss common at pressures in high 20s to mid 20s
Field defect above or below	Loss common at mid 20s to 20
Field defect above and below	Loss common at high teens

* These must be modified according to the individual patient. From W.M. Grant, J.F. Burke, Jr.: Why do some people go blind from glaucoma? Ophthalmology 89:991–998, 1982. By permission of the American Academy of Ophthalmology.

remains unknown. Although it has been realized for almost a century that faulty drainage of aqueous humor produces elevated intraocular pressure, microscopic examinations of the angle structures yield nonspecific findings. Many glaucomatous eyes show only an exaggeration of normal aging processes, and it is difficult to predict with accuracy which trabecular meshworks are those of glaucomatous eyes when a series of eyes are examined.

The secondary open-angle glaucomas are associated with specific and diagnostic ocular abnormalities.

Several ocular syndromes have been recognized in which glaucoma seems to occur in response to specific factors. These are of special interest because of the insight they provide into an understanding of the aqueous system and the pathogenesis of the glaucoma resulting from them.

Exfoliation syndrome (sometimes called "pseudoexfoliation") is a diffuse ocular condition with a high incidence of glaucoma. In this disorder, whitish flakes and sheets are seen on the surface of the lens and ciliary processes (Fig. 5–8). This material, which has the microscopic appearance of a filamentous, banded structure, can be found microscopically on the lens capsule, in blood vessel walls, and in the trabecular meshwork. The material is probably an abnormal basement membrane that is secreted in excess amounts, flows in the aqueous, and becomes deposited throughout the anterior portion of the eye. It may occlude the trabecular meshwork. The exfoliation syndrome can occur in one or both eyes and is associated with glaucoma in some populations (such as elderly Scandinavians) in up to 90% of cases followed for 10 years. Eyes with exfoliation syndrome are thus at high risk for developing glaucoma and should be examined periodically to detect any intraocular pressure elevations.

Pigment dispersion syndrome is another condition in which glaucoma seems to result from occlusion of the trabeculum by particles. Patients with this condition have an abnormally deep anterior chamber. Friction occurs between the posterior surface of the iris and the zonular fibers that suspend the lens as the pupil dilates and constricts. As a result, the zonular

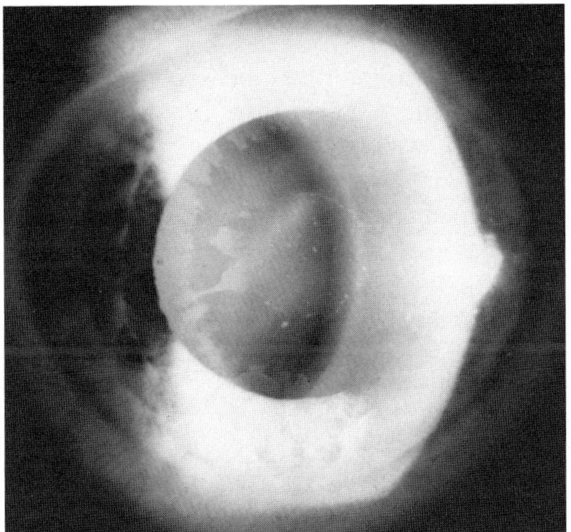

Fig. 5–8. Exfoliation syndrome. Characteristic accumulation of exfoliative material on anterior surface of lens. Central disc of exfoliative material corresponds to the size of the pupil before dilation. This central disc is surrounded by a clear zone in which exfoliative material has been rubbed away by movement of the iris during constriction and dilation of the pupil. A peripheral ring of exfoliative material surrounds the clear zone and actually extends out to the lens equator.

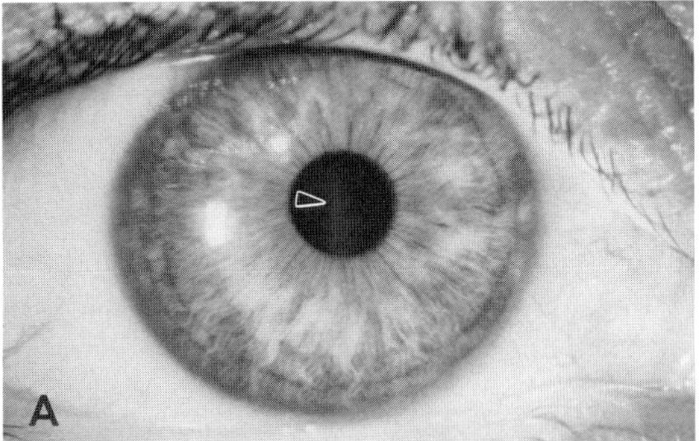

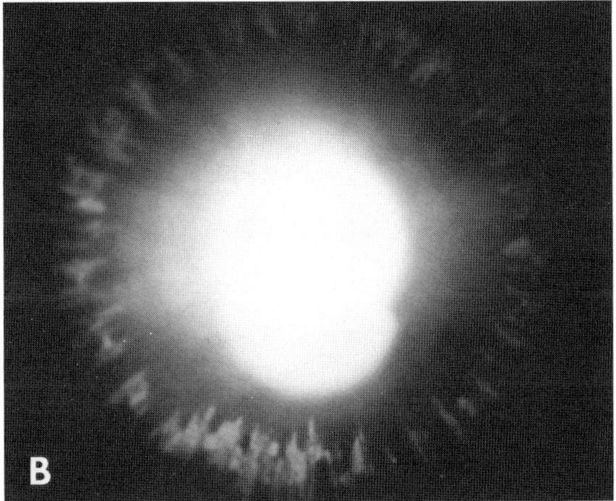

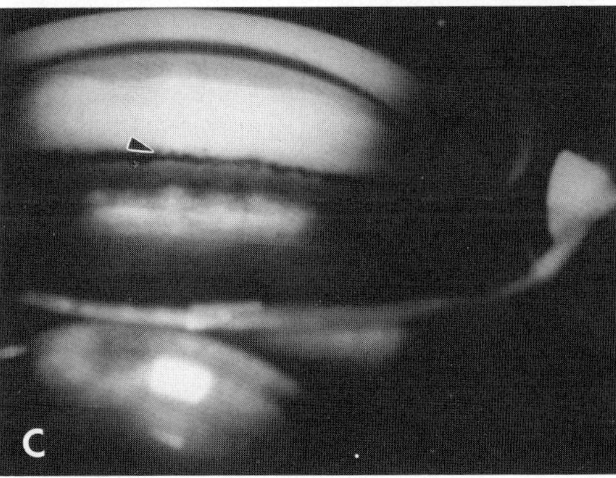

Fig. 5–9. Pigment dispersion syndrome. *A*, Krukenberg spindle (*arrowhead*). Deposit of pigment granules in a characteristic pattern on the corneal endothelium. This pattern is due to convection currents in the aqueous humor, which cools and sinks as it nears the cornea. *B*, Radial transillumination defects of iris. This characteristic finding is visible only if the clinician transilluminates the iris during slit-lamp examination, a step that can be done in less than 20 seconds. Each radial spoke is an area devoid of iris pigment epithelium and probably corresponds to a packet of zonular fibers. *C*, Heavy pigmentation of trabecular meshwork. A characteristic deposit of pigment appears in the meshwork over Schlemm's canal. This black "mascara line" (*arrowhead*) is a hallmark of pigmentary glaucoma.

fibers erode the delicate pigment cells of the posterior surface of the iris. Pigment granules are released from these spoke-like areas of iris damage (seen best with iris transillumination) and flow along with the aqueous humor (Fig. 5–9). The trabeculum may become so heavily covered with pigment that it appears as a black line (a "mascara line"). A vertically oriented deposition of pigment on the corneal endothelium (Krukenberg spindle) is another characteristic finding. Interestingly, glaucoma develops in only one-third of these patients, and why some patients with this syndrome escape glaucoma and others do not is unknown.

Angle-recession glaucoma is associated with blunt trauma to the eye. The trauma may cause a tear in the attachment of the ciliary body to the scleral spur and trabecular meshwork. Initially, such a patient may present with blurry vision from a hyphema after being struck in the eye with a tennis ball or other object. Such an injury has a high frequency of angle recession and predisposes the patient to glaucoma later in life. Angle recession usually involves a portion of the circumference of the eye, although it may extend for all 360°. The torn attachment of the ciliary body probably makes its contractions less effective in altering the shape of trabecular meshwork, and with time this is thought to lead to glaucoma.

Glaucoma can result from inflammation. The trabecular meshwork may become plugged with the debris of intraocular inflammation. Leukocytes, macrophages, erythrocytes, serum proteins, pigment, and other materials seen with iritis or uveitis may deposit in the meshwork and transiently elevate the intraocular pressure. Treatment should be aimed at eliminating the inflammation, although standard antiglaucoma medications also may be needed.

Corticosteroids can induce glaucoma. Prolonged use of corticosteroid eyedrops in some patients may cause a secondary glaucoma that mimics primary open-angle glaucoma. In susceptible patients, corticosteroid use four times a day for a month is usually required to cause the pressure elevation, although it may occur with shorter applications also. Clinical findings are nonspecific; aside from the elevated pressure the eyes appear normal. Histologic examination of the trabecular meshwork reveals the accumulation of an abnormal basement membrane-like collagen in this condition.

Low-tension glaucoma is characterized by cupping and field loss without evidence of elevated intraocular pressure.

A small number of patients may have optic disc cupping and progressive visual field loss characteristic of open-angle glaucoma yet never have a documented elevation of intraocular pressure. Care must be taken to obtain several pressure measurements at different times of the day and on different days because pressure may vary up to 10 mm Hg or more over these periods. Although aqueous humor dynamics may appear normal, often these patients have pressures at the upper end of the normal range. Also, if tested by tonography some of these patients have borderline high resistance to outflow of aqueous humor.

The mechanism of optic nerve damage in low-tension glaucoma is unknown, although several hypotheses exist. Some experts believe that these patients have an abnormally fragile optic nerve, making them susceptible to intraocular pressures that most other nerves could withstand. Others believe that the progressive damage to the disc occurs as a result of episodic or progressive vascular insufficiency. It is not known whether lowering the intraocular pressure will retard further damage in low-tension glaucoma, although most clinicians prescribe medications to attempt to lower the pressure. Such treatment might either lower the average intraocular pressure or limit pressure elevations that can occur diurnally or sporadically.

The clinical approach to glaucoma involves a careful history, clinical examination, sequential treatment, and consistent follow-up.

When the classic triad of elevated intraocular pressure, disc damage, and visual field loss is present, open-angle glaucoma is simple to diagnose. When only one or two of the findings are present, it is less easy to diagnose with confidence. Because optic nerve damage is irreversible, diagnosis should be made before extensive damage has occurred. Unfortunately, no single test can predict accurately which patients will develop optic nerve damage and which will not. For purposes of classification, patients with moderately elevated intraocular pressure but normal discs and fields are termed *"glaucoma suspects"* or *"ocular hypertensives."* Of patients with moderately elevated intraocular pressures (23 to 30 mm Hg; normal range, 10 to 22 mm Hg), approximately 1% per year will develop visual field defects. The decision to treat or not to treat must be made on the basis of a number of risk factors that together are of prognostic significance.

A careful history may disclose risk factors for open-angle glaucoma.

A family history of glaucoma increases the likelihood of glaucoma in a patient. If a parent has glaucoma, each child will have about a 20% chance of developing the disease. If a sibling has glaucoma, fellow siblings have about a 50% chance.

Age is known to play a significant role in the

appearance of glaucoma. Primary open-angle glaucoma is rare before the age of 40 years, but the incidence increases markedly thereafter. By age 80 years, 14% of people will have developed glaucoma.

Myopia is also a risk factor for the development of glaucomatous damage, perhaps because myopic eyes tend to be larger, with thinner sclera and thus weaker lamina cribrosa. Once intraocular pressure is brought under control, myopes lose their disadvantage and develop field loss at the same rate as do nonmyopic patients.

Diabetes mellitus is another risk factor for glaucoma. Diabetics have a three times greater chance than nondiabetics of developing glaucoma, perhaps because of the associated microvasculature disease.

Race is a factor in the development of glaucoma and of blindness from glaucoma; blacks have a significantly higher incidence than whites.

The clinical examination requires careful attention to the anterior segment, optic disc, and intraocular pressure.

Each structure of the anterior portion of the eye can yield clues to the pathophysiology of glaucoma and may also give an indication that glaucoma will develop in the future.

Cornea: Pigment deposition on the inferior endothelium in a linear fashion (Krukenberg spindle) may indicate pigmentary glaucoma (Fig. 5–9).

Keratic precipitates, a sign of intraocular inflammation, may be associated with elevated pressure if the meshwork is also involved in the inflammatory process.

Anterior chamber: The depth of the anterior chamber may indicate a propensity to angle-closure glaucoma (Fig. 5–7).

Inflammation (cells and flare) may have an associated elevated pressure.

Iris: Rubeosis iridis indicates a serious underlying problem and places the patient at grave risk for neovascular glaucoma.

Transillumination defects may indicate pigmentary glaucoma (Fig. 5–9).

Iris atrophy or a misplaced pupil may indicate the iridocorneal endothelial syndrome, in which glaucoma is frequent.

Heterochromia may indicate Fuchs' heterochromic cyclitis, which is accompanied by glaucoma in 20% of cases.

Lens: Exfoliation material on the anterior lens surface predisposes the patient to glaucoma (Fig. 5–8).

A hypermature cataract may be associated with phacolytic glaucoma.

Angle: Gonioscopy allows evaluation of the degree of angle narrowness and the potential for angle closure. Other clues may be found as well. Peripheral anterior synechiae may indicate chronic angle closure or prior inflammation. Diffuse heavy pigment deposition may indicate pigmentary glaucoma; heavy segmental pigmentation is often associated with exfoliation syndrome. Neovascularization of the angle seen on gonioscopy always means trouble and requires a search for the underlying cause.

Optic disc: The greatest single risk factor that is predictive of future damage is a large cup:disc ratio. This measurement is made ophthalmoscopically by estimating the overall diameter of the central cupped area of the optic disc in comparison with the overall diameter of the entire disc. The average cup occupies 30% of the optic disc surface; 99% of the normal population have optic cups occupying between 0 and 70% of the optic disc (Fig. 5–4). A cup larger than 70% of the disc should arouse suspicion of glaucoma, even if pressures are normal. A discrepancy in cup size between fellow eyes also is important. A difference in cup:disc ratios of more than 20% between the two eyes raises the question of glaucoma. Thus, although a 60% cup in one eye could be considered normal, the appearance of only a 10% cup in the fellow eye would arouse strong suspicion of disc damage and unilateral glaucoma in the widely cupped eye.

Glaucomatous optic disc cupping can occur both diffusely and in localized areas (Fig. 5–4). With damage from glaucoma, the optic cup enlarges and often becomes vertically elongated. As more axons are lost, the cup enlarges further and the lamina cribrosa becomes more prominent. The lamina begins to bow posteriorly, and the cup becomes deeper. At some sites around the perimeter of the disc, the cup can reach the rim of the scleral opening.

The superior and inferior poles of the disc are more susceptible to these changes. This anatomic weakness is the basis for the characteristic field defects that occur in the mid-stages of glaucoma. Further damage results in total loss of all optic disc tissue, leaving only a large, deep cup with prominent laminar markings.

The pattern and extent of visual field loss can be predicted from the location and degree of cupping. Because the retinal image is inverted, loss of inferior disc tissue results in visual field loss above fixation (a superior scotoma). By examination of the disc alone, an experienced observer is able to diagnose glaucoma in 85% of patients who have visual field loss and to identify correctly eyes with a normal field in about 90% of cases.

The occurrence of a splinter-shaped hemorrhage on the disc margin portends glaucoma in up to 70% of undiagnosed patients (Fig. 5–4 *B*). In patients with glaucoma, it may precede a localized worsening of the visual field by many months or longer. These hemorrhages may result from the shearing and stretching associated with the mechanism of glaucomatous cupping. When stretched too far the capillaries break, creating a local flame-shaped hemorrhage.

Accurate perimetry (visual fields) is essential for proper management of glaucoma.

Formal visual field examinations are essential for the diagnosis and management of glaucoma. Diagnostically, they may confirm a clinician's suspicion of glaucoma by showing a scotoma that correlates with observed disc cupping. A visual field deficit in an otherwise borderline glaucoma situation should weigh the balance of factors toward initiating treatment. Likewise, progressive field loss in a patient receiving glaucoma therapy is a sign that the glaucomatous damage is progressing and that further treatment is in order (Fig. 5–3).

Testing of the visual field has undergone revolutionary advances in recent years. The continued refinement of these tests has allowed early detection of field defects. The presence of optic nerve damage can be established long before the patient is aware of the loss. Loss of visual field encompasses either a loss of all vision in a geographic area of the field or, more subtly, a loss of sensitivity for functions such as color vision or sensitivity to dim light. The laborious task of plotting visual fields by hand has now been supplanted largely by computerized, semiautomated devices. However, many elderly and frail patients can be tested only by a skilled perimetrist who has cultivated the art through experience.

Tonography measures the resistance of the trabecular meshwork to aqueous outflow.

The measurement of the resistance of the trabecular meshwork to the outflow of aqueous humor is an additional piece of evidence in the evaluation of a glaucoma suspect. Although the technique is based on many assumptions and requires meticulous performance, it does give an estimate of trabecular meshwork resistance. It has long been known that external pressure applied to the eye forces aqueous from the eye and results in a temporarily lowered intraocular pressure. Tonography involves formal quantitation of this "ocular massage" (to obtain a measurement of the conductance of aqueous humor, known as a "C value") by applying a recording Schiøtz tonometer of known weight to the eye for 4 minutes. A normal meshwork allows aqueous to be forced from the eye during this time, resulting in a low intraocular pressure and a correspondingly high C value (0.28). A glaucomatous meshwork provides more resistance to the forced aqueous outflow, resulting in less aqueous leaving the eye, a correspondingly higher final pressure, and a low C value. A low C value, 0.13 or less, would be indicative of glaucoma. Values between 0.13 and 0.18 are suspicious for glaucoma.

Few absolute rules exist about when to initiate treatment in open-angle glaucoma, although guidelines are helpful.

1. *Clear-cut cases*: elevated pressure, disc cupping, field loss.

2. *Elevated pressure only*: Although there is no commonly agreed intraocular pressure above which glaucoma is assumed to exist,

most ophthalmologists use a pressure of 30 mm Hg or higher, found on serial examinations, as the basis for diagnosis and treatment. If the optic disc has suspicious cupping or other risk factors are involved, treatment is often started at pressures lower than 30 mm Hg.

3. *Cupping and field loss, but normal pressure*: The question of low-tension glaucoma arises, and repeated pressure measurements at various times of the day over several visits are needed. If cupping or field loss is marked, most ophthalmologists would institute therapy after obtaining diurnal pressure measurements (checking the pressure every 2 hours throughout the day).

4. *Suspicious cupping, but normal pressure*: The practitioner should obtain diurnal measurements as described above; perform visual field examination; and photograph, draw, or otherwise accurately record the exact appearance of the optic disc, including an estimate of the cup:disc ratio. If results of all tests are normal, the patient should be examined again in 6 to 12 months.

Treatment of open-angle glaucoma may involve medication, laser, or operation.

The ideal treatment for open-angle glaucoma would rectify the underlying pathophysiologic mechanism responsible for the elevated pressure. Until the underlying cause can be found, this goal remains elusive. Once the decision to treat has been made, the usual sequence of treatment is medications, followed by laser treatment, followed by filtration surgery. A β-adrenergic blocker is usually the first drug to be used, followed by the addition of a second agent (usually pilocarpine) and finally a third agent (usually an epinephrine derivative) as the situation demands. Clinicians are divided on the next step; some add a carbonic anhydrase inhibitor, and others perform laser procedures. If medications and laser therapy fail to lower the intraocular pressure adequately, they usually perform a filtration procedure.

The first-line treatment for open-angle glaucoma is eyedrops.

1. *Adrenergic agents*
   a. *β-Adrenergic blockers*: These decrease intraocular pressure by reducing aqueous humor flow up to 35%. *Timolol* (Timoptic) and *bunolol* (Betagan) are nonspecific β-adrenergic blockers (both β_1 and β_2), and *betaxolol* (Betoptic) is β_1-specific. These popular, widely used agents cause few ocular side effects. Their usage schedule of once or twice a day is convenient and encourages patient compliance. Systemic side effects may accompany use of these agents, including worsening of asthma (reportedly less so with the β_1-specific blocker betaxolol), congestive heart failure, and prolonging of atrioventricular conduction delays. Other side effects may also occur and are similar to those expected of the systemic β-adrenergic blockers.

   b. *Adrenergic agonists*:
      1) *Epinephrine* lowers intraocular pressure by several mechanisms, although they are not well understood. Classically, α-agonist activity was thought to cause vasoconstriction and thus decrease aqueous production; β-agonist activity was thought to increase aqueous outflow through the trabecular meshwork. More current research indicates that epinephrine may increase uveoscleral outflow and also may actually increase aqueous humor production in some cases. Up to 50% of patients may develop a chronic allergy to epinephrine, manifested by itchy, sore, red eyes or sometimes a contact dermatitis of the lids with dry, thickened, irritated skin. Dipivefrin (Propine) is a pro-drug of epinephrine and has a similar mode of action and side effects.

      2) *Apraclonidine* (Iopidine) is an α_2 agonist. It decreases aqueous flow by up to 35% and appears to be additive to other agents.

2. *Cholinergics.* Cholinergics stimulate ciliary muscle contraction, which increases aqueous outflow through the trabecular meshwork. Direct tendinous attachments from the ciliary muscle to the trabecular meshwork and canal of Schlemm exist, and tension on these appears to "open up" the meshwork. The small pupil associated with use of cholinergic drugs has no influence on the intraocular pressure and is an unwanted side effect of these agents. Other problems include the need for frequent application (four times a day), blur and dimness from the miotic pupil, brow ache, and induction of several diopters of myopia in younger patients.

a. *Direct-acting*: *pilocarpine, carbachol*.

b. *Indirect-acting*: cholinesterase inhibitors (*echothiophate iodide* [Phospholine Iodide], *physostigmine* [eserine]). By inhibiting the enzyme acetylcholinesterase, these agents prolong the action of endogenously released acetylcholine.

3. *Carbonic anhydrase inhibitors*. These include *methazolamide* (Neptazane) and *acetazolamide* (Diamox). Used systemically, these agents decrease aqueous humor flow by up to 35%. The medications may be associated with systemic side effects such as malaise, fatigue, depression, queasy stomach, gastrointestinal distress, kidney stone formation, and paresthesias in about a third of patients who use them on a long-term basis. Rarely, a blood dyscrasia such as aplastic anemia may occur.

Laser trabeculoplasty may be helpful in patients in whom eyedrops have not maintained adequate control of open-angle glaucoma.

Laser trabeculoplasty involves making a series of discrete laser applications to the trabecular meshwork over 180° or 360°. It is effective in approximately 70% of cases overall, although pressures may actually increase in 1% or 2% of patients. Current usage dictates that a full trial of medical therapy be used before laser therapy is considered. Laser trabeculoplasty improves aqueous outflow through the meshwork. The mechanism of this improvement is controversial. One theory holds that the heat and collagen shrinkage associated with laser treatment cause contraction of the trabecular lamellae in the vicinity of the laser site, which stretches and opens meshwork adjacent to the site. Evidence also exists for an alternative mechanism of action, trabecular cell activation and replication.

A surgical procedure may be required in refractory cases of open-angle glaucoma.

Three surgical methods are used for glaucoma.

1. In a *filtration procedure*, a new drainage route for aqueous is created surgically, allowing aqueous to enter the subconjunctival space. A full-thickness procedure creates a through-and-through hole into the anterior chamber at the limbus. A trabeculectomy first fashions a partial-thickness scleral flap and then creates the hole beneath the scleral flap. The scleral flap is designed to prevent excess run-off of aqueous, which often complicates full-thickness procedures. Fewer postoperative complications, such as hypotony, occur. A drawback to trabeculectomy, however, may be a resultant higher final postoperative pressure.

Certain cases may benefit from implantation of a *seton*, a tube, or other device to prevent scarring and closure of the sclerotomy and conjunctival drainage area created during the filtration operation. Some of these devices involve a plastic tube extending from the anterior chamber to porous plastic drainage chambers placed near the equator of the eye (the *Molteno implant*). Although they tend to have more complications than does standard filtration, they may work in eyes in which the standard operations have failed.

2. *Cyclodialysis* creates an alternative internal aqueous drainage route. By separating the ciliary body attachment from its insertion to the scleral spur, a cyclodialysis procedure allows aqueous to enter the suprachoroidal space, between sclera and choroid. Limited by a 40% success rate and the major complications of bleeding and cataract formation, cyclodialysis is usually not considered a "first-line" choice of operation and is rarely performed.

3. In a *cyclodestructive procedure*, whether done with the standard cryoprobe or with the laser, destruction of the ciliary body limits its production of aqueous and therefore reduces intraocular pressure. Major complications include pain, significant inflammation, cataract formation, and the risk of hypotony and phthisis. Because of these significant and potentially overwhelming complications, cyclodestructive procedures are used as a last resort when several other surgical procedures have failed. In some situations, however, cyclodestructive procedures may be the operation of choice, such as an eye with poor visual potential that may need a lowered pressure to alleviate pain.

Treatment for open-angle glaucoma requires a lifelong commitment for both patient and physician.

Management of glaucoma depends as much on careful observation and consistent follow-up as it does on treatment by medical, laser, and surgical techniques. The patient shares the responsibility for a satisfactory long-term program. Usually three or four examinations a year are required. A routine examination includes measurement of intraocular pressure, comparison of the disc with previous photographs, and review of the patient's medications. Periodic visual field tests are performed to detect advancement of the disease. Because intraocular pressure can follow a diurnal pattern, routine office visits should be scheduled at different times of day during the year.

Although the normal intraocular pressure range is from 10 to 22 mm Hg, an optic disc damaged from glaucoma seems more susceptible to further damage than is a nondamaged disc. As the cup enlarges, pressure must be brought lower and lower to avoid this further damage. An eye with a glaucomatous cup and "normal" pressure of 21 mm Hg may actually develop more damage because this pressure may be too high for that degree of cupping. Each patient's intraocular pressure must be viewed in light of the degree of disc damage. There is no arbitrary pressure below which all patients can be considered safe.

6

DISORDERS OF THE RETINA, VITREOUS, AND CHOROID

James P. Bolling
David C. Herman
John M. Pach

An understanding of the anatomy of the globe is important for studying diseases of the vitreous, retina, and choroid. The eye wall has three layers (Fig. 6–1). The outside layer is composed of the sclera, which anteriorly becomes the cornea. The middle layer is the uveal tract, composed of the choroid, ciliary body, and iris. The innermost layer of the eye wall is the retina.

The sclera maintains a constant ocular volume.

The *sclera* provides the tough outer coat of the eye; it protects the intraocular contents and helps maintain a constant intraocular volume. Sclera is composed largely of extracellular material and has a network of interlacing collagen fibrils. Scleral wounds heal very slowly, and in cases of scleral rupture or laceration, permanent sutures such as nylon or silk should be used. The sclera is thinnest immediately posterior to the insertion of the rectus muscles, and this portion of the sclera must be inspected carefully during the surgical repair of a suspected ruptured globe (Fig. 6–2). Posteriorly, the sclera is perforated by channels for the *short posterior ciliary nerves and arteries* and by the optic nerve.

Four to six openings in the sclera near the equator allow for the passage of the *vortex veins*, which drain the venous blood from the choroid. The sclera is also perforated near the equator at the 3 o'clock and 9 o'clock meridians by the *long ciliary nerves*, which innervate the cornea, iris, and ciliary body. The sclera is 0.3 to 0.5 mm thick in the thinnest areas and approximately 1 mm thick in the thickest areas near the optic nerve. In myopic individuals, the sclera is often thinner and may be especially thin and stretched in localized areas, which are termed *staphylomas*.

A rich sinus of blood vessels called the *choroid* lies inside the sclera. The choroid serves many important functions, including supplying oxygen and nutrients to the outer half of the retina, removing fluid from underneath the retina, and carrying heat away from the retina. The choroid may be difficult to appreciate when examining the fundus; large choroidal blood vessels, however, may be seen where the overlying pigment epithelium is thin (Fig. 6–3). Usually some variation in the pigment epithelium and often the large veins draining the choroid (vortex veins) may be seen near the equator in each of the quadrants. These vortex veins serve as important anatomic landmarks, both inside the fundus and on the outside of the globe.

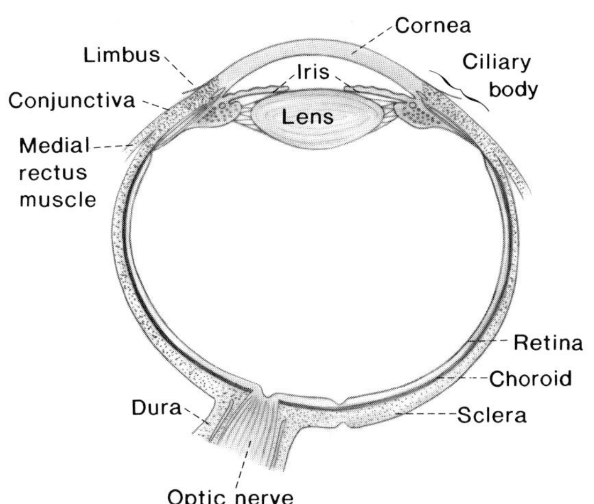

Fig. 6–1. Cross-section through the globe, showing the three layers of the eye wall. The sclera and cornea make up the outside layer. The middle layer of the eye is composed of the choroid posteriorly and the ciliary body and iris in the anterior portion of the globe. The retina lines the posterior two-thirds of the globe.

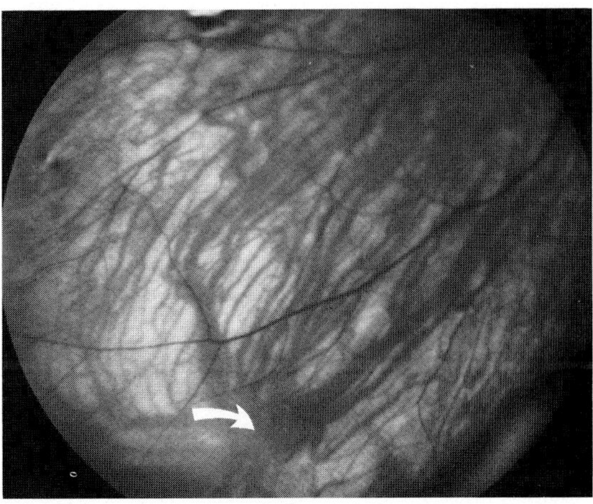

Fig. 6–3. Fundus view of the equator, showing a retinal vessel branch of the inferior temporal arcade and a large vortex vein draining the choroid (*curved arrow*).

Bruch's membrane separates the choroid and the pigment epithelium of the retina.

Bruch's membrane is a layer between the choroid and the pigment epithelium of the retina. It is partially composed of the basement membrane of the pigment epithelium and the basement membrane of the small blood vessels in the choroid (*choriocapillaris*). Between these two membranes is a layer composed of collagen and elastic tissue (Fig. 6–4). Damage to Bruch's membrane can lead to a typical degenerative response in which fibrovascular tissue grows under the retina from the choroid (choroidal neovas-

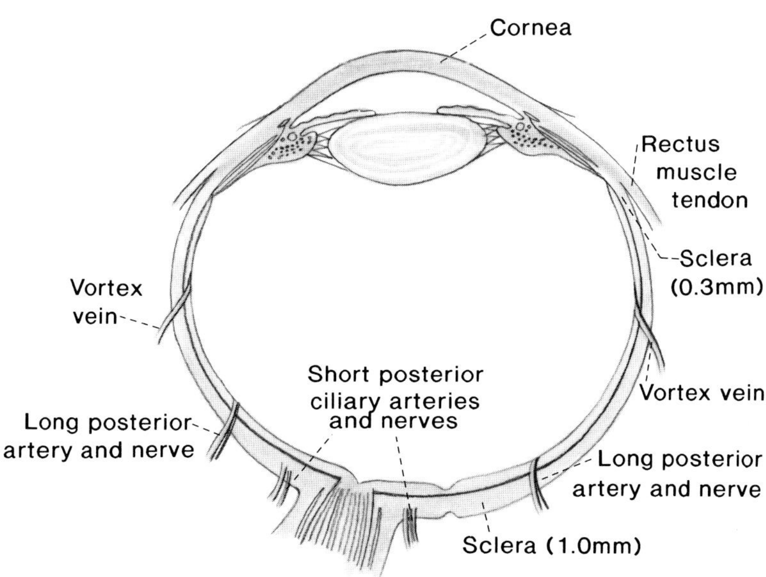

Fig. 6–2. The sclera is thickest posteriorly (1 mm) and thinnest just under the insertion of the rectus muscles (0.3 mm). The sclera is perforated posteriorly by the vortex veins, the long posterior ciliary arteries and nerves, and the short posterior ciliary arteries.

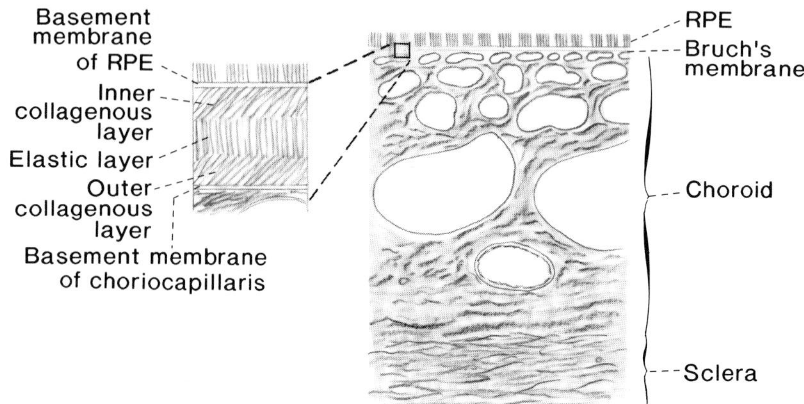

Fig. 6–4. Bruch's membrane lies between the retinal pigment epithelium (RPE) and choroid. It is composed of five layers: the basement membrane of the retinal pigment epithelium, an inner collagen layer, the elastic layer, an outer collagen layer, and the basement membrane of the choriocapillaris.

cularization). Inherent weakness in Bruch's membrane can lead to breaks known as *angioid streaks*. Angioid streaks may be associated with many different systemic conditions, such as pseudoxanthoma elasticum and Ehlers-Danlos syndrome.

The *pigment epithelium of the retina* is a monolayer of pigmented cells and blocks most of the choroid from ophthalmoscopic observation. The pigment epithelium has many important functions, including optical, mechanical, and nutritional support of the photoreceptors of the neurosensory retina. The pigment epithelium and photoreceptors are apposed but not physically attached; the potential space between the photoreceptors and the pigment epithelium is called the subretinal space.

The inner retina is horizontally oriented and the outer retina is vertically oriented.

The innermost layer of the eye wall is the *neurosensory retina*. This complex neural structure has been divided into several layers histologically (Fig. 6–5) and processes visual signals before transmitting impulses through the optic nerve to the lateral geniculate body. The outer

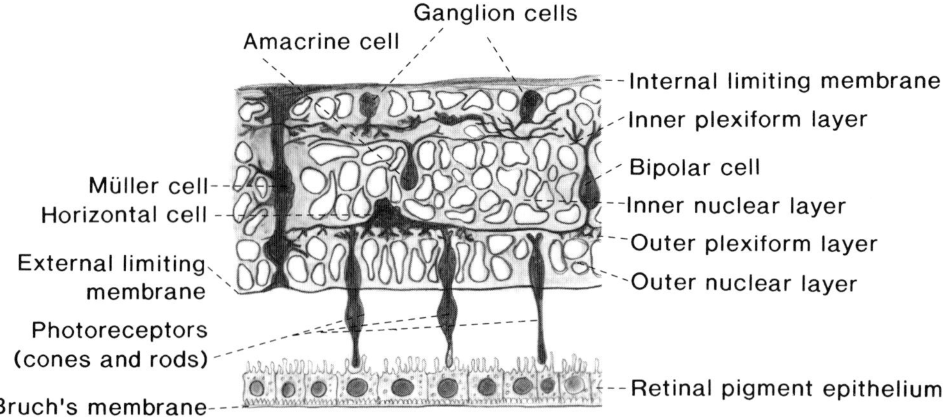

Fig. 6–5. The retina is divided into several layers histologically. Starting at the vitreous retinal interface, these layers include the internal limiting membrane, nerve fiber layer, ganglion cell layer, inner plexiform layer, inner nuclear layer, outer plexiform layer, outer nuclear layer, external limiting membrane, and the layer of rods and cones. Beneath the retina is the retinal pigment epithelium and Bruch's membrane.

layers of the retina have a vertical orientation. The inner layer of the retina (closest to the vitreous) is composed largely of the nerve fiber layer. Nerve fibers arc around the retina, transmitting information from photoreceptors. Nerve fibers do not cross the horizontal midline; damage to nerve fibers in various sections of the retina produces a characteristic visual field defect that stops at the horizontal raphe, as was discussed in Chapter 5.

The retina has its own layer of blood vessels that provide nutrition to its inner layers. This pattern of retinal blood vessels has a striking appearance when the fundus is viewed with an ophthalmoscope. The arteries can be differentiated from veins by size and color; arteries are thinner in caliber and brighter red. Arteries and veins intersect at many points in the fundus; it should be remembered, however, that arteries never cross arteries and veins never cross veins. This information may be helpful in analyzing vascular occlusions to determine whether a particular blood vessel is an artery or vein. Retinal vessels may serve as an indicator of the degree of atherosclerotic change in blood vessels elsewhere in the body.

Certain important fundus findings reflect the unique retinal anatomy. *Myelinated nerve fibers*, *cotton-wool spots*, and *flame-shaped retinal hemorrhages* (Fig. 6–6) are all found in the superficial (inner layers) of the retina. They have a distinctive feathered edge and obscure underlying retinal details. Hemorrhages deeper in the retina have a blot or dot appearance. Changes in the retinal pigment epithelium such as an increase or decrease in the density of the pigment can be observed to be under the neuroretina and are crossed over by the retinal vessels. Defects in Bruch's membrane may cause overlying changes in the pigment epithelium of the retina or changes in the vascular pattern of the choroid. Occlusion of a portion of the choroid results in atrophy of the overlying retinal pigment epithelium and neuroretina.

Diabetic retinopathy is a major retinal cause of blindness.

Diabetic retinopathy accounts for 7% to 20% of new cases of blindness each year, depending on the population studied. Diabetes

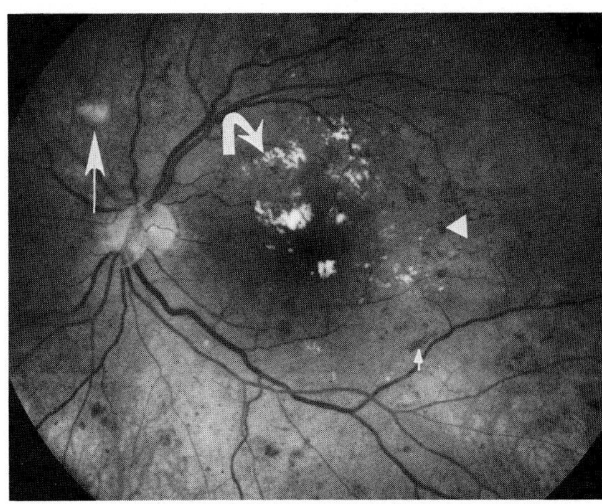

Fig. 6–6. Fundus in a diabetic patient reveals abnormalities of several layers of the retina. The *small arrow* shows a flame-shaped hemorrhage. The *large arrow* above the optic nerve indicates a cotton-wool spot. Exudates are present in the superior aspect of the macula, as indicated by the *curved arrow*. A dot retinal hemorrhage is designated by the *arrowhead*.

is becoming a more common cause of new cases of blindness despite the development of laser and vitrectomy procedures. Diabetes is becoming more frequent in the general population and, in addition, diabetics are living longer and have a greater chance of experiencing the long-term complications of the disease.

Diabetic retinopathy reflects the severity of the diabetes.

The incidence of retinopathy is correlated with the duration of the diabetes. Whereas 10% to 30% of diabetics who have had diabetes for 5 years may have some form of retinopathy, 75% to 95% of diabetics who have had diabetes for 15 years have retinopathy. Diabetic retinopathy is more common in hypertensive patients. Although a direct cause-and-effect relationship has not been established, theoretically hypertension would accelerate the course of diabetic retinopathy. Similarly, diabetic retinopathy is more common in patients who have diabetic nephropathy; although kidney disease might exacerbate retinopathy, a cause-and-effect relationship has not been proved.

Good control of hyperglycemia may delay the progression of diabetic retinopathy. Longitudinal and cross-sectional studies demon-

TABLE 6–1 Ophthalmoscopic Features of Diabetic Retinopathy

Venous dilation
Microaneurysms
Intraretinal hemorrhages
Macular edema
Hard exudates
Cotton-wool spots (nerve fiber layer infarcts)
Venous beading and loops
Intraretinal microvascular abnormalities
Neovascularization of the retina
Tractional retinal detachment
Vitreous hemorrhage
Macular dragging

strate that diabetics who have poor control are at greater risk for developing retinopathy. Although no prospective studies conclusively prove that poor control accelerates diabetic retinopathy in humans, research has shown that poor control hastens the onset of retinopathy in animals.

Diabetes may affect the entire eye. One common problem is a shift in refractive error associated with fluctuations in blood glucose concentrations. Diabetics may have reduced corneal sensation, a greater incidence of glaucoma and cataract, and pupils that are poorly reactive. Diabetic neuropathy may involve the third, fourth, or sixth cranial nerves and result in double vision. The most serious ocular complication of the disease is diabetic retinopathy. Diabetic retinopathy is classified as *nonproliferative* or *proliferative* on the basis of the absence or presence of neovascularization of the retina. Table 6–1 lists the fundus findings common in diabetes.

Diabetic retinopathy results from damage to small blood vessels.

Venous dilation is one of the early features of diabetic retinopathy. In otherwise normal fundi, diabetics have a 10% increase in vein width (measured on fundus photographs). As the changes of diabetic retinopathy become more severe, veins often become darker and irregular. With advanced retinopathy, venous loops and venous beading are frequent.

One of the more obvious fundus findings in diabetic retinopathy is *retinal hemorrhages*. These hemorrhages may occur deep in the retina (*dot/blot hemorrhages*) or may occur in the superficial retina and assume a *flame-shaped* appearance. Although retinal hemorrhages are sometimes striking in appearance, they may be present for years without significant visual loss.

Cotton-wool spots or *soft exudates* (Fig. 6–6) represent focal infarcts of the nerve fiber layer. These fluffy white patches in the superficial retina typically occur along the arcades and are considered a sign of retinal ischemia. They may also be present early in the course of diabetic retinopathy and do not necessarily indicate impending neovascularization, as once thought.

Microaneurysms are outpouchings in blood vessel walls. These vascular abnormalities are near the limit of resolution of the ophthalmoscope and may be visible only on fluorescein angiography. Two types of cells are present in retinal capillaries: endothelial cells and pericytes. Pericytes usually occur in a 1:1 ratio with endothelial cells. Microaneurysms sometimes occur where pericytes are lost. Changes in the permeability of the capillary walls allow serum to leak from the blood vessels into the retina. This accumulation of extracellular fluid in the retina can be observed clinically as a retinal thickening (edema). Commonly associated with retinal edema are hard exudates (Fig. 6–6) or bright-yellow lipoprotein condensations in the retina. These exudates frequently assume a circular arrangement in the retina centered about a cluster of microaneurysms or one very large microaneurysm.

Macular edema is an important cause of poor vision in diabetics.

Diabetic *macular edema* is found in about 10% of the diabetic population and directly correlates with the severity of the retinopathy. It is most common in patients with proliferative diabetic retinopathy. This is the result of abnormal leakage of macromolecules and ions from the retinal capillaries.

Macular edema can be categorized as *focal* or *diffuse*. Focal edema is characterized by clusters of microaneurysms with localized retinal thickening. Fluorescein angiography confirms that the major source of leakage is from the microaneurysms. Exudate rings may also be found around the areas of leakage. Large plaquelike lipid deposits within the fovea are associated with a poor prognosis and may lead to focal metaplasia of the retinal pigment epithelium.

Diffuse diabetic macular edema results from the generalized breakdown of the inner blood retinal barrier. It also has been suggested that retinal pigment epithelial dysfunction may contribute to diffuse edema.

Macular edema may improve spontaneously, but it is more likely to resolve in some cases if laser treatment is applied. The Early Treatment Diabetic Retinopathy Study (ETDRS) showed that laser treatment in selected cases of macular edema can reduce the risks of visual loss by one-half. Any patient with visual loss due to macular edema should be evaluated by an individual experienced in the treatment of diabetes.

Proliferative diabetic retinopathy indicates a poor prognosis.

Proliferative diabetic retinopathy is characterized by the growth of abnormal vessels between the retina and the posterior vitreous face. This may occur on the optic nerve (*neovascularization of the disc, NVD*) (Fig. 6–7) or away from the optic nerve (*neovascularization "elsewhere," NVE*) (Fig. 6–8). As the posterior vitreous face slowly collapses and pulls away from the retina, traction may be exerted on these fri-

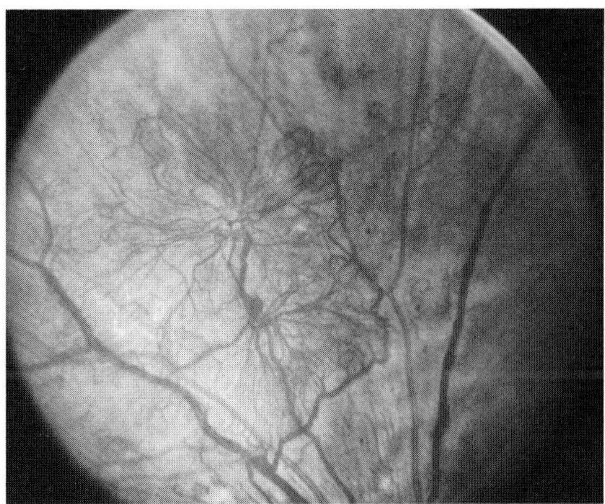

Fig. 6–8. Photograph from above the optic nerve in a patient with diabetes, showing neovascularization elsewhere (NVE) (away from the nerve).

able vessels, producing a preretinal or vitreous hemorrhage. The neovascularization may also fibrose and exert traction on the retina and cause a retinal detachment.

Neovascularization of the retina is a response to ischemia. It is believed that an *angiogenesis factor* is liberated by the retina in response to this ischemia. Fluorescein angiography may demonstrate retinal capillary nonperfusion (Fig. 6–9). Neovascularization of the retina and retinal capillary nonperfusion (on fluores-

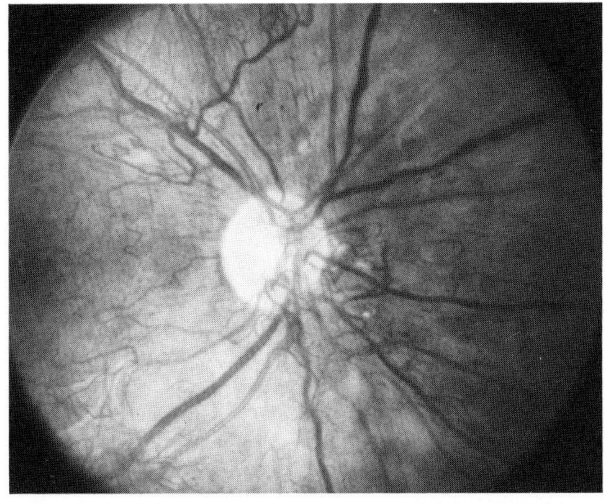

Fig. 6–7. The optic nerve of a patient with diabetes, showing extensive neovascularization of the disc (*NVD*).

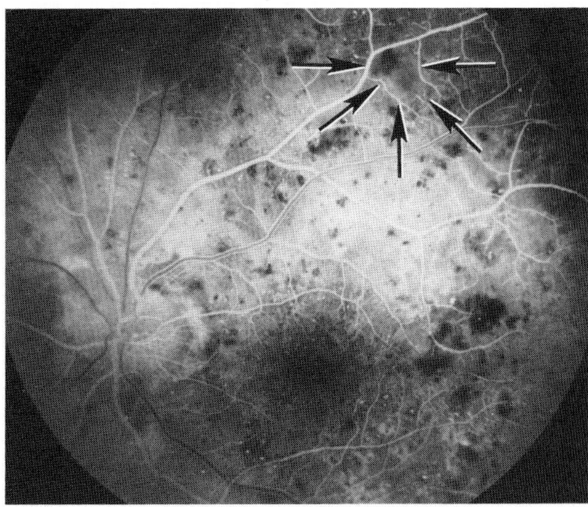

Fig. 6–9. Laminar venous phase of a fluorescein angiogram in a patient with diabetes, showing several areas of capillary nonperfusion; one of them is indicated by the *arrows*. The hyperfluorescent spots are microaneurysms.

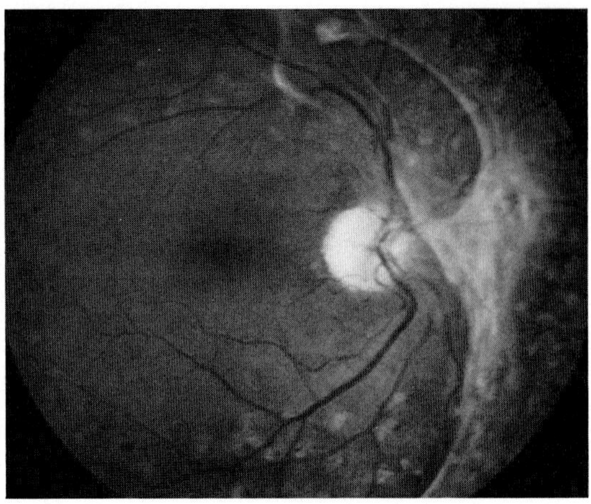

Fig. 6–10.   Right eye of a patient with diabetes; multiple laser spots (panretinal photocoagulation) are seen outside the arcades.

cein angiography) are signs of retinal ischemia, as is venous dilation.

As outlined in Table 6–2, visual loss due to proliferative diabetic retinopathy can be prevented in some cases with laser treatment (*panretinal photocoagulation*) (Fig. 6–10). Laser therapy may work by reducing the amount of ischemic retina or it may increase the delivery of nutrients to the retina.

TABLE 6-2   Usefulness of Panretinal Photocoagulation for Preventing Severe Visual Loss in Eyes with High-Risk Characteristics (3 Years After Treatment)

Characteristics of eyes	*Treated eyes, %*	*Control eyes, %*
Neovascularization elsewhere greater than 0.5 disc diameter in area and vitreous hemorrhage	7	30
Neovascularization of the disc less than 0.5 disc diameter in area and vitreous hemorrhage	4	26
Neovascularization of the disc greater than 0.5 disc diameter in area and no hemorrhage	9	26
Neovascularization of the disc greater than 0.5 disc diameter in area and vitreous hemorrhage	20	37

Neovascularization may lead to vitreous hemorrhage.

As traction is exerted on the neovascularization of the retina, a vitreous hemorrhage can occur. Patients usually experience a sudden onset of numerous floaters and loss of vision. If the visualization of the posterior segment is poor, ultrasonography can be used to determine the simultaneous presence of a retinal detachment.

Initial treatment of a vitreous hemorrhage is usually observation. Serial ultrasonography may be needed to monitor for the development of a retinal detachment. Most hemorrhages clear within 6 months. As the hemorrhage clears, the retina must be examined carefully to look for NVD or NVE. If neovascularization is present, panretinal photocoagulation should be performed. If the vitreous hemorrhage does not clear or if it is associated with a macular traction detachment, vitrectomy, membrane peeling, and photocoagulation may be considered.

A central retinal vein occlusion may be associated with systemic disease.

A *central retinal vein occlusion* has a characteristic history and fundus appearance (Fig. 6–11). Individuals usually complain of acute painless loss of vision in one eye. An afferent pupillary defect is typically present, and the fundus shows a pattern of scattered retinal hemorrhages, dilated and tortuous retinal veins, and retinal edema. Predisposing conditions include diabetes mellitus, glaucoma, hypertension, and abnormalities of blood viscosity, including polycythemia, sickle cell disease, and dysproteinemias.

There are two types of central retinal vein occlusion.

The visual acuity and prognosis after a central retinal vein occlusion are variable. The occlusion is classified as nonischemic or ischemic.

In *nonischemic central retinal vein occlusion*, patients usually complain of moderate visual loss. The visual acuity is usually 20/200 or bet-

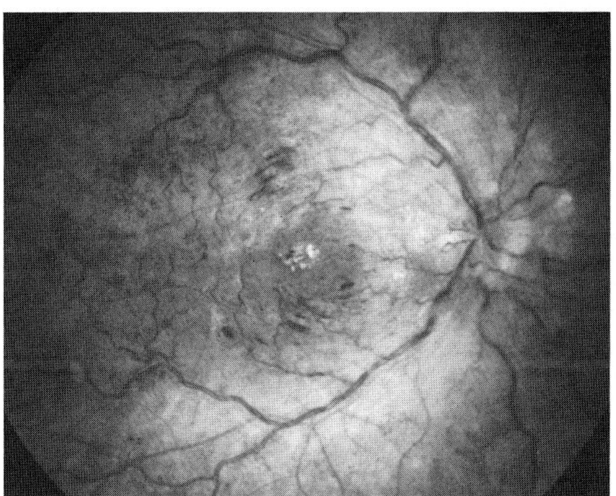

Fig. 6–11. Central retinal vein occlusion in the right eye. The nerve fiber layer and inner retina are thickened. Multiple flame-shaped retinal hemorrhages are present. A cotton-wool spot is present at nasal aspect of the optic nerve.

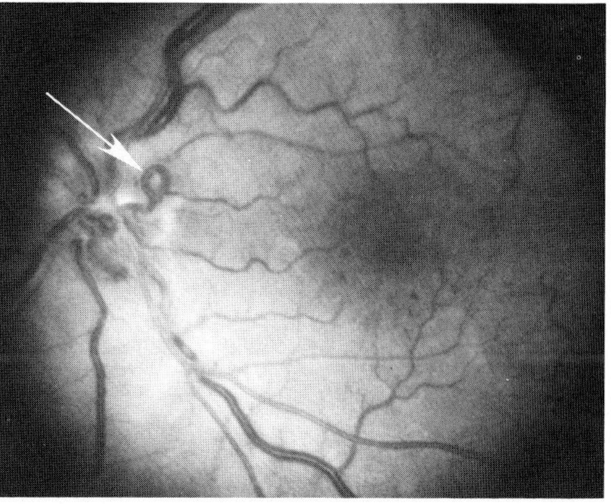

Fig. 6–12. Chronic central retinal vein occlusion. A venous collateral (*arrow*) is draining blood from the retinal veins into the choroidal circulation to bypass the obstruction at the disc.

ter. There may be mild optic disc swelling and dilated tortuous veins with scattered intraretinal hemorrhages. There are usually no cotton-wool spots. On fluorescein angiography, there is no evidence of capillary nonperfusion. Occasionally, these patients may improve spontaneously. A small percentage, however, may progress to the ischemic form.

Ischemic central retinal vein occlusion may lead to neovascular glaucoma.

Ischemic (hemorrhagic) central retinal vein occlusion is typified by a severe visual loss, usually worse than 20/200. Marked disc swelling, diffuse confluent intraretinal hemorrhages, cotton-wool spots, and diffuse retinal thickening with cystoid macular edema are seen. Fluorescein angiography reveals a delay in filling of the retinal circulation with severe capillary dropout. It is frequently difficult to visualize retinal vessels on fluorescein angiography because of the widespread intraretinal hemorrhages. Confluent retinal hemorrhages signify massive capillary damage.

Significant retinal ischemia may lead to retinal or iris neovascularization and neovascular glaucoma. Neovascular glaucoma usually occurs 3 months after the onset of the vein occlusion. Coexistent retinal arterial disease may ac-

count for the severity of this form of retinal vein occlusion.

The prognosis for vein occlusions depends on the degree of obstruction. Patients with a mild degree of obstruction may suffer minimal loss of vision and the fundus may return to its normal appearance. Others may have a more progressive course with permanent changes in visual acuity due to persistence of cystoid macular edema, macular ischemia, and retinal pigment epithelial changes. Peripapillary retinal-choroidal venous collaterals may form to bypass the obstruction (Fig. 6–12).

Management is aimed at identifying any underlying systemic disease and monitoring for neovascular glaucoma. Patients who exhibit a large degree of capillary dropout on fluorescein angiography may benefit from prophylactic panretinal photocoagulation. If the degree of ischemia cannot be determined, close follow-up is necessary. At the first sign of rubeosis (neovascularization of the iris), panretinal photocoagulation should be performed. If laser treatment cannot be performed because of opacities of the media, such as cataract, transconjunctival cryopexy may be considered.

Branch retinal vein occlusion occurs at arterial-venous crossings.

Branch retinal vein occlusion occurs most commonly at an arterial-venous crossing point.

The fundus appearance is diagnostic, with dilated retinal veins, microaneurysms, intraretinal hemorrhages, cotton-wool spots, and retinal thickening in the retinal sector drained by the affected vein (Fig. 6–13). The degree of visual loss is dependent on the extent of macular involvement. Macular edema, foveal hemorrhages, and dropout of the parafoveal capillaries contribute to the visual loss.

As the obstruction resolves, collaterals can be seen bridging the site of the occlusion and along the horizontal raphe. Although the visual acuity may improve spontaneously, vision may be permanently decreased because of the persistent macular edema. Retinal neovascularization may develop and lead to vitreous hemorrhage.

Medical treatment has not been shown to be of any benefit in branch retinal vein occlusion. Scattered laser photocoagulation in the distribution of the occluded vessel is necessary when neovascularization develops. If macular edema persists for more than 3 months and visual acuity is 20/40 or worse, macular laser photocoagulation can be considered. A grid pattern of burns is placed in the area of retinal edema and outside the foveal avascular zone in the distribution of the occluded vessel.

Retinal vein occlusion may rarely occur as a result of inflammation along the retinal veins. These veins appear sheathed. Such venous occlusions may occur in sarcoidosis or infectious retinitis.

Central retinal artery occlusion causes retinal whitening.

Occlusion of the central retinal artery or one of its branches can be caused by embolization or by thrombosis. Emboli are usually from the carotid artery and less commonly from the heart. The patient with a central retinal artery occlusion presents with a sudden monocular loss of vision. This may be preceded by episodes of amaurosis fugax. The visual loss is usually severe and an afferent pupillary defect is present.

Fundus examination reveals retinal arterial narrowing and segmentation of the blood column. Emboli may be visible on the optic nerve head or at distal bifurcations of the arterioles. The macula appears white or opaque except for a normal-appearing fovea. The fovea maintains its transparency because the retina is thin there. Other focal areas of the retina may be spared by a patent cilioretinal artery (Fig. 6–14). Within several weeks, the retina regains its normal transparency, but retinal atrophy and optic atrophy follow.

Irreversible retinal changes occur after 90 minutes of obstructed arterial blood flow. Immediate treatment, therefore, is imperative. A

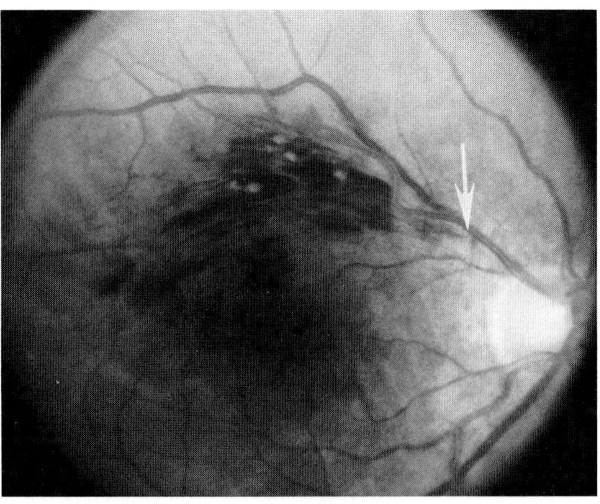

Fig. 6–13. Branch retinal vein occlusion in the right eye. The *arrow* indicates the point of obstruction. Five cotton-wool spots are present in the distribution of the retinal hemorrhages.

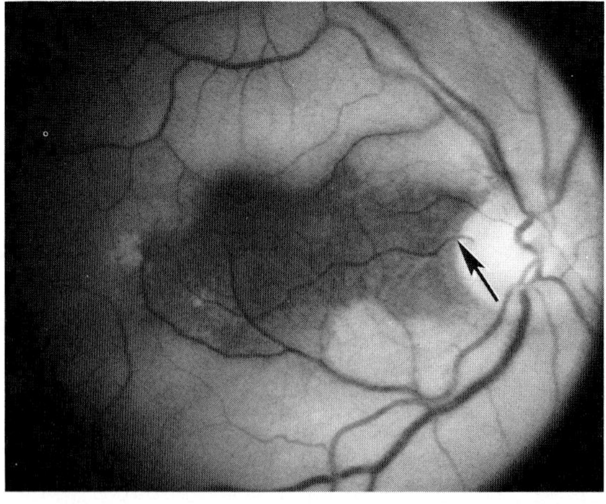

Fig. 6–14. Central retinal artery occlusion in the right eye. The remaining area of normal retina is supplied by a cilioretinal artery (*arrow*).

few patients have improved when treatment was given within the first day. Patients who present within 24 hours should be considered for treatment. Therapy is directed at lowering the intraocular pressure to restore blood flow and possibly moving the embolus distally. Digital massage, osmotic diuretics, and anterior chamber paracentesis are all methods of lowering the intraocular pressure. Inhaling a combination of 95% oxygen and 5% carbon dioxide (carbogen) has been recommended to produce arterial dilation. Even with heroic efforts, the prognosis for central retinal artery occlusion is dismal. Careful attention should be directed at finding the cause of the obstruction. The erythrocyte sedimentation rate should be determined without delay in all elderly patients to rule out the possibility of giant cell arteritis. A thorough medical evaluation is also indicated to identify a cardiac or vascular source of the embolus.

Obstruction of a branch of the central retinal artery produces a focal whitening of the retina that does not cross the horizontal raphe. An embolus may be noted at a bifurcation of a vessel. A branch retinal artery occlusion typically causes a visual field defect.

Carotid artery disease may simulate central retinal vein occlusion.

Atherosclerotic carotid artery disease may produce a picture similar to nonischemic central retinal vein occlusion (*venous stasis retinopathy*). Fundus examination reveals a normal disc with dilated veins and scattered intraretinal hemorrhages noted predominantly in the periphery (Fig. 6–15). The central retinal artery pressure can be measured in the office and is low; this characteristic is in contrast to central retinal vein occlusion, in which the central retinal artery pressure is normal. The veins are frequently irregular in caliber in addition to being dark and dilated. Microaneurysms occur similar to those that are found in diabetic retinopathy. Capillary nonperfusion may occur and is frequently most marked in the peripheral retina.

The retinal ischemia sometimes leads to neovascularization of the iris. This usually occurs with a high-grade carotid stenosis or carotid occlusion. Because a very low ophthal-

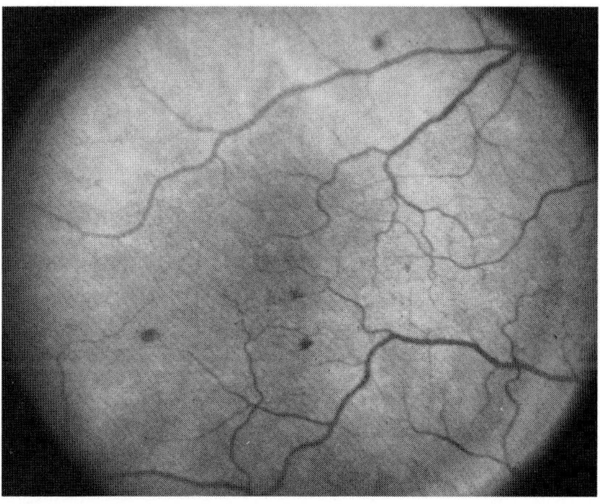

Fig. 6–15. An equatorial view in a patient with venous stasis retinopathy, showing scattered blot retinal hemorrhages.

mic artery pressure is required to produce this syndrome, it is usually seen with bilateral carotid disease. An intracranial blood flow "steal" is probably necessary to produce this syndrome in addition to the carotid stenosis.

Low ophthalmic artery pressure due to carotid artery disease can also lead to the development of a cataract, hypotony, and intraocular inflammation. The result of prolonged ocular hypoperfusion is neovascular glaucoma and phthisis (ocular ischemia syndrome).

Although frequently little can be done to improve the vision in an ischemic eye, laser treatment and cryotherapy may be helpful in preventing the eye from becoming painful. In addition, it is important to recognize the underlying vascular cause of the patient's problem because some patients are at significant risk of having a stroke.

There are three types of arterial emboli: cholesterol, calcific, and fibrin-platelet.

Cholesterol emboli (*Hollenhorst plaques*) may be a sign of carotid artery disease. These emboli are frequently asymptomatic and usually do not cause complete occlusion of the arteriole in which they lodge. Cholesterol emboli are highly refractile and yellow and have a typical appearance (Fig. 6–16). Although most cholesterol emboli originate in the carotid arteries, many patients also have associated coronary ar-

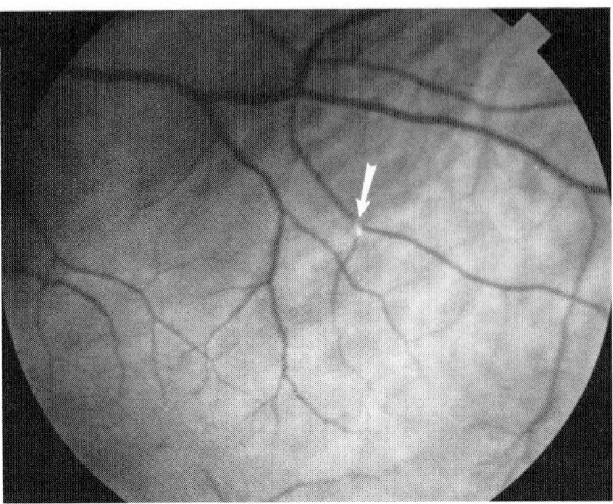

Fig. 6–16. Hollenhorst plaque (*arrow*) lodged at a branch point in a retinal arteriole.

tery disease. Patients with cholesterol emboli should have a thorough physical examination.

Calcific emboli are white, are typically much smaller than cholesterol emboli, and frequently result in an occlusion of the artery in which they lodge (Fig. 6–17). Calcific emboli originate in the great vessels, but they also may come from the valves of the heart.

Fibrin-platelet emboli are long, are dull in color, and frequently occlude the artery in which they lodge. They may come from the heart or great vessels.

Any of these findings of atherosclerotic vascular disease may be accompanied by the classic symptom of transient monocular blindness.

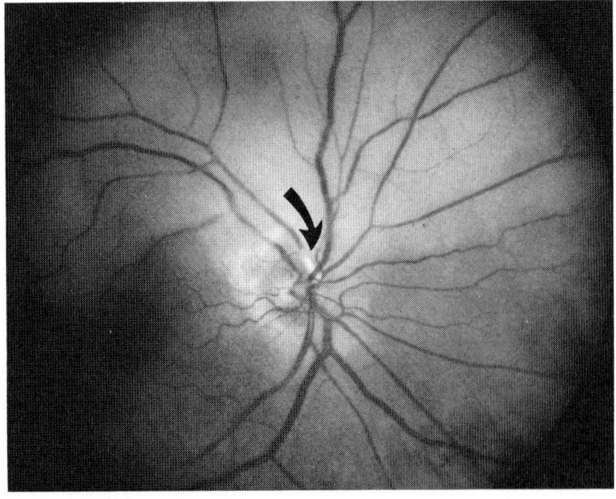

Fig. 6–17. A calcific plaque (*arrow*) at the disc causing a retinal artery occlusion.

This is termed *amaurosis fugax* and typically lasts from several minutes to 2 hours. It is helpful to elicit a history of covering the good eye to determine whether the symptoms were truly in one eye or were hemianopic (that is, corresponding loss of visual field in both eyes is indicative of a lesion posterior to the optic chiasm). A small number of patients with amaurosis fugax will proceed to develop a hemispheric stroke. The annual risk of stroke is only about 0.5% to 2% in patients with amaurosis fugax. Because patients with other symptoms of transient ischemic attacks such as transient hemiplegia are at a greater risk of stroke, all patients with amaurosis fugax should be questioned for other symptoms.

Systemic hypertension is associated with arterial narrowing.

Systemic hypertension leads to retinal arterial narrowing and arterial-venous crossing changes that parallel the severity of the disease. Focal constrictions in arterioles correlate with hypertension. Occlusion of the precapillary arterioles results in an ischemic infarct of the nerve fiber layer referred to as a cotton-wool spot. Abnormal vascular permeability leads to retinal hemorrhages, edema, and hard exudates. Malignant hypertension is characterized by optic nerve swelling and a macular star. Patients who present with bilateral disc swelling should be routinely screened for hypertension during the initial workup. Patients with hypertension are also more likely to develop ischemic optic neuropathy, branch vein occlusions, and arterial macroaneurysms.

Patients with forms of sickle disease are likely to develop proliferative sickle retinopathy.

Many diseases can lead to poor perfusion of the peripheral retina and segmental neovascularization. The classic example of a peripheral proliferative retinopathy is proliferative *sickle retinopathy*. Patients with sickle cell disease have an abnormal gene for hemoglobin (hemoglobin S or hemoglobin C). If patients have one normal gene and one S gene, they have sickle trait. Patients with sickle cell disease have both alleles for hemoglobin S. Patients with one S gene and one C gene have SC disease. Sickle retinopathy is common in patients with SC sickle cell disease. Patients with SS disease may develop proliferative sickle retinopathy, but less often than do patients with SC disease. Patients with sickle trait do not develop proliferative retinopathy unless diabetes is also present. Patients with both sickle trait and thalassemia trait are also at significant risk for developing a peripheral proliferative retinopathy (sickle cell thalassemia).

Sickle retinopathy develops as the peripheral arterioles become occluded. Arterial-venous anastomoses develop and eventually neovascularization occurs at the border between perfused and nonperfused retina. This may lead to vitreous hemorrhage and retinal detachment.

Hemorrhage can occur beneath the retina and promote retinal pigment epithelial hyperplasia (sunburst spots). Intraretinal hemorrhages may reabsorb with iridescent or refractile deposits. Other findings include conjunctival capillary stasis, central retinal artery or central retinal vein occlusion, perifoveal capillary obstruction, and angioid streaks. The peripheral neovascularization (sea fans) may spontaneously regress. Photocoagulation of poorly perfused retina or the feeder vessel may be effective in preventing vitreous hemorrhage.

Retinopathy of prematurity may progress to retinal detachment and blindness.

Retinopathy of prematurity is a disease of premature infants. Babies born at a very young gestational age frequently require oxygen, multiple drugs, and respiratory assistance for survival. These agents may have some effect on the retinal vessels, which are immature and incompletely developed in extreme prematurity. Many babies born before 36 weeks' gestation develop some form of retinopathy of prematurity. This usually regresses spontaneously, although a small percentage of infants proceed to develop a total retinal detachment.

Judicious limitation of oxygen to only the level necessary to ensure survival is suggested.

Most nurseries use pulse oximetry to maintain continuous monitoring of oxygen saturation in neonates. Other risk factors include low birth weight (less than 2,000 g), gestational age, xanthine administration, and the number of ventilator hours.

Retinopathy of prematurity has been *classified into five stages*. Stage 1 is characterized by a demarcation line that separates avascular from vascular retina. In stage 2 the demarcation line forms an elevated ridge. In stage 3 the ridge is present along with neovascularization of the retina, which extends into the vitreous cavity. Stage 4 is a retinal detachment in conjunction with the previous findings. Stage 5 is a total retinal detachment. In addition to the stage of active retinopathy, the location of the disease is important. The more posteriorly located the disease, the poorer the prognosis. In addition to the stage and location of the disease, *plus disease* (engorged posterior veins and tortuous arterioles) is a poor prognostic sign.

A cooperative multicenter prospective study has shown that cryotherapy of the peripheral avascular retina in retinopathy of prematurity is beneficial for patients who have extensive stage 3 disease and plus disease. Any premature infant whose birth weight was less than 2,000 g and any whose birth weight was between 2,000 and 2,500 g who received supplemental oxygen should be examined before dismissal from the nursery. The best time to examine a patient is a matter of controversy.

Other diseases that cause ischemia of the peripheral retina, such as carotid artery disease, multiple retinal emboli, diabetes, peripheral branch retinal vein occlusion, and inflammatory diseases of the peripheral retinal veins (sarcoidosis and syphilitic chorioretinitis), can all cause neovascularization of the peripheral retina (Table 6–3).

Retinitis pigmentosa causes night blindness.

Retinitis pigmentosa is a hereditary retinal dystrophy characterized by disc pallor, arteriolar narrowing, and clumping of pigment in the peripheral retina (Fig. 6–18). This pigment clumping causes the peculiar fundus appear-

TABLE 6–3 Diseases Associated with Peripheral Retinal Neovascularization

Sickle cell disease
Diabetes
Retinopathy of prematurity
Familial exudative vitreoretinopathy
Chronic retinal detachment
Multiple arterial emboli
Ocular ischemia (carotid artery disease)
Pulseless disease
Sarcoidosis
Pars planitis
Syphilis
Eales disease
Peripheral branch retinal vein occlusion

ance known as *"bone spicules."* Patients with retinitis pigmentosa usually present with complaints of poor night vision or a decreased visual field. The problem usually begins in the equatorial retina and proceeds posteriorly and anteriorly until the entire retina is involved. Patients with retinitis pigmentosa may have good central visual acuity for many years, although vision is usually poor in low light levels. Posterior subcapsular cataracts are frequent, and these patients may develop a particular macular finding suggestive of cystoid macular edema. Although monocular retinitis pigmentosa has been reported, typically retinitis pigmentosa is bilaterally symmetric.

Retinitis pigmentosa is a defect of the photo-receptors affecting primarily rods. Although the cause of retinitis pigmentosa is unknown, it may be associated with several systemic conditions. For example, retinitis pigmentosa occurring with deafness is called *Usher's syndrome.* The clinical entity of retinitis pigmentosa is most likely caused by many metabolic defects.

The ophthalmoscopic features of retinitis pigmentosa may be subtle in lightly pigmented individuals. The diagnosis can be confirmed with electrophysiologic testing, specifically electroretinography. Although no treatment for retinitis pigmentosa is known, patients should be evaluated for coexistent systemic disorders and genetic counseling should be offered.

Several conditions may simulate retinitis pigmentosa (*pseudoretinitis pigmentosa*). These conditions (Table 6–4) may often be differentiated from retinitis pigmentosa by electrophysiologic testing.

Stargardt's disease is a form of juvenile macular disease.

Stargardt's disease is a macular dystrophy that typically results in a perifoveal defect of the retinal pigment epithelium. The typical fundus appearance of a patient with Stargardt's disease is described as *bull's-eye maculopathy.* Stargardt's disease usually becomes symptomatic in the first or second decade of life, and visual acuity may vary from 20/30 to 20/200. Fluorescein angiography may be helpful in diagnosing the condition by displaying the typical pigmentary changes.

There is an accumulation of lipofuscin in the retinal pigment epithelium in Stargardt's disease. Stargardt's disease also may have a peripheral form associated with it in which flecks

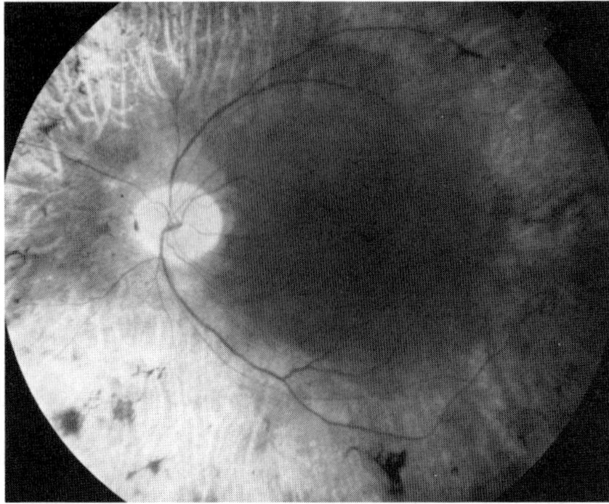

Fig. 6–18. Left eye of a patient with retinitis pigmentosa. Notice the optic atrophy, arteriolar narrowing, and pigmentary changes.

TABLE 6–4 Ocular Conditions That Can Mimic Retinitis Pigmentosa

Traumatic pigmentary retinopathy
Syphilitic chorioretinitis
Viral retinitis
Choroidal insufficiency
Extensive grouped hypertrophy of the retinal
 pigment epithelium
Chronic retinal detachment

of abnormal retinal pigment epithelium are found in the posterior pole and equatorial retina. This form gives a typical fundus appearance and is termed *fundus flavimaculatus.*

Macular degeneration is the most common cause of decreased vision in the elderly.

Macular degeneration is a degenerative eye disease found primarily in the elderly population. Some form of macular degeneration occurs in at least 20% of individuals older than 65 years. It is uncommon to find visually significant macular degeneration in an individual younger than 60 years. If findings suggestive of macular degeneration are present in a younger individual, an inherited retinal dystrophy such as Stargardt's disease or a form of acquired macular disease such as drug toxicity, trauma, myopic degeneration, or angioid streaks should be considered.

Macular degeneration usually presents with a decrease in central vision in one eye, although the disorder is always bilateral. The fellow eye usually experiences a similar loss of central vision within months or years. The cause of macular degeneration is unknown. Theories have been proposed suggesting that light toxicity, nutritional deficiencies, vascular insufficiency, and hereditary factors may play a role. Individuals with blue eyes are at higher risk for macular degeneration than those with brown eyes.

Drusen are an early sign of macular degeneration.

One of the early clinical signs of macular degeneration is the formation of drusen. *Drusen* are deposits located between the pigment epithelium and Bruch's membrane. Their location deep in the retina can be confirmed by the observation of retinal vessels coursing in front of these yellow spots (Fig. 6–19). Drusen are usually clustered in the macula, but they also may be found elsewhere in the fundus. Drusen may vary somewhat in appearance from a small white dot to a larger yellow dome-shaped lesion. Larger drusen have been characterized as "soft" and appear to be more commonly as-

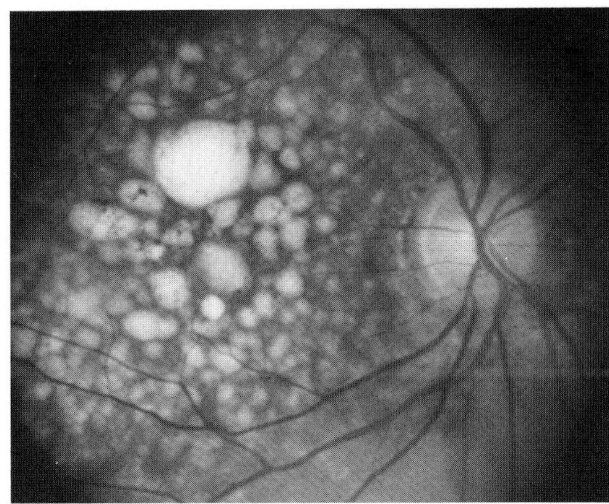

Fig. 6–19. Right eye with drusen.

sociated with visual loss due to neovascularization. Drusen are not usually visually significant, but they are important as a marker of potential visual loss due to more extensive macular degeneration. Drusen may sometimes affect the vision if they occur confluently or extend directly under the fovea. Most patients with drusen do not progress to the other sequelae of macular degeneration. Patients who have drusen should be cautioned, however, to seek medical attention if they notice a change in central vision.

The more visually disabling forms of macular degeneration can be divided into two categories: wet and dry.

Wet macular degeneration occurs when abnormal blood vessels (neovascularization) form under the retina. This complication of macular degeneration leads to rapid loss of central vision. Neovascularization can also occur in choroidal rupture, in angioid streaks, at the margin of laser scars, or in scars due to inflammation in the choroid, such as in the presumed ocular histoplasmosis syndrome (POHS).

The typical appearance of subretinal neovascularization is a gray-green area of pigment under the retina. In addition, retinal thickening (from macular edema) may occur over this area of pigment. A subretinal hemorrhage is frequently due to neovascularization. Retinal exudates may surround a neovascular membrane.

Although macular degeneration is always

bilateral, it is frequently asymmetric. A typical patient presents with blurred vision in one eye. Patients may complain of images appearing larger in one eye than in the other or of straight lines appearing curved with one eye. A gray area may occur in the central vision. Patients with known macular degeneration may notice a new scotoma on the Amsler grid chart when neovascularization develops.

Extrafoveal choroidal neovascularization may be treatable.

Neovascularization can be destroyed with laser photocoagulation. In a large multicenter prospective controlled study, this treatment has been shown to be effective when the neovascularization can be clearly identified and occurs at least 200 μm from the center of the foveal avascular zone. It is very important to recognize extrafoveal subretinal neovascularization because these new vessel membranes may later grow under the fovea and make treatment impractical (Fig. 6–20).

One must be familiar with the anatomy of the macula to understand the treatment of macular degeneration. On clinical examination, the macula is the area of the retina circumscribed by the superior and inferior temporal vascular arcades. The fovea is the area of retina corresponding to the highest level of visual acuity. It is located in the center of the macula and is darker in color. This dark area is

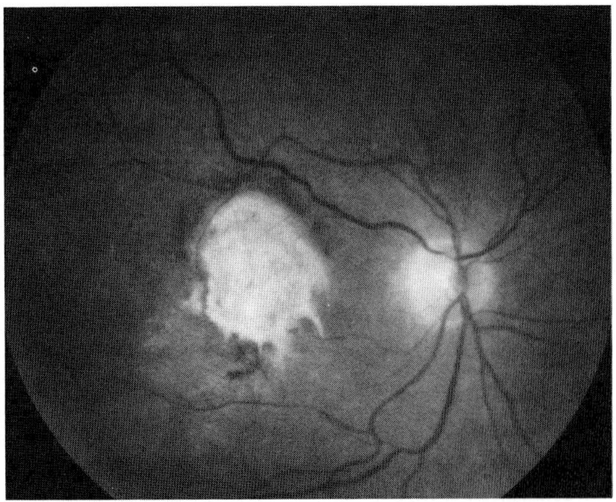

Fig. 6–20. The right eye of a patient with end-stage macular degeneration. A large subretinal scar (disciform scar) is present.

due to the increased height of the retinal pigment epithelial cells in the center of the macula and to the presence of xanthophyll in the macular retina. In addition, the fovea contains an area where no blood vessels are present (*foveal avascular zone*).

The fovea measures approximately 500 to 1,500 μm in diameter. The optic nerve may be used as a point of reference when the fovea is analyzed (Fig. 6–21). The optic nerve is 1.5 mm in vertical diameter (1,500 μm). The foveal avascular zone is approximately 300 to 500 μm in diameter and may be delineated by fluorescein angiography. The center of the fovea is located approximately 3 mm or 2 disc diameters from the temporal edge of the optic nerve. This is a helpful point to remember because patients with macular degeneration may have alteration of the pigment epithelium and the fovea may not be clinically obvious. If macular degeneration is suspected, a careful examination of the macula should be performed with the 90D lens and indirect slit-lamp biomicroscopy. The Hruby lens may also be used to study the detail of the macula. If an area of subretinal pigment, subretinal hemorrhage, or localized macular edema is present, the patient should be evaluated with fluorescein angiography. Fluorescein angiography is the definitive test for diagnosis of subretinal neovascularization (Fig. 6–22). After angiography is performed, the patient may then be examined with a fundus contact lens. A contact lens offers the best view of the fovea, but this examination should not be performed before fluorescein angiography because the quality of the photographs will be reduced temporarily after a contact lens examination.

A patient with suspected subretinal neovascularization should be evaluated for treatment immediately. Many institutions offer rapid fluorescein angiography service so that patients may undergo laser treatment the same day as their examination if neovascularization is present.

Dry macular degeneration is characterized by atrophy of the retinal pigment epithelium.

Dry macular degeneration is more common than the wet form and occurs when there is

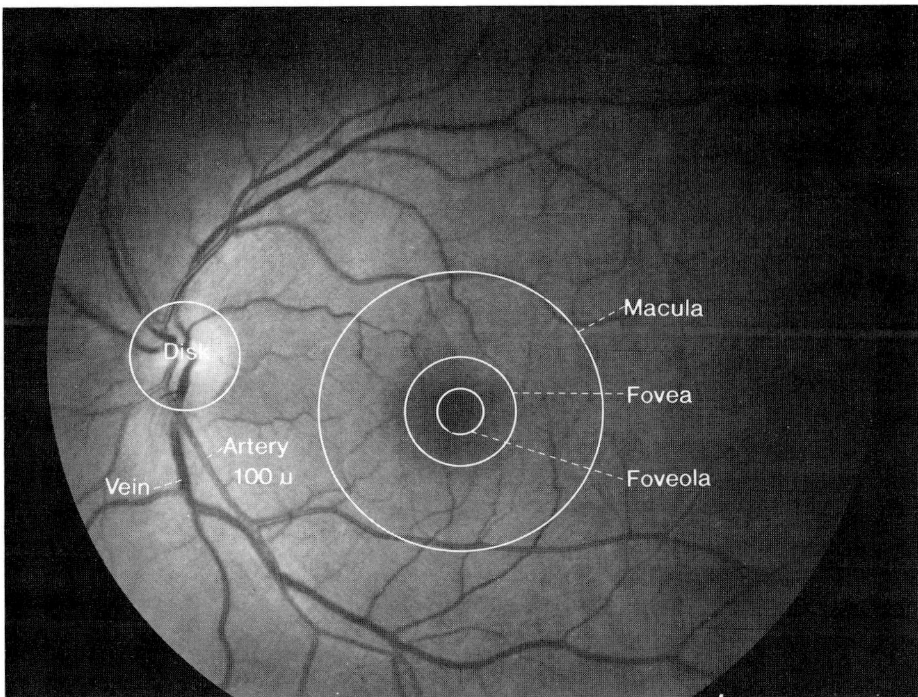

Fig. 6–21.   Anatomical divisions of the posterior pole. The average optic disc is 1,500 μm in diameter. The macula comprises 650,000 cones and is approximately 5,000 μm in diameter. Within the macula are the fovea (1,500 μm, with 100,000 cones) and the foveola (the central 350 μm, with 25,000 cones). The retinal arteries near the disc are about 100 μm in width, whereas the corresponding veins are approximately 150 to 175 μm in width.

complete atrophy of an area of retinal pigment epithelium and choroid. This creates a punched-out appearance in the retina. The irregular borders of an area of retinal pigment epithelium have led to use of the term *geographic atrophy of retinal pigment epithelium* (Fig. 6–23). Geographic atrophy (dry macular degeneration) usually leads to a progressive loss of central vision. No treatment has been proven effective for dry macular degeneration.

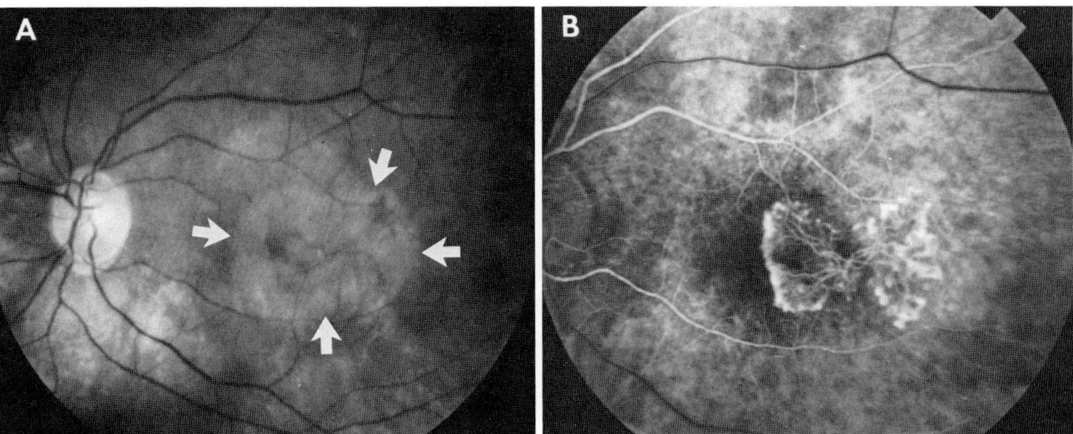

Fig. 6–22.   The left eye in a patient with macular degeneration, showing a choroidal neovascular membrane (*arrows*). *A*, Photograph. *B*, Fluorescein angiogram.

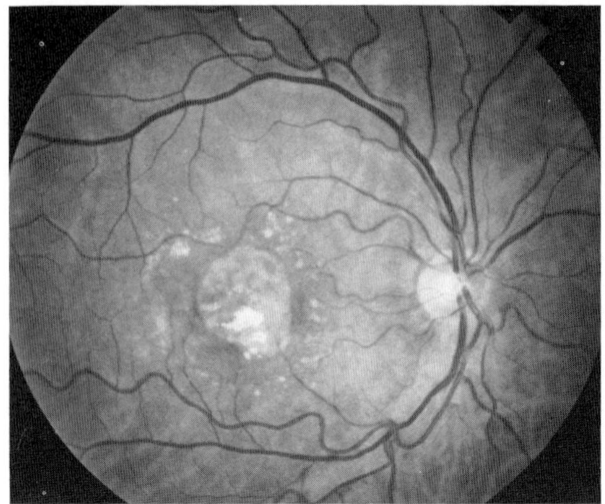

Fig. 6–23. Right eye in a patient with macular degeneration, showing geographic atrophy of the retinal pigment epithelium.

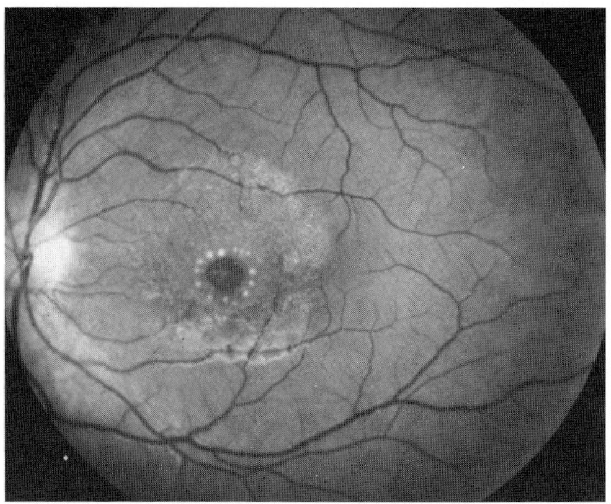

Fig. 6–24. Fundus photograph of the left eye in a patient with a macular hole. Notice the ring of subretinal precipitates at the margins of the retinal hole. A cuff of subretinal fluid is present.

Occasionally, the retinal pigment epithelium may lose its adhesion to Bruch's membrane and develop a shallow dome-shaped area (*retinal pigment epithelial detachment*). Pigment epithelial detachments may or may not be associated with detectable subretinal neovascularization and are generally considered not treatable with photocoagulation.

A macular hole has many different causes.

A *macular hole* is a full-thickness retinal break that occurs in the center of the macula (Fig. 6–24). It has the characteristic appearance of a round hole occurring where the fovea should be, and it is surrounded typically by a small cuff of subretinal fluid (a localized retinal detachment).

The most common type of macular hole occurs with no apparent cause (idiopathic macular hole). Macular hole may also occur as a result of long-standing macular edema due to any cause, including central retinal vein occlusion, branch retinal vein occlusion, and cystoid macular edema after cataract operation. A traumatic macular hole may develop immediately after a severe blow to the eye or as a delayed phenomenon. Epiretinal membrane, macular edema, and foveal cyst may all mimic a retinal hole.

Macular hole is usually diagnosed by careful fundus examination because the findings may be subtle. A macular hole may not be obvious on examination with an indirect ophthalmoscope, but it can usually be seen on indirect slit-lamp examination with a 90D lens, with a Hruby lens, or by examination with a fundus contact lens. Occasionally, a small area in the pigment epithelium may be abnormal near the hole, resulting in a hyperfluorescent "window defect" on fluorescein angiography. The main value of fluorescein angiography is to rule out other conditions such as cystoid macular edema or a retinal vein occlusion.

Idiopathic macular hole is often bilateral.

Idiopathic macular hole is almost exclusively seen in middle-aged women. The condition is frequently bilateral, although the development of a macular hole in one eye may occur months or years before that in the second eye. Several theories have been suggested as a cause to explain this phenomenon. A posterior vitreous detachment with a prominent vitreomacular adhesion is one possible cause. Vascular factors have also been suggested, and some examiners have noted that a large number of patients are taking estrogen replacements. One widely accepted theory is that a proliferation of fibroblast-like cells on the surface of the perifoveal region of the retina exerts a tangential traction force that causes thinning of the fovea and the development of a macular hole.

Often the progression from a normal fovea to a macular hole occurs over several weeks or months. This observation has led to the suggestion by some investigators that a pars plana vitrectomy performed in an eye with an impending macular hole may prevent further development of the macular hole. This treatment is not universally accepted and would be applicable only to a patient developing a macular hole in the second eye. Laser treatment around the margins of a macular hole to induce resolution of the small area of retinal detachment has been suggested; this treatment, however, is not universally accepted.

Central serous retinopathy usually resolves spontaneously.

Central serous retinopathy (also called central serous chorioretinopathy) is a self-limited disease causing a localized detachment of the retina. This produces the appearance of a small blister of fluid in the posterior pole. The disease occurs primarily in young to middle-aged adults and is more common in men than in women. Many investigators have noted that individuals with central serous retinopathy seem to have a "type A personality" (time conscious, tense, under stress). The symptoms of central serous retinopathy are usually described as monocular blurring or a focal gray area occurring in the central vision (a relative scotoma).

Examination of a patient with central serous retinopathy reveals an elevation of the retina and retinal vessels in a circular area in the posterior pole. Patients are symptomatic if the fovea is involved. This finding may be subtle and is best seen with the slit lamp with a contact lens. It may also be seen with an indirect ophthalmoscope if one is careful to notice the light reflexes on the surface of the retina. Fluorescein angiography is diagnostic in central serous retinopathy. A pinpoint area of hyperfluorescence usually becomes larger and brighter through the early phases of angiography (Fig. 6–25). In the late phases, a vertical plume of hyperfluorescence extends from the pinpoint leak. This finding is seen only on very late views 10 to 30 minutes after the injection and is called a "smokestack sign." It is important to perform fluorescein angiography in cases of suspected central serous retinopathy, not only to confirm the diagnosis but also to rule out the possibility of choroidal neovascularization, which has a much more serious prognosis and may require photocoagulation.

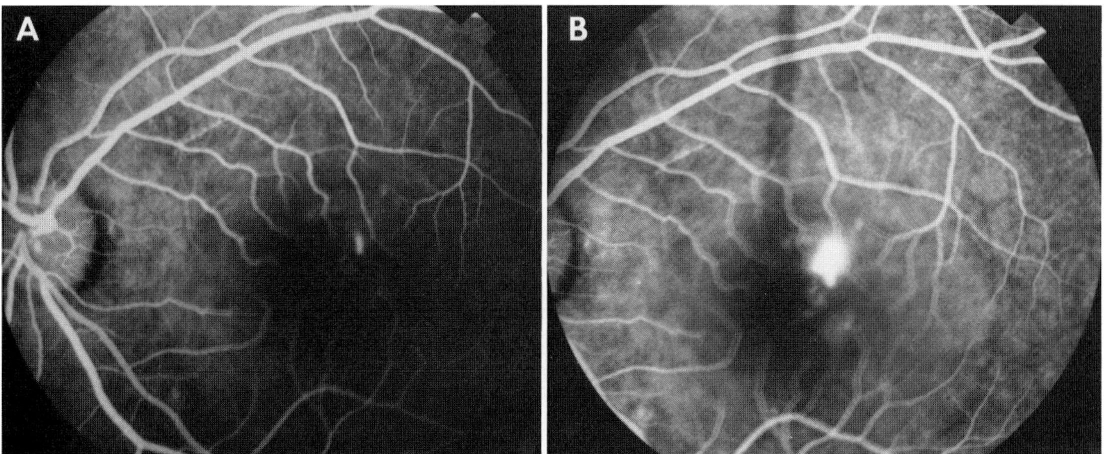

Fig. 6–25. Fluorescein angiogram of left eye with central serous retinopathy. *A*, Early view with a pinpoint leak. *B*, Later view, showing enlargement of the hyperfluorescent spot (smokestack sign).

Focal defects in the retinal pigment epithelium allow fluid to leak into the subretinal space.

Central serous retinopathy is important not only as a clinical syndrome but also in understanding the function of the retinal pigment epithelium. The retinal pigment epithelium presents a barrier to the movement of fluid from the choroidal extravascular space into the neurosensory retina. Under normal circumstances, fluid between the neurosensory retina and pigment epithelium flows actively and passively into the choroid. In central serous retinopathy, a focal defect in the pigment epithelium allows movement of fluid in the opposite direction and fluid accumulates in the subretinal space. Understanding the forces that move fluid in and out of the subretinal space is essential to an understanding of retinal detachment.

Because central serous retinopathy usually resolves spontaneously in 1 to 3 months, various treatments have been suggested as effective. Most ophthalmologists agree that for a primary episode of central serous retinopathy in one eye, observation is the preferred treatment. However, if the patient has recurrences or persistent subretinal fluid, one should consider laser treatment.

Central serous retinopathy may result in a bullous, highly elevated retinal detachment on rare occasions. It is important to distinguish this disease from the more common retinal detachment due to a retinal hole (rhegmatogenous retinal detachment). Patients with bullous retinal detachments in both eyes due to central serous retinopathy have been described.

Macular pucker is due to proliferation on the retinal surface.

Macular pucker is a distortion of the macula caused by a layer of fibroblast-like tissue on the surface of the retina. This condition is also referred to as *preretinal fibroplasia, surface wrinkling retinopathy,* or *cellophaning.* Macular pucker is usually idiopathic, but it may occur after retinal detachment, with trauma, in association with diabetic retinopathy, or after intraocular inflammation.

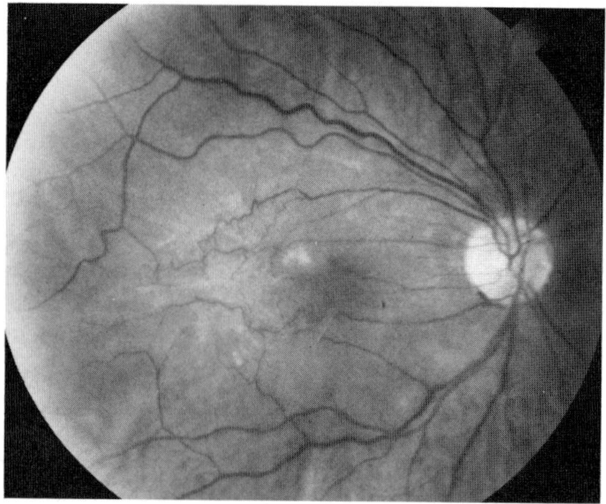

Fig. 6–26. Macular pucker in the right eye. Notice the distortion of the retinal vessels.

Patients with macular pucker usually complain of distortion in vision. They may also notice blurring and decreased visual acuity. The symptoms are usually progressive over time, but in a large percentage of patients the symptoms seem to stabilize. Idiopathic macular pucker usually occurs in one eye, but it may be binocular in 5% to 10% of patients.

Examination of the macula usually reveals a fine glistening membrane on the surface of the retina. The retinal vessels are often distorted and retinal folds may be seen extending from an area of macular pucker (Fig. 6–26). Fluorescein angiography can be helpful to rule out other retinal diseases such as macular hole or macular degeneration. Occasionally, other macular disease may coexist with macular pucker and may indicate a poor prognosis for surgical repair.

Cystoid macular edema may develop several weeks after uncomplicated cataract operation.

The *cystoid macular edema* syndrome may cause decreased vision after cataract operation. This poorly understood entity is less common with extracapsular cataract procedures and phacoemulsification than with intracapsular cataract operation. Many patients develop macular edema for no apparent reason approximately 4 to 6 weeks after cataract surgery. Fortunately,

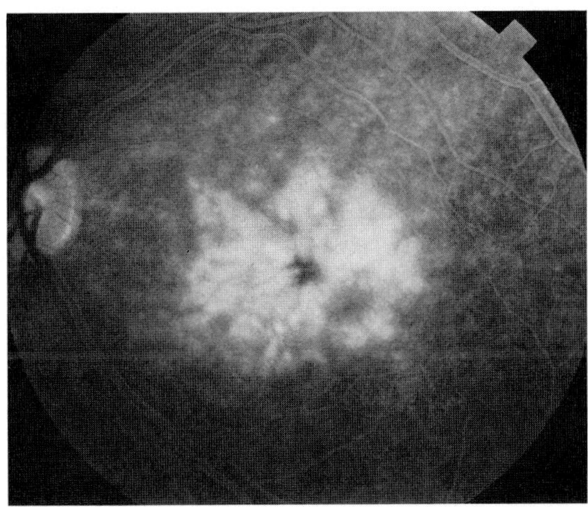

Fig. 6–27. Fluorescein angiogram of the left eye in a patient with cystoid macular edema, showing a typical cystoid pattern. This is a late angiographic view.

macular edema usually resolves spontaneously. The incidence of persistent cystoid macular edema is as high as 50% after complicated cataract operations (vitreous loss, rupture of posterior capsule, choroidal effusion or hemorrhage) and only 0.5% after uncomplicated procedures. If the macular edema persists for more than 6 months, a permanent decrease in vision may result from glial proliferation. When suspected, the diagnosis of cystoid macular edema is confirmed with fluorescein angiography (Fig. 6–27).

Abnormal vitreoretinal adhesion occurs at the margin of lattice degeneration.

There are several common degenerations of the peripheral retina, including lattice degeneration, cobblestone degeneration (paving stone degeneration), and cystoid degeneration. These usually require the use of an indirect ophthalmoscope to examine adequately.

Lattice degeneration can have a variable appearance, but it is usually a circular or elongated oval area in the peripheral retina between the equator and the ora serrata (Fig. 6–28). Lattice degeneration may occur as a small spot approximately a third of a disc diameter in size or may run circumferentially (parallel to the ora serrata) as a linear strip for 3 to 4 clock hours.

Lattice degeneration has a glistening or granular refractile appearance. Sometimes white lines can be seen crisscrossing the length of the lattice degeneration and, when examined in profile by scleral depression, the areas of lattice are noticeably thinner than the surrounding normal retina. Reactive pigmentation is often present at the borders of an area of lattice degeneration. Extensive lattice degeneration is usually associated with degenerative changes in the vitreous such as liquid (optically empty) spaces, condensation of vitreous fibrils, and posterior vitreous detachment.

Lattice degeneration is associated with a slightly increased risk of retinal detachment. When an eye suffers blunt trauma, the retina may tear at an area of lattice degeneration. Occasionally, atrophic round holes may develop in the center of an area of lattice degeneration; these holes are unlikely to lead to retinal detachment. A much more dangerous finding is tearing of the retina at an edge of lattice degeneration. Such a tear is much more likely to lead to a retinal detachment.

Histologically, lattice degeneration appears as a marked thinning of the neurosensory retina with an overlying liquefaction of the overlying vitreous. In addition, there are usually dense vitreoretinal adhesions at the margin of a lattice degeneration area. A retinal tear at the

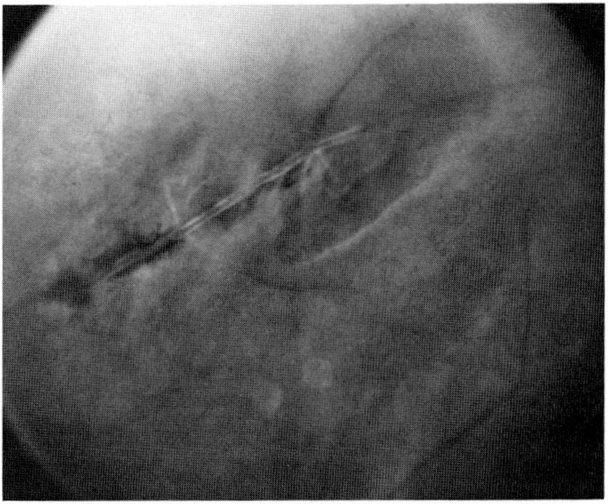

Fig. 6–28. An area of peripheral retina shows a blood vessel crossing an area of lattice degeneration. Notice the sheathed appearance of the vessel.

margin of a lattice lesion with the edge of the hole lifted up and a surrounding cuff of subretinal fluid usually requires treatment with cryotherapy or laser to prevent progression to a retinal detachment. Round atrophic retinal holes are not usually treated prophylactically.

Cobblestone degeneration represents choroidal insufficiency.

Cobblestone degeneration is usually easy to detect as a circular or oval white area at the ora serrata. Cobblestone degeneration may occur as one or two isolated spots or may be extensive with many punched-out white areas.

Histologically, cobblestone degeneration represents a loss of the choroid and retinal pigment epithelium. The white area in the center of a cobblestone lesion is actually the sclera seen through the transparent overlying layer of neurosensory retina.

Because the retina is intact with no overlying vitreoretinal abnormalities, patients with cobblestone degeneration are not at increased risk for retinal detachment. Cobblestone degeneration can be a manifestation of choroidal ischemia, or it may occur at the anterior margin of a choroidal mass lesion such as a malignant melanoma. In the absence of other ocular signs or symptoms, cobblestone degeneration alone does not warrant further evaluation.

Peripheral cystoid degeneration is usually benign.

Peripheral cystoid degeneration of the retina is very common and present to some degree in almost all older individuals. This finding is much more subtle than cobblestone degeneration or lattice degeneration. It appears as a fine bubbly appearance in the peripheral retina. The cysts are very tiny and close to the limit of resolution of the indirect ophthalmoscope.

Cystoid degeneration is much more obvious in a retina that is detached and gives the retina a frosted appearance. Histologically, cystoid degeneration appears as a collection of extracellular fluid in the outer plexiform layers of the peripheral retina. The cystic space takes up most of the space of the retina with compressed nerve fibers separating each cyst.

Retinoschisis may simulate retinal detachment.

Occasionally, the peripheral cystic spaces may coalesce and actually split the retina into an inner and outer layer. This finding is called degenerative *retinoschisis* and is quite common. Retinoschisis may be seen as a subtle thickening of the peripheral retina noticed with scleral depression or may be extensive and simulate a retinal detachment.

Differentiating an area of retinoschisis from retinal detachment is a common dilemma. Retinoschisis is almost always greatest in the inferior temporal quadrant. It is usually bilateral, although it may be asymmetric. Retinoschisis usually has a tense blister-like appearance, whereas a retinal detachment often has a billowing, loose appearance. A diagnostic feature of retinoschisis is the "internal frosting" seen in the center of a schisis cavity on the inner layer of retina. These tiny spots represent the broken compressed strands that previously joined the inner and outer layer of retina.

Occasionally, retinoschisis and retinal detachment may coexist. In order for retinoschisis to develop into a retinal detachment, a hole must occur in the outer layer of the schisis cavity. These areas are usually large, circular, atrophic areas with a rolled margin. Fluid from the schisis cavity may dissect through the outer layer break and collect in the space between the retinal pigment epithelium and retina; this accumulation causes a retinal detachment.

Retinal detachment occurs when flow into the subretinal space is greater than flow out of the subretinal space.

A *retinal detachment* is an accumulation of fluid between the neurosensory retina and the retinal pigment epithelium. Under normal circumstances, fluid is constantly pumped out of the subretinal space into the choroid. If a hole is present in the retina, an abnormal flow of fluid may occur from the vitreous cavity into the subretinal space. If the flow of fluid into the subretinal space is greater than the flow of fluid out from the subretinal space into the choroid, fluid will accumulate under the retina and cause a retinal detachment (Fig. 6–29). A reti-

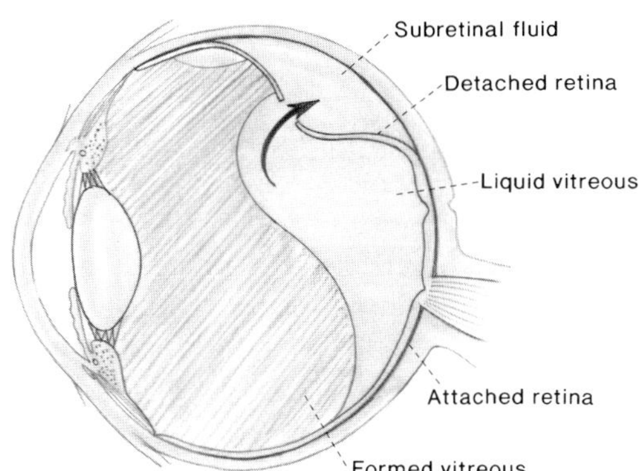

Fig. 6–29. Cross section of the globe, showing detachment of the vitreous and a torn retina leading to retinal detachment.

nal detachment due to a hole in the retina is called a *rhegmatogenous retinal detachment*. Fluid produced in the ciliary body flows posteriorly into the vitreous cavity and then through the retinal hole into the choroid. This increased posterior uveal outflow may cause a low intraocular pressure in a patient with a retinal detachment.

Vitreous detachments are common but may cause a retinal tear.

Other factors important in the development of a retinal detachment are a vitreous detachment, traction on the retinal hole, and eye movement. As people age, the vitreous undergoes degenerative changes that lead to vitreous detachment and *syneresis* (change from a formed vitreous to a separated vitreous of partially formed and partially liquid vitreous). *Vitreous detachment* occurs when the formed vitreous moves anteriorly and separates from the retina. This happens spontaneously with age but may be very symptomatic if it occurs suddenly. The patient may notice the sudden occurrence of floaters or flashing lights. Approximately 10% of patients with an acute vitreous detachment will develop a hole in the retina where the vitreous is firmly adherent. This tearing may liberate some retinal pigment epithelial cells into the vitreous cavity. These cells ("*tobacco dust*") can be seen at the slit lamp as pigmented specks floating in the anterior vitreous and are pathognomonic for a retinal tear. In addition

to causing a retinal tear, the vitreous detachment may allow the more liquid syneretic portion of the vitreous to migrate through the open retinal break. In addition, the vitreous may be attached to the retina on one side of a retinal hole, elevating this edge of the hole. This configuration allows fluid to be directed more easily through the retinal hole into the subretinal space when the eye moves. The first step in treating a rhegmatogenous retinal detachment is to identify the retinal break.

Occasionally, a retinal detachment may occur without a hole in the retina. This is due to a flow of fluid into the subretinal space from the choroid (reverse flow, leak). This situation (*nonrhegmatogenous retinal detachment*) arises in central serous retinopathy or other disorders that cause dysfunction of the retinal pigment epithelium (such as choroidal tumor) (Table 6–5).

Treatment of a rhegmatogenous retinal detachment usually involves indenting the wall of the eye over the area of the retinal tear with a *scleral buckle*. In recent years, interest has developed in alternative methods of repairing retinal detachments without a permanent scleral buckle. These techniques use either a temporary balloon buckle (which is later removed) or an injection of a high-molecular-weight inert gas into the vitreous cavity that will not pass through the retinal hole (*pneumatic retinopexy*).

Retinal detachment may be prevented by recognition of a retinal hole.

Patients with symptoms of a vitreous detachment must be examined carefully to rule out a retinal hole. For diagnosis of a retinal hole, it is important to do a careful slit-lamp examina-

TABLE 6–5   Causes of Nonrhegmatogenous Retinal Detachment

Central serous retinopathy
Harada's disease (Vogt-Koyanagi-Harada syndrome)
Sympathetic ophthalmia
Choroidal tumor
Posterior scleritis
Optic pit

tion to look for pigmented cells in the anterior vitreous and to examine the vitreous with the aid of a Hruby lens or 90D lens to detect separation. Posterior vitreous detachment frequently can be confirmed by noting an operculum (*Fuchs' ring*) floating over the optic nerve. Next, the fundus is examined with an indirect ophthalmoscope. Before scleral depression is begun, it is important to scan the entire fundus carefully because many retinal breaks can be identified without the aid of scleral depression, especially large posterior breaks. Once the peripheral, equatorial, and posterior regions of the retina have been carefully scanned in a methodical fashion, scleral depression to detect retinal holes can be performed.

When the eye wall is indented with a scleral depressor, the choroid under the retina changes color. The retina is also less transparent when viewed obliquely, and therefore retinal holes can be observed more easily when viewed at an angle than when viewed perpendicular to the retinal surface. Scleral depression enhances the identification of vitreous attachments to the retina because they stand out on the apex of the area of depressed retina.

The peripheral retina is studied with scleral depression.

The technique of *scleral depression* with indirect ophthalmoscopy takes time to master. A cotton-tipped applicator, thimble-type scleral depressor, or straight scleral depressor may be used to indent the globe. A methodical approach is important to ensure that all areas of the retina are scanned. It is usually best to start in the inferior temporal quadrant, where the eyelids are most lax. To depress the inferior temporal quadrant of the right eye, the examiner stands at the patient's left side while the patient is reclining. The scleral depressor is held in the left hand and the condensing lens in the right hand. First, the patient looks up and the depressor tip is applied to the temporal aspect of the lower eyelid near the lid crease (Fig. 6–30). The patient then looks down and to the right slightly, and the examiner should be able to visualize the indentation created by the scleral depressor tip (Fig. 6–31). After the

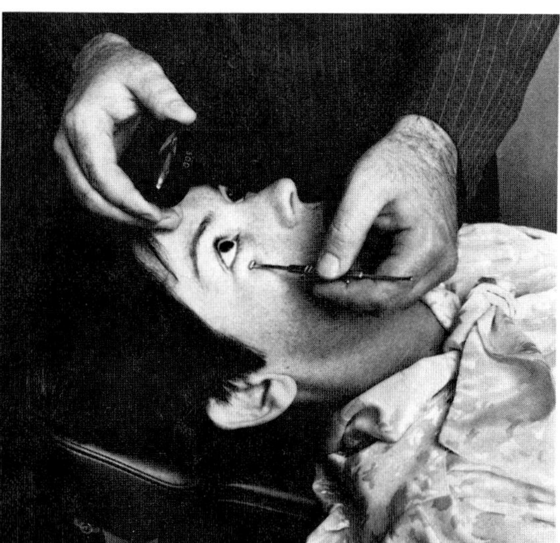

Fig. 6–30. The right eye of a patient is about to be examined with scleral depression. The patient is asked to look up and the depressor is placed at the lid crease. The condensing lens is in the right hand, and the scleral depressor is held in the left hand. The examiner is standing at the patient's left side.

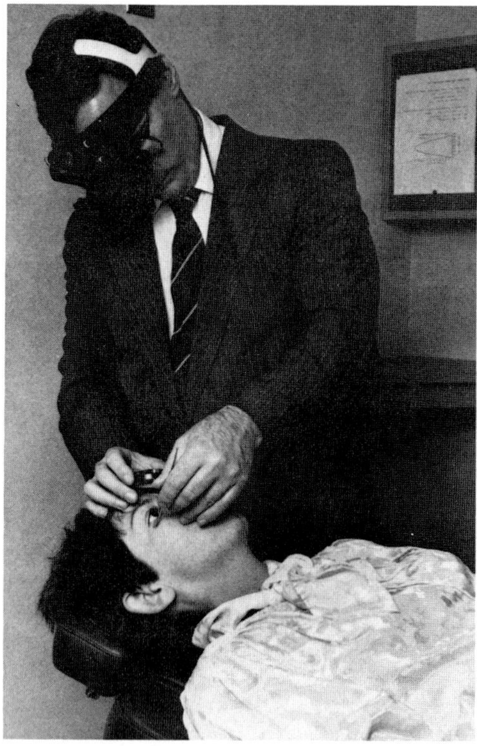

Fig. 6–31. Scleral depression of the inferior temporal quadrant of the right eye. The scleral depressor is held in the left hand.

depression is visualized, the depressor is slowly moved up to the 9 o'clock meridian and down to the 6 o'clock meridian, and the entire inferior temporal quadrant is inspected. The examiner then proceeds to the superior temporal quadrant and holds the scleral depressor in the right hand and the condensing lens in the left hand (Fig. 6–32). After the entire superior temporal quadrant has been inspected, the superior nasal quadrant of the right eye is inspected from the patient's right side (Fig. 6–33). Finally, the inferior nasal quadrant is inspected; the examiner holds the depressor in the right hand and stands at the patient's right side (Fig. 6–34).

Contact lens examination may aid in locating retinal holes.

For any case in which a retinal hole is suspected but not identified, an alternative approach is to proceed with a *three-mirror (Goldmann) contact lens* examination. Occasionally, small retinal breaks may be identified with the contact lens which may be missed with scleral depression. The eye is anesthetized with a drop of proparacaine or tetracaine. The patient is positioned at the slit lamp and asked to look up while the contact lens is applied to the cornea. A small amount of methylcellulose solution is

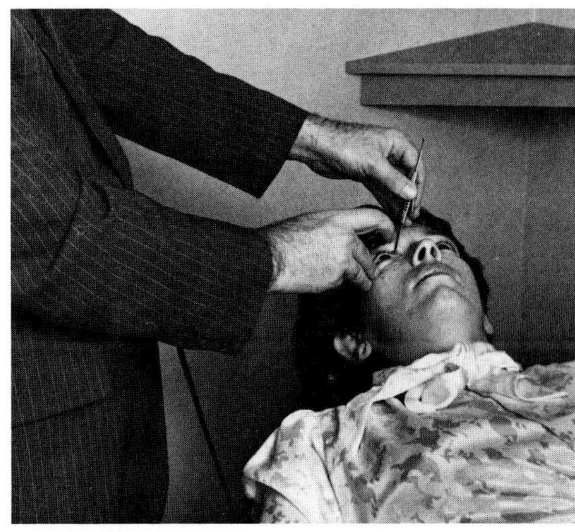

Fig. 6–33. Scleral depression of the superior nasal quadrant of the right eye. The scleral depressor is held in the left hand. The examiner is now at the patient's right side.

used to make good contact with the cornea. The two largest mirrors on the Goldmann lens will give the best views of the peripheral retina. Each of these mirrors should be rotated to inspect the peripheral retina for 360°.

If no retinal breaks are identified, it must be assumed that the patient has a vitreous detachment without a retinal break. Even though a

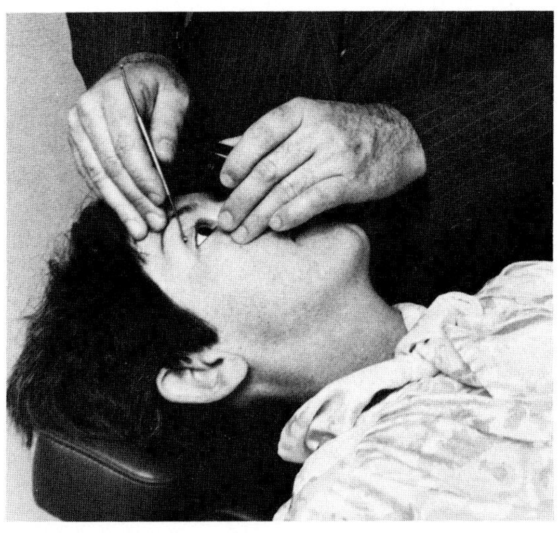

Fig. 6–32. Scleral depression of the superior temporal quadrant of the right eye. The scleral depressor is held in the right hand.

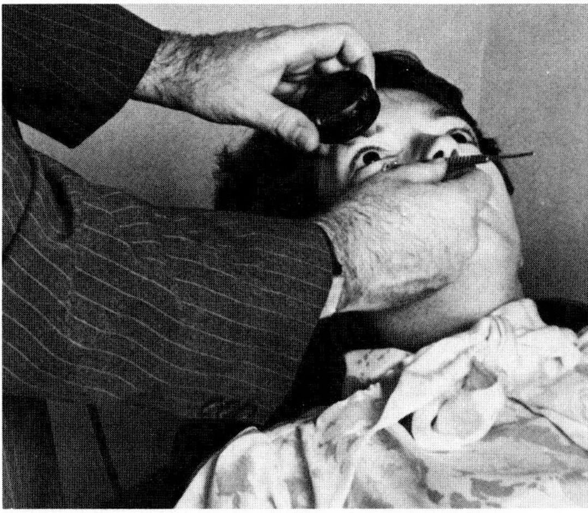

Fig. 6–34. Scleral depression of the inferior nasal quadrant of the right eye. The scleral depressor is held in the right hand, and the examiner stands at the patient's right side.

retinal break may not be present at the time of the examination, there is no guarantee that one cannot develop one in the future. Therefore, it is very important to advise the patient to watch for any increase in symptoms such as new floaters, increased flashing lights, or a visual field defect. In addition, it is a good idea to re-examine the patient in 1 month to determine whether any new retinal holes have developed. If no retinal holes have developed at the second examination and the symptoms have stopped, then the patient can be reassured and advised to return if symptoms recur or if symptoms develop in the other eye. However, if flashes and floaters persist, another examination in several weeks or months should be planned. If pigmented cells are present in the vitreous indicating a retinal break, but no retinal break is identified, it is appropriate to refer the patient to a retinal specialist. If vitreous hemorrhage obscures the fundus, ultrasonography may be used to rule out a retinal detachment and the patient may be confined to bed to speed settling of the vitreous hemorrhage.

Not all patients with a retinal break develop retinal detachment.

Once the retinal break has been identified, the examiner must determine whether the retinal break places the individual at a substantial risk of developing a retinal detachment. Retinal breaks are not uncommon and occur in approximately 5% of the population. Retinal detachments occur in about 1 in 10,000 individuals per year. Obviously, not all patients with a retinal break develop a retinal detachment. Treatment to prevent progression to a retinal detachment, however, has relatively few risks. If an individual is at significant risk for developing a retinal detachment, the area of the retinal break may be outlined with laser treatment or cryotherapy to produce a chorioretinal adhesion and prevent retinal detachment.

In general, asymptomatic holes rarely require treatment. Holes in the superior aspect of the fundus are more likely to lead to a retinal detachment than are holes in the inferior aspect of the fundus. *Horseshoe-shaped tears* occur because of traction at the edge of the retinal break and almost always require treatment.

These are usually surrounded by a cuff of subretinal fluid. *Round holes* rarely produce retinal detachment and frequently do not require any treatment. If a patient has had a retinal detachment in the other eye or there is a history of retinal detachment in an immediate family member, the risk of developing a retinal detachment may be greater and treatment should be considered.

Retinal breaks are caused by abnormalities of the vitreous.

Two groups of people are at greatest risk for developing retinal detachment: young people (usually men) exposed to blunt trauma or penetrating ocular trauma and elderly people, especially those who have had cataract operation.

Patients who suffer severe ocular trauma are at great risk for developing a retinal break. In blunt trauma, the anterior to posterior compression of the globe results in a stretching of the peripheral retina and traction at the insertion of the vitreous base. These changes can lead to avulsion of the vitreous base and a linear break at the anterior or posterior margin of the vitreous base. This linear smooth tear is called a *dialysis* and is the most common retinal break found in retinal detachment associated with trauma. If the vitreous base is avulsed, it may be seen draped through the pupil with a small amount of pigment on its border like a pigmented ribbon. Detecting an avulsion of the vitreous base at the slit lamp must lead one to look carefully for a retinal dialysis. A dialysis can easily be missed because of its peripheral location and also because it may occur in the superior nasal quadrant where scleral depression is difficult to perform. The retinal detachment associated with a dialysis may have a subtle appearance and may progress slowly because the vitreous in a young individual is usually not syneretic and thus the retina has a less elevated detachment. The patient may develop a retinal detachment due to a dialysis months or years after the injury. Persistent traumatic iritis should heighten one's suspicion to look for a retinal dialysis.

When a penetrating injury occurs and the vitreous is disturbed, occasionally a proliferative response will result with traction bands occurring within the vitreous cavity. This proliferative vitreoretinopathy may cause a traction retinal detachment or tear of the retina. This response has been studied extensively and is predictable. Because of this, patients who have suffered lacerations of the sclera frequently require vitrectomy to relieve vitreous traction.

Blunt trauma causes retinal whitening.

Commotio is a whitening or loss of transparency of the retina produced immediately at the time of blunt trauma (see page 283, Fig. 11–13). This trauma may also be associated with retinal hemorrhage, choroidal rupture, and other findings of trauma. Commotio is associated with visual loss, which may recover or may persist and evolve to a traumatic pigmentary retinopathy with permanent loss of vision. Animal studies have shown that this initial loss of retinal transparency due to trauma is a result of damage to the photoreceptors. These damaged portions of rods and cones may be engulfed by the underlying retinal pigment epithelium and repaired and may eventually return to completely normal architecture. If the damage to the photoreceptors is severe, however, clumps of abnormal pigment epithelial cells develop (traumatic pigmentary retinopathy).

Choroidal rupture is a break in Bruch's membrane.

A *choroidal* rupture is pathognomonic of blunt ocular trauma (see page 283, Fig. 11–14). This is a white line that occurs concentric to the optic nerve and may be associated with decreased central vision if the fovea is involved. Multiple choroidal ruptures may occur.

A choroidal rupture occurs when stretching of the layers of the eye wall results in a breaking or rupture of Bruch's membrane. Bruch's membrane is relatively elastic tissue and retracts when a break in continuity occurs. The overlying pigment epithelium also separates, as do the inner layers of the choroid in many cases. Frequently, subretinal hemorrhage is associated with a choroidal rupture. Individuals with a choroidal rupture are at risk for the development of neovascularization occurring within this break in Bruch's membrane. The new vessels may not appear for months or years after the injury.

The vitreous is composed of hyaluronic acid and collagen fibrils.

The vitreous is composed of a mixture of hyaluronic acid solution and collagen-like fibrils. Hyaluronic acid is a large polysaccharide molecule with unique characteristics. Because hyaluronic acid molecules can bond loosely to a large number of water molecules, a very weak solution of hyaluronic acid in water can have a very high viscosity.

The vitreous fibrils give the vitreous a definite structure. These fibrils run through the vitreous in a large interlacing network and are anchored to the retina in very specific points. There is a firm attachment of the vitreous fibrils to the margin of the optic nerve. When the vitreous separates from the optic nerve posteriorly, often some tissue from the surface of the optic nerve is pulled anteriorly into the vitreous (Fuchs' ring). The vitreous may also be attached at the fovea and in a band that overlaps the ora serrata for several millimeters on each side. This circumferential insertion of the vitreous into the peripheral retina and pars plana of the ciliary body is called the *vitreous base*.

The most common abnormalities of the vitreous are vitreous syneresis and asteroid hyalosis.

The most common abnormality of the vitreous is *syneresis*, or degenerative changes in the vitreous. In syneresis, cavities of liquid vitreous develop. At the same time, vitreous fibrils may form condensations in the vitreous and may be noted by the patient as floaters. Frequently, this change can be detected at the slit lamp in an elderly individual.

Another finding frequently encountered is *asteroid hyalosis*. This is a condition in which white, yellow, or gold refractile deposits appear dispersed through the vitreous. Although they may make the view of the fundus difficult with the direct or indirect ophthalmoscope, they rarely affect vision. The abnormalities in asteroid hyalosis are composed of calcium salts and are attached firmly to the vitreous fibrils. Although these areas may move around with the vitreous fibrils, they stay in relatively the same position because of their attachment to the vitreous fibrils.

Bergmeister's papilla and Mittendorf's dot are residual primary vitreous.

The embryonic development of the vitreous is relatively complicated. Early in the development of the eye, the primary vitreous includes a column of blood vessels that originate from the optic nerve and run through the center of the vitreous to the posterior surface of the lens. This network of blood vessels envelops the lens as the *tunica vasculosa lentis*. Later in embryonic development, this vascular network (hyaloid vessels) regresses. Occasionally, persistent hyaloid vessels may be detected in the adult state. This condition of *persistent hyperplastic primary vitreous* consists of a fibrovascular canal extending from the optic nerve to the posterior lens surface and presents as a white retrolental mass. The abnormality is often associated with an abnormally small eye (*microphthalmos*). In addition, one may detect the ciliary processes pulled toward the center of the retrolental mass. Occasionally, an incomplete form of persistent hyperplastic primary vitreous may occur with a small stalk extending just from the optic nerve and ending in the mid-vitreous. This abnormality, termed *Bergmeister's papilla*, represents a remnant of the hyaloid system. Another remnant may occur coming from the posterior surface of the lens. This white dot-like opacity on the posterior surface of the lens is called a *Mittendorf dot*. These limited forms of persistent primary vitreous are often present with normal vision and are usually incidental findings.

Uveitis means intraocular inflammation.

When the inside of the eye is inflamed, typical symptoms include pain, light sensitivity (photophobia), floaters, and decreased vision. Although the uvea is the middle layer of the eye just inside the sclera (iris, ciliary body, choroid), uveitis may involve other intraocular structures such as the retina, vitreous, or aqueous.

Patients with uveitis may or may not have a red eye; inflammatory cells, however, will be detected inside the eye. These may be deposited on the endothelium of the cornea (*keratic precipitates*) (Fig. 6–35), floating in the anterior chamber or vitreous, or localized in the retina or choroid. It is important to do a complete eye examination on a patient with suspected uveitis and to search for cells floating in the anterior chamber or vitreous. The cellular reaction in the anterior chamber is usually graded from 1 to 4. Grade 1 indicates only a few cells detected floating in the anterior chamber. Grade 4 indicates a hypopyon. In addition to cells floating in the anterior chamber, increased protein in the aqueous may be detected by a decrease in clarity of the aqueous (*flare*).

Uveitis is often classified according to which area of the eye is most inflamed (iris, ciliary body, or choroid). Some uveitis syndromes typically produce one type of intraocular inflammation (for example, ankylosing spondylitis usually produces iridocyclitis). Some uveitis syndromes such as sarcoidosis may produce inflammation in the anterior segment (iritis, iridocyclitis) or in the posterior segment (choroiditis, vasculitis). Occasionally, the entire intraocular contents are involved equally. In such cases, the term "panuveitis" may be appropriate.

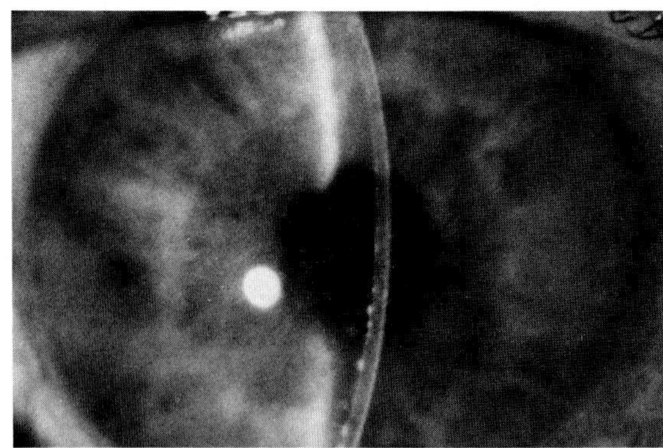

Fig. 6–35. Keratic precipitates on the corneal endothelium of a patient with uveitis.

Uveitis may be endogenous or exogenous.

Uveitis is generally divided into endogenous uveitis and exogenous uveitis. *Endogenous uveitis* describes ocular inflammatory disorders with no infectious or other exogenous causes. Systemic diseases with unknown causes such as sarcoidosis and Behçet's syndrome fall into this category. *Exogenous uveitis* is used to describe uveitis arising from factors outside the body. Infectious uveitis and traumatic uveitis are two examples of exogenous uveitis.

Endogenous uveitis is generally thought of as an autoimmune phenomenon. The primary cause or causes of endogenous uveitis have not been discovered; however, a number of uveitis syndromes can be recognized. If a specific syndrome is identified, the prognosis may be given and the appropriate level of treatment recommended.

Recurrent anterior uveitis may be a manifestation of ankylosing spondylitis or Reiter's syndrome.

Ankylosing spondylitis is a form of arthritis affecting the spine and sacroiliac joints. Recurrent anterior uveitis occurs in approximately 20% of cases. Men are affected three times more frequently than women, and 90% of patients are HLA-B27 positive.

Attacks of anterior uveitis are characterized by pain, redness, and photophobia. Anterior segment inflammation is seen, and patients may occasionally even develop a hypopyon (Fig. 6–36). A marked cellular response may also occur in the vitreous. Patients with ankylosing spondylitis should be treated aggressively to prevent the development of acute glaucoma or adhesion of the iris to the lens (*posterior synechiae*).

Reiter's syndrome is a triad of arthritis, urethritis, and uveitis. Conjunctivitis is found in one-third to two-thirds of patients. Symptoms may include mild discomfort, blurred vision, and occasional redness and photophobia. The course is usually benign, self-limited, and less severe than in ankylosing spondylitis. HLA-B27 antigen is present in approximately 90% of patients with Reiter's syndrome.

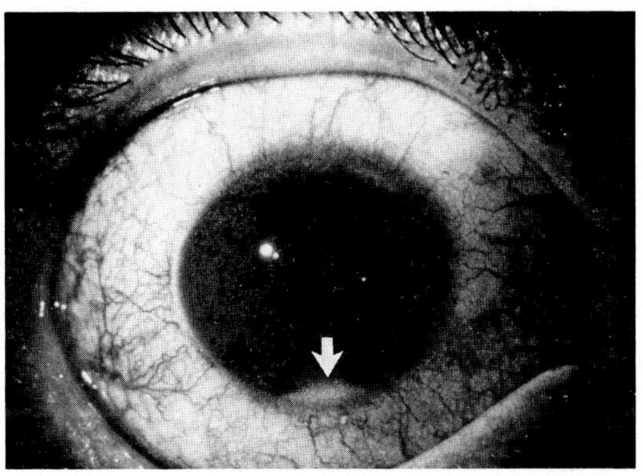

Fig. 6–36. A hypopyon (*arrow*) in the right eye of a patient with ankylosing spondylitis.

Fuchs' iridocyclitis eyes includes heterochromia and small keratic precipitates.

Fuchs' heterochromic iridocyclitis classically includes a lighter iris on the involved eye (heterochromia), atrophy of the iris surface, minimal cell and flare in the anterior chamber, and widely scattered, small, round, nonconfluent keratic precipitates. Conjunctival injection is usually absent, and patients may develop cataract in the affected eye at an early age. Often, Fuchs' iridocyclitis is asymptomatic, and, as a general rule, patients should not be treated with corticosteroids.

Fuchs' heterochromic iridocyclitis has a varied presentation and is more common than was appreciated in years past. In an individual with brown eyes, atrophy of the iris may be difficult to detect. Although Fuchs' heterochromic iridocyclitis is usually unilateral, it may be bilateral in as many as 10% of cases, and occasionally the involved iris may appear darker than the fellow eye instead of lighter. In a small percentage of patients, the inflammation may be more severe than in typical cases and may involve the vitreous and choroid. Involvement of the ciliary body may produce an intermediate uveitis (pars planitis, cyclitis).

Juvenile rheumatoid arthritis may be associated with uveitis.

Juvenile rheumatoid arthritis affects young girls most frequently and is usually pauciarticular (four joints or fewer). Antinuclear antibody is present in approximately 80% of patients with juvenile rheumatoid arthritis and iridocyclitis.

Iridocyclitis occurs in the teenage years and is usually bilateral. Patients have cell, flare, and keratic precipitates. Frequently, cataract and band keratopathy may develop. In severe cases, vision may be severely affected.

Topical corticosteroids are usually the treatment of choice. Often, cycloplegic agents are required to reduce posterior synechiae formation. Cataract operations may be complicated in patients with juvenile rheumatoid arthritis.

Posner-Schlossman syndrome may cause mild inflammation and high intraocular pressure.

Posner-Schlossman syndrome (glaucomatocyclitic crisis) is an inflammatory disease of the anterior segment of unknown cause. Patients have fine keratic precipitates, high intraocular pressure (often more than 40 mm Hg), and a dilated pupil. The inflammation is suspected to involve the trabecular meshwork and cause the pressure to increase. Patients usually respond well to cycloplegic drops and topical corticosteroids. Medications that reduce aqueous production may also be required. The response to topical therapy is usually rapid (complete resolution in several days). Patients may be subject to recurrent episodes.

Pars planitis may cause cystoid macular edema.

Pars planitis is a uveitis of unknown cause that involves primarily the pars plana and anterior vitreous. This disease typically is in young adults and is bilateral. Involvement is usually symmetric and may resolve spontaneously after several years ("burnout").

Patients with pars planitis usually present with floaters. Cells are seen in the vitreous and possibly the anterior chamber. Inflammation in the ciliary body may be detected as a layer of white cells on the pars plana (snowbank). It is necessary to perform scleral depression to detect this change. Occasionally, small abscesses may be seen floating in the dependent portion of the vitreous (snowballs). Patients are usually comfortable without injection or photophobia.

The cause of pars planitis is unknown; however, patients with toxoplasmosis, sarcoidosis, or toxocariasis may present with a form of inflammation that resembles pars planitis. There is a mild association between pars planitis and multiple sclerosis. Treatment of pars planitis should be deferred unless there is decreased vision with documented cystoid macular edema. Fluorescein angiography is necessary to make this diagnosis. Treatment then will require depot steroid injections (peribulbar injections) or systemic corticosteroids. In general, the prognosis for pars planitis is good.

Behçet's syndrome is a triad of iritis, mouth ulcers, and genital ulcers.

Behçet's syndrome is a rare form of uveitis that may present with recurring hypopyon, sheathing around retinal arterioles, and retinal and vitreous hemorrhages. Patients may have arthritis, and central nervous system involvement has been described. Behçet's syndrome characteristically recurs and may cause blindness due to posterior segment involvement. The treatment of choice for Behçet's disease is corticosteroids. Chlorambucil or cyclosporine may be necessary for patients who respond poorly to corticosteroids.

Inflammatory bowel disease may be associated with inflammation in any part of the eye.

Ulcerative colitis and Crohn's disease can be associated with iritis or iridocyclitis in 5% to 10% of patients. Occasionally, episodes of colitis may be predicted by preceding intraocular inflammation. Patients may also have involvement of the choroid or optic nerve. Inflammatory bowel disease may also be associated with scleritis or episcleritis. Topical corticosteroids and cycloplegics are used for iritis. Optic neuritis or choroidal involvement, however, may require systemic corticosteroids. Patients with ulcerative colitis may experience improvement in their intraocular inflammation if the colon is removed or if the bowel symptoms can be controlled with sulfonamides.

Sympathetic ophthalmia and Vogt-Koyanagi-Harada syndrome cause inflammation in the choroid.

Sympathetic ophthalmia is a bilateral form of choroiditis that occurs after a penetrating injury to the globe or, rarely, even after intraocular operation. Large keratic precipitates are present, as well as yellow nodules in the choroid (*Dalen-Fuchs nodules*). Sympathetic ophthalmia carries a poor prognosis. The incidence of sympathetic ophthalmia has dropped dramatically with careful repair of scleral lacerations. In cases of severe eye trauma with no hope of any vision, enucleation of the traumatized eye may be recommended to prevent the development of sympathetic ophthalmia in the fellow eye. Uveitis does not occur for at least 14 days, although sympathetic ophthalmia may develop years after trauma.

Harada's disease is a bilateral choroiditis that presents with nonrhegmatogenous retinal detachments. Inflammation may also be seen in the vitreous and anterior chamber. Harada's disease may affect only the eye or may be part of a larger syndrome that includes meningitis and uveitis. Patients with choroiditis, meningitis, decreased hearing, and poliosis (vitiligo around the eyes and mouth) have the Vogt-Koyanagi-Harada syndrome. The prognosis is variable depending on how long the retinal detachment persists. Treatment with systemic corticosteroids is usually adequate to control the inflammation; however, the possibility of an infectious disease such as tuberculosis, syphilis, or fungal meningitis must be ruled out before treatment with steroids is given.

Sarcoidosis may involve the anterior or posterior segment.

Sarcoidosis is a disease of unknown cause characterized by noncaseating granulomas. Patients may present with large keratic precipitates and iritis. This form of intraocular inflammation is often complicated by posterior synechiae. Inflammation may occur in the choroid or along the retinal vessels. Sarcoidosis may also involve the orbit with inflammation of the lacrimal gland, conjunctiva, or lids. Occasionally, the diagnosis can be made by a biopsy of the conjunctiva.

Presumed ocular histoplasmosis syndrome never has associated vitreous or anterior chamber inflammation.

Presumed ocular histoplasmosis syndrome is a chronic choroidal inflammatory disease characterized by round, punched-out areas approximately one-quarter to one-half disc diameter in size (Fig. 6–37). These may have some associated reactive pigmentation at the margin or may simply appear as atrophic round areas in the choroid. The characteristic finding in this syndrome is the distribution of the chorioretinal scars. They occur around the optic nerve (peripapillary), around the fovea (perifoveal) (Fig. 6–38), and near the equator (peripheral). The syndrome is thought to be related to infection with the histoplasmosis organism because the fundus findings are seen primarily in endemic areas; the actual relationship to histoplasmosis, however, is not well understood. Histoplasmosis is usually asymptomatic, but it may become symptomatic if the perifoveal scars serve as a site of choroidal neovascularization. In this instance, patients with histoplasmosis may benefit from laser therapy, similar to patients with macular degeneration.

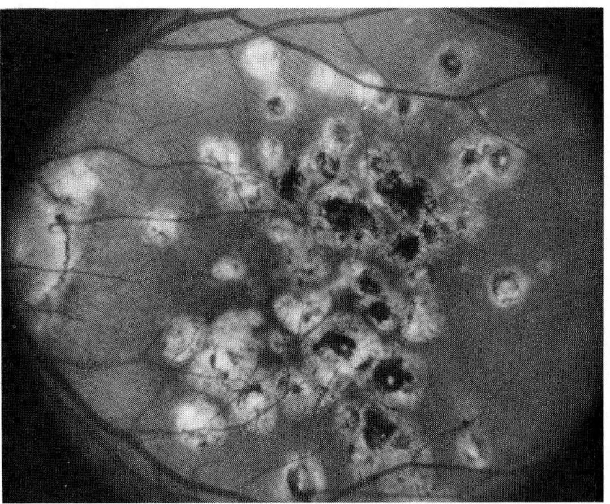

Fig. 6–37. Many round, atrophic "histo spots" in the perifoveal region and around the optic nerve in the left eye of a patient with the presumed ocular histoplasmosis syndrome.

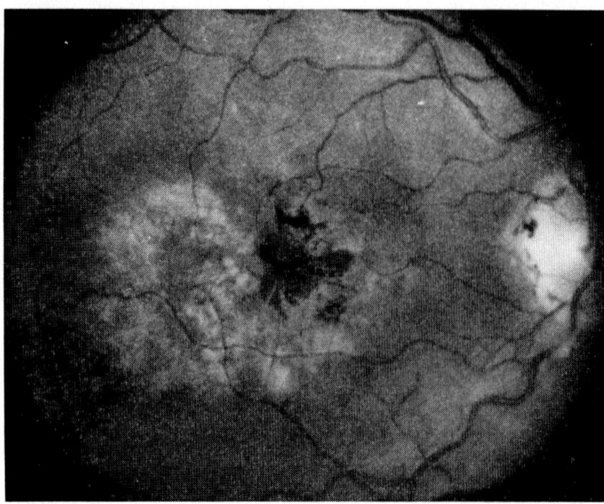

Fig. 6–38. Subretinal scarring extending under the fovea in a patient with presumed ocular histoplasmosis syndrome.

Endophthalmitis is a serious intraocular infection.

Endophthalmitis is an infection of the contents of the globe. Organisms can proliferate with little resistance once the vitreous is involved. Most cases of endophthalmitis occur after ocular operations such as cataract extraction. Postsurgical endophthalmitis is usually a bacterial infection and can be caused by gram-positive or gram-negative organisms. In rare cases, a chronic form of endophthalmitis may occur many months after a cataract operation. This is usually due to *Propionibacterium acne* (an anaerobic bacteria) or *Staphylococcus epidermidis*.

The eye is often red and painful and the vision is greatly impaired when endophthalmitis occurs. On examination, there are large numbers of cells in the anterior chamber and vitreous. Often, the retina may not be visible. A hypopyon may be present in the anterior chamber.

Endophthalmitis may occur after penetrating trauma. It is advisable to take samples for culture from edges of the wound during repair of a scleral laceration. Patients should be treated with prophylactic intravitreal antibiotics after penetrating trauma. With any history of ocular penetration in a "dirty" or rural environment (penetration with a stick or piece of metal), patients should receive anaerobic coverage with intravenous clindamycin. Traumatic endophthalmitis is due to *Bacillus cereus* in 10% to 20% of cases. This organism causes a fulminant endophthalmitis that can cause loss of the eye in 24 hours.

Treatment of suspected endophthalmitis includes an intraocular specimen sent for culture and smear followed by broad-spectrum coverage with intensive topical antibiotics. After culture results are received, antibiotic therapy may be modified accordingly. The greatest intraocular concentrations of antibiotics are achieved with direct intravitreal injection. Although intravitreal injections may cause some retinal toxicity, in severe endophthalmitis the risk is warranted. Less severe cases of endophthalmitis may be treated with fortified topical antibiotic drops applied every 30 minutes. Subconjunctival injections and intravenous antibiotics boost intraocular concentrations slightly over those with frequent topical administration. A vitreous operation may be beneficial in severe cases of endophthalmitis. Vitrectomy provides adequate material for culture and may remove inflammatory debris from the vitreous cavity.

Metastatic endophthalmitis is usually fungal.

Fungal endophthalmitis may occur after trauma or by direct extension from a corneal ulcer; a large percentage of fungal endophthalmitis, however, occurs through hematogenous spread from a systemic fungal infection. The organism most likely to cause metastatic endophthalmitis is *Candida albicans*. Intravenous drug abusers and patients with chronic indwelling venous catheters are at risk for fungal endophthalmitis. In addition, immunosuppressed patients with superficial fungal infections are also susceptible. Curiously, patients with acquired immunodeficiency syndrome rarely develop fungal endophthalmitis.

Cytomegalovirus retinitis is seen in immunodeficiency and neonates.

Infection of the retina with cytomegalovirus occurs in immunosuppressed patients and infants. Recent experience with patients who have acquired immunodeficiency syndrome has shown a high incidence of cytomegalovirus retinitis. Cytomegalovirus retinitis has a hemorrhagic appearance on the leading edge with atrophic retina behind it (Fig. 6–39). It can be suppressed, but not eradicated, with ganciclovir, a congener of the antiviral acyclovir.

Toxoplasmosis causes a punched-out retinal scar.

Toxoplasmosis gondii is a parasite that has a reservoir in the common house cat. Human infections occur, and the retina is a common site for infection with this protozoan. The current understanding of this infection is that most individuals acquire the infection before birth in transmission across the placenta. This occurs when a pregnant woman has an acute infection with toxoplasmosis acquired through the respiratory route. It may cause a mild flulike illness after inhalation of toxoplasmosis organisms from infected cat feces. The organism may cause only a transient systemic infection and is rapidly brought under control by the immune system. If, however, cysts cross the placenta and infect the neonate, the infection may not be totally eradicated. Also of some concern is that ocular toxoplasmosis may result from the eating of infected meat or through respiratory infections in immunocompromised individuals.

The typical appearance of a toxoplasmosis lesion varies depending on whether the infection is in an active state or whether the organ-

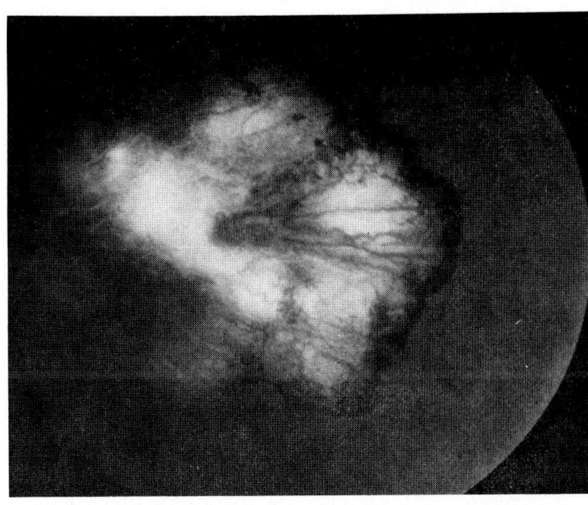

Fig. 6–40. An inactive toxoplasmosis scar with a scalloped margin created by multiple recurrences.

isms are inactive in the encysted form in the retina. A common fundus finding is a punched-out chorioretinal scar with necrosis of the overlying retina and the choroid producing a white lesion with a black hyperpigmented reactive ring around the punched-out appearance. The white area is actually the underlying sclera. This appearance is typical for a focus of previous toxoplasmosis infection and is often asymptomatic. Toxoplasmosis chorioretinitis often becomes inactive without treatment.

Occasionally, patients may notice floaters or blurred vision associated with activity of a toxoplasmosis lesion, typically during episodes of reactivation. In such an occurrence, a white area of retina occurs at the margin of a toxoplasmosis scar. A series of episodes such as this can result in a scalloped area of necrotic retina, indicating multiple episodes of previous toxoplasmosis infections (Fig. 6–40).

Treatment for toxoplasmosis is not uniform. The standard treatment has included sulfonamides. More recently, clindamycin has been suggested as a more effective treatment because the drug may have more effect on the encysted organisms. Tetracycline has also been suggested in some cases.

Toxocara canis *produces an intraocular granuloma.*

Toxocara canis is a parasite that may enter the eye and cause a chronic inflammatory lesion.

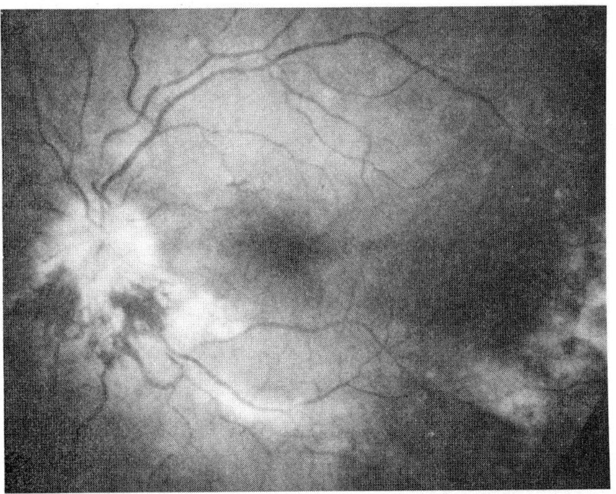

Fig. 6–39. Hemorrhages on the optic nerve and some white areas of retina in a patient with cytomegalovirus retinitis. Sheathing is present along the inferior temporal vein.

The infection is acquired by ingesting organisms that have come from the parasite's reservoir in dogs. Dogs, especially puppies, are not fastidious with their bowel habits, and the parasites released in the feces may be recovered from the fur of puppies. These can be transmitted to children by direct contact with the dog or by playing in an area of soil that has been contaminated. The eye is only one site that may be infected with *Toxocara*. Other areas include the liver and the brain.

In the eye, the organisms cause a chronic inflammatory lesion that may result in subretinal fibrosis and dragging of the retina. Such a lesion often has a typical appearance of subretinal strands extending from the optic nerve to an intraocular granuloma. In the past, *Toxocara canis* has been mistaken for retinoblastoma; however, awareness of this misdiagnosis and effective examination techniques can usually prevent such an error. The enzyme-linked immunosorbent assay for *Toxocara canis* can be helpful in confirming the diagnosis.

Malignant melanoma of the choroid is the most common primary intraocular malignancy.

Melanomas arise from melanocytes that are present in the uveal tract (choroid, ciliary body, or iris). These melanocytes are similar to those found in the skin. Most intraocular melanomas arise from the choroid or ciliary body; iris melanomas are uncommon.

Malignant melanomas of the choroid can be diagnosed clinically.

The diagnosis of uveal melanoma can usually be made with noninvasive techniques. Although some reports in the older literature show a high error rate in the diagnosis of malignant melanoma, studies from large centers where patients with melanoma are frequently seen show that the diagnosis of melanoma can be at least 98% specific. To make the diagnosis, a careful complete eye examination is necessary in combination with special techniques such as photography, fluorescein angiography, ultrasonography, and transillumination. Malignant melanoma may arise de novo, although it usu-

ally develops in an area of a pre-existing nevus. A *nevus* is a pigmented melanocytic choroidal mass that is less than 2 mm thick. It is important to be able to recognize suspicious nevi and melanomas and to differentiate them from other pigmented fundus lesions.

Thickness is a characteristic of melanoma.

A melanoma has a typical appearance of a steeply elevated nodule with a narrow base in the center of a nevus (Fig. 6–41). This pattern of growth is called a *collar button lesion* and is very important to recognize. Although histologically melanomas always contain pigment, clinically they may appear hypopigmented or amelanotic in some cases. Two factors that should strongly suggest the possibility of malignancy are growth and thickness.

Observing lesions for growth is a basic principle in evaluating pigmented fundus lesions. It is important to document these areas as carefully as possible. The first choice in documenting such a lesion is a fundus photograph. Occasionally, if the media are cloudy or the lesion is located in a very anterior location such as the ciliary body, one may have to rely on transillumination and ultrasonography to document the size of the lesion.

Any pigmented fundus lesion more than 1 mm in thickness should be characterized as

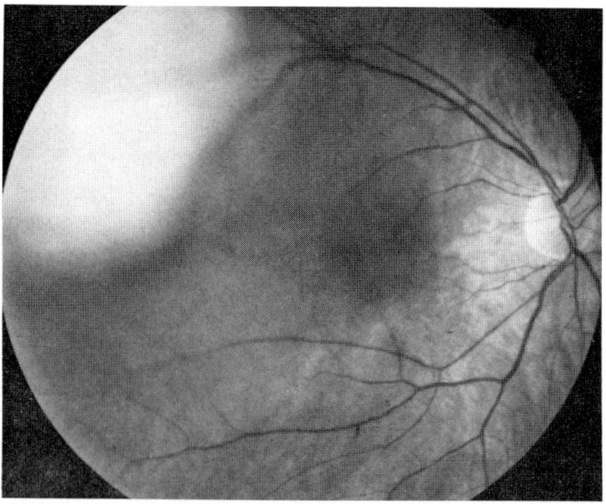

Fig. 6–41. The right eye of a patient with a minimally pigmented malignant melanoma of the superior temporal choroid in the superior temporal aspect of the macula.

suspicious. Such a lesion should be carefully documented and reexamined every 3 months.

Many common pigmented fundus lesions may simulate malignant melanoma. The most difficult lesions to differentiate from melanoma include other intraocular tumors such as metastases or adenomas and adenocarcinomas of the retinal pigment epithelium. One fairly common *"pseudomelanoma"* is a choroidal hemorrhage or choroidal effusion. This should readily be differentiated by history and ultrasonography; however, in selected instances actual biopsy may be necessary. Table 6–6 lists common pseudomelanomas.

Treatment of malignant melanoma is controversial.

The treatment of malignant melanoma is a matter of considerable controversy. Historically, the treatment of choice has been enucleation (removal of the tumor-containing eye). However, in the 1970s, with improved diagnostic techniques, it became obvious that enucleation of malignant melanoma did not produce a clear improvement in survival. In fact, some studies even suggested a transient increase in the number of tumor-related deaths in the first year after enucleation. This information, in addition to the need to offer alternative therapies to patients who have tumors in their only functioning eye, has led to the development of alternative treatments of malignant melanoma. Several large groups have shown that survival after malignant melanoma treated with radiation approximates that after enucleation. The effect on survival of irradiation for malignant melanoma is the topic of a cooperative prospective randomized study. It will be several years before this controversy is settled. Treatment of malignant melanoma with radiation requires high doses of radiation because melanoma is not a radiosensitive tumor. Radiation is applied by a proton beam that can be highly focused or with brachytherapy by applying radioactive material to the eye wall.

Retinoblastoma is the second most common primary intraocular malignancy.

Retinoblastoma arises from the precursor cells of the photoreceptors (retinoblasts). This highly malignant tumor is found almost exclusively in patients younger than 4 years. Retinoblastoma is the most common primary intraocular tumor in blacks because of the low frequency of malignant melanoma in the black population.

Retinoblastoma requires emergency treatment.

Retinoblastoma is a highly malignant tumor that is nearly 100% fatal without treatment. With early treatment and recognition, the death rate from retinoblastoma may be as low as 2%. It is therefore very important to be aware of this malignancy and to avoid delay in diagnosis or treatment.

Retinoblastoma usually presents as a whitish pupillary reflex (*leukocoria*). Familiarity with the differential diagnosis of leukocoria is essential (Table 6–7). It is absolutely necessary for any child presenting with leukocoria or strabismus to have a careful fundus examination.

TABLE 6–6 Fundus Lesions that May Mimic Malignant Melanoma

Choroidal nevus
Hemorrhagic choroidal neovascularization
Congenital hypertrophy of the retinal pigment
    epithelium
Reactive hyperplasia of the retinal pigment
    epithelium
Melanocytoma of the optic nerve
Choroidal detachment
Carcinoma metastatic to the choroid

TABLE 6–7 Differential Diagnosis of Leukocoria

Retinoblastoma
Retinopathy of prematurity
Congenital cataract
Toxocara canis
Old organized vitreous hemorrhage
Endophthalmitis
Retinal detachment
Persistent hyperplastic primary vitreous

Other less common presentations of retinoblastoma include pain, decreased vision, exophthalmos, or redness.

Retinoblastoma may occur as an isolated tumor or may be multicentric. The multicentric variety of tumor is hereditary. Because the tumor may be multicentric, regular follow-up of a patient who had retinoblastoma is important to monitor for the development of additional tumors.

Retinoblastoma may be treated with enucleation or radiation. The tumor has also been treated with photocoagulation and cryotherapy. The exact combination of therapies to be used in retinoblastoma requires individual consideration.

Angiomatous malformations may indicate a phakomatosis.

Several angiomatous malformations found in the fundus deserve mention. Although they are not malignant tumors, they do have some associations with systemic disease. The angiomatous malformations include retinal capillary hemangioma, cavernous retinal hemangioma, and cavernous hemangioma of the choroid.

A *capillary retinal hemangioma* may occur as an isolated lesion or in conjunction with the *von Hippel-Lindau syndrome*. This lesion has a strawberry color and may occur anywhere in the retina. There is typically a large feeder arteriole and a draining venule. Occasionally, this lesion may decompensate and have retinal edema and exudates associated with it.

If a retinal capillary hemangioma becomes visually significant by producing exudate and edema extending into the macula, the tumor may be treated with cryotherapy or intense photocoagulation to reduce the amount of leakage from such a lesion. The von Hippel-Lindau syndrome is one of the phakomatoses and may be associated with tumors of the kidney, adrenal gland, and central nervous system.

A *cavernous retinal hemangioma* appears as saccular dilatations of retinal veins grouped in the retina. They do not decompensate and leak and do not require treatment. Cavernous retinal hemangioma may be associated with cavernous hemangiomas of the central nervous system, liver, and skin.

Cavernous hemangioma of the choroid may occur in isolation or as part of the *Sturge-Weber syndrome*. Typically, choroidal cavernous hemangiomas that occur without systemic findings are discrete and may simulate other choroidal tumors such as malignant melanoma or choroidal metastases. In Sturge-Weber syndrome, the choroidal cavernous hemangioma is diffuse and usually involves the entire fundus. The appearance has been described as a "tomato ketchup" fundus.

Arteriovenous malformations may be associated with *Wyburn-Mason syndrome*. Malformations of the midbrain may be present.

Patients with *neurofibromatosis* sometimes develop a retinal tumor known as an *astrocytic hamartoma*. This lesion is white or light in color, is several millimeters in diameter, and has a bumpy berry-like configuration.

7

NEURO-OPHTHALMOLOGY

Thomas J. Liesegang
Thomas J. McPhee

Patients with neuro-ophthalmic problems may present with vague symptoms that require a thorough history.

Patients with neuro-ophthalmic problems frequently present with *vague symptoms*, and it is important that a thorough and careful history elaborate the chief complaint. Specific features to record are the patient's own descriptive words, the circumstances of the complaint, progression or remission of the problem, and any associated signs or symptoms. A detailed past medical history, the medications currently being taken, and the nutritional, social, and family history are general historical facts that build on the chief complaint. Deliberations with a careful history will usually yield a diagnosis that the examination merely confirms; failure to obtain a careful history may result in the missed diagnosis of a potentially significant neurologic disease. Prompted by this working diagnosis, the examiner may use several specific neuro-ophthalmic tests.

Special techniques are used during the neuro-ophthalmic examination.

Some form of *confrontation visual field* testing should be performed on every patient who presents for ophthalmologic examination. These tests can be performed on virtually any patient, even those with limited cognition (Fig. 7–1). There are several more refined levels of testing that may be necessary, depending on the chief complaint, the visual acuity, and the ability of the patient to cooperate. The threshold or sensitivity of the visual field varies; the central 30° of the retina is dominated by retinal cone cells capable of discriminating fine detail, whereas the peripheral portions of the retina are dominated by retinal rod cells capable of sensitivity in low lighting conditions but with poor discrimination of detail (Fig. 7–2).

Visual field testing may be kinetic or static. In *kinetic* testing (for example, Goldmann or tangent screen), the stimulus is moved to different areas and the point at which it is first seen by the patient is marked. The line connecting these points (isopter) outlines a geographic area outside of which the stimulus is not detected (Fig. 7–3 *Top*). Several isopters may be defined by the use of different-sized stimulus objects. Specific areas of depressed sensitivity (scotomas) within the isopter may be present. Normal kinetic visual fields can be defined to 90° temporally, 60° nasally, 60° superiorly, and 70° inferiorly.

In *static* (stationary) perimetry, a specific point is chosen for examination and the stimulus is increased until its threshold is determined (Fig. 7–3 *Bottom*). Other points are examined similarly until a profile of retinal sensitivity is established for the entire visual field. *Octopus, Humphrey,* and other automated and computerized machines or the Goldmann perimeter in

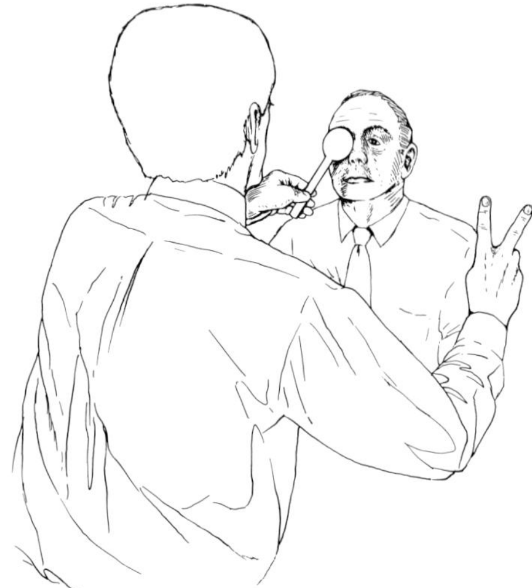

Fig. 7–1. The technique of visual field testing by confrontation. The patient fixates on the examiner's nose with one eye while the other eye is covered by the examiner. The four quadrants of vision are tested with one, two, or no fingers. This test is easily performed even on children.

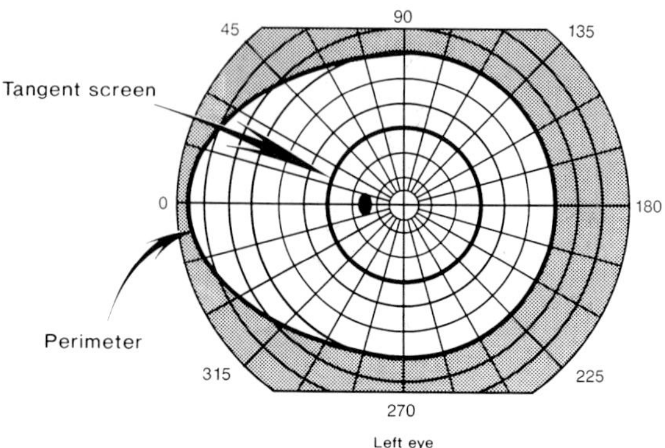

Fig. 7–2. The tangent screen tests the central 30° of the visual field, whereas the entire visual field can be tested with a perimeter (either automated or manual).

the static mode can accomplish this type of visual examination.

The *tangent screen test* at 1 or 2 m, a standard test for evaluating the central 30° of the visual field, is invaluable for verifying the physiologic characteristics of the visual field (that is, the normal blind spot) and for excluding functional or factitious visual field defects (Fig. 7–4). The *Amsler grid* is a rapid screening test for central visual field defects (Fig. 7–5). The subjective description of the occurrence and localization of visual field defects is possible with little equipment at a bedside examination (Fig. 7–6). Small visual defects, however, may be difficult to demonstrate. The value of *colored objects* in visual field examination has been debated for years. Optic nerve lesions are more readily detected with a red object, whereas retinal lesions are more easily detected with a blue object. In clinical practice, confrontation testing reveals subtle changes perceived in the brightness of the color red in depressed areas compared with simultaneous testing in normal areas of the visual field.

Acquired color vision abnormalities usually indicate optic nerve disease.

Acquired *color vision* abnormalities generally indicate a diffuse disease of the optic nerve, especially compressive or demyelinating lesions.

Fig. 7–3. *Top,* The kinetic method of visual field testing, in which various-sized targets are moved in from the periphery until they are first recognized. Smaller targets will have to get closer to the macula before being recognized. This defines the contour of the "island of vision." *Bottom,* The static method of visual field testing, in which a target is stationary but increased in size or intensity until it is recognized. This describes the profile of the "island of vision" in a different fashion. (Modified from F.J. Bajandas, L.B. Kline: Neuro-Ophthalmology Review Manual. Second edition. Thorofare, New Jersey, Slack, 1987, pp. 1–42.)

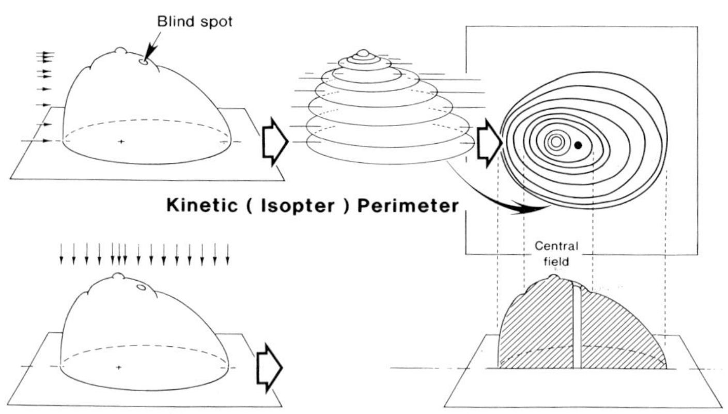

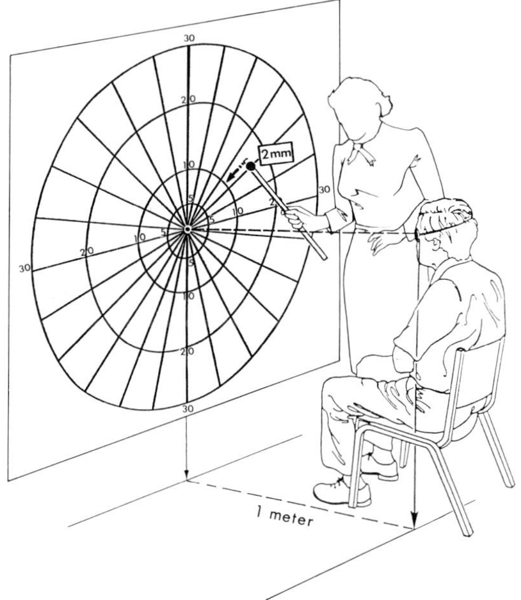

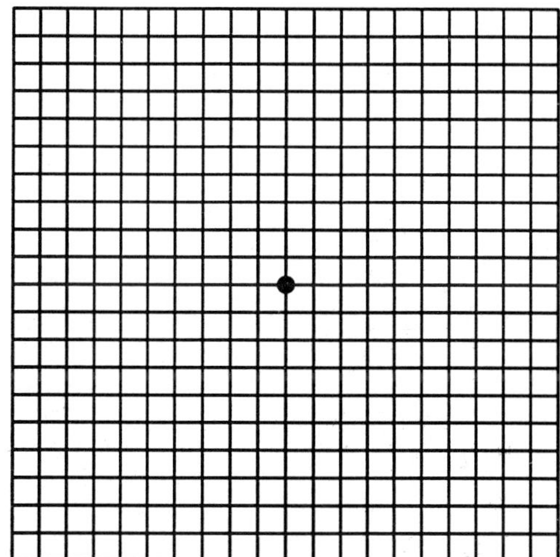

Fig. 7–4. The tangent screen test at 1 m evaluates the central 30° visual field with a high degree of accuracy. It is most helpful for verifying the normal blind spot, for identifying lesions that "obey" the midline, and for confirming functional visual field defects. (Modified from D.R. Anderson: Testing the Field of Vision. St. Louis, C.V. Mosby Company, 1982, pp. 44–45.)

Fig. 7–5. The Amsler grid. All the lines should appear clear and straight when no central visual field defect is present. The patient must maintain central fixation on the dark, large, central point of the grid.

Color vision abnormalities may be present in optic nerve disease despite normal visual acuity and normal results of visual field testing, or they may be detected in various retinal diseases not easily apparent by ophthalmoscopy. Patients with reduced visual acuity to the level of 20/100 from refractive error or from cornea, lens, or vitreous abnormalities usually maintain normal color perception. Moreover, in patients with evident optic nerve disease, the preservation of normal color vision virtually excludes a compressive lesion of the nerve. The simplest screening test is the Hardy-Rand-Rittler series of plates comparing the normal eye with the involved eye.

The photostress test has abnormal results in retinal disease.

The *photostress* test may help to distinguish unilateral visual loss with macular disease from that with optic nerve disease. After the visual acuity is measured, a bright light is shown direct-

ly into one eye for 60 seconds and the other eye is occluded. The examiner then records the length of time (in seconds) required to read the same visual acuity chart. The other eye is tested in a similar fashion. In optic nerve disease, the time required for retinal readaptation should be the same in both eyes, whereas with retinal disease, the readaptation time in the affected eye is prolonged compared with that in

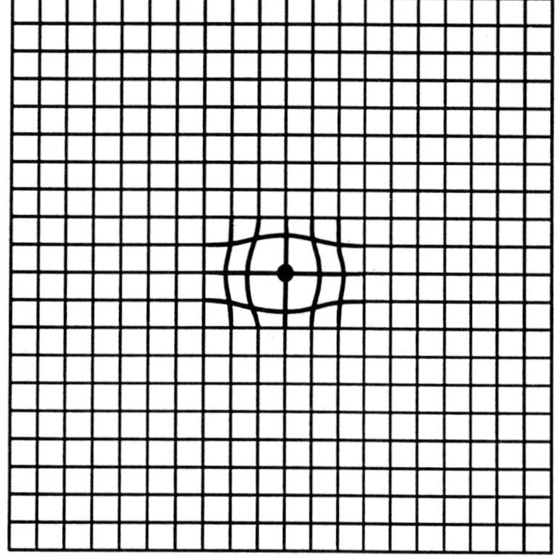

Fig. 7–6. A central defect in the Amsler grid, caused by a small lesion in the macular area that has distorted both the horizontal and the vertical lines.

the normal eye because of the slower recovery time of the retinal photoreceptors.

Optokinetic nystagmus confirms intact saccade and pursuit gaze mechanisms.

Optokinetic nystagmus defines the movement of the eyes as the patient views a succession of regularly presented figures or stripes. The usual stimulus for eliciting this nystagmus is a rotating drum with regularly spaced, alternating patterns or dark and light stripes or a similarly constructed tape (Fig. 7–7). There is an initial slow movement of both eyes followed by a rapid reflex movement to the next figure. The direction of the nystagmus (slow phase) is determined by the direction the figure is moved with the re-fixation movement (fast phase) occurring in the opposite direction. Optokinetic nystagmus is present in both horizontal and vertical directions in all patients with normal visual acuity and normal ocular motility. Optokinetic nystagmus is proof of some degree of vision (at least 20/200) and is also proof of the presence of an intact pursuit and saccade gaze system. Optokinetic nystagmus testing is important in the localization of cortical brain abnormalities.

Ophthalmodynamometry measures the ophthalmic artery pressure.

Ophthalmodynamometry is a technique for measuring the ophthalmic artery (not central retinal artery) blood pressure. The ophthalmodynamometer is a spring gauge calibrated to reflect pressure applied perpendicular to the scleral wall of the globe. The optic nerve is visualized with an ophthalmoscope; the pressure at which the central retinal artery begins to pulsate is the diastolic pressure, and the pressure at which the central retinal artery collapses is the systolic pressure. Conversion tables are used to express the values in millimeters of mercury. The intraocular pressure must be normal and fairly symmetric for meaningful ophthalmic artery pressure determinations and comparisons. The systolic blood pressure of the ophthalmic artery is approximately 80% of the brachial artery systolic pressure, and the diastolic pressure is 70% of the brachial artery diastolic pressure.

Ophthalmodynamometry is important for evaluating occlusive vascular disease of the ophthalmic or carotid arteries, especially if there is an asymmetric pressure between the two eyes in persons with appropriate symptoms and signs. The interpretation of symmetrically decreased values is a more complex and debated topic and usually requires more sophisticated testing. The measurement of *ophthalmic artery pressure* may have application in the evaluation of low-tension glaucoma and vascular disease of the optic nerve or in monitoring patients after carotid artery operation.

The retinal nerve fiber layer can be viewed and correlated with nerve damage.

The normal retinal *nerve fiber layer* is seen with the ophthalmoscope in red-free (green) light as a homogeneous, slightly opaque layer of regular striations (see Fig. 5–2). Defects in

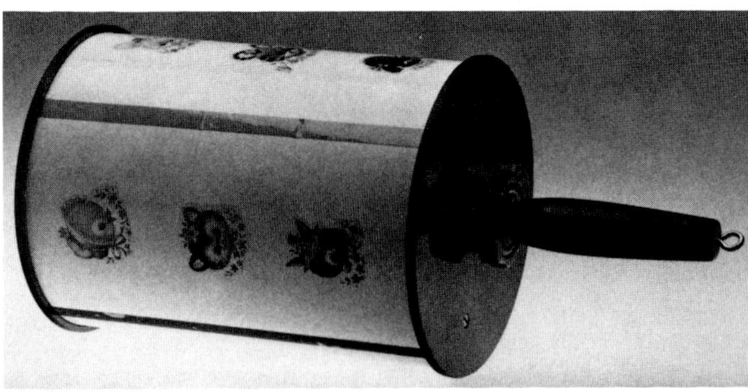

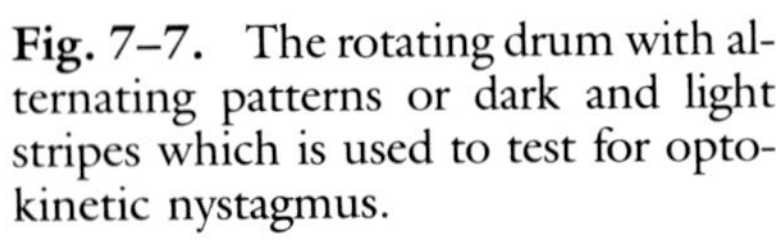

Fig. 7–7. The rotating drum with alternating patterns or dark and light stripes which is used to test for optokinetic nystagmus.

the retinal nerve fiber layer may be slit-like in an arcuate area in glaucoma, or there may be multiple slit-like defects in multiple sclerosis. Diffuse defects can be seen after severe optic nerve damage, or segmental defects can be seen in branch artery occlusion. Normal peripapillary striations are lost in papilledema but are retained in anomalous elevations of the optic disc (that is, pseudopapilledema). The observation of normal striations in a patient with profound visual field loss suggests a functional (nonorganic) problem.

Neurologic examination of the cranial nerves may localize a lesion.

During the course of motility evaluation, the *third*, *fourth*, and *sixth cranial nerves are assessed*. Impairment of cranial nerves may be important in identifying diseases or localizing neurologic defects. *Fifth nerve* function is tested by checking sensation in all three divisions of the trigeminal nerve (that is, the forehead and cornea, the cheek, and the angle of the jaw and under the jaw). A peripheral *seventh nerve* lesion causes paresis of the muscles on one side of the face and forehead. A seventh nerve lesion of the central brainstem spares the brow because of bilateral innervation. The absence of tearing on the side of a seventh nerve defect suggests a lesion of the parasympathetic fibers to the lacrimal gland, which travel for a short distance with the seventh nerve. Hearing loss in association with a seventh nerve palsy suggests a lesion in the cerebellopontine angle, where the acoustic nerve also may be involved.

Electrophysiologic testing is useful in selected circumstances.

The generation of the A wave of the *electroretinogram* depends on an intact choroidal circulation, and the generation of the B wave depends on an intact retinal circulation. Electroretinography (ERG) is a method of studying the choroidal and retinal circulations and may supplement information obtained with fluorescein angiography. ERG is essential for identifying early tapetoretinal disease or other photoreceptor dystrophies, especially early in their course before the distinctive pigmentary, vas-

cular, and optic nerve changes are present. ERG is especially helpful for detecting ophthalmic (retinal) disease in a child (such as Leber's congenital amaurosis) before significant ophthalmoscopic changes are present. A flat ERG correlates with loss of photoreceptor activity. The ERG may occasionally be abnormal in some neurologic diseases.

The *visual-evoked response* (or *visual-evoked potential*) is an electrical activity appearing in the electroencephalogram associated with the presentation of a visual stimulus. After the eye receives a stimulus, the electrical activity generated is accumulated and averaged on a computer to produce an evoked response. The latency, amplitude, and conduction of the evoked response are recorded and compared with the results in normal patients. Each optic nerve is tested separately and then the nerves are tested together. The stimulus can be projected onto the macula or other area of the retina so that selected areas can be examined or compared. The visual-evoked response is useful for identifying diseases of the optic nerve, localizing diseases along the visual pathway, or monitoring optic nerve function during surgical procedures near the optic nerve. Optic neuritis produces a characteristically increased latency period and decreased amplitude compared with the normal eye. Other types of optic nerve disease may produce other patterns on the visual-evoked response.

Fluorescein angiography may define the retinal disease.

Fluorescein angiography is useful in a few selected neuro-ophthalmic problems. Papilledema can be distinguished from pseudopapilledema by fluorescein angiography because true papilledema shows capillary dilatation and telangiectatic changes of the disc capillaries, and the early photographs show leakage of fluorescein from the capillaries. Control photographs obtained before angiography may reveal optic nerve drusen, a common cause of pseudopapilledema, from autofluorescence.

Fluorescein angiography may demonstrate choroidal or retinal circulatory abnormalities, which may be associated with small vessel disease affecting the optic nerve or be part of a more generalized vascular disease (such as collagen disease). Fluorescein angiography helps to distinguish subtle forms of retinal diseases when the cause of decreased visual acuity is obscure.

Neuroradiologic procedures usually conclude the neurologic examination.

Multiple *radiologic procedures* are available that further define neuro-ophthalmic diseases. These include skull radiography, polytomography, angiography, pneumoencephalography, computed tomography, and magnetic resonance imaging. The indications for each test vary, and selection of the correct evaluations helps to conclude the neuro-ophthalmic evaluation expediently.

The anatomy of the visual sensory system comprises the retina, optic nerves, optic chiasms, optic tracts, lateral geniculate bodies, optic radiations, and the occipital cortex.

Careful examination of the visual field may allow accurate localization and identification of the causes of disease within the visual system. Understanding visual field topography depends on an understanding of the organization of the visual sensory system pathway, which includes the retina, optic nerve, optic chiasm, optic tract, lateral geniculate body, optic radiation, and the occipital cortex (Fig. 7–8).

Most retinal *nerve fibers* entering the optic disc originate from the *papillomacular bundle*. The remainder of nerve fibers originate from the peripheral portion of the retina (Fig. 7–9). Fibers from the *peripheral retina* originate both temporally and nasally to the fovea and arch around the papillomacular bundle to enter the optic disc at its superior and inferior poles. Fibers from the peripheral retina nasal to the optic nerve pass in a straight line to the optic disc. Nerve fibers are also distinguished into superior and inferior depending on an irregular line (the horizontal raphe) that separates upper and lower peripheral fibers.

As the nerve fibers pass posteriorly in the optic nerve, the papillomacular fibers become centrally located and the peripheral retinal fibers are located on the periphery. The *optic nerve* has intraocular (1 mm), intraorbital (25 mm), intracanalicular (4 to 10 mm), and intracranial (10 mm) portions until it reaches the *optic chiasm*. Within the optic chiasm, central and

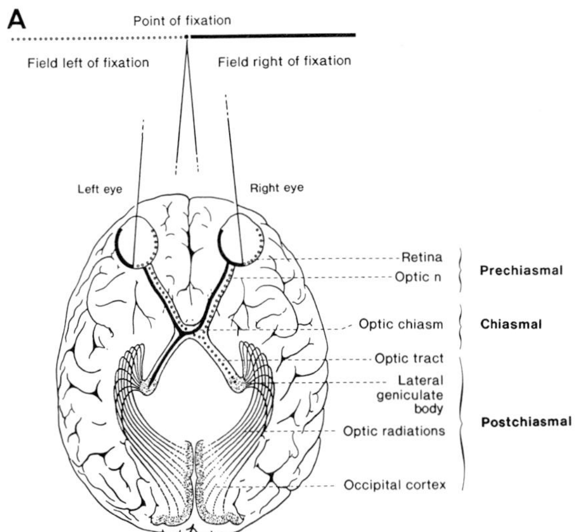

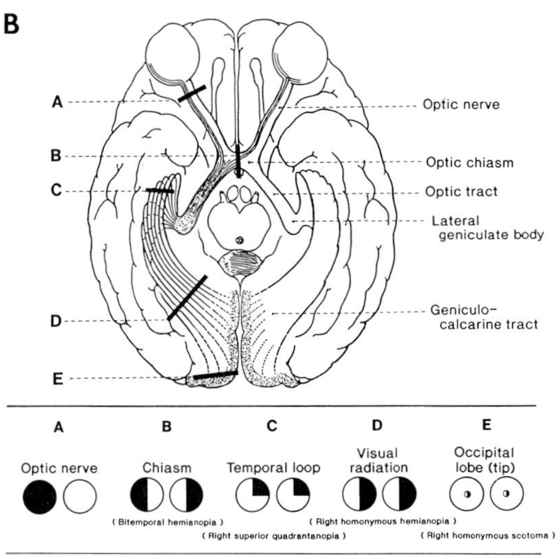

Fig. 7–8. *A*, The visual sensory system, showing the origin of the stimulus in the retina, the passage of the impulse through the optic nerve, the crossing of the nasal fibers in the optic chiasm, the optic tract made up of temporal nerve fibers from the same eye and nasal nerve fibers from the opposite eye, and the sweep of the optic radiations through the temporal lobe, the parietal lobe, and finally the occipital cortex. *B*, The corresponding visual field defects for various lesions along the pathway, shown in the accompanying visual fields.

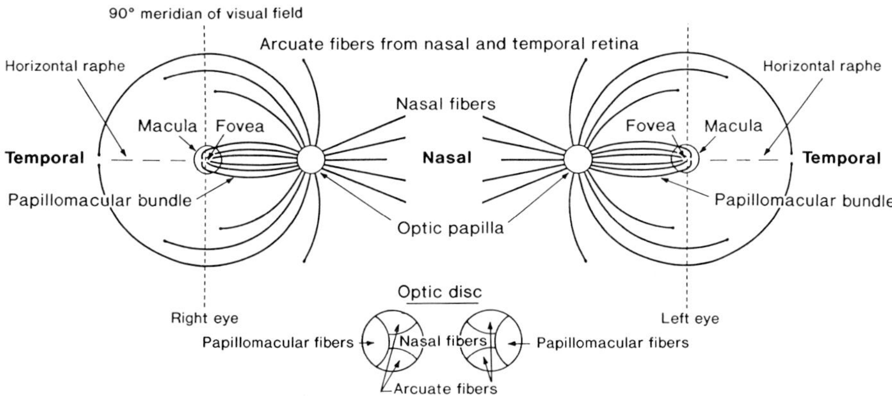

Fig. 7–9. The organization of the nerve fiber layer in the retina, emphasizing the origin of the fibers within the retina and their course toward the optic nerve.

peripheral fibers originating temporally to the fovea do not cross but pass to the optic tract on the same side. Nasal retinal fibers cross in the chiasm and pass to the contralateral optic tract. The retinal nerve fibers that pass in the nerve, chiasm, and optic tract terminate and synapse in the *lateral geniculate body*, which is a triangular, multilaminated structure with crossed and uncrossed fibers represented in specific layers of the structure. The *optic radiation* then loops forward in the temporal lobe anterior to the tip of the lateral geniculate body (Meyer's loop) and then passes posteriorly to the occipital cortex (Brodmann's area 17). The fibers from the macula and from the inferior and superior retinal quadrants follow a specific route in this visual pathway, resulting in predictable patterns of nerve loss associated with specific lesions. When the nerve fibers reach the cortex, the macular representation is at the tip of the occipital lobe, whereas the peripheral field representation is spread over the medial portion of the occipital lobe within the calcarine fissure. The *visual cortex* receives its blood supply from the posterior cerebral artery and from the middle cerebral system. The optic radiation also is supplied by the middle and posterior cerebral arteries.

Visual field defects correspond predictably to the area of the visual system that is damaged. Damage to the nerve fiber layer in the retina or optic nerve produces altitudinal defects or scotomas (areas of decreased visual sensitivity surrounded by an area of normal sensitivity). Most neurologic lesions affecting the optic chiasm or the visual structures posterior to the chiasm cause field defects that are oriented along the vertical meridian. A *hemianopic field defect* involves the temporal or nasal half of the visual field of one or both eyes. A *quadrantanopic field defect* involves roughly one quarter of the visual field (Fig. 7–8 *B*). *Homonymous defects* affect corresponding fields in each eye. *Congruity of visual field defects* refers to the similarity of the field defect in one eye to the defect in the other eye. The visual field defect may also be described in terms of its density and the contour of its borders. The *density* of the defect can be defined in terms of the size or brightness of the stimulus that can or cannot be seen. The *contour* of the visual field is defined by the abruptness in the transition from the normal visual field to the defect measured.

In combination with a knowledge of the anatomy of the visual system and the type of visual defect observed, interpretation of field defects usually predicts the location of a lesion (Fig. 7–8 *B*). Retinal lesions cause corresponding defects in the visual field (that is, supratemporal retinal lesions produce infranasal field defects). The depth of the field defect depends on the degree of destruction of the retinal receptors. In some instances the overlying retinal nerve fibers in transit to the optic disc are also damaged, and this damage causes a field defect in these additional nerve fibers, usually giving an arcuate appearance to the field loss (for fibers that travel from the peripheral portion around the papillomacular bundle) or a sector defect (for fibers that run in a straight course from the nasal portion of the retina).

Optic nerve disease can cause several different types of visual field defects. *Central scotomas* (Fig. 7–10 *A*) are seen with lesions that affect the optic nerve diffusely, such as optic neuritis and compressive lesions. A *cecocentral scotoma* (Fig. 7–10 *B*) is a field defect in which a central scotoma is connected to the blind spot with an area of depressed visual field in between. This scotoma is seen with toxic amblyopias (such as from vitamin B_{12} deficiency or tobacco or alcohol abuse) or with hereditary forms of optic neuropathy (Leber's optic neuropathy). *Paracentral scotomas* (Fig. 7–10 *C*) are often associated with early glaucoma or lesions around the macula. An *arcuate scotoma* (Fig. 7–10 *D*) occurs from lesions of the optic nerve that interrupt the entering fibers that arc around the papillomacular bundle. Arcuate defects are most common from glaucoma or vascular disease (such as temporal arteritis, collagen disease, migraine). An *altitudinal defect* affects either the upper or the lower half of the visual field and is an extreme example of an arcuate-type defect. Although this defect has been clinically correlated with vascular causes, there is no known anatomic basis in the vascular or nerve fiber system to explain this phenomenon.

Disease in the area of the optic chiasm characteristically produces a *bitemporal hemianopia* (Fig. 7–11 *A*). The visual defect is more apparent in the central than the peripheral portion because the central portion is the most sensitive. The bitemporal visual field defect sometimes may be detected earlier with red-colored testing objects than with white objects. A lesion in the optic nerve just anterior to the junction with the optic chiasm causes a typical pattern of field defect described as a *junctional scotoma* (Fig. 7–11 *B*). This consists of a central scotoma in one eye and a superior temporal field defect in the contralateral eye that lines up in the vertical meridian. The anatomic basis for this defect is that it is related to the inferior nasal retinal fibers, after crossing in the chiasm loop, coursing anteriorly for a short and variable distance into the contralateral optic nerve before passing posteriorly into the tract. This loop is termed von Willebrand's knee.

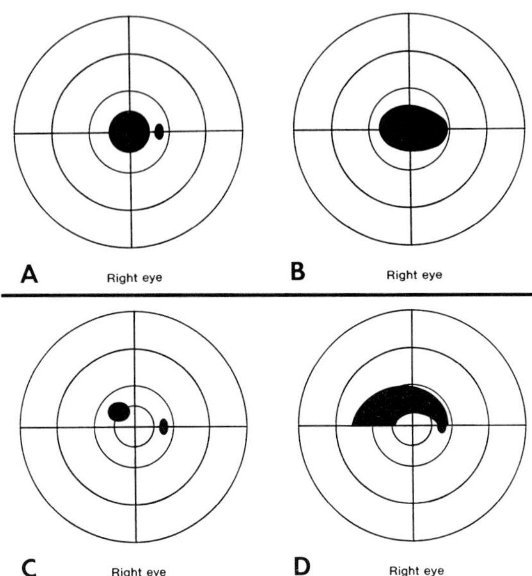

Fig. 7–10. Various types of depression within the central field of vision (scotomas) caused by disease of the retina or the optic nerve. *A*, Central scotoma. *B*, Cecocentral scotoma. *C*, Paracentral scotoma. *D*, Arcuate scotoma.

Disease of the optic tract or geniculate ganglion produces a *homonymous hemianopia* that may be incongruous or may be complete (Fig. 7–11 *C*). Lesions in the optic radiation cause a fairly congruous homonymous superior quadrantanopia with a lesion in the temporal lobe (Fig. 7–11 *D*) or an inferior quadrantanopic defect with a lesion in the parietal lobe (Fig. 7–11 *E*), or they may produce a total homonymous hemianopia if the lesion is extensive. Lesions of the occipital cortex are usually extremely congruous but may or may not spare the macula (Fig. 7–11 *F* and 7–11 *G*). *Sparing of the macula* is characteristic of occipital lesions and may be related to the vast macular representation in the occipital cortex, to the dual blood supply from the middle and posterior cerebral circulation, or to the possibility of double innervation.

Other functions of the cerebral cortex allow more accurate localization of neurologic defects. *Temporal lobe dysfunction* is associated with psychomotor seizures, olfactory and gustatory sensations, and hallucinations. *Parietal lobe dysfunction* in the dominant hemisphere produces inability to read (alexia), to write (agraphia), and to calculate (acalculia). Lesions of the non-

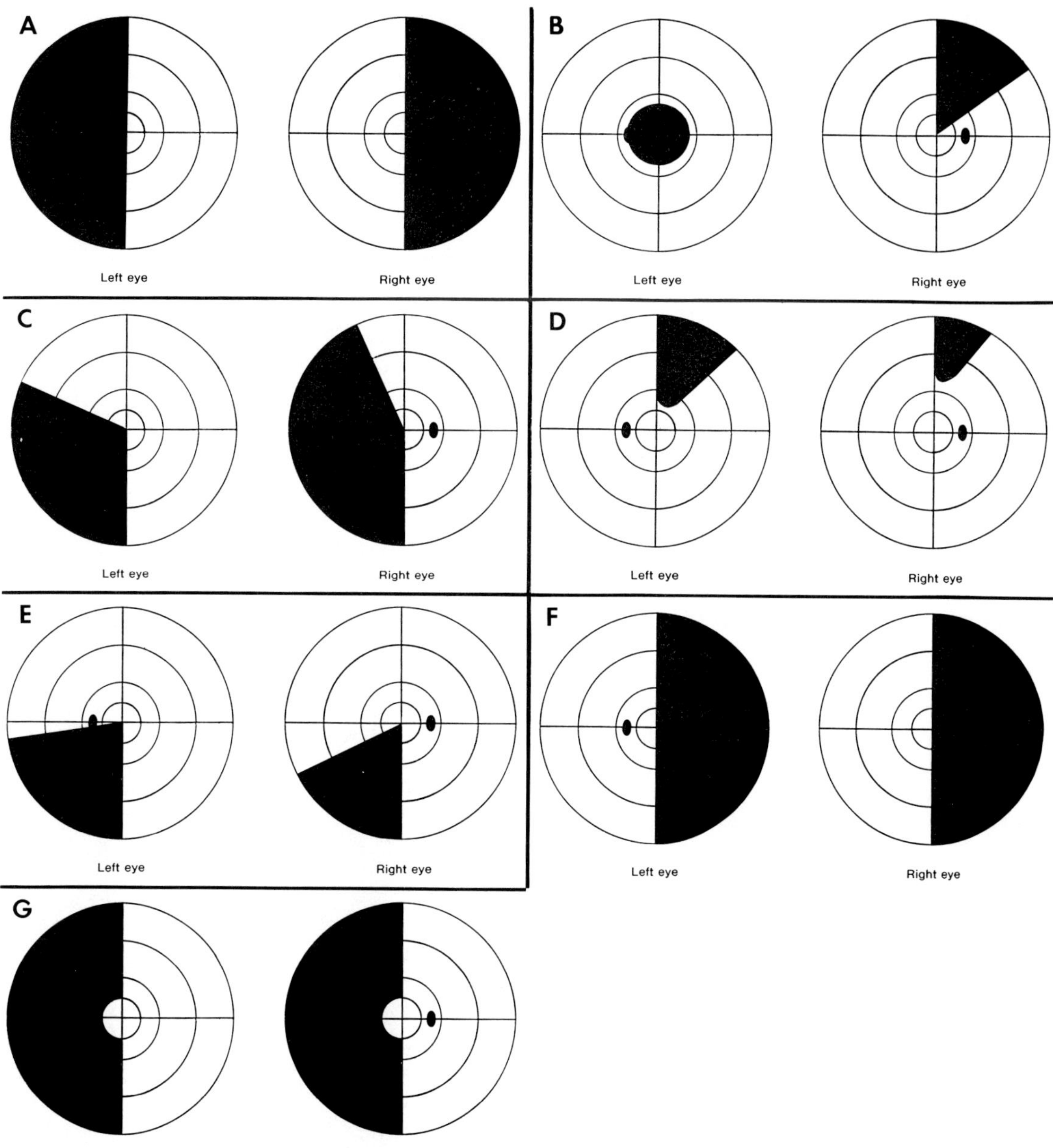

Fig. 7–11. *A*, A complete bitemporal visual field defect characteristic of a lesion in the optic chiasm. *B*, Junctional scotoma is characteristic of a lesion in the left optic nerve just before the junction with the optic chiasm. *C*, An incomplete and incongruous left homonymous hemianopia due to a right optic tract lesion. *D*, A fairly congruous right homonymous superior quadrantanopia ("pie in the sky") caused by an anterior lesion of Meyer's loop in the left temporal lobe. *E*, A left inferior quadrantanopic defect from a lesion in the right parietal lobe. *F*, A complete right homonymous hemianopia with macular splitting associated with a lesion in the left occipital lobe. Complete homonymous defects are in themselves nonlocalizing. *G*, A left homonymous hemianopia with macular "sparing" associated with a lesion in the right occipital lobe.

dominant parietal hemisphere produce disturbances in body awareness, denial of hemiparesis, or abnormal posturing of the affected extremities. Disorders of the *occipital lobe* produce primarily visual field defects, although visual hallucinations with unformed images are of diagnostic significance. The optokinetic response is usually normal in optic nerve lesions but abnormal in parietal lobe lesions.

A *constricted* visual field is one of the more common defects and may be caused by opaque media (for example, cataract), glaucoma, chronic disc edema, or more distinct patterns in association with specific optic nerve damage. Functional field loss (hysteria or malingering) produces *contraction* of the visual field, which characteristically does not expand as expected when the tangent screen examination is performed at 2 m compared with 1 m.

The afferent pupillary fibers leave the optic tract to enter the brain.

Light stimulates the retinal photoreceptors and also the associated pupillomotor fibers, which subsequently regulate the size of the pupil. The pupil constricts through the stimulation of the parasympathetic system (iris sphincter) and dilates with stimulation of the sympathetic system (iris dilator). The *pupillary fibers* are transmitted by way of the optic nerve through the chiasm and then leave the optic tract before the lateral geniculate body to enter the brainstem (Fig. 7–12). After synapse in the *pretectum*, the fibers are distributed to the ipsilateral and contralateral *Edinger-Westphal nucleus* by an intercalary neuron. The efferent pupillary fibers (parasympathetic system) exit at the midbrain along with the third cranial nerve with a final synapse at the *ciliary ganglion.* Postganglionic fibers are then distributed to the iris sphincter and ciliary body by way of the short ciliary nerves. The sympathetic pathway for pupil dilation originates in the hypothalamus, descends through the brainstem to the lower cervical region, and exits the spinal cord to ascend by way of the sympathetic chain to synapse in the superior cervical ganglion (Fig. 7–13). The sympathetic fibers enter the cranial vault with the carotid plexus to join the ophthalmic division of the trigeminal nerve and

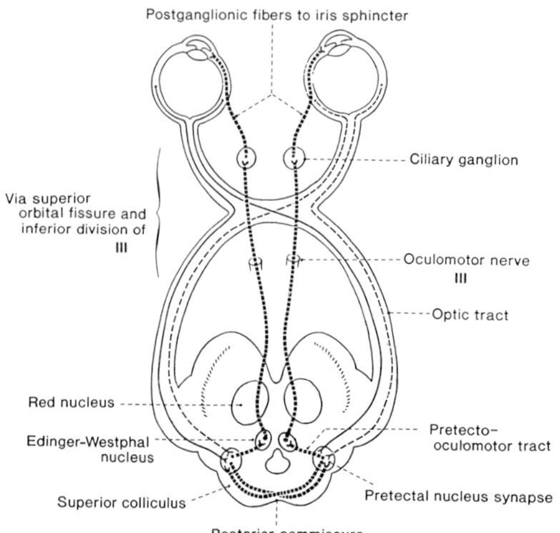

Fig. 7–12. Pathway of the pupillary light reflex. Light stimulates the retinal photoreceptors and initiates the visual and also the pupilloconstrictor reflex. Pupillary fibers travel with the visual nerve fibers via the optic nerve and decussate at the chiasm. Pupillary fibers exit from the optic tract before the lateral geniculate body and enter the brainstem by way of the brachium of the superior colliculus. After synapse in the pretectum, the fibers are distributed to the ipsilateral and contralateral Edinger-Westphal nucleus by an intercalary neuron. The efferent pupillary fibers of the parasympathetic system exit the midbrain with the third nerve to synapse finally at the ciliary ganglion. Postganglionic fibers are then distributed to the iris sphincter and ciliary body by way of the short ciliary nerves.

later join the nasociliary and long ciliary nerves to reach the ciliary body and the dilator fibers of the iris.

This complex anatomic pattern results in the symmetry of the *direct* and *consensual pupillary response* (Fig. 7–14). A direct pupil response refers to the normal brisk pupillary response when light is shone in the eye as the patient is fixating at a distant target. The consensual pupillary response refers to the normal brisk pupillary response that occurs in the opposite eye at the same time. In a normal pupillary response, if a light is moved every second back and forth between the two pupils, both pupils remain constricted with a slight dilation between swings. In a *Marcus Gunn (afferent) pupillary defect*, the pupillary response becomes unequal because there is a lack of constriction or even a dilatation when the involved eye is stimulated. For practical purposes, a Marcus Gunn pupil indicates a lesion of the optic nerve

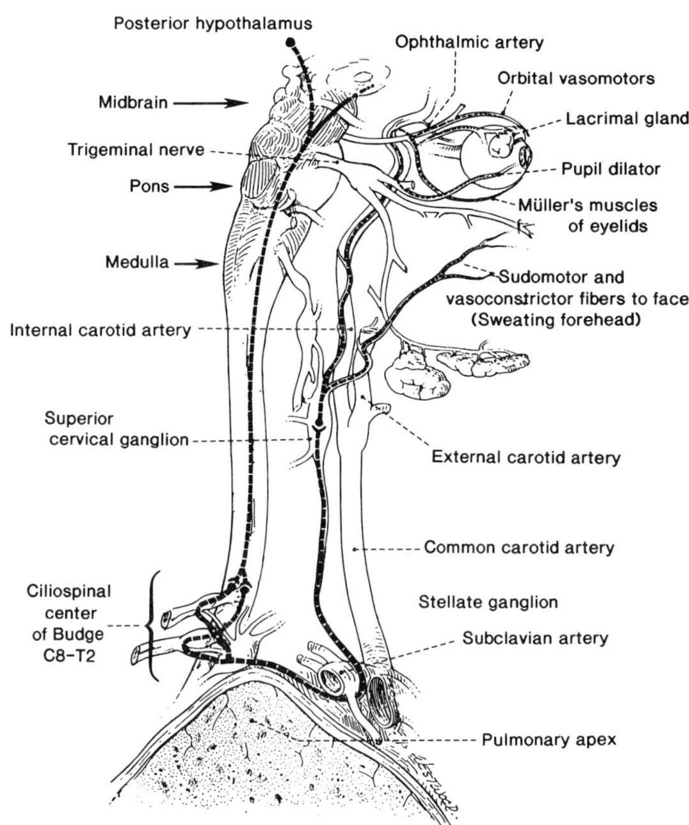

Fig. 7–13. Pathway of the sympathetic system for pupillary dilatation. The hypothalamic sympathetic fibers compose a polysynaptic system. The intra-axial tract is considered the "first-order" neuron. The "second-order" neuron has a circuitous course through the chest and ascends with the carotid system into the neck. The "third-order" neuron originates in the superior cervical ganglion and is distributed to the orbit by way of the ophthalmic artery and the ophthalmic division of the trigeminal nerve and to the face with branches of the external carotid artery.

or extensive retinal disease. If there is no Marcus Gunn pupil and ophthalmoscopy is normal in a patient with claimed unilateral visual loss, there is a strong probability that the visual loss is functional (that is, not organic). In a patient with an amaurotic pupil (no light perception), the pupils are of equal size in ambient light but the pupil of the blind eye does not react to direct light and the opposite pupil does not show a consensual response; when the light is shone in the good eye, however, there is a normal pupil response on that side and a good consensual response in the blind eye. This reaction confirms that the afferent

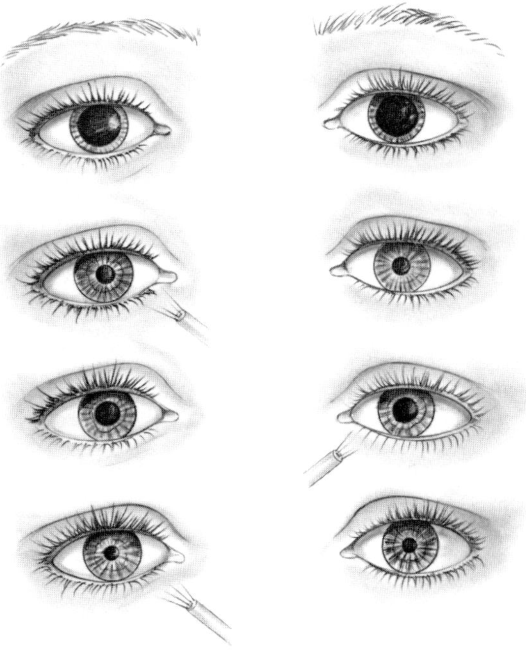

Fig. 7–14. An afferent pupillary defect in the left eye, demonstrated with the swinging flashlight test. Both pupils constrict when the light is shined in the right eye. When the light is swung back to the left eye, both pupils dilate. When the light is swung back to the right eye, both pupils again constrict. This reaction indicates a defect along the course of the afferent pupillary fibers from the left eye.

TABLE 7-1 Characteristics of Pupil Abnormalities in Neuro-ophthalmology

Abnormality	General characteristics	Responses to light and near stimuli	Room condition in which anisocoria is greater	Response to mydriatics	Response to miotics	Response to pharmacologic agents
Essential anisocoria	Round, regular	Both brisk	No change or darkness	Dilates	Constricts	Normal and rarely needed
Horner's syndrome	Small, round, unilateral	Both brisk	Darkness	Dilates	Constricts	Cocaine 4%, poor dilation Hydroxyamphetamine 1%, no dilation if third-order neuron damage
Tonic pupil syndrome (Holmes-Adie syndrome)	Usually larger* in bright light; sector pupil palsy, vermiform movement Unilateral or, less often, bilateral	Absent to light, tonic to near; tonic redilation	Light	Dilates	Constricts	Pilocarpine 0.1% or 0.125%, constricts Methacholine 2.5%, constricts
Argyll Robertson pupils	Small, irregular, bilateral	Poor to light, better to near	No change	Poor	Constricts	–
Midbrain pupils	Mid-dilated; may be oval; bilateral	Poor to light, better to near (or fixed to both)	No change	Dilates	Constricts	–
Pharmacologically dilated pupil	Very large,[†] round, unilateral	Fixed[‡]	Light	–	None[‡]	Pilocarpine 1%, will not constrict
Third cranial nerve palsy, nonischemic	Mid-dilated (6 mm–7 mm), unilateral (rarely bilateral)	Fixed	Light	Dilates	Constricts	–

* Tonic pupil may appear smaller after prolonged near-effort or in dim illumination; affected pupil is initially large, but with time it becomes smaller.

[†] Atropine-dilated pupils have diameters of 8 to 9 mm. No tonic, midbrain, or oculomotor palsy pupil is ever this large.

[‡] Pupils may be weakly reactive, depending on interim after instillation.

pathway is involved (the optic nerve) but the efferent system (sympathetic and parasympathetic system) is normal. There are several characteristic pupillary abnormalities in neuro-ophthalmology (Table 7–1).

There are many causes of a light-near dissociation of the pupillary response.

The *near synkinesis* consists of *convergence of the eyes*, *miosis of the pupils*, and *accommodation of the lens*. The exact anatomic pathway for pupillary constriction to near effort is not well known, but there are several abnormalities in which the pupils respond poorly to light but do respond to near effort.

The classic *Argyll Robertson pupils* of syphilis have the following specific criteria: 1) the vision is normal; 2) one or both pupils are affected; 3) there is no reaction to light, but there is a brisk reaction to near stimulation; and 4) the pupils are miotic and irregularly shaped and respond poorly to cycloplegic drugs (Fig. 7–15 *A*). In clinical practice, not all of these criteria are present in syphilitic pupils. The pathologic defect is thought to be between the pretectal nucleus and the Edinger-Westphal subnucleus. Other causes of a *light-near dissociation* are diabetes mellitus, Parinaud's syndrome, and Adie's tonic pupil. In diabetes, the pupils are slightly large; the poor response to light may be related to severe retinopathy or to selective neuropathy of the pupillomotor fibers. In Parinaud's syndrome there is a compressive lesion in the area of the posterior third ventricle of the midbrain; the pupils are slightly dilated with poor or no response to light but a brisk response to near fixation.

Adie's tonic pupil usually is diagnosed in an asymptomatic young woman.

Adie's tonic pupil is a benign condition, found in females, that is most commonly unilateral, has a slightly larger pupil that has minimal or no reaction to light stimulation, and has a slow tonic constriction and redilation in response to an accommodative (near) stimulus (Fig. 7–15 *B*). Under the slit lamp, pupillary constriction is segmental and wormlike (vermiform). The

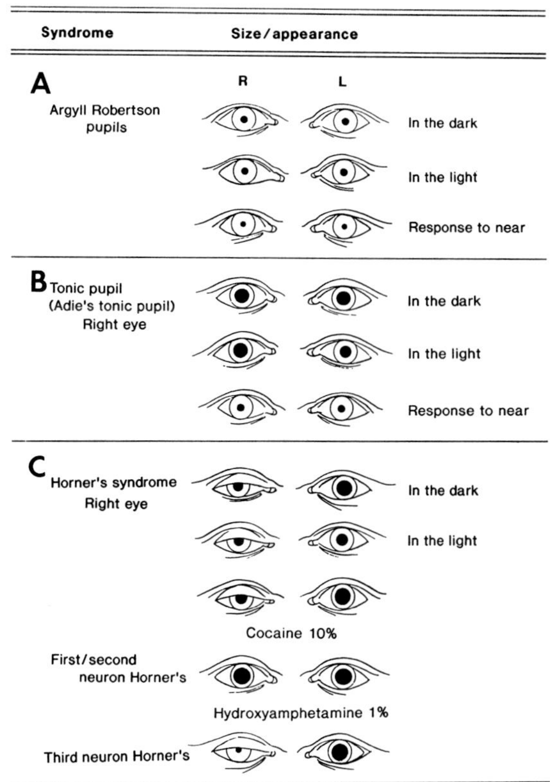

Fig. 7–15. The pupil size and reaction in the clinical syndromes of the Argyll Robertson pupil (*A*), Adie's tonic pupil (*B*), and Horner's syndrome (*C*).

cause is presumably related to damage to the ciliary ganglion. Accommodative abnormalities accompany a tonic pupil; the patient may describe slow accommodation in changing fixation between a near and a distant object (Table 7–2).

TABLE 7–2 Characteristics of Tonic Pupil Syndrome (Adie's Tonic Pupil)

Relative mydriasis in bright illumination
Poor to absent light reaction*
Slow contraction to prolonged near effort
Slow redilation after near effort
Iris sphincter sector palsy*
Segmental vermiform movements of iris border*
Defective accommodation
Pupil constricts with methacholine 2.5%, pilocarpine 0.1% (normal pupil does not)
Associated with diminished deep tendon reflexes

* Slit-lamp examination is helpful.

Horner's pupil is due to a disruption along the sympathetic innervation.

Any abnormality that disturbs the sympathetic innervation from the brainstem to the pupil may cause *Horner's syndrome* on the involved side. Horner's pupil is smaller, and the difference is accentuated in dim illumination, which allows the normal pupil to dilate (Fig. 7–15 C). Ptosis (due to loss of Müller's muscle function), apparent but not true enophthalmos (due to narrowed fissure), a lower lid that is usually slightly higher than normal ("reverse ptosis"), hyperemia (due to loss of vascular tone), absence of facial sweating, and increased amplitude of accommodation complete the clinical picture.

Isolated Horner's syndrome may be observed, but associated symptoms may suggest other vascular or neoplastic processes. The first neuron runs from the hypothalamus to the spinal cord (C8-T2), the second neuron runs from the spinal cord to the superior cervical ganglion near the carotid bifurcation, and the third neuron runs to the peripheral innervation of the ocular structures. The association with other nerve damage, a history of neck trauma or operation, carotid vascular disease, or cervical bony abnormalities establish disease of the third neuron in the sympathetic chain (Table 7–3). A lesion in the apex of the lung (especially a carcinoma) is associated with the second neuron of the sympathetic chain.

Topical cocaine (2% to 10%) blocks the nerve terminal uptake of norepinephrine, potentiating its effect and causing dilation of the pupil—but only if the sympathetic innervation is intact. Although cocaine confirms the presence of Horner's pupil, topical hydroxyamphetamine (Paredrine) can determine which neuron is involved. Hydroxyamphetamine causes release of norepinephrine from the nerve endings and stimulates the dilator muscle. It thus causes dilation of the pupil in Horner's syndrome if the first- or second-order neuron is involved but not if the third-order neuron is interrupted.

The ocular motor control system has four subsystems.

The ocular motor control system has four basic subsystems: *saccades, smooth pursuits, vestibular-ocular movements,* and *vergence movements* (Fig. 7–16). *Saccades* are rapid eye movements in which the eyes move in unison to fix on a target or in response to a command. These movements are precise, predetermined, and not very sensitive to systemic drugs. A saccade is probably generated in the frontal cortex and

TABLE 7–3 Diseases at Various Locations Causing Horner's Syndrome

First-order neuron*
  Stroke (brainstem)
  Trauma
  Spinal cord tumors
Second-order neuron
  Trauma (neck)
  Vertebral metastases
  Apical lung lesions
Third-order neuron
  Migraine
  Cavernous sinus lesion*
  Carotid disease
    Trauma (angiography?, endarterectomy, neck manipulation)
    Atherosclerosis (general disease process, carotid aneurysmal dissection, carotid thrombosis)

* Site of possible Horner's and sixth cranial nerve palsy.

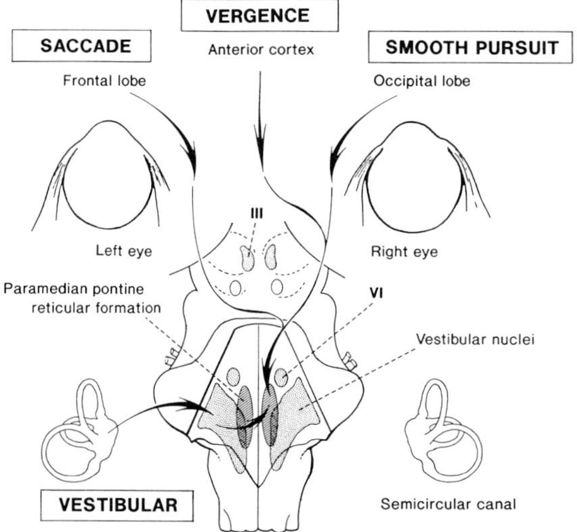

Fig. 7–16. The subsystems of the ocular motor control system (saccades, smooth pursuit, vestibular, and vergence systems) and their influence on the brainstem and eye movements.

passes through the internal capsule to the pontine reticular formation, to the pretectal area, and then to the third, fourth, and sixth cranial nerve nuclei.

Smooth pursuit movements are slow, continuous, accurate movements of the eye to follow a slowly moving object. These movements are very sensitive to drugs. Smooth pursuit movements are generated in the occipital area and travel through the internal capsule to the paramedian pontine reticular formation and the pretectum.

Vestibular eye movements maintain eye fixation during changes in body or head position. The sensory organs for vestibular eye movements are the semicircular canals, utricle, and saccule. Movements generated here travel through the vestibular nuclei through the eighth nerve to the paramedian pontine reticular formation and then to the third, fourth, and sixth cranial nerves. This system can be tested clinically by actively moving the head in the "doll's eye maneuver" or by caloric stimulation.

The *vergence system* controls normal dysconjugate eye movements such as convergence or divergence. The stimulation for these movements is a disparity in retinal images between the two eyes. This is probably generated in the anterior cortex and travels to the pretectal area.

Two centers in the brainstem control eye movements.

The *gaze center* for controlling horizontal eye movements is in the *paramedian pontine reticular formation*. The *gaze center* for controlling vertical gaze movements is in the *central pretectal area* of the mesencephalon (midbrain). Impulses from the cortical centers terminate in these gaze centers, and then appropriate signals are sent to the third, fourth, or sixth nerve nuclei to stimulate the appropriate eye movements by way of the medial longitudinal fasciculus (Fig. 7–17).

The third oculomotor nerve nucleus lies inferior to the sylvian aqueduct within the brainstem and is composed of two adjacent masses of cells divided into subnuclei. A midline subnucleus innervates both levator muscles of the eyelids, and another midline group supplies parasympathetic innervation to the eye. The medial rectus, inferior rectus, and inferior oblique muscles receive their innervation from the appropriate ipsilateral subnuclei, whereas the superior rectus receives its innervation from the contralateral superior rectus subnucleus. The oculomotor nerve runs through the parenchyma of the midbrain and exits on the ventral side of the brainstem as a series of

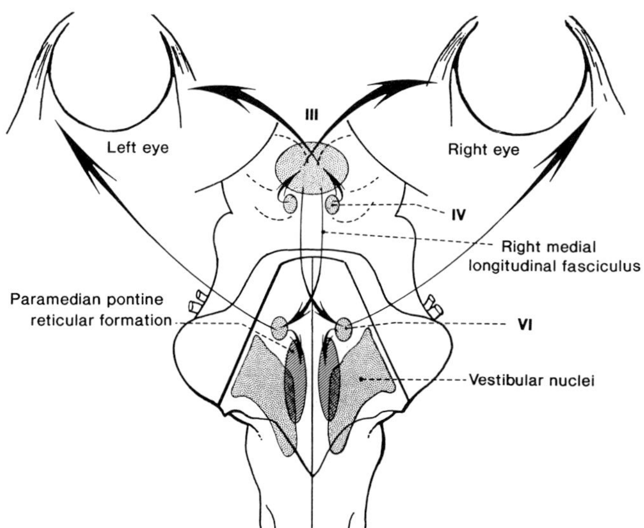

Fig. 7–17. The brainstem control of ocular eye movements with the interconnection of the third, fourth, and sixth nerve nucleus by means of the median longitudinal fasciculus and the paramedian pontine reticular formation.

discrete rootlets before coalescing into the main nerve trunk (Fig. 7–18). The nerve passes into the cavernous sinus (Fig. 7–19) and then into the orbit through the superior orbital fissure. Within the orbit the nerve divides into a superior division (which innervates the levator and superior rectus muscles) and an inferior division (which innervates the medial rectus, inferior rectus, and inferior oblique muscles). The parasympathetic pupillary fibers run within the inferior branch of the oculomotor nerve.

The fourth (trochlear) nerve nucleus lies inferior to the sylvian aqueduct within the brainstem just caudal to the third nerve nucleus. The fourth nerve exits the dorsal surface of the brainstem, crosses to the other side, and then passes ventrally around the brainstem, through the cavernous sinus, and then into the orbit through the superior orbital fissure. It innervates the superior oblique muscle. The trochlear nerve, unlike the oculomotor and abducens nerves, does not pass through the annulus of Zinn to enter the orbit. This anatomic arrangement is evident clinically during cataract operation—the retrobulbar anesthetic, which is injected with the muscle cone, paralyzes all of the extraocular muscles rapidly except the superior oblique.

The sixth (abducens) nerve nucleus is located in the pons, inferior to the floor of the fourth ventricle and close to the paramedian pontine reticular formation and the medial longitudinal fasciculus. The sixth nerve exits from the ventral surface of the pons and enters the cavernous sinus inferior to the third and fourth nerves. It is the most medial cranial nerve in the cavernous sinus and is closest to the carotid artery. The nerve enters the orbit through the superior orbital fissure and terminates in the lateral rectus muscle.

Horizontal gaze abnormalities can occur with cortical or brainstem lesions.

Horizontal gaze abnormalities may manifest in several ways, such as inability to sustain gaze in one direction, inability to move the eyes rapidly, or a gaze-induced nystagmus. Ablative lesions involving the frontal lobe usually result in a gaze paralysis to the side opposite the lesion. Stimulative tumors can drive eyes to the opposite side. Lesions involving the parietal or occipital lobe produce an abnormality of smooth pursuit to the same side.

The most common location of gaze palsy due to brainstem lesions is in the paramedian pontine reticular formation with a gaze paralysis to the same side. *Internuclear ophthalmoplegia* is a failure of adduction or slowed adduction of an eye on the side of the lesion in combination with nystagmus of the abducting (contralateral) eye. This is due to a lesion of the medial longitudinal fasciculus. Bilateral internuclear ophthalmoplegia is seen in a young person with demyelinating disease (multiple sclerosis); a unilateral internuclear ophthalmoplegia usually occurs in older patients with a brainstem stroke.

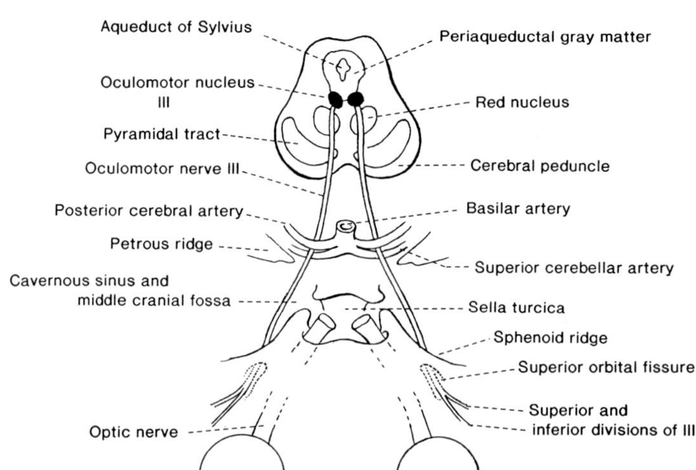

Fig. 7–18. The course of the third cranial nerve from the third nerve nucleus in the brainstem to its destination in the extraocular muscles within the orbit.

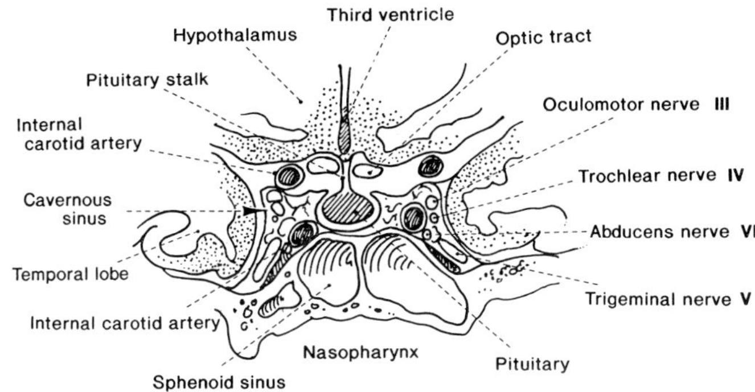

Fig. 7–19. A coronal section through the cavernous sinus, demonstrating the association of the third, fourth, fifth, and sixth cranial nerves, the internal carotid artery, the pituitary, and the sphenoid sinus.

If the brainstem lesion affects the paramedian pontine reticular formation and the medial longitudinal fasciculus on the same side, the patient is not able to gaze with either eye toward the side of the lesion (gaze palsy) and is not able to adduct the eye on the side of the lesion (internuclear ophthalmoplegia). This constellation of signs is called paralytic pontine exotropia or the "one and one-half syndrome" (one and half of another) and has precise localizing value.

Congenital ocular motor apraxia is an uncommon childhood neurologic disorder with selective loss of horizontal saccades and pursuit. Head thrusts are used to stimulate the vestibulo-ocular reflex, which slowly drives the eyes toward the direction of gaze. Horizontal gaze movements are the most severely disturbed. The disorder becomes less evident as the child matures and learns to "hide" the head thrusts.

Vertical gaze abnormalities usually occur with midbrain lesions.

Parinaud's or sylvian aqueduct syndrome involves lesions of the pretectal or tectal area of the mesencephalon (midbrain) with features including disturbance of vertical gaze (upgaze more than downgaze), convergence insufficiency, lid retraction, retraction nystagmus, disturbances in accommodation, and pupillary abnormalities. A lesion in or near the posterior third ventricle (such as pinealoma) with hydrocephalus is the most common cause, although vascular disease and demyelinating disease have also been reported. Upward gaze is usually affected more than downward gaze. The pupillary light reflex is sluggish, although the near stimulation may be intact. Lid retraction (Collier's sign) is due to loss of normal synkinesis between superior rectus and levator palpebral muscles in the upper lid. Retraction nystagmus is elicited by the optokinetic stimulus moving downward; both globes retract into the orbit and converge slightly.

Progressive supranuclear palsy (Steele-Richardson-Olszewski syndrome) is a degenerative neurologic condition that begins with a vertical gaze paresis and later manifests a horizontal gaze paresis along with various degrees of pseudobulbar palsy, rigidity of the neck and upper part of the trunk, and dysarthria. Dementia and respiratory failure develop in the final stages.

Skew deviation is an acquired dysconjugate vertical deviation of the eyes resulting from lesions anywhere in the pathway of vertical gaze. It implicates a posterior fossa or brainstem lesion.

Several supranuclear oculomotor disorders may have some localizing value.

Ocular bobbing is characterized by irregular, unpredictable, and spontaneous downward jerks of the eyes followed by a slower, upward movement toward the primary position. It occurs in comatose patients with severe pontine disease due to hemorrhage, infarct, or tumor.

Cerebellar disease may produce several supranuclear oculomotor disorders, including ocular dysmetria, ocular flutter, and opsoclonus. *Ocular dysmetria* describes an overshooting or undershooting of gaze during changes in fixation in either a horizontal or a vertical meridian. *Ocular flutter* is a rapid horizontal pendular oscillation in primary gaze of small amplitude that occurs spontaneously during or after a change in fixation. *Opsoclonus* is an involuntary repetitive, irregular, and chaotic multidirectional conjugate eye movement that even persists during sleep.

Ocular myoclonus is a rapid oscillation of the eyes in any direction. It is similar to nystagmus except that the movements are irregular, vary in amplitude, and may be associated with myoclonic movements in other parts of the body. It indicates severe brainstem disease and may have associated palatal myoclonus. *Oculogyric crisis* is a conjugate spasmodic deviation of the eyes upward and may be tonic or clonic. There are recurring episodes that last about 30 seconds and then abate. It is associated with epilepsy, or postencephalitis, or overdose of chlorpromazine.

Nystagmus is a rhythmic, repetitive oscillation of the eyes.

Nystagmus is characterized by a rate (rapid or slow), amplitude (coarse or fine), direction (horizontal, vertical, or rotational), and type of movement (jerk or pendular). In *pendular nystagmus* the eye movements in each direction are equal, whereas in *jerk nystagmus* there is a slow component in one direction and a fast compo-

nent (or jerk) in the opposite direction. The direction of the fast phase defines the nystagmus as downbeating, upbeating, left-beating, and so on. In most cases, the movements are conjugate and equal in both eyes. The patterns of nystagmus that have localizing value are present in the primary position, whereas various nystagmoid movements (which are nonspecific and nonlocalizing) are not present in the primary position. When there are symptoms of *oscillopsia* (perception of environmental movement), the nystagmus is acquired. Most types of nystagmus can be diagnosed by a thorough office examination and by fitting the pattern to the classic description.

Several forms of nystagmus are specific, recognizable, and of localizing value (Fig. 7–20 and Table 7–4).

Latent nystagmus occurs only when one eye is covered and consists of a bilateral jerk nystagmus with the jerk (fast) component away from the covered eye. Vision is diminished when the eyes are tested separately but normal when the eyes are uncovered. Latent nystagmus is congenital and may be seen in association with strabismus or with congenital nystagmus. It is more pronounced when the dominant eye is covered.

Congenital nystagmus is noted shortly after birth and is horizontal and pendular but may be vertical, circular, or elliptical and may occa-

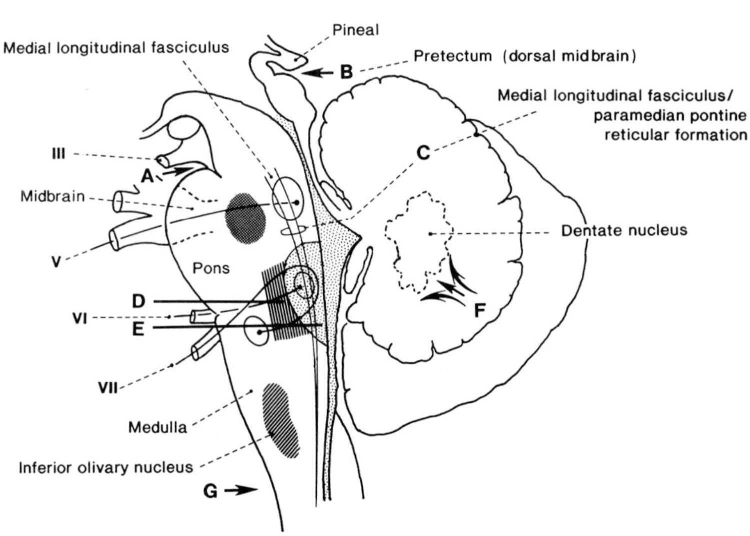

Fig. 7–20. Brainstem regions associated with pathologic eye movements of localizing significance. *A,* Seesaw nystagmus; *B,* convergence retraction nystagmus; *C,* internuclear ophthalmoplegia; *D,* gaze paretic ocular bobbing; *E,* periodic alternating nystagmus, vestibular; *F,* upbeat nystagmus; *G,* downbeat nystagmus.

TABLE 7-4 Localization of Nystagmus

Type	Localization
Downbeat	Craniocervical junction
Periodic alternating	Craniocervical junction
Gaze-evoked	Vestibular, cerebellum (?)
Upbeat	Vermis cerebellum, medulla
Seesaw	Diencephalon, mesencephalon
Torsional	Central vestibular
Convergence-retraction	Dorsal midbrain
Rebound	Cerebellum

sionally be jerk-type. It is usually less pronounced in convergence so that affected children can have good near vision and do well in school. The afferent visual system is normal, and the patient may have a "null zone" of gaze (with a head turn) that minimizes the nystagmus and gives the best visual acuity. High astigmatism is frequently found. An essential characteristic of congenital nystagmus is that it remains horizontal during vertical gaze. The nystagmus is absent during sleep.

Spasmus nutans is a nystagmus that appears at about 18 months of age and disappears by 36 months of age. It is a horizontal or vertical, pendular, low-amplitude but high-frequency nystagmus. The most important features are the head turn and head nodding.

Downbeat nystagmus consists of a fast-phase downward jerk when the eyes are in the primary position. It is associated with long-standing disease at the cervical medullary junction, such as Arnold-Chiari malformation, spinocerebellar degeneration, and brainstem stroke.

Upbeat nystagmus consists of a fast-phase upward jerk when the eyes are in the primary position. It is associated with intrinsic brainstem disease or cerebellar disease.

Convergence-retraction nystagmus is due to co-contraction of extraocular muscles on attempted convergence and in upward gaze; it is best demonstrated during optokinetic testing. The defect is seen in dorsal midbrain disease (sylvian aqueduct, Parinaud's syndrome) and is seen in association with other findings, including poor upward gaze, lid retraction, light-near dissocia-tion of pupils, and abnormalities of accommodation and convergence.

Seesaw nystagmus is a pendular and rotary torsion nystagmus with a dissociated vertical vector in which the intorting eye rises and the extorting eye falls. The defect is most frequently associated with chiasmal suprasellar lesions and bitemporal hemianopia.

Periodic alternating nystagmus is a jerk nystagmus that undergoes rhythmic changes in amplitude and direction. The cycle alternates from left to right continuously with a short rest period in between. It is acquired in association with a vascular or demyelinating disease in the brainstem.

Vestibular nystagmus is a horizontal rotary form of jerk nystagmus in the primary position. With peripheral (labyrinthine) vestibular disease, the jerk is in the same direction in all fields of gaze. In central vestibular disease, the jerk may alter direction with change in position of gaze.

Gaze paretic nystagmus is a coarse, large-amplitude, irregular, jerk nystagmus associated with recovering paresis of gaze in one direction. The eyes can move in the direction of gaze but cannot maintain gaze and quickly slip back toward the primary position. Horizontal gaze paretic nystagmus is associated with cerebellar or pontine lesions. Vertical gaze paretic nystagmus occurs with lesions in the pretectal area.

Gaze-evoked nystagmus is a rapid, regular nystagmus that occurs with attempted gaze away from the primary position. This may indicate a lesion in the posterior fossa, but it is not more specific. It most commonly occurs in association with use of drugs, such as anticonvulsants, sedatives, or tranquilizers.

Disorders of cranial nerves have multiple causes.

The most common causes of palsies of the third, fourth, and sixth cranial nerves are microvascular disorders (diabetes, hypertension), trauma, tumor, and aneurysm; a certain proportion remain idiopathic. The diagnosis is frequently made on the basis of accompanying neurologic signs and symptoms.

The third cranial nerve innervates the levator muscle, superior, inferior, and medial rectus muscles, the inferior oblique muscle, and the pupil.

Multiple entities can affect the third nerve in its long course to the orbit (Fig. 7–18 and Table 7–5). Involvement of the third cranial nerve nucleus in the brainstem is rare but is characterized by bilateral ptosis and bilateral limitation of upgaze. The fascicular portion of the nerve is frequently involved with vascular, neoplastic, or demyelinating diseases of the brainstem with specific neurologic features depending on the involved area (Table 7–6). *Benedikt's syndrome* consists of ipsilateral third nerve palsy and contralateral ataxia. *Weber's syndrome* consists of ipsilateral third nerve palsy with contralateral hemiparesis. *Nothnagel's syndrome* consists of ipsilateral third nerve palsy and cerebellar ataxia.

In its course toward the cavernous sinus, the third nerve travels alongside the posterior communicating artery. An aneurysm at the junction of the posterior communicating artery and the internal carotid artery causes an isolated third nerve palsy with pupillary involvement. The cavernous sinus syndrome usually involves the third, fourth, and sixth cranial nerves along with the first and second branches of the fifth cranial nerve (Fig. 7–19). Orbital involvement of the third cranial nerve may result in selective paresis of structures because the nerve splits into two divisions before entering the orbit. The superior division innervates the superior rectus and levator palpebrae, and the inferior division innervates the inferior rectus, medial rectus, inferior oblique, the pupil, and accommodation. The orbital apex syndrome (ophthalmoplegia from multiple cranial nerve palsies, decreased vision, and decreased sensation from trigeminal nerve involvement) may be associated with masses within the orbit or extension from masses in the paranasal sinus or intracranial cavity.

TABLE 7–5 General Causes of Oculomotor (Third Nerve) Palsies

Nuclear
  Infarction
  Demyelination
  Metastatic tumor
Fascicular
  Infarction
  Demyelination (rare)
  Tumor
Interpeduncular
  Aneurysm (involves third more frequently than
    fourth, and sixth is the least commonly
    involved)*
  Trauma: lumbar puncture, concussion
  Meningitis
Cavernous sinus
  Carotid-cavernous fistula or dural cavernous fistula
  Granulomatous inflammation (Tolosa-Hunt
    syndrome)
  Intracavernous aneurysm*
  Extension of pituitary tumor (such as
    macroadenomas)
  Meningioma
  Sphenoid sinus carcinoma
  Metastatic tumor
  Mucormycosis (other fungus)
  Herpes zoster
Orbit
  Inflammation (pseudotumor) and apex syndromes
  Trauma
  Tumor
  Sinus processes
Ischemic (nonlocalizing)
  Diabetes
  Hypertension
  Collagen vascular arteritides
Miscellaneous
  Polyneuritis (Guillain-Barré-Fisher syndrome)
  Cyclic oculomotor palsy (Bielschowsky)
  Migraine

* Note several locations for aneurysms, which can cause up to 30% of third cranial nerve palsies, 4% of fourth cranial nerve palsies, and 2% of sixth cranial nerve palsies.

TABLE 7–6 Brainstem Syndromes with Third Cranial Nerve Palsy

Nothnagel's syndrome
  Ipsilateral third
  Cerebellar ataxia
  Lesion at superior cerebellar peduncle
Benedikt's syndrome
  Ipsilateral third
  Contralateral hemitremor lesion near red nucleus
Weber's syndrome
  Ipsilateral third-nerve contralateral hemiparesis
  Third nerve involved at cerebral peduncle
    ventrally
Claude's syndrome
  Features of Nothnagel's and Benedikt's syndromes

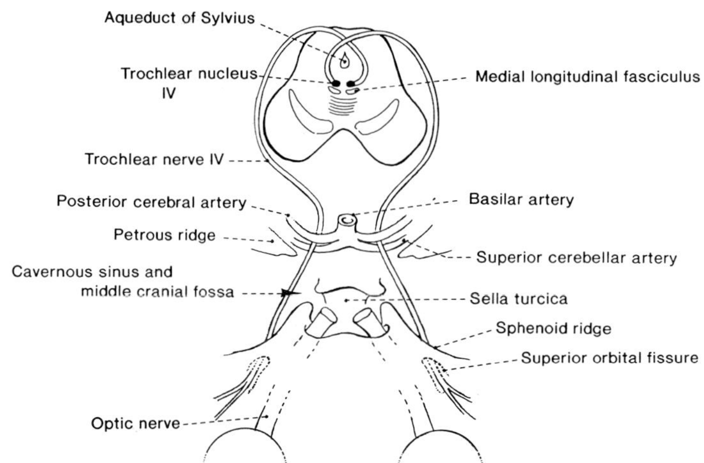

Fig. 7–21. The long course of the fourth cranial nerve, which exits the brainstem on the dorsal surface, crosses to the opposite side, and travels to the superior oblique muscle in the orbit.

Oculomotor palsy with normal pupils (a "pupil-sparing third") is usually caused by intrinsic microvascular disease such as diabetes, hypertension, or giant cell arteritis. Presumably the more peripheral parasympathetic fibers of the nerve are spared the ischemia. The opposite is true with compressive masses.

The fourth cranial nerve innervates the superior oblique muscle.

Closed head trauma with contrecoup forces transmitted to the brainstem by the free tentorial edge is the most common cause of *fourth nerve palsy* (Fig. 7–21). Other causes of palsy include diabetes, neoplasms, meningitis, decompensation of a congenital fourth nerve paresis, aneurysms or vascular anomalies, and hydrocephalus (Table 7–7). Bilateral fourth nerve palsy may be associated with severe head trauma with coma.

Congenital fourth nerve paralysis may present with a long-standing head tilt and a large vertical fusional amplitude, which help maintain binocular vision. It is not uncommon and may be asymptomatic until a later age or until a significant illness causes decompensation.

The fourth nerve may be involved with other cranial nerves by lesions within the cavernous sinus or the superior orbital fissure. In the presence of a third nerve palsy, the fourth nerve function can be detected by intorsion of the eye in downgaze. A recently acquired fourth nerve palsy is best confirmed by a three-step Parks-Bielschowsky test, which defines the maximal hypertropia in primary gaze, in gaze right or left, and in a position of head tilt right or left (Fig. 7–22).

The sixth cranial nerve innervates the lateral rectus muscle.

Abducens paralysis is the most common ocular motor palsy. Lesions of the *sixth nerve* nucleus in the brainstem cause an ipsilateral gaze palsy because of the proximity to the paramedian reticular formation (Fig. 7–23). The fascicular portion of the seventh nerve loops over the sixth nerve nucleus so that concomitant involvement of the sixth and seventh

TABLE 7–7 Causes of Superior Oblique Paresis

Fourth nerve palsy (true palsy)
  Trauma (may be bilateral)
  "Vascular"
  Diabetes
  "Decompensated congenital paresis"*
  Posterior fossa tumor (rare)
  Cavernous sinus/superior orbital fissure syndromes
  Neurosurgical procedures
  Herpes zoster
Myasthenia
Orbital: pseudotumor, injury to trochlea (sinus surgery), Graves' myopathy (fibrotic inferior oblique, superior rectus)

* Fusional vertical amplitudes help make this common diagnosis.

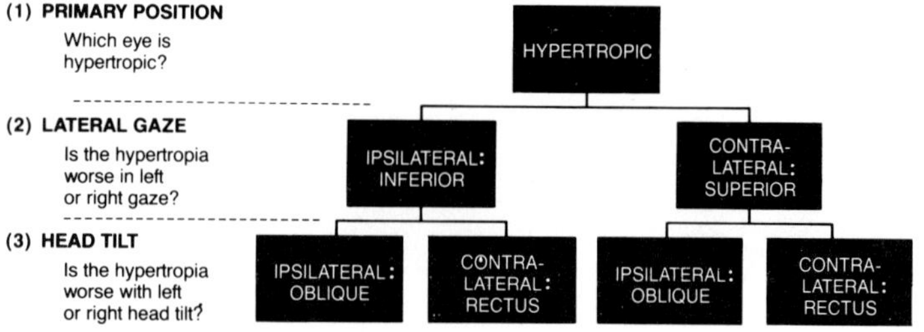

Fig. 7–22. The Parks-Bielschowsky three-step test, which helps to find the paretic muscle in an acute-onset vertical muscle deviation.

nerves suggests a lesion in the pons. Involvement of the fascicular portion of the sixth nerve may be part of several syndromes (Table 7–8). *Millard-Gubler syndrome* is characterized by ipsilateral sixth and seventh nerve palsy and contralateral hemiplegia. *Foville's syndrome* is characterized by paralysis of gaze, deafness, facial palsy, loss of taste from the anterior tongue, Horner's syndrome, and analgesia of the face all on the side of the lesion.

In the subarachnoid space, changes in intracranial pressure may cause downward displacement of the brainstem with subsequent stretching of the sixth nerve, which is tethered at its exit from its pons. This is a nonlocalizing sign associated with increased intracranial pressure in pseudotumor cerebri or related to a mass lesion. Other causes of a sixth nerve palsy within the subarachnoid space include hemorrhage after lumbar puncture, meningeal infection, inflammation, or infiltration. Because of its proximity to the petrous bone, an abscess in the petrous apex after complicated otitis media

may yield the clinical findings of *Gradenigo's syndrome*. This consists of sixth nerve palsies along with facial paralysis, facial pain, and decreased hearing on the side of the lesion. *Pseudo-Gradenigo's syndrome* can be seen with a cerebellopontine angle tumor or with a nasopharyngeal tumor that has obstructed the eustachian tube and invaded the cavernous sinus. Findings include defects in the fifth, sixth, seventh, and eighth nerves along with ataxia and papilledema.

Lesions in the cavernous sinus rarely produce isolated sixth nerve palsy; usually the third and fourth cranial nerves and the first division of the fifth nerve are involved along with Horner's syndrome. Orbital involvement of the sixth nerve is usually associated with proptosis. It may be difficult to distinguish between a paresis and a mechanical muscle restriction unless a forced duction test is performed.

An isolated sixth nerve palsy may be seen as a postviral syndrome in young patients or as an ischemic mononeuropathy in older adults (especially those with diabetes and hypertension). These improve over time. A sixth nerve palsy in a young individual which does not clear is

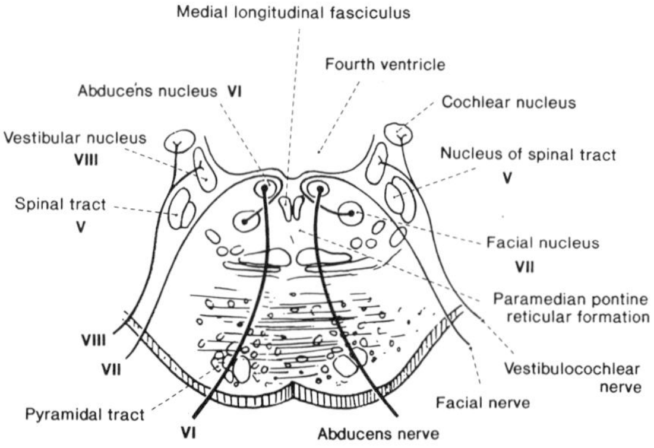

Fig. 7–23. The relationship of the sixth cranial nerve nucleus and fasciculus to other structures in the brainstem as the nerves exit from the ventral surface of the brainstem.

TABLE 7–8   Brainstem Syndromes of Sixth Cranial Nerve Palsy

Millard-Gubler syndrome (ventral pontine peduncle)
  Sixth nerve paresis
  Seventh nerve paresis
  Contralateral hemiparesis
Raymond syndrome (peduncle)
  Sixth nerve paresis
  Contralateral hemiparesis
Foville's syndrome (dorsal pontine)
  Horizontal conjugate gaze palsy
  Ipsilateral fifth, seventh, eighth cranial nerve palsy
  Ipsilateral Horner's syndrome

suggestive of a brainstem lesion. Some of the causes of a sixth nerve palsy are listed in Table 7–9, which differentiates the localizing from the nonlocalizing types.

Deficits of fifth cranial nerve function often have neurologic significance.

The *trigeminal nerve* supplies sensation to the face by way of its three main branches: the *ophthalmic*, the *maxillary*, and the *mandibular.* Testing for somatotrophic hypesthesia (with a cotton wisp) may suggest the specific localization depending on whether the ophthalmic, maxillary, or mandibular division or multiple divisions are involved (Fig. 7–24 and Table 7–10). Facial or ocular pain may be associated with

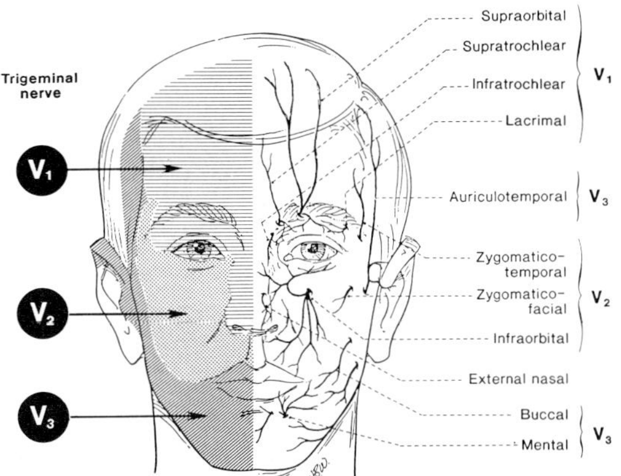

Fig. 7–24. The sensory distribution of the three divisions of the trigeminal nerve in the face and the scalp. (Modified from N.R. Miller: Walsh and Hoyt's Clinical Neuro-Ophthalmology. Vol 2. Fourth edition. Baltimore, Williams & Wilkins, 1985, pp. 999–1043.)

multiple inflammatory conditions of the fifth cranial nerve or may be referred to the trigeminal nerve from local processes in the dura or neck.

TABLE 7–9 Causes of Sixth Nerve Palsies

Pontine syndromes: infarction, demyelination, tumors, contralateral hemiplegia, ipsilateral facial palsy, ipsilateral horizontal gaze palsy (with or without ipsilateral internuclear ophthalmoplegia), ipsilateral facial analgesia

Cerebellopontine angle lesions (acoustic neuroma, meningioma): in combination with disorders of the eighth, seventh, and ophthalmic-trigeminal nerves (especially corneal hypesthesia), nystagmus, and dysfunction of the cerebellum

Middle fossa disorders (tumor, inflammation of medial aspect of petrous): facial pain/numbness, with or without facial palsy

Cavernous sinus or superior orbital fissure (tumor, inflammation, aneurysm): in combination with disorders of the third, fourth, and ophthalmic-trigeminal nerves (pain, numbness); carotid-cavernous or dural arteriovenous fistula

Orbit
  Sinus processes (infection, inflammation, mucocele, mucopyocele)
  Trauma (typically, zygomatic arch causes hematoma?)
  Graves' ophthalmopathy (medial rectus restriction)

Nonlocalizing
  Increased intracranial pressure
  Head trauma
  Lumbar puncture or spinal anesthesia
  "Vascular hypertension"
  Diabetes
  Migraine
  Parainfections (postviral; middle ear infections)
  Basal meningitis
  Sarcoidosis

TABLE 7–10 Differential Diagnosis of Diminished Sensation in the Various Divisions of the Fifth Cranial Nerve

Ophthalmic division
  Neoplasm (orbital apex, superior fissure, cavernous sinus, and middle fossa)
  Aneurysm of the cavernous sinus
Maxillary division
  Orbital floor fracture
  Maxillary anterior carcinoma
Mandibular division
  Nasopharyngeal carcinoma
  Middle fossa tumor
All divisions
  Nasopharyngeal carcinoma
  Cerebellopontine angle tumors
  Intracavernous aneurysm
  Demyelinating disease
  Brainstem lesion
  Meckel's cave or middle fossa tumor
  Trigeminal neurofibroma
  Tentorial meningioma
Corneal only
  Herpes simplex
  Ocular surgery
  Cerebellopontine angle tumors
  Dysautonomias

The facial nerve may be involved in neurologic syndromes seen by the ophthalmologist.

The *seventh cranial nerve* leaves the pons and travels with the eighth cranial nerve and along with the nervus intermedius (tearing, salivation, taste) through the auditory canal and then through the stylomastoid foramen to supply the movements of the face and eyelids (Fig. 7–25). The various muscle groups of the seventh cranial nerve are tested by having the patient smile, close the lids forcibly, and wrinkle the forehead. The sensory portion can be tested by taste sensation on the anterior tongue or by cutaneous sensation along the external auditory canal. Autonomic function of salivation or lacrimation can be assessed. Lesions that involve the facial nerve from the pons to the geniculate ganglion impair all the functions of the nerve, whereas lesions that are distal to the geniculate ganglion affect only certain functions of the seventh nerve. A *cerebellopontine angle tumor* affects all functions of the seventh nerve, causing unilateral facial paralysis, decreased hearing, hyperacusis, and decreased taste. Associated neurologic deficits may include fifth, sixth, and eighth cranial nerve deficits with Horner's syndrome, gaze palsy, nystagmus, papilledema, and cerebellar dysfunction.

Bell's palsy is a common unilateral facial palsy possibly related to edema within the bony canal during the course of the seventh nerve. Pain and facial numbness have been reported. Most patients have a total or partial recovery. The resulting corneal exposure is the most serious potential complication.

Ramsay Hunt syndrome is a herpes zoster infection of the geniculate ganglion presenting with vesicles on the tympanic membrane, the external auditory canal, or the external ear associated with ipsilateral facial weakness, decreased tearing, hyperacusis, and decreased taste in the anterior two-thirds of the tongue.

Blepharospasm is a bilateral uncontrolled spasm of the eyelids. The spasm may be strong and prolonged to a degree that patients become functionally blind even with normal visual function. The spasms do not occur when the patient is asleep. The cause is unknown, but the disorder probably is related to a central nervous system cause. *Meige's syndrome* is a variant in which the lower facial musculature is also involved in the spasm.

Many disorders involve only the extraocular muscles themselves or the neuromuscular junction.

In addition to ocular motility disorders related to the supranuclear areas of the brain, the brainstem nuclei or their connections, and the lesions along the course of the third, fourth, and sixth cranial nerves, several other disorders may involve the extraocular muscles themselves or their neuromuscular junctions.

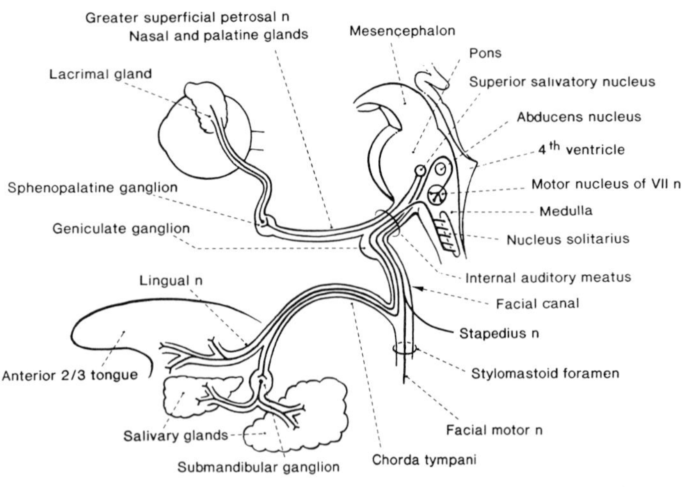

Fig. 7–25. The course of the seventh cranial nerve. The seventh nerve has both motor function (facial muscles) and sensory and autonomic function.

These are generally multisystem disorders that can involve peripheral skeletal muscles and also other organ systems.

Myasthenia gravis is characterized by muscle weakness and fatigue. It involves skeletal muscles; thus, the pupillary and ciliary muscles, which are smooth, are unaffected. The major ophthalmic complaints are ptosis and diplopia. Ocular involvement occurs in 90% of patients, but up to 20% may have only ocular complaints. Clinical characteristics include variability of muscle function within minutes, hours, or days with remissions and exacerbations. The ptosis is variable, and the extraocular muscle pattern of involvement shows no specific consistent pattern but may mimic any oculomotor cranial nerve palsy or gaze disturbance (Table 7–11). The disease can occur at any age; concomitant thyroid disease, a thymoma, or collagen vascular disease is occasionally seen. The impaired neuromuscular transmission in myasthenia is due to the presence of antibodies to acetylcholine receptors in the motor end plate of striated muscles. The clinical diagnosis is confirmed by the presence of acetylcholine antibody levels, specific electromyographic findings, or a clinical response to a test dose of edrophonium chloride (Tensilon).

Chronic progressive external ophthalmoplegia is a group of disorders characterized by slowly progressive, symmetric immobility of the eyes, orbicularis oculi weakness, and ptotic lids, but sparing of the pupil. The patients seldom complain of diplopia. The disorder may occur in an isolated ocular form or may be part of several clinical entities. *Kearns-Sayre syndrome* has an onset in childhood and consists of chronic progressive external ophthalmoplegia, cardiac conduction defects, and pigmentary retinopathy. *Oculopharyngeal dystrophy* is found in families with a history of ptosis, ophthalmoplegia, and dysphagia, and usually with French-Canadian ancestry. *"Ophthalmoplegia plus"* consists of chronic progressive external ophthalmoplegia plus a wide variety of neurologic disorders associated with this disease, including spinocerebellar degeneration, myotonic dystrophy, and hematologic disorders. Muscle biopsy demonstrates mitochondrial accumulations beneath the plasma membrane and between myofibrils.

TABLE 7–11 Ophthalmic Signs of Myasthenia Gravis

Ptosis (most common)
Quiver movements of eyelid or eye, eyelid twitch
Orbicularis weakness
Extraocular muscle palsy
Gaze palsies
Convergence paresis
Internuclear ophthalmoplegia
Nystagmus
Skew deviation

Myotonic dystrophy is an autosomal dominant disease with ophthalmic signs of ptosis, progressive external ophthalmoplegia, orbicularis weakness, myotonia of lid closure, and polychromatophilic cataracts and retinal pigmentary degeneration. Myotonia is the phenomenon in which muscle fibers have persistent contraction when they should be relaxed. Multiple systemic findings include baldness, myotonic cardiomyopathy, myopathy of the face, neck, and limbs, and testicular atrophy.

Thyroid ophthalmopathy is associated with Graves' disease, but it may also occur in patients who show no laboratory evidence of thyroid dysfunction. The pathologic characteristics are mucopolysaccharide deposition and inflammatory cell infiltration of orbital tissues, including the ocular muscles. The extraocular motility disturbances are secondary to restriction, infiltration, or fibrosis of the extraocular muscles. The most common ocular motility pattern is a limitation in elevation due to involvement of the inferior rectus and an abduction weakness due to involvement of the medial rectus muscle. Double vision is a common chief complaint. Additional ocular findings include proptosis, lid retraction, lid lag, conjunctival and lid edema, corneal exposure, and optic neuropathy from muscle compression at the orbital apex. The diagnosis usually takes place in the appropriate clinical setting, but forced duction muscle testing (confirming the restrictive nature of the muscle problem), computed tomography scanning, or ultrasonography can confirm extraocular muscle involvement.

Orbital myositis is an inflammatory process

affecting one or more of the extraocular muscles. The patients complain of pain and diplopia. The disorder is probably a subset of idiopathic orbital pseudotumor, which affects multiple tissues within the orbit. The inflammation usually responds dramatically to systemic corticosteroids. Careful follow-up is essential to distinguish these idiopathic inflammatory processes from lymphoma, systemic collagen vascular disease, or Wegener's granulomatosis.

The ocular examination and other neurologic signs may reveal findings that localize brain tumors.

Some specific visual sensory or visual motor abnormalities allow accurate localization of brain tumors or masses. Correlation with other neurologic abnormalities frequently pinpoints the diagnosis before other testing is performed. Large brain lesions produce *papilledema*, which is a nonlocalizing ophthalmic finding.

Occipital lobe tumors usually are fairly large before they are recognized. Visual field defects are the main features, with the majority demonstrating congruous or complete hemianopia with either splitting or sparing of the macula. Quadrantic visual field defects are usually vascular in origin. Visual hallucinations with unformed images (sparkling colorful lights, flashes, flickering) may occur as a solitary phenomenon or as an aura of a major convulsion. There are no typical neurologic features of occipital lobe tumors. Vascular insults (vertebrobasilar disease) are much more common than tumors in this location.

Parietal lobe tumors involve the sensory-motor cortex, the language centers, and the association areas of body and visual orientation. Features vary depending on whether the dominant or nondominant lobe is involved. Visual disturbances may consist of alexia (inability to identify letters on the visual chart), inattention to objects in the opposite visual field, or constructional apraxia (inability to perform a purposeful motor act). The patients are usually unaware of these visual abnormalities. A homonymous inferior quadrantanopia is the classic visual field. Tumors deep within the parietal lobe may interrupt the smooth pursuit system, with inability to pursue objects in the direction

of the tumor; therefore, they produce an asymmetric optokinetic nystagmus response. Vascular insults and tumors occur with equal frequency in the parietal lobe.

Frontal lobe lesions may produce progressive monocular visual loss with a central scotoma from compression. Further enlargement may involve the optic chiasm with a bitemporal visual field defect. Horizontal deviation of the eyes away from the side of the tumor may be a part of a seizure phenomenon. Papilledema may result from overall increased intracranial pressure or from local compression of the optic nerve. The main features of frontal tumors are mental symptoms such as irritability, apathy, and unusual behavior.

Temporal lobe tumors damage the optic radiations with variable morphologic characteristics. The most common type of defect is an incongruous superior homonymous hemianopia with sloping margins (complete or incomplete). Tumors in the anterior tip of the temporal lobe produce either no field defect or a contralateral upper homonymous field defect. Formed visual hallucinations (people or places) are a hallmark of temporal lobe lesions.

Meningiomas commonly arise below the frontal lobe, especially the sphenoid ridge and olfactory groove. With sphenoid ridge meningiomas, the most common ophthalmic findings are monocular proptosis and visual loss, which is insidious in onset and progressive. The optic nerve defect may be subtle with a small central scotoma, color vision defects, and a small afferent pupillary defect. Over time, optic atrophy and optociliary shunt vessels (connecting central retinal veins and peripapillary choroidal vessels) develop. Proptosis and ophthalmoplegia result from extension of tumor through the superior orbital fissure. Plain skull radiographs show diagnostic new bone formation (hyperostosis).

Tumors in the area of the sella turcica may result in visual loss and endocrine abnormalities.

The sella turcica (roof of the sphenoid sinus), the pituitary gland, the optic chiasm, the circle of Willis, and the cavernous sinus are intimately related within the parasellar area. Tumors within this area produce visual loss with optic atrophy, bitemporal field defects, endocrine abnormalities, and ophthalmoplegia in various combinations.

Pituitary adenomas usually do not secrete hormones; instead they destroy pituitary function. The chromophobe adenoma compresses the remaining normal pituitary tissue, causing hypopituitarism. Eosinophilic adenomas secrete growth hormones, prolactin-secreting adenomas result in galactorrhea and amenorrhea, and basophilic adenomas secrete ACTH and produce Cushing's syndrome. Pituitary adenomas produce characteristic radiographic findings.

Headaches are a common neurologic symptom of pituitary tumors, and visual loss is the predominant ocular symptom. The visual loss is usually gradual and asymmetric. Bitemporal visual field loss can usually be demonstrated on careful examination. Although bitemporal hemianopia is the pathognomonic visual field defect of an intrasellar tumor, a wide range of visual field defects are possible depending on the anatomic relationship of the chiasm to the pituitary gland and the direction of growth of the tumor. The optic disc becomes pale over time. Ocular motor palsies occur typically with cavernous sinus invasion.

Craniopharyngiomas are congenital in origin from squamous epithelial cell rests with probable neoplastic transformation. Most are suprasellar, but they may originate within the sella. Symptoms vary with the age at onset. Headache and endocrine abnormalities are usually conspicuous in children, whereas in adults the chief complaints are headache and decreased vision. The ophthalmic signs vary with the location of the tumor, direction of growth, involvement of the chiasm, and obstruction of the third ventricle. Optic atrophy is usually present, although papilledema is occasionally seen. Prechiasmal (central scotomas) or chiasmal (bitemporal hemianopia) visual field defects are demonstrated in most patients. Cranial nerve palsies are uncommon, although sixth nerve palsy may result from increased intracranial pressure. Suprasellar calcification on plain skull radiographs is the characteristic finding.

Tuberculum sella meningiomas present with gradually decreased vision, usually in one eye and later progressive involvement of the second eye. The junctional scotoma in the second eye is highly characteristic of a suprasellar meningioma; other chiasmal defects are possible. Bilateral optic atrophy is usually present. Headache and pituitary dysfunction are late symptoms. Hyperostosis of the tuberculum sella on plain radiographs is diagnostic.

Gliomas of the optic nerve, chiasm, and hypothalamus may occur as a benign childhood tumor (frequently associated with von Recklinghausen's disease or neurofibromatosis type I) or malignant glioma in adults. Intraorbital gliomas in children present with proptosis, visual loss, optic disc swelling, and ophthalmoplegia. They may be stationary or slowly progressive and may be congenital. Chiasmal gliomas cause hydrocephalus by invasion of the third ventricle, resulting in spastic weakness of the legs and urinary retention; extension into the hypothalamus results in dwarfism and other endocrine disturbances. Ocular symptoms are unilateral or bilateral visual loss, optic atrophy, apparent "congenital" nystagmus, and field defects. Malignant gliomas in adults behave more aggressively than do childhood gliomas, often with a rapidly progressive, fatal course.

The *empty sella syndrome* is not a tumor but causes visual symptoms that mimic those of an intrasellar tumor. The primary empty sella develops spontaneously, whereas the secondary empty sella develops after removal of an intrasellar tumor. In the primary empty sella syndrome, the suprasellar subarachnoid space is pushed into the pituitary fossa and flattens the pituitary gland, resulting in intractable headaches; endocrine and visual field defects are rare.

Tumors below the tentorium usually cause predominantly oculomotor disturbances.

Whereas the supratentorial tumors discussed above produce primarily visual sensory abnormalities, the tumors arising below the tentorium cause predominantly oculomotor disturbances. The major infratentorial tumors involve the cerebellum, cerebellopontine angle, fourth ventricle, and brainstem.

The symptoms and signs of *cerebellar tumors*

vary depending on whether the tumor arises from the midline or lateral hemisphere. Midline cerebellar tumors cause truncal and gait ataxia. Hemispheric tumors produce ataxic signs on the same side. The neuro-ophthalmic signs of cerebellar disease are usually the result of damage to the cerebellum and disruption of its connections to the brainstem (Table 7–12). Symptoms that result include instability of fixation, nystagmus, ocular dysmetria and flutter, gaze paresis, and defective pursuit. Nonspecific signs include papilledema and fourth and sixth nerve paresis resulting from increased intracranial pressure. Vision and visual fields are usually normal.

Cerebellopontine angle tumors are usually schwannomas of the eighth nerve (acoustic neuromas). Bilateral vestibular schwannomas are associated with neurofibromatosis 2. Tinnitus, decreased hearing, and vertigo are early symptoms. Later, fifth and seventh nerve compression occurs, followed by hemispheric cerebellar symptoms. Large tumors may compress the lower brainstem. Vestibular nystagmus is a constant feature. This is a horizontal and rotary, primary position jerk nystagmus with increased amplitude of the excursion during attempted gaze in the direction of its fast phase. The diagnosis is made on the basis of clinical manifestations, audiologic findings, and the neurologic and neuro-ophthalmic abnormalities.

Cerebrovascular disease is probably the most common cause of adult neuro-ophthalmic dysfunction.

Ophthalmologists are frequently consulted to evaluate visual field defects, diplopia, amau-

TABLE 7–12 Common Findings in Various Cerebellar Diseases

Ocular dysmetria

Ocular flutter

Ocular myoclonus

Opsoclonus

Nystagmus

Retinal degeneration (inherited diseases)

Skew deviation

Square-wave jerks

rosis fugax, or other ophthalmic deficits in patients with cerebrovascular disease. Among the causes are occlusive or hemorrhagic cerebrovascular disease, vascular malformations and intracranial aneurysms, vascular inflammatory conditions, and vascular spasm (migraine).

On the route to supplying the cerebral hemisphere, the *internal carotid artery* travels through the cavernous sinus and has branches, including the ophthalmic artery (to the retina, choroid, and the orbit), the posterior communicating artery (to the vertebrobasilar system), the trigeminal and anterior meningeal arteries and the hypophyseal arteries (to the pituitary and optic chiasm), and the anterior choroidal artery (to portions of the internal capsule and temporal lobe) (Fig. 7–26). The internal carotid artery ends by dividing into the anterior and middle cerebral arteries, which supply the majority of the cerebral hemispheres. The *vertebral arteries* ascend from the subclavian artery and join together at the lower end of the pons to form the *basilar artery*. The brainstem, cerebellum, occipital lobes, and medial temporal lobe

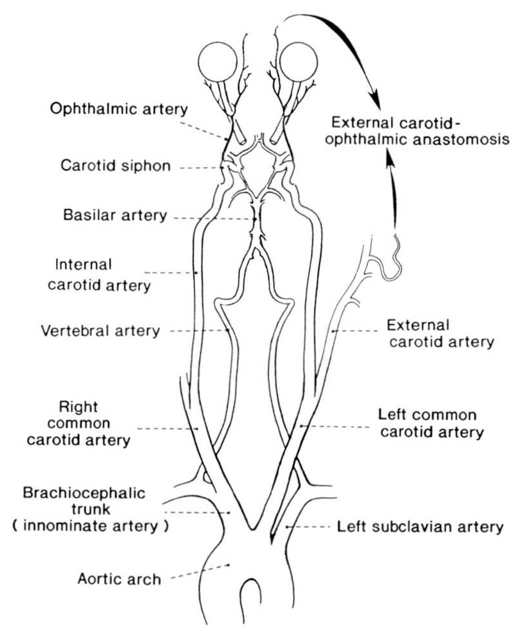

Fig. 7–26. The major arteries and their branches that supply the brainstem, cerebellum, and cerebrum. There are extensive anastomotic connections between these systems.

are supplied by the vertebrobasilar arterial system. There are abundant anastomotic channels between the external and internal carotid systems (maxillary branch of the external carotid and the ophthalmic artery), between the two internal carotid artery systems (anterior communicating artery), and between the carotid and vertebrobasilar systems (posterior communicating artery). These anastomotic pathways help to explain the presence or lack of neurologic symptoms in various disorders.

Arterial occlusive disease of the central nervous system is most commonly caused by thrombosis and embolism.

Occlusion of an artery by a thrombus or an embolus causes ischemia and infarction of the distal tissue. *Arteriosclerosis* is the most common cause of occlusion, but other causes include vascular inflammation, osseous obstruction of the circulation, cardiac and other emboli, and blood coagulation disorders. The extent of the neurologic deficit depends on the size of the vessel occluded and whether prompt collateral flow or recanalization occurs.

Transient ischemic attacks are temporary focal cerebral deficits caused by a momentary interruption of the blood supply. Most are related to microemboli of atheromatous debris, fibrin, and platelets from either the carotid or the vertebrobasilar arteries. Neurologic symptoms of a transient ischemic attack of the carotid system consist of motor and sensory defects on one side of the body and aphasia; ophthalmic symptoms include transient blindness (amaurosis fugax) and homonymous hemianopia. Neurologic symptoms of a transient ischemic attack of the vertebrobasilar system consist of sensory and motor deficits in one to four extremities with ataxia and dysequilibrium. Ophthalmic symptoms consist of transient blindness, bilateral altitudinal defects, or partial or complete homonymous defects. Transient ischemic attacks usually last less than 15 minutes, but a significant number progress to a full cerebral infarction within days to weeks.

A *cerebral infarction (stroke)* has various neurologic or ophthalmic symptoms depending on which vessel has been occluded. Vertebro-basilar ischemia is associated most frequently with bilateral simultaneous blurring or dimming of vision because of ischemia of the occipital visual cortex from blockage of the terminal branches of the basilar artery. The attacks are spontaneous or can be precipitated by head turning if degenerative cervical osteophytic processes compress the vessels. Other brainstem symptoms may occur simultaneously, such as vertigo, facial numbness or dysarthria, or transient diplopia. Severe ischemia results in stroke with permanent neurologic abnormalities.

Amaurosis fugax is associated with a high incidence of atheromatous carotid disease.

Amaurosis fugax is a temporary monocular visual loss related to reversible ischemia in the ophthalmic circulation. Patients may describe a haze or curtain that involves the upper, lower, or all of the visual field. Atheromatous carotid disease is frequently associated, but the exact pathogenesis is debated. It is probably caused by microemboli that have lodged in small bifurcations, although these are rarely seen because the attacks are so brief. Bright cholesterol plaques, creamy glistening fibrin-platelet emboli, or calcium emboli have been seen between attacks (Table 7–13). There are inconclusive data at present to allow prediction of retinal infarction or cerebral stroke subsequent to amaurosis fugax. The risk of subsequent cerebral infarction is higher in patients older than 50 years, with a carotid bruit, with reduced retinal artery pressure, with venous stasis retinopathy, and with previous transient ischemic attacks.

Patients with amaurosis fugax need a careful medical and neurologic evaluation. The ophthalmologist should assess risk factors for vascular disease and perform a careful ophthalmic examination to detect any vascular abnormalities, and an internist or neurologist should evaluate blood pressure, carotid pulses, temporal artery pulse, and pulse rate. Several non-invasive studies are available that can evaluate the carotid artery bifurcation (Doppler ultrasonography, ultrasonographic imaging) or assess the hemodynamics of the carotid circulation distal to the carotid bifurcation (ophthalmo-

TABLE 7–13 **Neurologic and Neuro-ophthalmic Signs Associated with Occlusions of Important Arteries**

Artery obstructed	*Clinical signs*
Internal carotid or common carotid	May be asymptomatic if collateral flow from contralateral internal carotid and the vertebrobasilar system is adequate Contralateral hemiplegia, hemisensory loss, homonymous hemianopia, aphasia, agraphia, alexia if dominant hemisphere involved
Anterior cerebral	Contralateral paralysis and hemisensory loss
Middle cerebral	Contralateral hemiplegia, hemianesthesia Homonymous hemianopia Language disturbance if dominant hemisphere involved
Basilar	Coma and often death Quadriparesis or hemiplegia, dysarthria, dysphagia, third, fourth, sixth, or seventh cranial nerve palsy, Horner's syndrome, horizontal gaze paralysis, pupillary abnormalities
Anterior-inferior cerebellar	Unilateral facial palsy, deafness, cerebellar deficit leg and arm, contralateral loss of pain and temperature sensation, Horner's syndrome
Superior cerebellar	Ipsilateral cerebellar deficit, contralateral hemiplegia, hemisensory deficit arm/leg
Posterior cerebral	Hemisensory loss, contralateral ataxia, choreoathetosis, tremor, alexia without agraphia, contralateral homonymous hemianopia, visual agnosia, hemiplegia

dynamometry, ocular plethysmography, fluorescein appearance time). Digital subtraction angiography or formal arteriography is indicated in some patients.

Retinal artery occlusion, venous stasis retinopathy, and ocular ischemia are signs of ocular circulatory disease.

Retinal arterial occlusions cause painless and abrupt visual loss. The occlusion can be segmental with quadrantic or altitudinal visual loss or central with diffuse retinal edema and a cherry-red appearance of the macula. The visual field defect corresponds to the clinical appearance. Most retinal artery occlusions are embolic. Examination may reveal cholesterol or fibrin-platelet emboli associated with atherosclerotic extracranial internal and common carotid arteries, calcific emboli from endocardial vegetations, fat emboli from bone fractures, septic emboli during septicemia, or emboli associated with mitral valve prolapse. Inflammatory closure of the arteries may also occur in association with collagen vascular disease or temporal arteritis. Patients with these retinal strokes have a lower survival rate, most commonly related to coronary artery disease.

Chronic ischemia of the eye from atheromatous occlusive disease of the carotid arteries may lead to either venous stasis retinopathy or the chronic ocular ischemia syndrome. Venous stasis retinopathy is due to decreased profusion pressure as a result of occlusive disease of the carotid system. There are unilateral microaneurysms, small retinal hemorrhages, punctate areas of capillary dilatation, and irregularity in the caliber of retinal veins; the vascular abnormalities are generally most prominent in the equatorial fundus. Ophthalmodynamometry confirms a low ophthalmic artery pressure. Carotid endarterectomy may be indicated.

More severe ocular ischemia produces an anterior chamber inflammatory response with poor vision, ocular pain, corneal edema, and a red eye. Over a variable period (days to months), iris rubeosis, synechiae, cataract, mid-dilated pupil, retinal hemorrhages, retinal edema, narrowed arterioles, and dilated veins develop. The intraocular pressure may be high (from chronic angle closure related to neovascularization) or low (if the eye is pre-phthisical and hypotonic).

The anatomic location of an aneurysm determines the neuro-ophthalmic symptoms.

Aneurysms are local dilatations of the arterial walls and may be saccular or fusiform. Saccular aneurysms are berry-like outpouchings and tend to rupture, whereas fusiform aneurysms are more likely to thrombose. *Aneurysms of the internal carotid artery* occur in the intracavernous portion, supraclinoid artery, posterior communicating artery, anterior cerebral artery, middle cerebral artery, and ophthalmic artery (Fig. 7–27). Visual symptoms vary with the location but may include loss of central and peripheral vision, facial pain, ophthalmoplegia, Horner's syndrome, and exophthalmos.

Vertebrobasilar aneurysms are usually located at the bifurcation of the basilar artery close to the exit of the oculomotor nerve. The third nerve is vulnerable to these aneurysms; other cranial nerve palsies and corticospinal and spinothalamic tract signs may also occur.

Various inflammatory diseases of the cranial arteries are probably autoimmune reactions.

Although some inflammatory diseases involve the large cerebral arteries (Takayasu's dis-

ease), most affect the medium-sized and small arteries (lupus erythematosus, temporal arteritis, Wegener's granulomatosis). The common cause may be an autoimmune process. *Giant cell (temporal) arteritis* involves all layers of the arterial wall with infiltration of plasma cells, lymphocytes, and giant cells. The posterior ciliary arteries, the ophthalmic artery, and the central retinal artery are typically involved. This disease is seen in the elderly (older than 60 years) in association with constitutional symptoms (polymyalgia rheumatica) and frequently ophthalmic symptoms. Visual loss is the most common ophthalmic symptom and may be the presenting complaint. Amaurosis fugax or transient gray patches of vision may precede permanent visual loss. Ischemic infarction of the optic nerve can be confirmed by the pale edema of the optic disc and hemorrhages of the nerve fiber layer. Other patients may demonstrate a central retinal artery occlusion. The finding of a thickened, pulseless, and painful temporal artery is diagnostic. Determining the erythrocyte sedimentation rate remains the most important and reliable laboratory test for diagnosis and for monitoring disease activity. If the disease is suspected, temporal artery biopsy is indicated to confirm the diagnosis.

Wegener's granulomatosis has a characteristic necrotizing granulomatous vasculitis of the respiratory tract, kidneys, and various other tis-

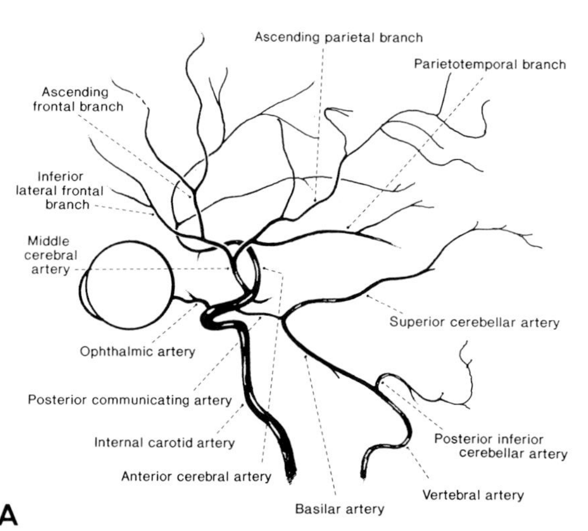

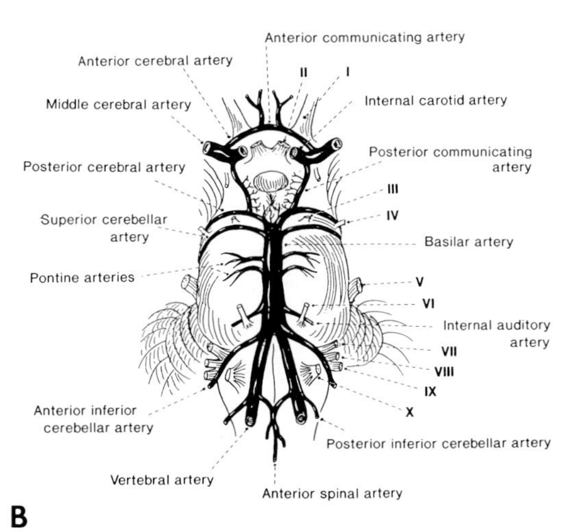

Fig. 7–27. Common location of aneurysms along the cerebral and vertebrobasilar artery system, in the lateral (*A*) and basal (*B*) views.

sues. Ophthalmic symptoms arise from granuloma formation and invasion of the orbital and chiasmal area. *Periarteritis nodosa* affects medium-sized arteries, causing small infarcts throughout the central nervous system or intracerebral hemorrhages. Neuro-ophthalmic symptoms are variable and related to the area of the brainstem or cerebral cortex involved. The retinal vessels may be visibly involved with the arteritic process. *Disseminated lupus erythematosus* causes cerebral microinfarctions with focal neurologic symptoms and occasionally an occlusive retinal arteritis.

Migraine may occur in a classic, common, or ophthalmic form.

Classic migraine is a clinical syndrome with an aura of neurologic disturbance (usually visual, but occasionally motor or sensory) preceding the development of severe hemicranial pain (Table 7–14). When visual, the aura consists of a rather typical pattern of scintillations and fortifications (Fig. 7–28). The headaches and visual symptoms of classic migraine tend to diminish as a patient becomes older. *Common migraine* consists of less well-defined symptoms (nausea, light-headedness, depression, and gastrointestinal upset) associated with a headache. *Acephalgic migraine* (without headache) may be seen in some patients who may manifest only ophthalmic or neurologic symptoms and signs. *Ophthalmoplegic migraine* is associated with transient ocular motor abnormalities. *Cluster headache* is probably a migraine variant in which severe unilateral head pain may occur daily for a period of days or weeks in association with tearing, nasal congestion, and conjunctival hyperemia.

The clinical signs and symptoms of migraine can be attributed to changes associated with vasoconstriction and vasodilatation of the blood vessels. This spasm may also affect the optic nerve and retinal vessels and, in an occasional patient, may cause permanent ischemic damage to the optic nerve, retina, or cerebrum (*complicated migraine*). A careful history is of utmost importance in confirming this diagnosis. The neurophysiologic basis of migraine remains unknown, although heredity, stress, and

TABLE 7–14 Transient Neurologic and Ophthalmic Accompaniments of Migraine

Paresthesia
Dysarthria
Hemiplegia
Deafness
Confusion
Recurrence of stroke
Cyclic vomiting
Car sickness
Scintillations with or without fortification
Blurring or blindness
Hemianopia
Transient blindness
Diplopia
Mydriasis
Horner's syndrome

other psychic factors have been implicated. The disease usually appears before age 40 years: in patients older than 40, other causes of cerebral ischemia must be considered.

There is a wide range of normal variation of the optic disc.

There are many *abnormalities of the optic disc*. Some of these are developmental abnormalities with coloboma, tilting, crescents, or abnormal vessels; in others, the disc is small or the optic cup is large, round, deep, or slightly tilted. In myopia, the globe is enlarged with a tilted or oblique exit of the optic nerve from the eye with a temporal peripapillary depigmentation (*myopic crescent*). *Hypoplasia* is a small optic disc, often with a yellowish peripapillary halo; there may be a decreased number of axons with a stable visual impairment. Hypoplasia may be unilateral or bilateral and may be associated with other central nervous system disorders. An *optic pit* (variation of coloboma) is a round or oval hole in the temporal portion of the disc that is occasionally connected with serous detachment of the sensory retina. The visual symptoms vary depending on the size of the pit and the detachment.

Vascular anomalies of the disc include remnants of the unresorbed hyaloid artery system. This includes *Bergmeister's papilla*, which is a central vascular core or surrounding fibroglial

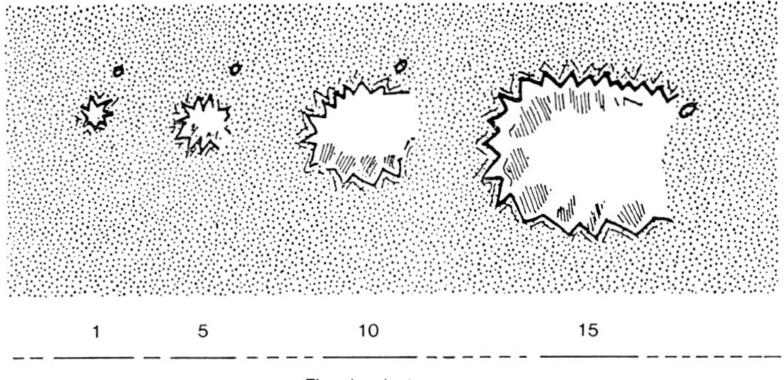

Fig. 7–28. The scintillating scotoma and fortification pattern of ophthalmic migraine. (From R.M. Burde, P.J. Savino, J.D. Trobe [eds.]: Clinical Decisions in Neuro-Ophthalmology. St. Louis, C.V. Mosby, 1985, pp. 91–115. By permission of the publisher.)

sheath. In extreme instances, the hyaloid vascular system and primary vitreous may persist, causing a "tenting up" of the peripapillary retinal tissue.

There are several causes of optic disc edema.

Edema of the optic disc is caused by a disturbance in the normal pressure gradient across the lamina cribrosa between the intraocular pressure and the cerebrospinal fluid pressure. The edema involves only the portion of the disc anterior to the lamina cribrosa. The various causes of optic disc swelling can be categorized into ocular, orbital, intracranial, or systemic types.

Optic disc swelling associated with increased intracranial pressure is termed *papilledema* (Fig. 7–29). It is seen in association with neoplasms, hemorrhage, edema, or an increased volume of cerebrospinal fluid (such as hydrocephalus). The increased pressure in the optic nerve sheath is probably transmitted from the subarachnoid space. Axoplasmic stasis occurs, resulting in vascular congestion and extracellular fluid accumulation in the disc and later in the retina. The ophthalmoscopic characteristics of papilledema include dilatation of the optic nerve capillaries, venous distention, retinal hemorrhages, loss of spontaneous venous pulsation, and preservation of the central optic cup. The visual symptoms in papilledema are usually mild, with only transient obscurations of vision and a slightly enlarged blind spot. The pupillary reactions, color vision, and central vision are usually normal. Long-standing papilledema leads to a secondary optic atrophy with progressive visual defects, usually beginning in the periphery.

Pseudotumor cerebri (benign intracranial hypertension) refers to the findings of increased cerebrospinal fluid pressure in the absence of an expanding intracranial lesion. Neurologic findings are absent, except that a nonlocalizing sixth nerve palsy may be associated with the increased intracranial pressure. This clinical setting usually occurs in young, overweight females, in patients with certain metabolic disorders (diabetes mellitus, sarcoidosis, chronic pulmonary disease), or in association with some systemic medications (corticosteroids, vitamin A, tetracycline).

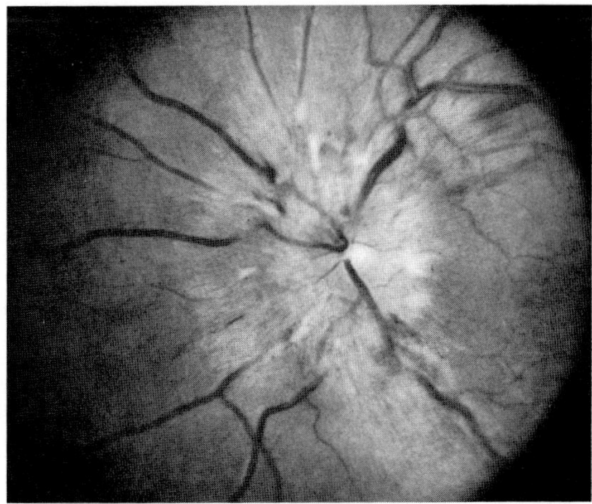

Fig. 7–29. Papilledema of the left optic nerve with elevation and blurring of the disc margin, disc hyperemia, small splinter hemorrhages, and white nerve fiber defects (cotton wool spots) and engorged and dusky veins. The vision was normal.

Unilateral disc edema may be seen in local orbital disease, usually in association with proptosis. The orbital lesion is usually a tumor impinging on the optic nerve causing stagnation of axonal flow and subsequent disc edema.

Malignant hypertension is associated with increased intracranial pressure and bilateral optic disc edema. Other vascular signs of hypertension—including narrowing of the retinal arterioles with retinal hemorrhages and exudates—are present.

Optic disc edema is also associated with conditions in which there are a low intraocular pressure and a normal pressure in the cerebrospinal fluid. There are numerous causes of ocular hypotony, including trauma, surgery, and ocular inflammation (Irvine-Gass syndrome, pars planitis). Frequently, other ocular abnormalities (choroidal detachments, corneal edema) preclude good visualization of the optic disc. These conditions are all associated with slowing of the axoplasmic flow through the optic nerve.

Prolonged optic disc swelling from whatever cause may eventuate in optic atrophy with loss of central and peripheral vision. Ophthalmoscopically, the optic disc gradually changes from a reddish discoloration to gray-white associated with proliferation of glial connective tissue within the optic disc. The retinal vessels may be sheathed and the disc margins permanently blurred.

Optic neuropathy is caused by inflammatory, degenerative, and ischemic factors.

Optic neuropathy is a disease process that impairs nerve conduction and manifests with loss of visual acuity and changes in the visual field. It is helpful to categorize the different causes of optic nerve damage into inflammatory optic neuritis, degenerative (inherited or acquired) optic neuropathy, and ischemic optic neuropathy. Involvement of the optic nerve by these entities may be visible ophthalmoscopically with a papillitis, or the process may occur in the retrobulbar portion of the nerve with no visible intraocular signs. The same functional defects occur whether the process is at the optic disc or in the retrobulbar optic nerve. The inflammatory causes of optic neuritis tend to damage the periaxial portion of the nerve, whereas degenerative processes tend to affect the central portion of the nerve.

The optic nerve may be affected by various inflammatory disorders.

Inflammatory optic neuritis is associated with many ocular inflammatory conditions. Infections within the eye such as endogenous or exogenous endophthalmitis, nematode endophthalmitis (*Toxocara*), cryptococcosis, and toxoplasmosis cause optic disc swelling from the production of toxic products that alter the vascular permeability of the disc vessels. Viral infections of the retina or brain may be complicated by optic neuritis, as seen in herpes simplex, herpes zoster, cytomegalovirus, or acute sclerosing panencephalitis. Neuroretinitis, retinal vasculitis, and papillitis have been observed in Behçet's disease and in collagen vascular disease. Sarcoidosis may cause a nodular papillitis from infiltration of the optic nerve and retina.

Certain forms of uveitis may be associated with inflammation of the optic disc with leakage of the vessels. The profound visual loss usually is an indication of an optic neuritis rather than optic disc edema from hypotonia. Meningitis and subsequent optic nerve sheath and nerve involvement may be associated with blood-borne infection from bacteria, fungi, tuberculosis, or syphilis. Local orbital infections, especially with mucormycosis or *Aspergillus*, may spread to involve the optic nerve.

The optic nerve is vulnerable to toxic, nutritional, and demyelinating disorders.

A multitude of factors may act in concert to produce *toxic degenerative optic neuritis. Tobacco amblyopia* is the most common recognized cause, usually occurring in older pipe-smoking men with a cecocentral scotoma and decreased central and color vision. *Nutritional amblyopia* presents with the same clinical findings in patients with chronic alcoholism. Tobacco and alcohol amblyopia may have a similar pathophysiology that causes damage to the optic nerve. Methyl alcohol (methanol or wood alcohol) ingestion causes an acute symptom complex, including blindness, delirium, convulsions, and circulatory collapse; chronic exposure causes cecocentral scotomas. Lead poisoning, certain drugs (chloramphenicol, disulfiram, digitalis, quinine), and the vitamin B_{12} deficiency of pernicious anemia can cause an optic neuropathy. Thyroid optic neuropathy results from compression of the nerve within the narrow confines of the orbital apex by thickened rectus muscles.

Multiple sclerosis is the most prominent among the *demyelinating optic nerve diseases* (diseases in which myelin is lost throughout the central nervous system). Multiple sclerosis is a chronic affliction that has an extremely variable course and may last many years before spontaneous remission. The spinal cord is the most common site of early involvement with symptoms of numbness and tingling. Optic neuritis is a clinical diagnosis of transient visual loss lasting weeks to several months with variable recovery of vision. Up to 50% of patients with idiopathic optic neuritis may ultimately develop multiple sclerosis. Probably a third of patients with multiple sclerosis have a clinical history of optic neuritis at some time in their course, but more than 90% have evidence of optic nerve damage.

The visual loss is usually unilateral and profound with loss of color perception and a dense central scotoma. There is an afferent pupillary defect with mild pain (lasting several weeks) on movement of the eye. Although the optic nerve may be swollen, initially its appearance is normal in the retrobulbar form of optic neuritis, but later optic nerve pallor becomes evident. The visual and other neurologic symptoms may be exacerbated by heat or exercise (Uhthoff's sign). Magnetic resonance imaging is highly sensitive in detecting these plaques in the central nervous system. The visual-evoked potential test shows a conductive delay. The visual loss in idiopathic optic neuritis or that associated with multiple sclerosis is usually progressive over 2 to 5 days with visual recovery beginning within a few weeks in the vast majority of cases. Chronic progressive visual loss im-

plies a compressive lesion rather than optic neuritis (Fig. 7–30). The cause of multiple sclerosis remains unclear.

Devic's disease (neuromyelitis optica) and acute disseminated encephalomyelitis may be variants of multiple sclerosis with an acute and severe course. Bilateral acute papillitis may be seen in both of these conditions. The leukodystrophies are a group of diseases characterized by progressive demyelination of the cerebral white matter. They are genetically determined inborn errors of metabolism; some of the variants are Schilder's disease, Krabbe's disease, and metachromatic leukodystrophy.

Ischemia to the optic nerve can cause various visual symptoms and have various causes.

Ischemia to the optic nerve occurs when the profusion pressure in the posterior ciliary arteries is inadequate. This may occur from hemodynamic factors (systemic hypotension, hyperviscosity) or from occlusion of the posterior ciliary arteries caused by arteriosclerosis, hypertension, diabetes, collagen vascular disease, temporal arteritis, or occlusion of the carotid arteries or the aortic arch. Some glaucoma specialists believe that acute or long-term elevation of intraocular pressure causes ischemic damage to the optic nerve with subsequent optic disc changes.

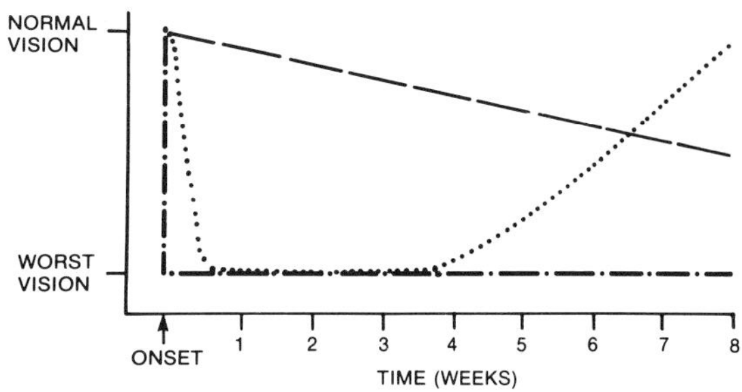

Fig. 7–30. The clinical course of the visual loss and recovery in optic nerve disease depends on whether the disease is caused by an optic neuritis ($\cdot\,\cdot\,\cdot\,\cdot\,\cdot$), an ischemic optic neuropathy ($\cdot-\cdot-\cdot$), or an infiltrative compressive nerve lesion ($-\,-\,-$). (From S. Lessell: Current concepts in ophthalmology: optic neuropathies. N Engl J Med 299:533–536, 1978. By permission of the journal.)

Ischemia to the optic nerve may manifest with amaurosis fugax or with transient altitudinal, sectoral, or arcuate defects that may become permanent. The altitudinal defects have a predilection for the lower half of the field of vision. The optic nerve ischemia may be evident at the disc but may occur in the retrobulbar portion, in which case no abnormalities may be observed ophthalmoscopically. When the disc is involved (anterior ischemic optic neuropathy), it is usually swollen with a pale pink or even hyperemic appearance and may be confined to a segmental portion of the disc. Later, optic atrophy appears. Temporal arteritis is a specific form of ischemic optic neuropathy.

Optic atrophy is the final result of many insults to the optic nerve or may occur in hereditary forms.

Optic atrophy is characterized by loss of axons and a chalky white appearance to the disc. It can be the result of any process that damages the retinal ganglion cells and axons, such as optic neuritis or degenerative, vascular, or toxic optic neuropathy. Optic atrophy can occur from various drug toxicities, poisons, or certain vitamin deficiencies. Infiltration of the optic nerve from cancer, leukemia, lymphoma, or sarcoid may result in optic atrophy, as may radiation necrosis after treatment of brain tumors. Identifying optic atrophy requires a search for the underlying cause.

Several hereditary optic atrophies appear early in life with insidious, bilateral, and symmetric loss of central vision. *Leber's optic atrophy* affects primarily males (X-linked); it is characterized by sudden bilateral visual loss in the second or third decade of life with cecocentral scotomas. During the acute neuritic stage, optic disc hyperemia, edema, and swelling of the nerve fiber layer are evident; optic atrophy occurs later with permanent visual loss. Another example is Behr's hereditary optic atrophy (recessive), which begins in infancy and progresses for several decades with a moderate visual defect. Other neurologic abnormalities may be present, including cerebellar ataxia, spasticity, and pyramidal tract abnormalities. *Infantile hereditary optic neuropathy* occurs in a dominant or recessive form. In the recessive form, optic atrophy occurs shortly after birth with profound visual loss. The dominant form is milder, although it may be progressive into early adult life. The peripheral fields usually remain intact.

8

DISORDERS OF THE ORBIT
James A. Garrity

Orbital disorders are often difficult to diagnose, and a systematic approach is essential. The orbit is a pear-shaped bony socket that contains the globe, the extraocular muscles, nerves, blood vessels, orbital fat, and the lacrimal gland (Fig. 8–1). The volume of the orbital socket is approximately 30 mL. The retrobulbar and peribulbar tissues contribute 70% to the orbital volume and the globe itself accounts for the remaining 30%. Several of the vessels and nerves originating in the apex of the orbit are destined to supply the areas of the face around the orbital aperture. The orbit is surrounded on three sides by sinuses: the frontal sinus above, the ethmoid and sphenoid sinuses medially, and the maxillary sinus below. The evaluation and treatment of orbital disease fall within the therapeutic reach of many specialties (ophthalmology, neurosurgery, otorhinolaryngology, and plastic surgery); we advocate a team approach for the management of complex orbital problems.

The chief signs and symptoms of orbital disease are proptosis, diplopia, ptosis, and visual loss.

Because so many important structures inhabit such a relatively confined area, any or all of the cardinal signs and symptoms of orbital disease can be produced by a small but critically placed lesion (Table 8–1).

The most obvious cardinal sign of orbital disease is *proptosis.* Because of the rigid confines of the orbital walls, a disease process within or adjacent to the orbit usually displaces the globe forward or in a direction opposite to the lesion (Fig. 8–2). A patient with proptosis must be evaluated to determine whether it is true proptosis or one of the many causes of pseudoproptosis.

An accurate history can assist the examination by historically documenting previous ocular trauma or inflammation; either can ultimately lead to an atrophic (phthisical) globe with resultant enophthalmos and a pseudoproptosis of the contralateral eye. Patients, surprisingly, may be unable to recall past trauma that has "blown out" the floor or medial wall of the orbit. Another example of apparent proptosis caused by contralateral enophthalmos is one from metastatic scirrhous adenocarcinoma (breast, lung, or stomach) to the orbit. This restrictive orbitopathy is secondary to the generalized contraction that the tumor promotes. An easily overlooked cause of pseudoproptosis is a large globe from unilateral high myopia. Lid retraction can also give the appearance of ipsilateral proptosis (Fig. 8–3).

Diplopia may be associated with an orbital process. Forced ductions are helpful in determining whether the double vision is from a mechanical (restrictive) or a neurogenic cause. Topical anesthesia is achieved by applying a cotton swab soaked in 5% cocaine or 4% lidocaine against the muscle insertion. With this anesthesia, a fine-toothed forceps can be used to grasp the muscle tendon and rotate the globe.

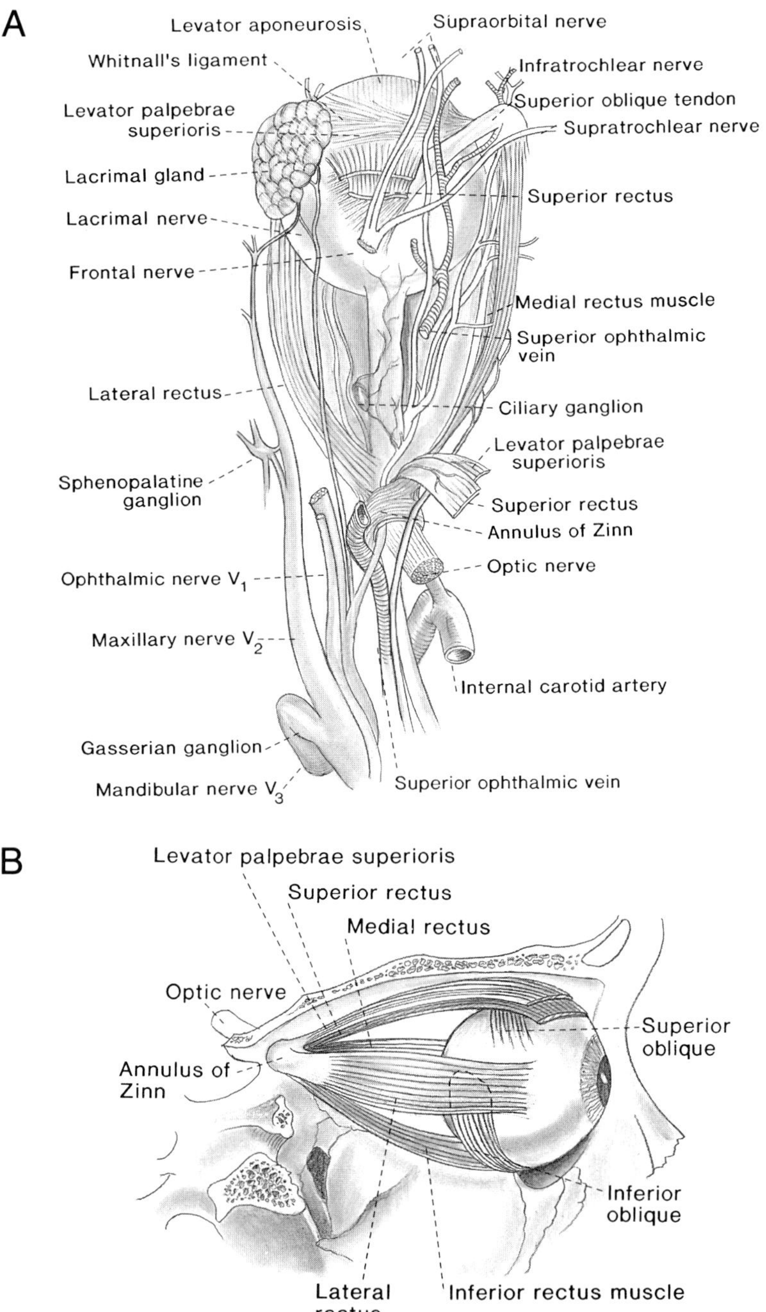

Fig. 8–1.   Anatomy of orbit.

Results of this test are subjective but can be helpful.

One should also evaluate ocular alignment to determine whether a pattern suggestive of a cranial nerve weakness or multiple cranial nerve palsies are present. In the latter situation, the lesion is most likely located in the cavernous sinus. Documenting decreased corneal sensation with either a wisp of cotton or an esthesiometer may be helpful in providing confirmatory evidence of a cavernous sinus abnormality.

A unilateral external ophthalmoplegia typi-

TABLE 8–1 Signs and Symptoms of Orbital Disease

Proptosis
Diplopia
Ptosis
Visual loss

cally produces 2 to 3 mm of proptosis secondary to relaxation of the tethering effect of the extraocular muscles. This finding may give the false impression of an orbital mass when in fact the actual lesion is located in the cavernous sinus. One must always evaluate critically any motility imbalance, especially if the pattern is unusual, the findings are variable, ptosis is present, and the pupil is normal. Myasthenia gravis should be suspected and the Tensilon (edrophonium) test should be considered. A positive response can be determined from the lid elevation if it is ptotic, or by observation of a change in ocular alignment with either Maddox rod or Lancaster red-green testing.

Like diplopia, *ptosis* in association with an orbital disorder can be either neurogenic or mechanical. Perhaps the most important aspect of the ptosis evaluation from an orbit standpoint is palpation beneath the superior orbital rim for the detection of superior orbital masses. Neurogenic ptosis displays other features of a palsy or partial palsy of cranial nerve III. An additional cause of ptosis, a myogenic cause, should be considered, and, as mentioned

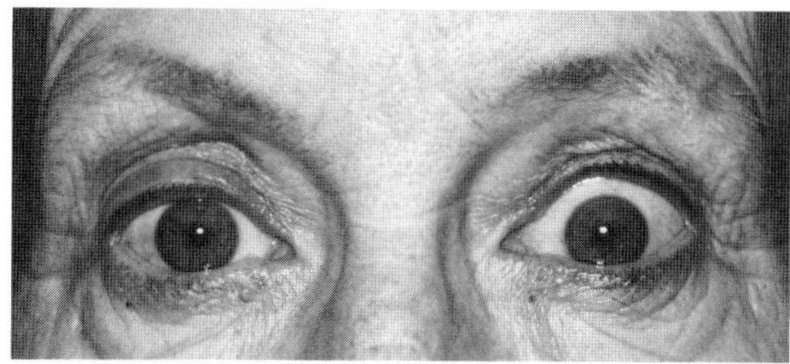

Fig. 8–3. Pseudoproptosis of the left globe caused by unilateral lid retraction from Graves' ophthalmopathy. There was no demonstrable proptosis with the Krahn exophthalmometer.

above, Tensilon testing for suspected myasthenia gravis should be considered, especially if the ptosis is variable.

Visual loss is a nonspecific sign and, if present, tends to be gradual and progressive. Evidence of an optic neuropathy may be present, as demonstrated by acquired color vision defects, an afferent pupillary defect, or a visual field defect. Acquired hyperopia, a correctable form of visual loss, can be caused by an intraconal tumor indenting the posterior portion of the globe; the refractive change usually resolves after the mass has been removed. One type of episodic visual loss is fairly specific for orbital disease, namely, gaze-evoked amaurosis. This phenomenon has been described in cases of orbital cavernous hemangioma and optic nerve sheath meningioma; in certain positions of gaze, the tumor presumably occludes the blood supply and transient visual loss occurs.

The orbit can be imaged by plain radiography, computed tomography, magnetic resonance imaging, and ultrasonography.

Plain radiography is helpful for delineating fractures or the bony destruction that may be caused by some tumors. Modern *computed tomography (CT)* can produce 1.5-mm axial cuts through the orbit, enabling sophisticated evaluation of soft tissues. The data collected from these thin-cut axial images can then be used to reconstruct images in the coronal or sagittal planes. Alternatively, direct scanning of the orbit in both the axial and the coronal planes can be performed (Fig. 8–4).

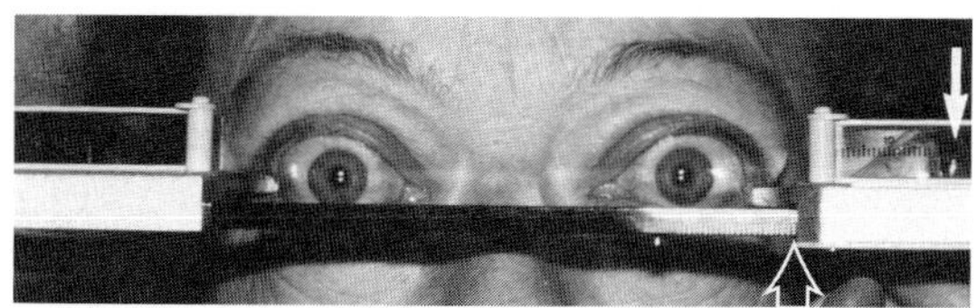

Fig. 8–2. Exophthalmometry with the Krahn exophthalmometer (the Hertel type can also be used). The footpieces are placed against the lateral orbital rim. The base measurement (*open arrow*) is noted (100 mm) and used for all subsequent measurements. The position of the cornea is then read off the scale (*closed arrow*), which is 23 mm for the left eye. (From R.S. Bahn, J.A. Garrity, G.B. Bartley, C.A. Gorman: Diagnostic evaluation of Graves' ophthalmopathy. Endocrinol Metab Clin North Am 17:527–545 Sept 1988. By permission of W.B. Saunders Company.)

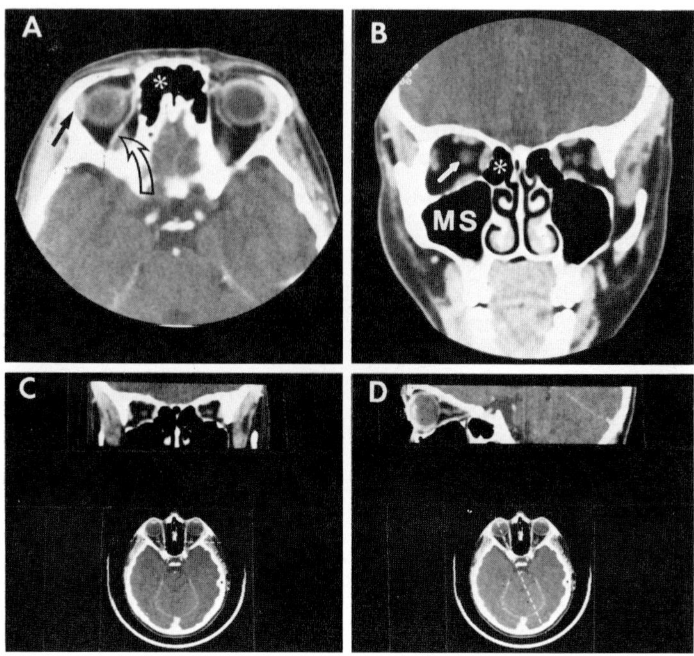

Fig. 8–4. Series of normal CT scans from the same patient. Scans in *A* and *B* are direct 3-mm axial and coronal views. Scans in *C* and *D* are reconstructed coronal and sagittal views obtained by computer reformatting of 1.5-mm axial data. A, Axial view through the superior orbit. Note the globes, ethmoid sinus (*asterisk*), superior ophthalmic vein (*open arrow*), and lacrimal gland (*solid arrow*). View is asymmetric because patient's head was slightly tilted. B, Direct coronal view: maxillary sinus (*MS*), ethmoid sinus (*asterisk*), medial rectus, inferior rectus, lateral rectus, superior rectus, and optic nerve (*arrow*). C, Reconstructed coronal view, corresponding to same level as direct scans in *B*. D, Reconstructed sagittal view. These sagittal and coronal views can be used to advantage in the evaluation of floor fractures.

The orbit is best evaluated by scans no thicker than 3 mm in both the axial and the coronal plane. One can obtain reconstructed coronal scans from 3-mm axial scans that are of good quality but offer less resolution than 1.5-mm cuts. For patients who are unable to extend their necks or who have extensive metallic dental work or for sedated children, reformatted coronal images are a better option. Coronal imaging is important in the evaluation of orbital disease, particularly with lesions along the roof or floor. Orbital CT scanning is the current imaging standard, although orbital *magnetic resonance imaging* (*MRI*) holds much promise, particularly as experience is gained with this technique (Fig. 8–5). One notable advantage of MRI over CT is that MRI can sometimes offer histologic clues not available with CT scanning. In addition, the patient is not exposed to ionizing radiation. Relative disadvantages of MRI are the cost and the relatively long scanning time required.

Ultrasonography is a valuable ancillary test for orbital diagnosis (Fig. 8–6). High-frequency sound waves are propagated through soft tissue, and the differential reflection of these waves by tissues in the path of the beam is recorded. *A-scan* sonograms produce a one-dimensional tracing that can provide specific comparisons of tissue reflectance as well as accurate measure-

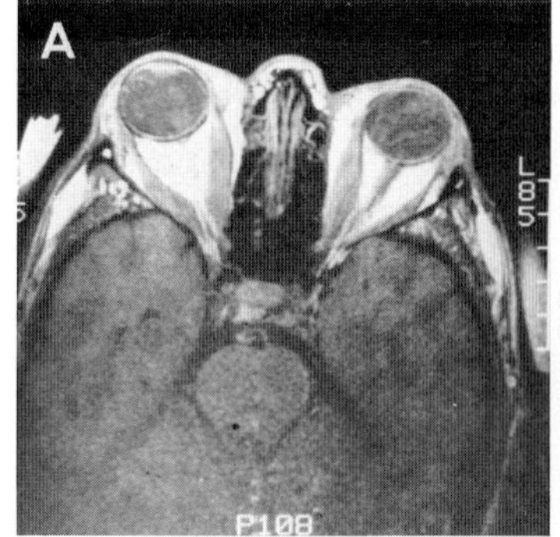
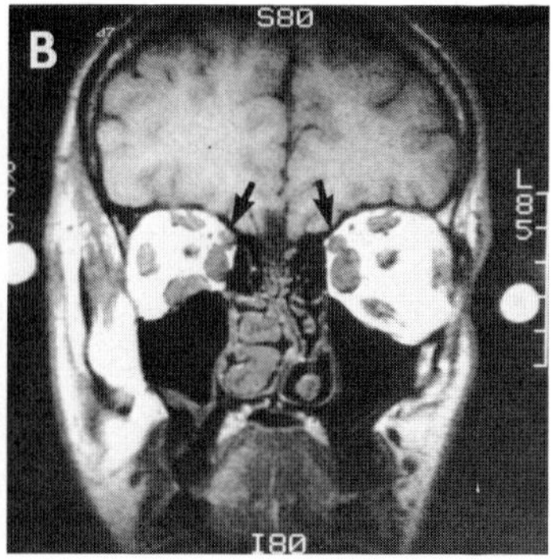

Fig. 8–5. MRI scans in a patient with Graves' ophthalmopathy. T1-weighted images display anatomic features to better advantage. *A*, Axial view, showing enlarged medial and lateral rectus muscles with characteristic fusiform muscle enlargement and sparing of the muscle insertions. *B*, T1-weighted coronal image, clearly demonstrating that all extraocular muscles are enlarged. Note superior oblique muscles (*arrows*).

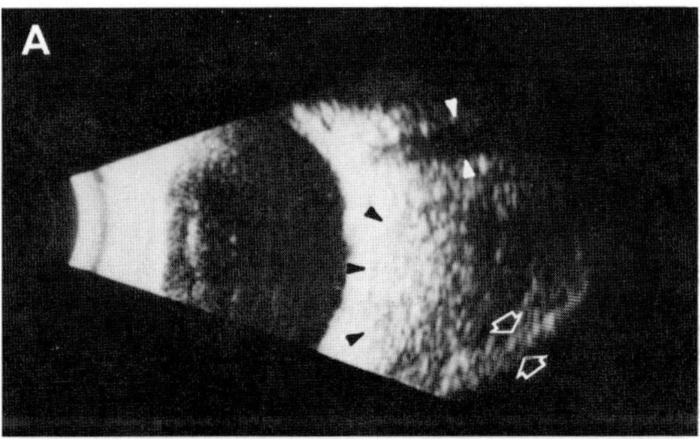

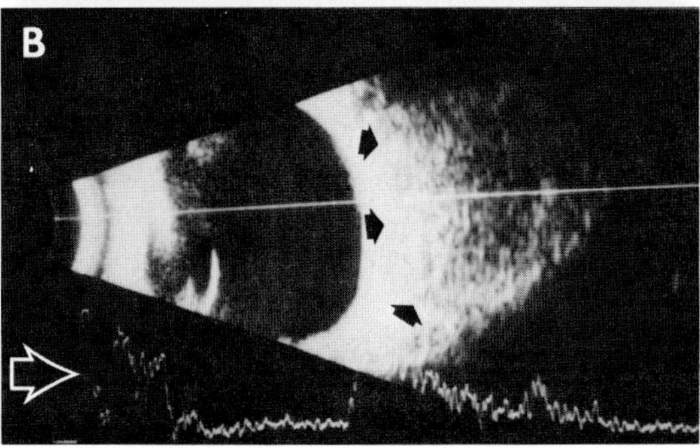

Fig. 8–6.   B-scan ultrasonography of large orbital cavernous hemangioma (*black arrowheads* on *A* and *black arrows* on *B*). *A*, Probe placed horizontally, optic nerve medially (*white arrowheads*), and lateral rectus laterally (*open arrows*). *B*, Same view as in *A* with superimposed A-scan vector (*open arrow*), showing typical kappa pattern associated with a cavernous hemangioma (*black arrows* outline anterior border of tumor).

ments of tissue dimensions. *B-scan* sonograms display a two-dimensional cross section of the eye and orbit. The transducer can be used with either a water bath or a contact method. The contact B-scan technique is most likely to be used in a general office setting. Its advantages are its low cost, noninvasive technique, and ready availability. Disadvantages include the high levels of technical and interpretive skills needed by the operator. In addition, the posterior orbit is not seen reliably and lesions located along the orbital roof or floor may be missed, particularly with the contact B-scan. The water bath B-scan technique is not as readily available and is more cumbersome to use, although it does offer better resolution than the contact method. In most centers, CT and MRI have essentially replaced ultrasonography, but ultrasonography still proves helpful in certain situations, most notably in orbital lymphangiomas.

The orbital disease mnemonic is VEIN.

When the evaluation has determined that a "true" proptosis exists, we have found the mnemonic *VEIN* (*v*ascular, *e*ndocrine, *i*nflammation/infection, *n*eoplasm) helpful in terms of clinical classification (Table 8–2). Clinically significant proptosis is regarded as a difference of 2 mm or more as measured by either the Krahn or the Hertel exophthalmometer.

"V" is for vascular exophthalmos.

Vascular causes of proptosis are from either the venous circulation (varix) or the arterial circulation (dural shunt or carotid cavernous fistula). A *varix* has a characteristic history of either positional (dependent) proptosis or proptosis induced by Valsalva maneuvers (Fig. 8–7). A long-standing varix, because of eventual orbital fat atrophy, can produce enophthalmos in the primary position until a Valsalva maneuver reveals its true identity. Suspicion of a varix should alert the radiologist to perform CT either with jugular compression or during a Valsalva maneuver. Operative intervention for varices can be fraught with difficulty, and observation is usually the most prudent form of therapy.

The *dural sinus fistula* or *low-flow shunt* can masquerade as unilateral red eye or glaucoma (Fig. 8–8). Because of its insidious onset, a high index of suspicion is necessary, particularly if the globe is not injected or if proptosis is minimal. The symptoms of headache or tinnitus need not be present. Orbital CT scanning or B-scan ultrasonography may reveal a slightly enlarged superior ophthalmic vein with either enlarged muscle(s) or normal-sized muscle(s). Observation and antiglaucoma therapy may be the only required treatment. In addition to being diagnostic, selective carotid angiography is

TABLE 8–2   Clinical Classification of Proptosis

V	Vascular
E	Endocrinologic (dysthyroid)
I	Inflammatory/infectious
N	Neoplastic

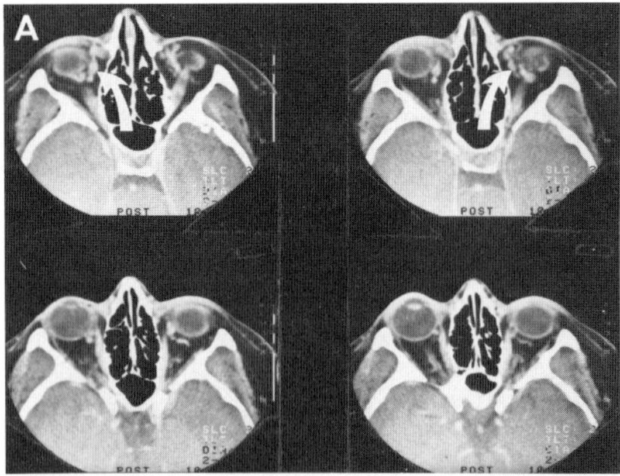

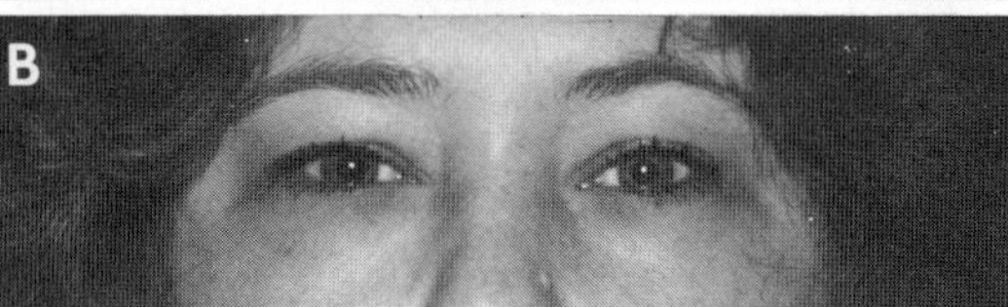

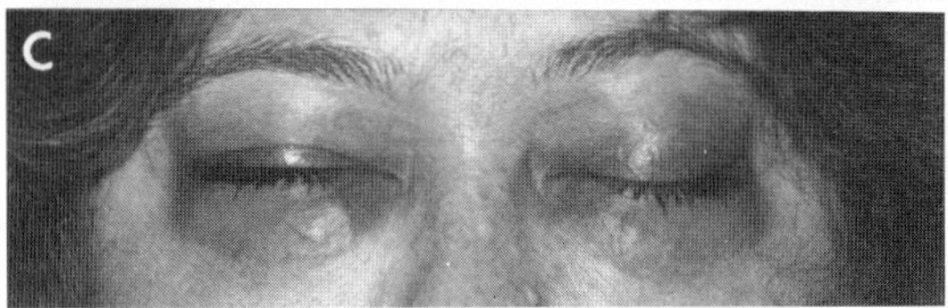

Fig. 8–7. *A*, Axial CT scans, showing varix of each superior ophthalmic vein (*arrows*). *B*, Pre-Valsalva appearance. *C*, Post-Valsalva appearance, with proptosis and mechanical ptosis.

often therapeutic. Frequently, the fistula will close spontaneously. Embolization with polyvinyl alcohol and small detachable balloons are other therapeutic options.

Carotid-cavernous fistulas (high-flow shunts) (Fig. 8–9) that arise either spontaneously or after trauma are symptomatic in terms of subjective bruits, proptosis, or visual loss. Objectively, the proptosis, chemosis, and various degrees of ophthalmoplegia are related to the congested orbit. Arterialized conjunctival vessels that approach the limbus in a corkscrew fashion are characteristic of this condition. CT scanning and B-scan ultrasongraphy will reveal both symmetrically enlarged extraocular muscles and a dilated superior ophthalmic vein. Fistulas with a spontaneous onset have a better chance of spontaneous resolution, although many times the shunt must be closed with either a detachable balloon or a carotid ligation.

"E" is for endocrine exophthalmos.

The following case report illustrates many of the important features of dysthyroid orbitopathy.

A 66-year-old woman first noticed vertical diplopia 8 months before evaluation. The vision in the left eye had become progressively blurred over the same period. Hyperthyroidism had been diagnosed 3 years previously and was treated with radioactive iodine.

The best corrected visual acuity was 20/40 in the right eye and 20/400 in the left eye. The pupillary responses and color vision were normal. Ocular ductions were severely restricted in upgaze in the left eye. In primary gaze there were 35 prism diopters of left hypotropia that decreased to 4 prism diopters of left hypotropia in the reading position. Krahn exophthalmom-

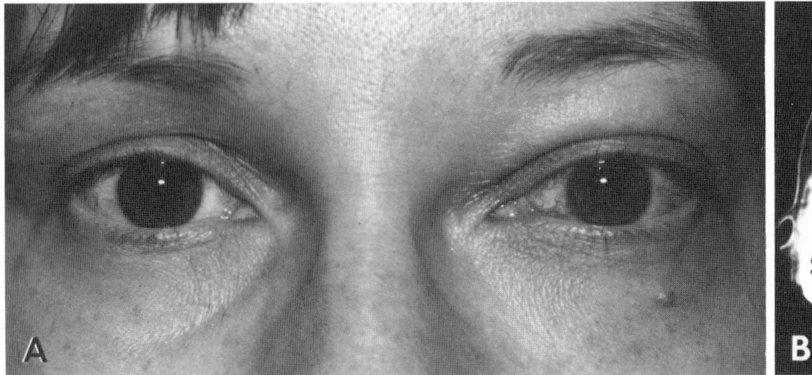

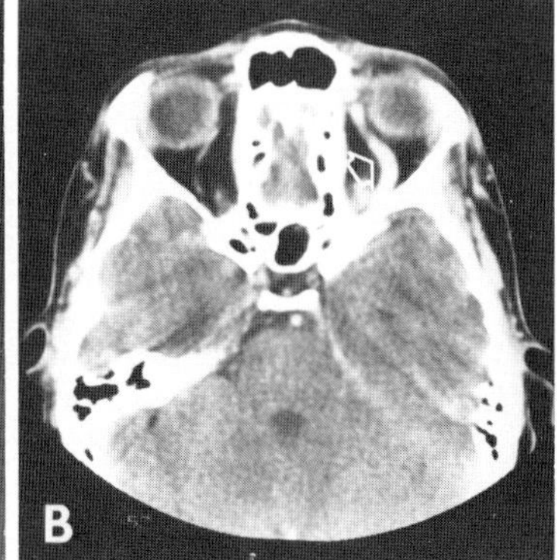

Fig. 8–8. *A*, A 30-year-old woman with dural sinus fistula. She noted a red left eye 1 month post partum. The vision was normal, although the left eye was injected and had 2 mm of proptosis. Intraocular pressures were 15 mm Hg in the right eye and 30 mm Hg in the left eye. *B*, Orbital CT scan, axial view. Note the grossly enlarged superior ophthalmic vein (*open arrow*).

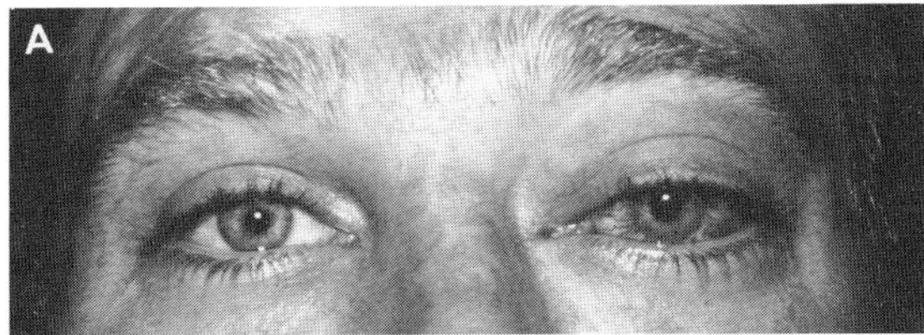

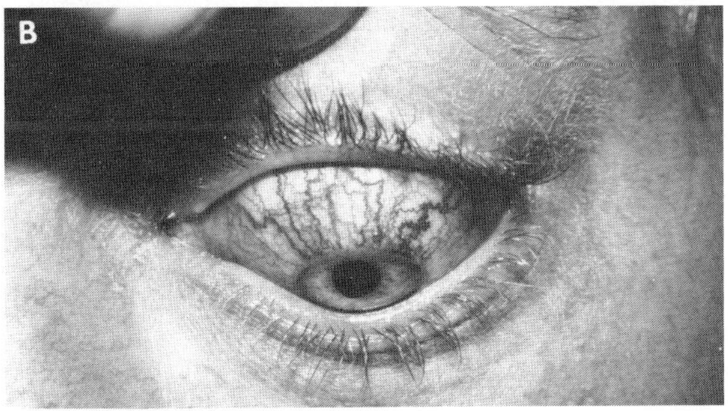

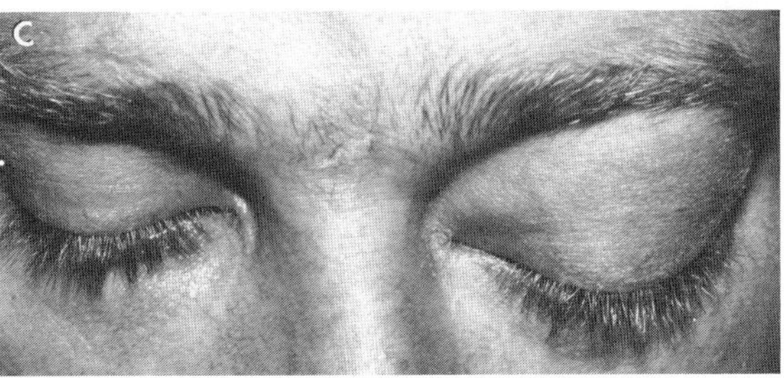

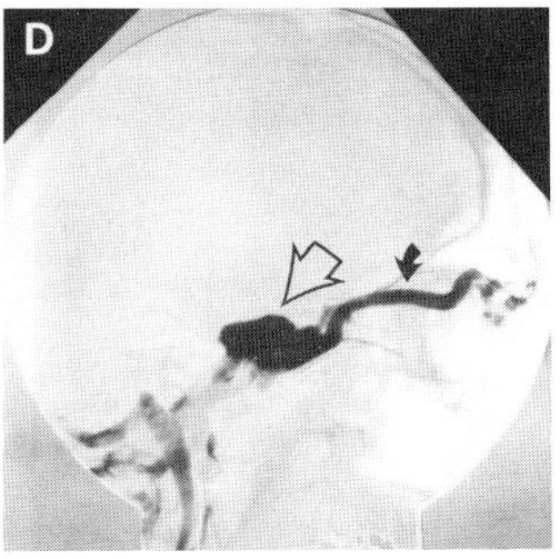

Fig. 8–9. *A,* A 30-year-old man with traumatic carotid-cavernous fistula. He was involved in a motor vehicle accident, sustaining a closed-head injury with a 15-hour loss of consciousness. The left eye had normal vision, slightly impaired abduction, and arterialization of conjunctival vessels. The intraocular pressure in the left eye was increased (15 mm Hg right eye and 25 mm Hg left eye). The fistula was treated with balloon occlusion and proximal ligation of the internal carotid artery. *B,* Arterialization of the conjunctival vessels. Typical corkscrew vessels approaching the limbus. *C,* Proptosis, 8 mm, of the left globe. *D,* Traumatic carotid-cavernous fistula. Left lateral subtraction view of internal carotid angiogram, demonstrating collection of contrast material within cavernous sinus (*open arrow*) and major vascular decompression in retrograde direction through superior ophthalmic vein (*small curved arrow*).

etry was 20 mm right eye and 21 mm left eye. The lid fissures were 12 mm right eye and 13 mm left eye. Cataracts were noted, greater in the left eye than in the right eye, and the ophthalmoscopic evaluation was normal. Goldmann and tangent screen visual fields showed generalized depression without evidence for an optic neuropathy (Fig. 8–10).

Graves' ophthalmopathy with restriction of the left inferior rectus muscle and cataracts were diagnosed. Results of examination 3 months later were unchanged. The left inferior rectus muscle was recessed 5 mm, and postoperatively the patient had single vision. Two months later the left cataract was removed and an intraocular lens was inserted. Visual acuity was restored to 20/20 in the left eye.

Six months later the patient noted an insidious loss of vision affecting the right eye. Examination revealed vision of finger counting in the right eye and 20/30 in the left eye. A moderate right afferent pupillary defect was present. The patient was unable to see any Ishihara color plates with the right eye, but she correctly identified all the color plates with the left eye. The lid fissures were 13 mm for the right eye and 16 mm for the left eye (Fig. 8–11). There was no lid edema, chemosis, or injection. Each orbit was firm to retropulsion. The ophthalmoscopic evaluation was normal. A tangent screen visual field showed an inferior cecocentral scotoma (Fig. 8–12). CT scanning of the orbit demonstrated enlarged extraocular muscles with apical crowding typical of Graves' ophthalmopathy (Fig. 8–13). A bilateral transantral orbital decompression was performed,

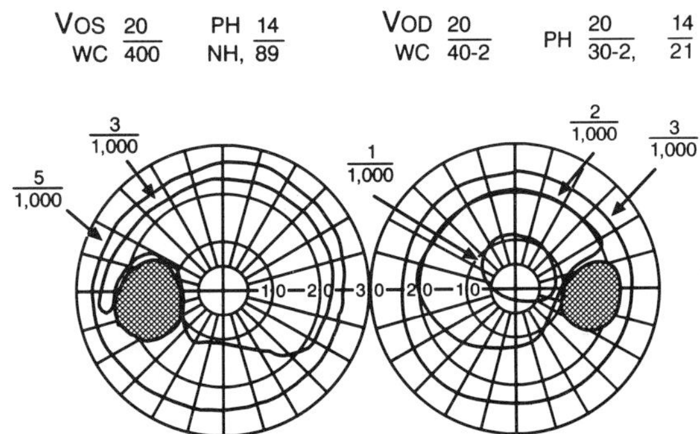

Fig. 8–10. Tangent screen visual fields, demonstrating generalized depression from cataracts. NH, no help (from pinhole, PH); WC, with correction.

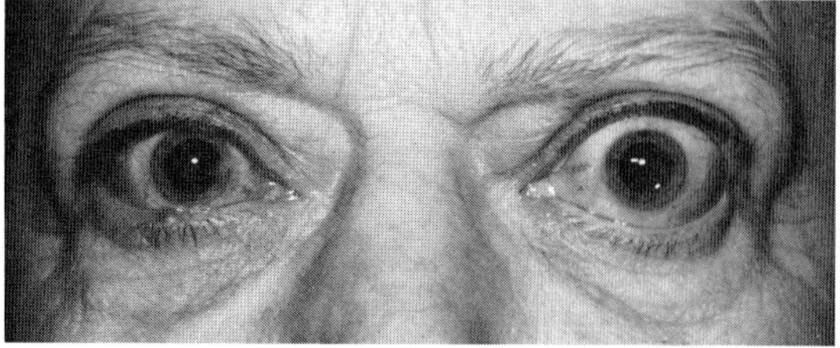

Fig. 8–11. Profound dysthyroid optic neuropathy affecting the right eye. Note the presence of bilateral lid retraction and the absence of any inflammatory features of Graves' ophthalmopathy.

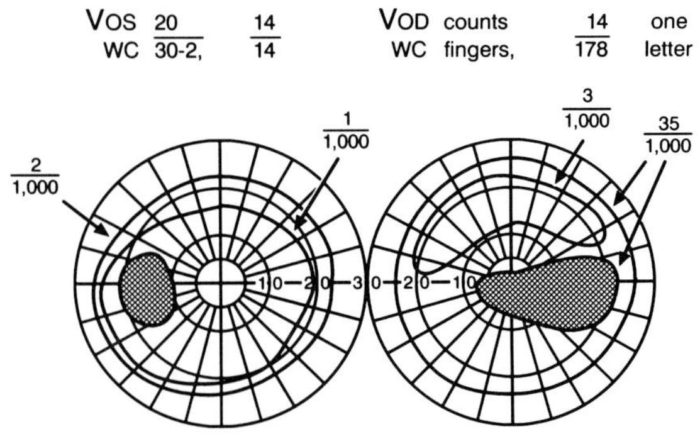

Fig. 8–12. Tangent screen visual fields, demonstrating a dense inferior cecocentral scotoma in the right eye. V, visual acuity; WC, with correction.

and postoperatively the vision returned to normal as the visual field defect gradually resolved.

The instructive features of this case are the diplopia and the loss of vision. The most frequently affected extraocular muscles in thyroid orbitopathy are the inferior and medial rectus muscles. The diplopia arises because of restriction (that is, the inferior rectus still functions in downgaze but does not "relax" to allow the globe to rotate upward). When this affects the medial rectus muscle, it resembles a lateral rectus palsy.

Visual loss in the setting of Graves' ophthalmopathy must be reconciled. A cataract was the obvious source on the initial examination. The optic neuropathy of Graves' disease was not so obvious on the subsequent examination. The insidious onset is typical, and the relatively "quiet" external appearance also may be typical. The clues to the correct diagnosis were the visual loss, afferent pupillary defect, color vision defect, and the visual field defect, which as a rule tends to affect the inferior portions of the visual field. The fundus evaluation, as this case demonstrates, may be entirely normal. Another source of visual loss in Graves' ophthalmopathy is corneal exposure, which was easily excluded on examination.

Endocrine exophthalmos (dysthyroid orbitopathy) is usually related to hyperthyroidism but can also be seen in euthyroidism or hypothyroidism. The diagnosis seldom presents a challenge in patients with classic orbital changes and overt hyperthyroidism, but in chemically euthyroid patients with asymmetric proptosis the diagnosis can be elusive. The most helpful and consistent signs are eyelid retraction and eyelid lag. Another subtle but characteristic clinical finding is temporal flare of the upper lid. Other features of thyroid eye disease include orbital congestion with proptosis, injection and chemosis of the conjunctiva and eyelid fullness, myopathy, and optic neuropathy. None of the signs indi-

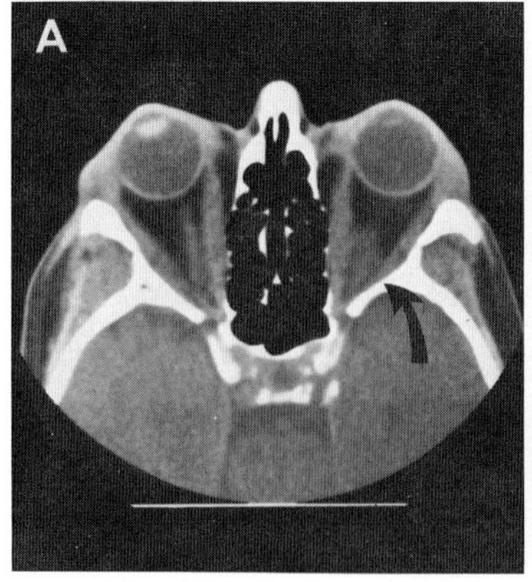

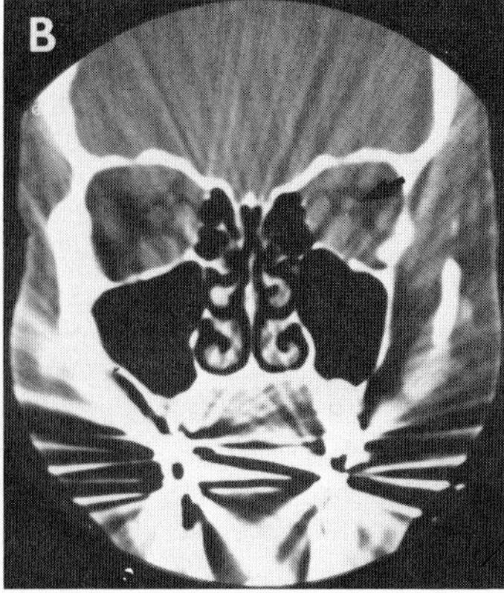

Fig. 8–13. Orbital CT scans. *A*, Axial view. The left orbital apex (*arrow*) is more "crowded" than the right. *B*, Coronal view. The left optic nerve (*arrow*) is beginning to be compressed by the enlarged extraocular muscles.

vidually is pathognomonic of thyroid eye disease. An important supportive laboratory test is the thyroid-releasing hormone suppression test for subclinical hyperthyroidism. A relatively new laboratory test is the sensitive thyroid-stimulating hormone assay, which is also capable of identifying early or subtle hyperthyroidism on the basis of a single serum analysis.

Orbital imaging techniques may show enlarged extraocular muscles (Table 8–3). Characteristically, the inferior rectus is affected first, followed in decreasing order of frequency by the medial rectus, superior rectus, and lateral rectus muscles (Fig. 8–5). Because of venous congestion at the orbital apex by the enlarged muscles it is possible to image a dilated superior ophthalmic vein in some cases of dysthyroid orbitopathy. The fusiform enlargement of the muscles with sparing of the tendinous insertions, in combination with the characteristic pattern of muscle enlargement, distinguishes dysthyroid orbitopathy from other entities such as myositis and carotid-cavernous fistula. A bulging orbital septum from prolapsed fat is also a useful finding on CT or MRI scans.

Therapy for the proptosis may require only simple observation or lubricating eyedrops. Orbital decompression is indicated for corneal exposure, for compressive optic neuropathy, and in advanced cases of proptosis before extraocular muscle surgery (muscle recessions exacerbate proptosis by releasing the tethering effect of the muscles and allowing the globe to come forward). Contemporary surgical decompressive techniques also allow safe and effective surgical options for certain cases of impaired cosmesis. Orbital decompression can be accomplished transantrally, transorbitally, or transcranially and can be performed on one, two, three, or all four orbital walls, depending on the amount of proptosis (Fig. 8–14). The presence of an optic neuropathy from apical compression requires inclusion of either a medial wall decompression into the ethmoid sinus or removal of the orbital roof because these are the only two walls that allow for decompression of the apex of the orbit. Other therapeutic options include eyelid surgery for exposure and corticosteroids or radiation therapy for acute congestive orbitopathy and compressive optic neuropathy.

"I" is for inflammatory/infectious exophthalmos.

Inflammatory causes of proptosis include idiopathic inflammatory orbital "pseudotumor" (nonspecific orbital inflammation) and infections. Both entities develop rapidly and are associated with discomfort. The *inflammatory*

TABLE 8–3 Differential Diagnosis of Enlarged Extraocular Muscles

Dysthyroid orbitopathy
Inflammation (orbital pseudotumor or myositis)
Lymphoma
Vascular malformation (carotid-cavernous or dural sinus fistula)
Metastatic tumor
Orbital cellulitis
Sphenoid wing meningioma
Plexiform neurofibroma
Amyloidosis
Sarcoidosis
Trichinosis

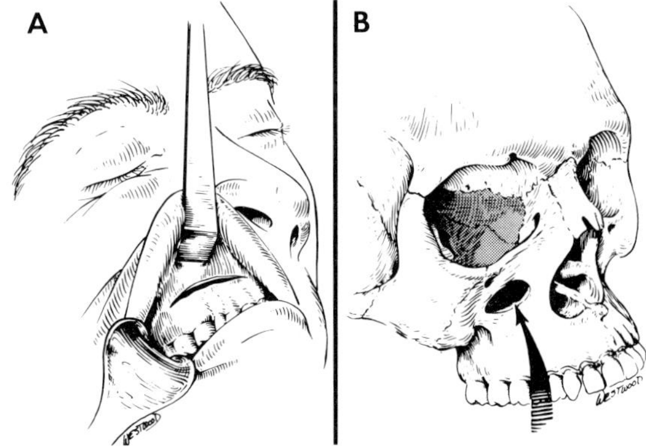

Fig. 8–14. Transantral orbital decompression. Operation begins with a gingivobuccal incision (*A*). The maxillary sinus is entered, and, through this sinus, the ethmoid sinus is then exenterated. The medial wall and floor of the orbit (shaded area in *B*) are then removed. The periorbita is incised, and orbital fat prolapses into the sinuses. (From C.A. Gorman, L.W. DeSanto, C.S. MacCarty, F.C. Riley: Optic neuropathy of Graves's disease: treatment by transantral or transfrontal orbital decompression. N Engl J Med 290:70–75, 1974. By permission of the journal.)

pseudotumors generally have an explosive onset with eyelid and conjunctival erythema, swelling, pain, and impairment of vision and motility (Fig. 8–15). The inflammation can be diffuse or located in either the anterior or the posterior portion of the orbit. The inflammation can also be localized to certain areas or tissues within the orbit, such as myositis, dacryoadenitis, and perioptic neuritis. Clinically, affected patients do not appear "toxic" and are not febrile, as are many patients with infectious proptosis. A patient with *myositis* can have involvement of one or more extraocular muscles and present with pain, proptosis, diplopia, lid erythema, swelling, chemosis, and injection over the involved muscle(s). Radiographically, the involved muscle(s) is enlarged, often with involvement of the tendinous insertion, a differential point in favor of myositis and in contrast to Graves' disease.

Acute *dacryoadenitis* presents with pain, erythema, and swelling of the upper lid. Proptosis and globe displacement are minimal. The upper outer lid is tender to palpation, and swelling in this area produces a characteristic S-shaped lid (Fig. 8–16). CT scanning shows an enhancing mass in the lacrimal fossa with edema extending into Tenon's space. The importance of coronal views in the evaluation of lacrimal fossa masses cannot be overemphasized.

The last form of localized orbital inflammation is *perioptic neuritis*. This simulates optic neuritis, but proptosis and pain with retropulsion of the globe are present. The optic nerve is enlarged on CT scan evaluation.

These inflammatory entities share a common feature: an exquisite response to corticosteroids. Most episodes resolve after a short course of prednisone; however, for the cases that advance into a chronic stage, one should

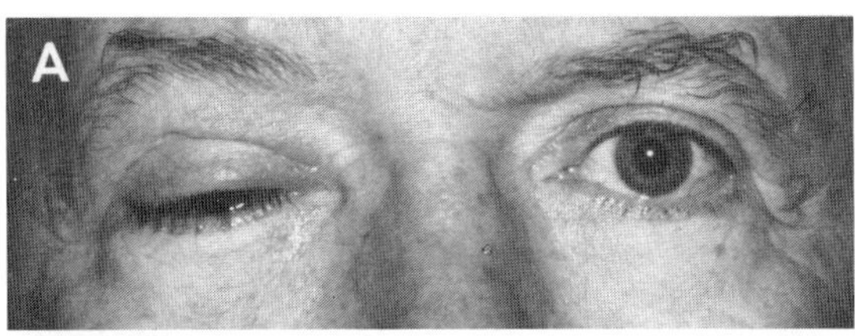

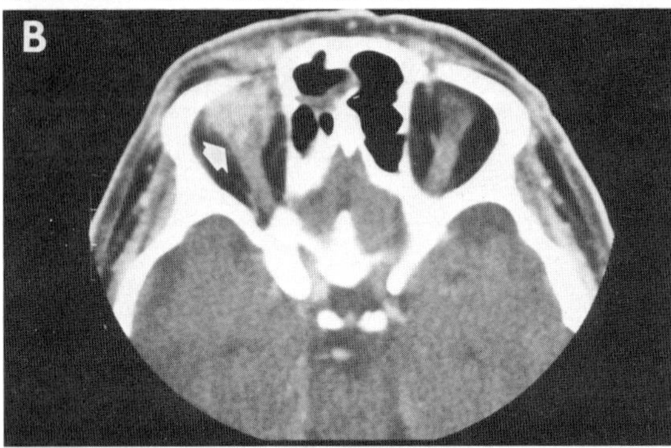

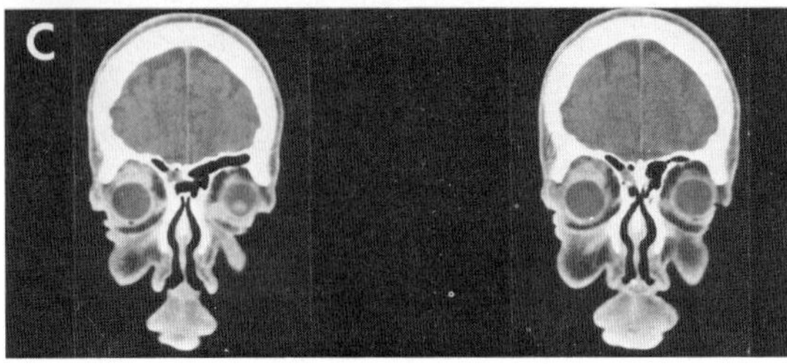

Fig. 8–15. *A*, A 56-year-old man with a 2-week history of progressive pain, ptosis, and impaired ductions of right eye. The globe was injected and chemotic. *B*, Axial CT scan, demonstrating an infiltrative process superiorly in the right orbit (*arrow*). *C*, Coronal CT scans better define the infiltrative process. The orbital inflammation clinically resolved after 36 hours of high-dose oral corticosteroids.

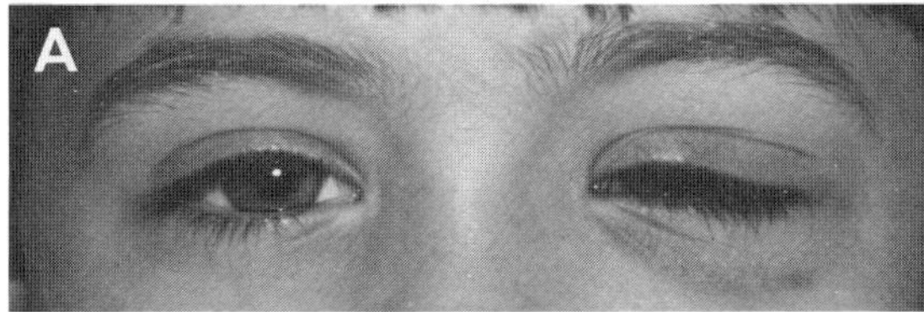

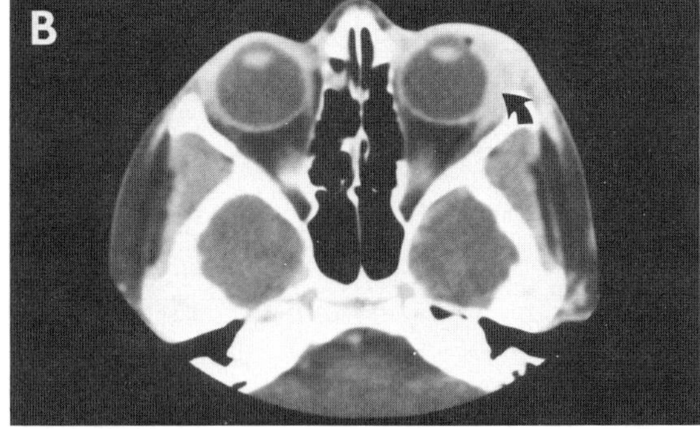

Fig. 8–16. *A*, A 6-year-old girl with left inflammatory dacryoadenitis with an erythematous S-shaped upper eyelid. *B*, Axial CT scan, showing infiltrative process affecting the left lacrimal gland (*arrow*). Note how the inflamed gland conforms to the globe (neoplastic processes, in contrast, often indent the globe).

consider biopsy and possibly radiation therapy, particularly for inflammatory pseudotumors and dacryoadenitis. If the biopsy reveals a vasculitis, cytotoxic therapy such as cyclophosphamide may be required. Radiation therapy is not advised in this setting.

Infectious causes of proptosis include orbital cellulitis or abscess (Fig. 8–17). Patients with *orbital cellulitis* are usually febrile and have a "toxic" appearance, although some patients with an orbital abscess may lack systemic manifestations. The time course of infectious proptosis is usually not as rapid as the inflammations but is progressive in nature. Initial evaluation of cellulitis in pediatric cases should include blood cultures because this age group frequently has bacteremia. Broad-spectrum antibiotics with initial coverage for *Haemophilus influenzae* in children and *Staphylococcus aureus* in adults should be selected. Antibiotic therapy alone may suffice; however, if proptosis increases, if ocular motility decreases, or if there is intervening visual loss, surgical drainage of the orbit and sinus must be considered.

CT scanning will define the orbital involvement and demonstrate concomitant sinus disease. Orbital foreign bodies, an important consideration with an infection, may or may not be imaged. MRI scanning in cases of suspected metallic foreign bodies is not recommended.

"N" is for neoplastic exophthalmos.

Most orbital tumors are associated with proptosis, some more than others. Optic nerve sheath meningiomas take up little room in the orbit and produce minimal proptosis, as do some compressible vascular lesions. Alternatively, orbital tumors with firm tissue consistency, such as neurinomas or optic nerve gliomas, are associated with more pronounced proptosis. Tumors within the muscle cone produce axial proptosis (protrusion directly forward), whereas extraconal tumors displace the eye out and in a direction opposite that of the lesion. One other important clinical feature of orbital neoplasms is their usual lack of associated pain. Adenoid cystic carcinoma of the lacrimal gland is a notable exception to this observation because of perineural invasion with

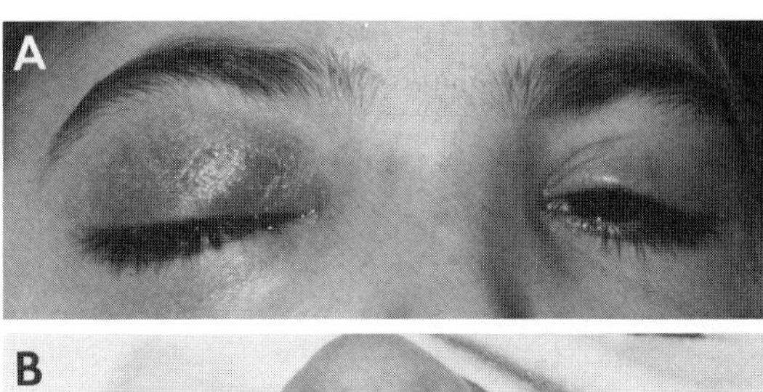
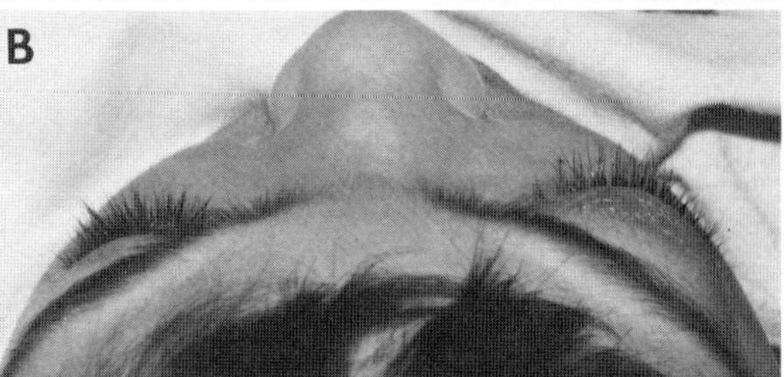
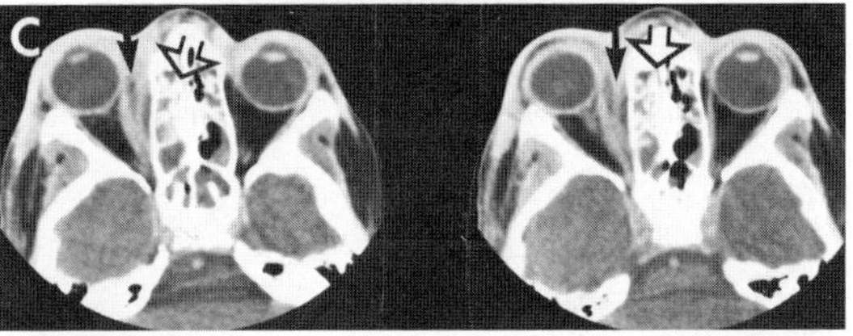
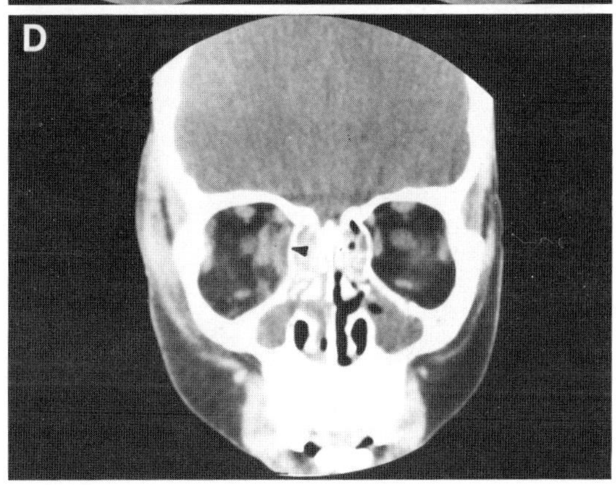

Fig. 8–17. *A,* An 8-year-old boy with a 1-week history of upper respiratory infection noted erythema, ptosis, proptosis, and impaired ocular ductions over 8 hours. *B,* Proptosis, 6 mm, of right globe. *C,* Axial CT scans. Ethmoid sinusitis (*open arrows*) is evident, along with an orbital cellulitis (*closed arrows*). *D,* Coronal CT scan. Sinusitis is apparent in both maxillary and ethmoid sinuses. Note subperiosteal fluid collection on right (*arrowhead*). Entire process resolved with parenteral antibiotics.

characteristic deep-seated orbital pain early in the course.

Selected types of orbital tumors categorized as benign, malignant, and metastatic are described below.

Cavernous hemangioma is the most common benign primary orbital tumor in adults.

The most frequent benign primary orbital tumor is a *cavernous hemangioma* (Fig. 8–18). This encapsulated tumor is found predominantly in females, and the average age at onset of symptoms is 42 years. Because the tumor grows slowly, its presence is tolerated well until the inevitable effects of its mass become apparent. The tumor may be located in the intraconal or extraconal space, and choroidal folds may be seen by ophthalmoscopy. An intraconal tumor indenting the globe directly behind the macula will shorten the anterior-posterior diameter of the globe, producing a hyperopic shift in the refractive error. Treatment of a cavernous hemangioma is excision, which is facilitated in some cases by the use of an ophthalmic cryoprobe to manipulate the tumor. Complete excision is curative.

Capillary hemangiomas, alternatively, characteristically affect the pediatric population and become evident within the first few weeks of life. If the superficial dermis is involved, the typical strawberry hemangioma is apparent; deeper lesions typically have a blue appearance. Crying or a Valsalva maneuver accentuates the lesion. Superficial hemangiomas bear a resemblance to a nevus flammeus, but the latter is a flat lesion and does not blanch on pressure, as does a capillary hemangioma.

Capillary hemangiomas may grow fairly rapidly during the first year of life (Fig. 8–19). Although most capillary hemangiomas regress spontaneously, this change tends to occur later in the first decade. Treatment is indicated if visual function is threatened by amblyopia. Mass effects can induce an astigmatic refractive error or cause the lid to become ptotic and occlude the visual axis. Amblyopia thus may result from either anisometropia or sensory deprivation. Unsightly cosmetic deformities can be psychologically disabling to the patient or the parents, and treatment may be justified.

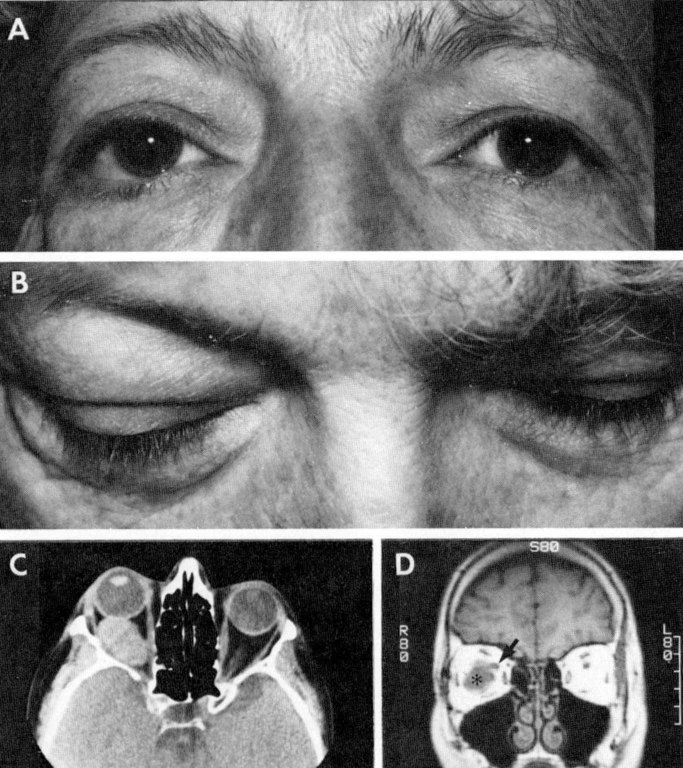

Fig. 8–18. A 60-year-old woman with an orbital cavernous hemangioma. Initial symptom was visual blurring in right eye. *A*, Normal external appearance. *B*, Proptosis, 5 mm, of the right globe is apparent. *C*, Axial CT scan, showing large intraconal tumor. The optic nerve could not be imaged even with coronal views. *D*, Coronal T1-weighted MRI scan. The mass (*asterisk*) is easily seen to be separate from the optic nerve (*arrow*).

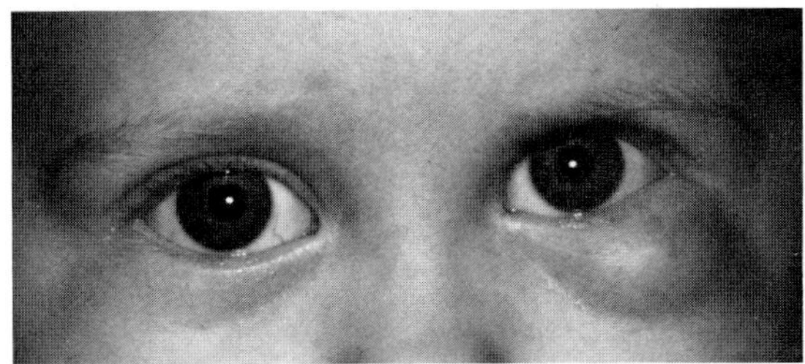

Fig. 8–19. A 15-month-old girl with typical-appearing capillary hemangioma of the left lower eyelid and anterior orbit. This was first noted at 3 months of age. Lesion had purple-blue appearance that intensified with crying. Because the mass did not indent the globe (which might cause amblyopia from astigmatism or anisometropia) and because capillary hemangiomas may involute spontaneously, no treatment was required.

Treatment of eyelid or orbital capillary hemangiomas includes intralesional injection of corticosteroids or systemically administered oral corticosteroids. The precise therapeutic mechanism of action is unknown, although vascular occlusion is hypothesized. Advantages of intralesional injection include delivery of a large dose to the desired area with minimal sys-temic side effects. Adverse ophthalmic complications may include intraocular arterial occlusions from drug emboli, sloughing of the lid, and subcutaneous atrophy. Low-dose radiotherapy (200 to 500 rads) has also been advocated as a means of treatment.

The lacrimal gland is the site of epithelial and lymphoid neoplasms.

The *lacrimal gland* is a modified salivary gland and can give rise to a benign epithelial neoplasm termed a *benign mixed tumor* or *pleomorphic adenoma* (Fig. 8–20). This lesion predominantly affects men, and the mean age at presentation is 39 years. Clinically, symptoms are usually present for at least a year, with proptosis and globe displacement being the cardinal features. A CT scan will show a lacrimal fossa mass, which may indent the globe. In contrast, a lacrimal fossa mass conforming to the shape of the globe is an important feature of inflammatory (Fig. 8–16) or lymphoid infiltration of the lacrimal gland (Fig. 8–21). Pressure thinning of the lateral orbital wall may

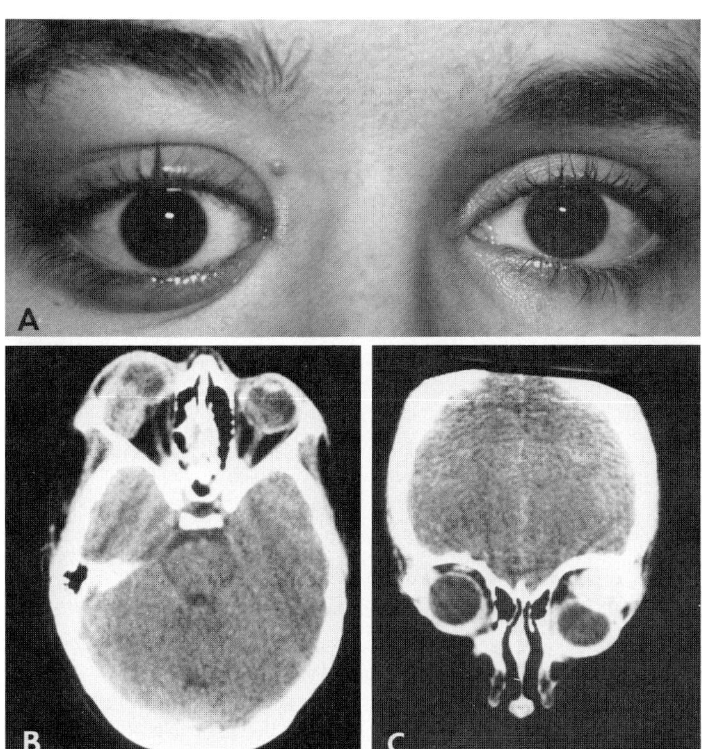

Fig. 8–20. *A*, Benign mixed tumor of the lacrimal gland in a 26-year-old woman with a 1-year history of progressive proptosis and displacement of the right globe. There were 2 mm of proptosis, 2 mm of downward displacement, and 1 mm of inward displacement of the right globe. *B* and *C*, CT scans, axial (*B*) and coronal (*C*) views, showing well-demarcated lacrimal fossa mass indenting the globe. (Courtesy of J.S. Kennerdell, M.D.)

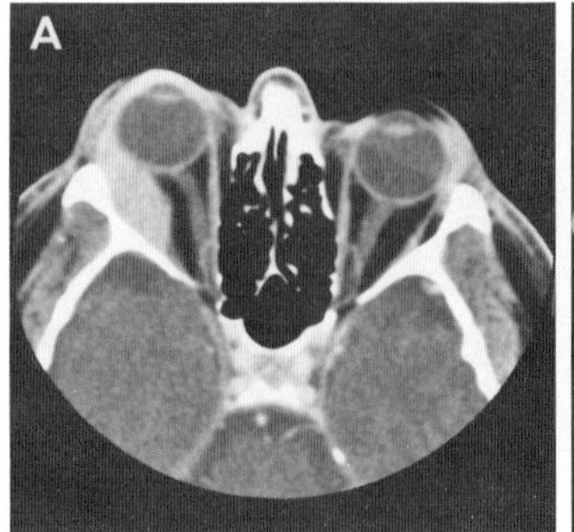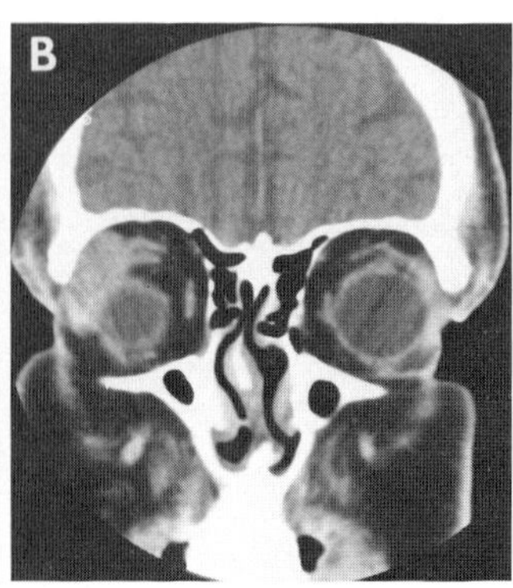

Fig. 8–21. Lymphoma of the right lacrimal gland in a 45-year-old man with a 2-month history of right upper lid ptosis. Mass conforms to shape of globe. CT scans, axial (*A*) and coronal (*B*), show a well-demarcated mass molding to the shape of globe. Adjacent bone was normal. A systemic evaluation showed that the lymphoma was confined to the orbit. The lacrimal gland was treated with radiation.

be seen on plain skull radiographs or computed tomograms. The tumor is best removed by a lateral orbitotomy, delivering the tumor with its "capsule" intact. The "capsule" is actually a condensation of surrounding tissue incorporated by the enlarging tumor. Incomplete removal or rupture of the "capsule" will lead to a recurrence in one-third of cases. Unfortunately, recurrences may behave more aggressively than the primary lesion.

Optic nerve gliomas are frequently seen in association with neurofibromatosis.

Juvenile pilocytic astrocytomas, more commonly referred to as *optic nerve gliomas,* may affect any or all portions of the anterior visual pathway. Those involving the system distal to the chiasm are appropriately termed "optic nerve glioma." This lesion should be suspected in any child with unexplained visual loss and a pale optic disc (Fig. 8–22). The peak incidence of optic nerve glioma is between 2 and 6 years of age, and 90% of the lesions will become apparent by the end of the second decade. Most of the tumors are unilateral; when bilateral, neurofibromatosis is more likely. Up to 15% of patients with neurofibromatosis may have a glioma involving the anterior visual pathways. Some of these may be asymptomatic. However, if a glioma is present there is a 25% chance that the patient has neurofibromatosis. The di-

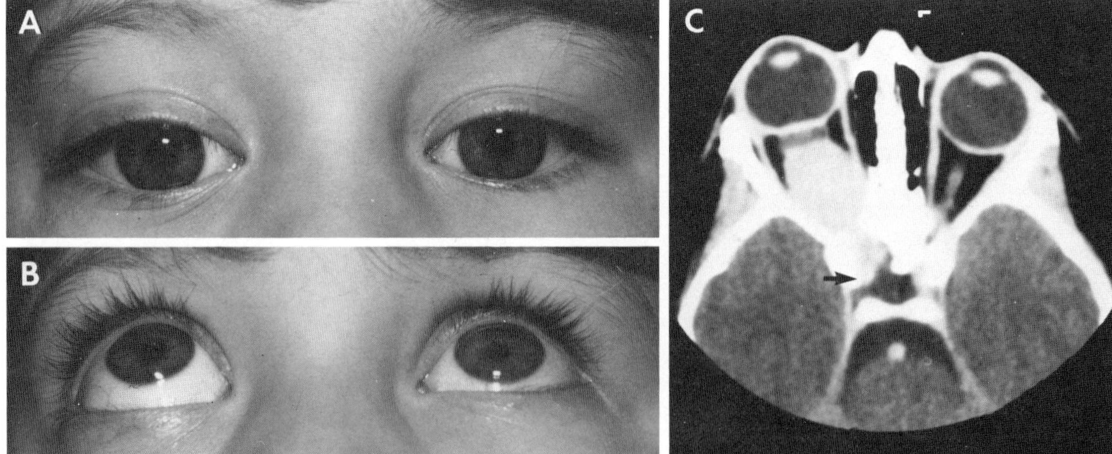

Fig. 8–22. Optic nerve glioma in a 3-year-old girl. *A*, Proptosis of the right eye at presentation. *B*, Proptosis was more evident when viewed from below. Visual acuity in the right eye was 20/200 and a prominent afferent pupillary defect was present. The optic disc was edematous. *C*, Axial CT scan, demonstrating optic nerve glioma with typical cystic appearance of the distal end of optic nerve. The bone windows (not shown) revealed an enlarged optic canal. Intracranial extension is apparent (*arrow*). The chiasm was also involved. (Courtesy of J.S. Kennerdell, M.D.)

agnosis can be fairly certain with the neuroradiologic techniques available today, although atypical cases require biopsy for definitive diagnosis. Management is controversial; however, if vision is lost and the glioma is confined to the orbit and spares the chiasm, there is uniform agreement that the glioma should be excised from the chiasm to the globe. Other therapeutic options include radiation, and recently there has been interest in chemotherapy.

When a child has evidence of an optic nerve tumor, consideration should also be given to the possibility of an optic nerve meningioma.

Meningiomas in childhood are rare but can be clinically aggressive, in contradistinction to the more common optic nerve sheath meningioma of adulthood.

Optic nerve sheath meningiomas are more commonly diagnosed in women than in men (Fig. 8–23). Subjective visual complaints (visual loss or transient visual obscurations) are most frequent, although vision may be relatively well preserved despite evidence of gross tumor radiographically. The ophthalmoscopic appearance of a chronically swollen optic disc or optic atrophy is invariably present. The appearance

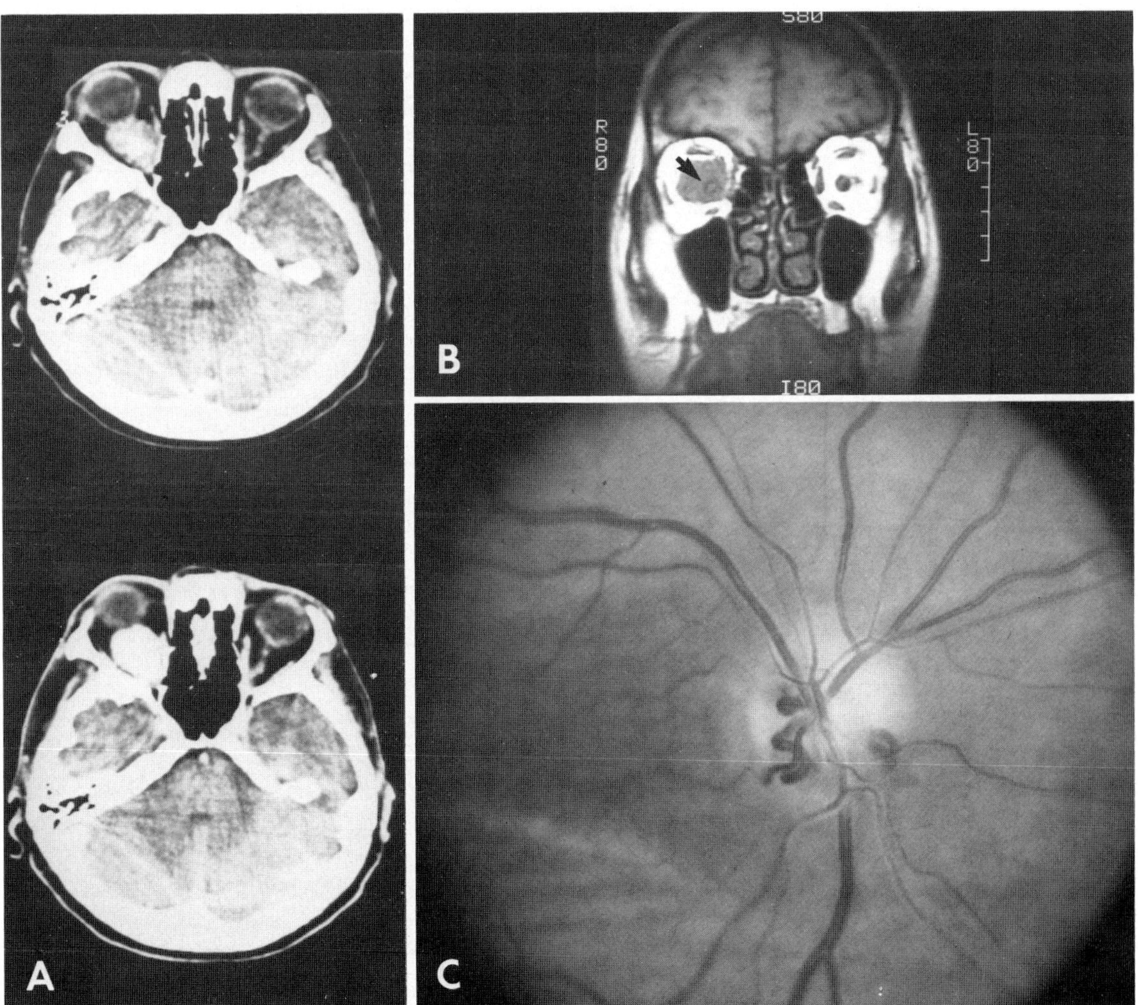

Fig. 8–23. Optic nerve sheath meningioma in a 65-year-old woman. *A,* Axial CT scans (without contrast on top scan and contrast-enhanced on bottom scan), showing a contrast-enhancing calcium-containing mass in or near the optic nerve. *B,* MRI scan, coronal T1-weighted view, clearly demonstrates an optic nerve sheath mass surrounding the optic nerve (*arrow*). *C,* Fundus photograph, demonstrating a pale optic nerve with optociliary shunt vessels.

of optociliary shunt vessels on the disc is suggestive of an optic nerve sheath meningioma, although this is nonspecific and can also be seen with other conditions, most notably a sphenoid wing meningioma. Contrast-enhanced thin-section CT is probably the best radiographic technique currently available. Calcium within the lesion is a helpful differential diagnostic feature in favor of meningioma. MRI was initially relatively insensitive to the presence of a meningioma, although contrast enhancement with gadolinium and chemical shift fat suppression appears to obviate this problem.

As with optic nerve gliomas, treatment is controversial and should be individualized. If vision is lost and the meningioma is confined to the orbit, surgical excision is an option. Although meningiomas are usually radioresistant, there are some reports of favorable responses to treatment.

Adenoid cystic carcinoma is the most aggressive malignant orbital tumor.

The lacrimal gland may give rise to several malignant tumors, of which the most aggressive is *adenoid cystic carcinoma*. Symptoms are generally present for a shorter period than with the benign mixed tumor, but pain may be present early in the course because of perineural invasion and bone destruction. There is no consensus concerning the best management; exenteration, en bloc excision, and radiation are options.

The lacrimal gland is the site of lymphoid infiltration, and CT often demonstrates molding of the lacrimal gland to the globe (Fig. 8–21). *Lymphomas* can also infiltrate any structure within the orbit, including orbital fat, extraocular muscles, and even the optic nerve. Systemic evaluation for lymphoma is indicated. Lymphoma isolated to the orbit usually responds to radiation in doses of 2,500 to 3,000 rads.

Rhabdomyosarcoma is the most common primary orbital malignancy in children.

Rhabdomyosarcoma is the most frequent primary orbital malignancy of childhood and must be suspected in any child with acute proptosis (Fig. 8–24). The average age at presentation is 7 years, and boys are affected slightly more often than girls. If this diagnosis is suspected, a biopsy should be performed without delay. Biopsy specimens may reveal a very poorly differentiated tumor that requires immunocytochemical or electron microscopic evaluation for final diagnosis. Combination radiotherapy and chemotherapy has led to an 80% survival rate, although the prognosis is worse if there is extension into the surrounding sinuses.

Metastatic orbital disease is usually seen in patients in their sixth or seventh decade of life.

Orbital involvement can occur long after a primary tumor has been treated, especially

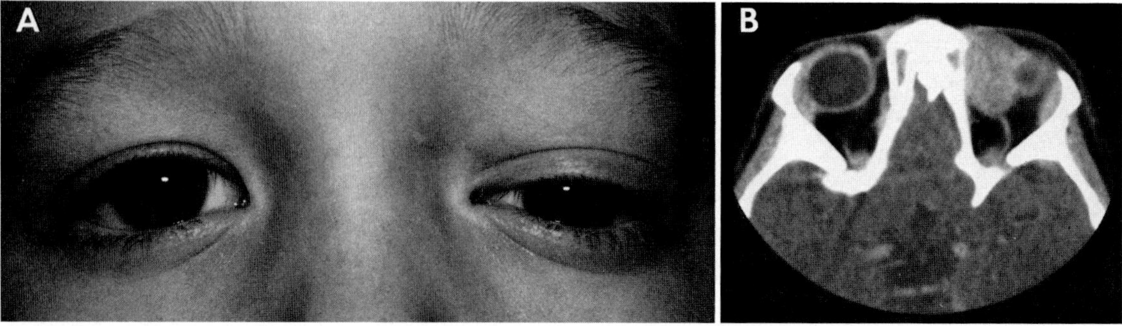

Fig. 8–24.   A 4-year-old boy with rhabdomyosarcoma of the orbit. *A*, Fullness in the superonasal left orbit, ptosis of the left upper eyelid, and proptosis and inferior displacement of the left eye. The evolution of the clinical course was rapid, characteristic of this tumor. *B*, Axial CT scan, showing rhabdomyosarcoma in the left superior orbit.

with breast or prostate carcinomas. Alternatively, metastatic renal or lung carcinomas may present before the primary tumor has been detected. Treatment is generally nonsurgical with the exception of a biopsy.

Orbital involvement as an extension from an adjacent site constitutes a secondary orbital tumor.

The orbit is surrounded on three sides by paranasal sinuses. Of the sinuses, the maxillary and ethmoid sinuses are most likely to give rise to a secondary orbital tumor. *Squamous cell carcinoma* is the most frequent type. The globe is displaced away from the offending area. These tumors can be difficult to treat and, despite radical treatment, often lead to death.

Various tumors of the lids may spread posteriorly, and when these lesions became fixed to the underlying rim or surface of the bony orbit one may infer orbital involvement. *Basal cell*, *squamous cell*, and *sebaceous gland carcinomas* are the most likely offenders. In addition, squamous cell carcinomas and especially sebaceous cell carcinomas carry the added threat of metastatic disease.

The last type of tumor to be considered in this category is the secondary orbital *meningioma*. The neoplasm most frequently arises from the sphenoid wing, and its presence is suggested by the appearance of unilateral "myxedematous" lids with proptosis, especially in a middle-aged woman. The "en plaque" variant may be associated with hyperostosis of the posterior lateral wall of the orbit and the orbital roof (Fig. 8–25). Vision may be reduced if the optic foramen is compromised. Visual loss, an atrophic optic disc, and optociliary shunt vessels define the Spencer-Hoyt triad in spheno-

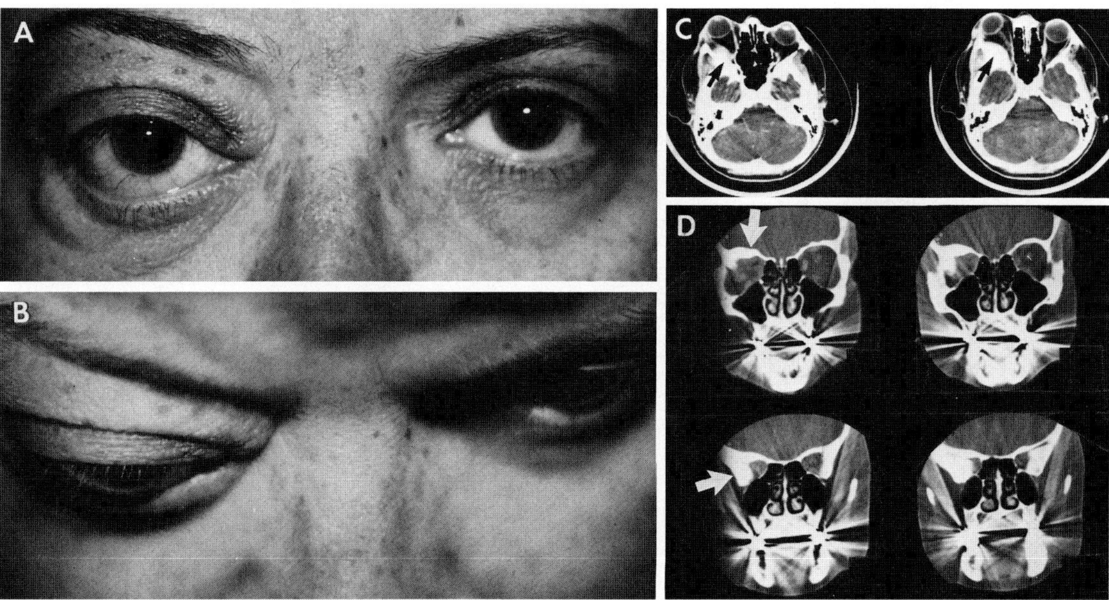

Fig. 8–25. Sphenoid wing meningioma with secondary orbital invasion in a 38-year-old woman. She initially presented with visual loss in the right eye (20/100 with an afferent pupillary defect, acquired dyschromatopsia, a faintly pale optic disc, and choroidal folds) and proptosis (10 mm of proptosis and 3 mm of downward displacement of the globe). *A*, Proptosis and downward displacement of right globe. *B*, More apparent proptosis. The radiologic differential diagnosis included fibrous dysplasia (unlikely because of her age) and metastatic prostate carcinoma (impossible because of her gender). She was treated with a frontotemporal craniotomy. Most of the hyperostotic bone was removed. The lacrimal gland was infiltrated with tumor and removed. The lateral rectus muscle was biopsied and found to be infiltrated. The optic canal was unroofed. Postoperatively, the vision returned to 20/20 and there was a proptosis reduction of 5 mm. *C*, Axial CT scans. Hyperostosis of the right sphenoid wing (*arrows*) with optic nerve compression. The right lateral rectus muscle is enlarged. *D*, Coronal CT scans. Note the thickened posterior lateral orbital wall and roof (*arrows*).

orbital meningiomas. This constellation of findings may also be seen with optic nerve sheath meningiomas.

Orbital fractures are most likely to involve the floor, medial wall, and roof.

The lateral wall of the orbit is the strongest and is rarely subject to the types of fractures that may affect the other three walls. Fractures affecting the floor are commonly known as *"blowout" fractures*. They are caused by objects larger than the globe striking the anterior orbit and causing a fracture of the orbital floor (direct ocular trauma by smaller objects tends to rupture the globe). The fracture can be generated either by hydraulic forces transmitted through the globe, which blow out or fracture the floor into the maxillary sinus, or by a force directed primarily to the inferior rim, which

causes the floor to buckle and fracture (Fig. 8–26).

The importance of a thorough ocular examination cannot be overemphasized. Approximately 10% of patients with blowout fractures have an associated injury to the eye. As part of this evaluation, baseline Hertel or Krahn exophthalmometry measurements along with motility and Maddox rod measurements should be noted. Follow-up examinations during the following 10 to 14 days should entail comparative measurements. If there is persistent diplopia in primary gaze or reading position or if significant enophthalmos is developing, a more detailed radiologic evaluation is recommended. CT with coronal views (and sagittal if possible) may define the fracture and even show the entrapment to better advantage (Fig. 8–27 *A*).

If there is diplopia, the globe is most often restricted in upgaze (Fig. 8–27 *B*). However, restriction in downgaze is possible, particularly with more posteriorly situated fractures. The inferior oblique/inferior rectus complex may be entrapped in the fracture or the orbital fat alone may be entrapped. Because of the various connective tissue septae within the orbital soft tissues, the muscle itself does not need to be incarcerated in order to produce clinical evidence

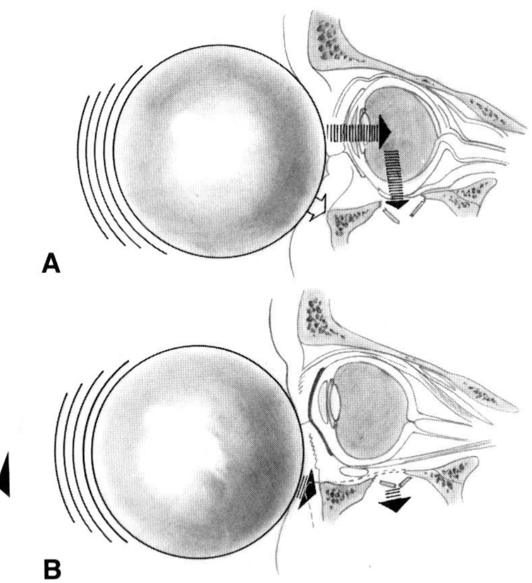

Fig. 8–26. The two popular theories of orbital floor (blowout) fractures. *A*, The hydraulic theory presumes that pressure delivered to the anterior orbit is transmitted equally throughout the orbit. The transmitted pressure blows out the floor of the orbit. It is intuitively apparent from this illustration how the eye may be "deformed" from this type of blunt trauma. This may account for an associated hyphema, angle recession, retinal dialysis, or choroidal rupture, just to name a few of the possible injuries. *B*, The buckling-floor theory presumes delivery of the major force to the inferior orbital rim and floor, which causes it to buckle and subsequently fracture.

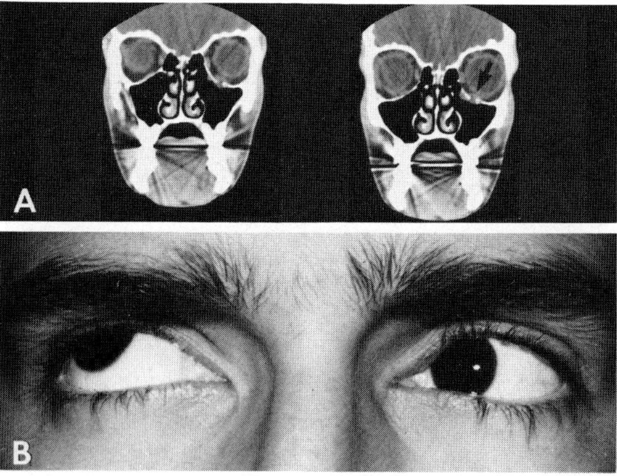

Fig. 8–27. *A*, Coronal CT scans demonstrating fracture of left orbital floor with entrapment of inferior rectus muscle *(arrow)*. *B*, Clinical effects of entrapped orbital tissue are apparent in upgaze. The left orbital floor was surgically explored and the entrapped tissues were freed.

of entrapment. Simply reducing the prolapsed fat from the fracture may be curative in this situation. Alternatively, a silicone (Silastic) plate or a bone graft can be placed across the fracture. Diplopia may also arise from contusional injury to the inferior rectus/inferior oblique muscles or their supplying nerves. A hematoma or edema in the muscle may also account for a similar motility disturbance. These disturbances will generally improve during a 2-week observation period. The use of corticosteroids or prophylactic antibiotics during this period is optional.

Because the medial orbital wall is paper-thin (hence the term "lamina papyracea"), it is the wall most prone to fracture. Fortunately, there are few instances in which this is clinically significant. It is occasionally necessary to reduce this fracture and remove pieces of bone that have impaled the medial rectus muscle. The use of a Silastic or collagen plate is optional. One must remember that the medial wall of the orbit travels straight back to the optic nerve and foramen, so it is possible to injure the optic nerve during insertion of such an implant or by posterior migration after insertion. Implants placed along the orbital floor may also injure the optic nerve.

The least frequent fracture involves the orbital roof. This type of fracture may result from direct trauma to the brow or forehead, such as from a diving injury (striking the top of the head on the bottom of a swimming pool). Generally, a mechanical ptosis is present and there may be difficulty with upgaze or downgaze because bone fragments have impaled the superior rectus/levator complex or there is mechanical restriction to upgaze.

Roof fractures are generally approached by a neurosurgeon because of potential involvement of the dura, brain, and frontal sinus. In addition to the usual thorough ophthalmic examination, the evaluation also needs to establish whether cerebrospinal fluid rhinorrhea is present. CT with axial and coronal views should be performed. The films should be studied carefully, with special attention given to ascertain the presence of a fracture into the frontal sinus, a fracture through the inner table of the skull, or pneumocephalus. In selected circumstances, one may consider reducing the fracture from the orbital side.

9

OPTICS, REFRACTION, AND CONTACT LENSES

Jay C. Erie

Refractive error is the most common cause of poor vision, and neutralization of refractive error restores useful visual function to more patients than does any other form of ophthalmic therapy. Because of advances in pseudophakia (intraocular lenses), contact lenses, and new surgical modifications of myopia and astigmatism, visual optics is becoming increasingly important in the clinical practice of ophthalmology.

OPTICS

The study of optics can be divided into two areas: physical optics and geometric optics.

Physical optics is the study of the physics of light. It is concerned with the basic nature of light, its properties, and its behavior. In physical optics, the theories of light as a particle (photon) and light as a form of wave motion are united to explain optical phenomena.

Geometric optics, however, is much more useful to the ophthalmologist in understanding refractive error and its correction. With geometric optics, optical problems can be solved on the basis that light is represented by *rays* that travel in straight lines, and both the particle and the wave-like characteristics of light are not considered.

All naturally occurring light sources are divergent; lenses can create convergence.

Vergence represents the direction of a ray of light perpendicular to the wave front. In geometric optics it is represented by drawing a straight line (Fig. 9–1). By convention, *divergence* is represented by minus numbers. In nature, light always diverges and has negative (−) vergence. We can distinguish various degrees of vergence. As the light wave front moves farther from its source, it becomes less curved and the rays become less divergent. At an infinite distance, the rays become parallel and have zero vergence. Conversely, *convergence* is represented by plus numbers and has positive (+) vergence (Fig. 9–2). It should be apparent that for rays to converge they must be acted on by an optical system that changes their vergence.

The unit of convergence and divergence is the diopter.

The unit of measurement of vergence is the *diopter.* At a distance of d meters from a point light source, there is a vergence of D diopters (D = 1/d). Therefore, the greater the distance from a point light source, the smaller the vergence. The concept of vergence is useful because the effect of lenses can be described in terms of their action on vergence of light. The

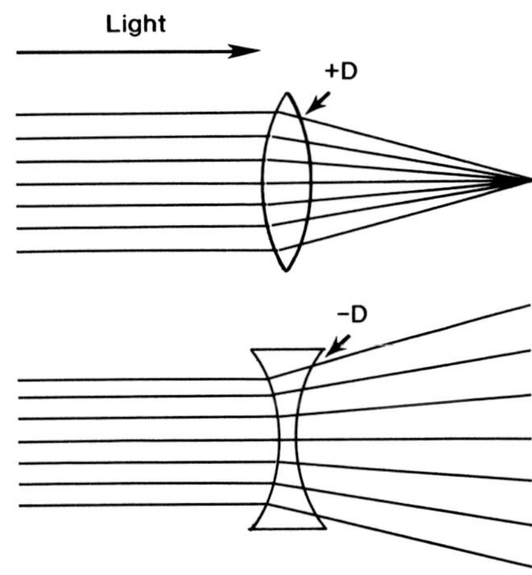

Fig. 9–3. Plus and minus lenses. A plus lens (convex) adds vergence by converging light rays; it has plus power (+D). A minus lens (concave) subtracts vergence by diverging light rays; it has minus power (−D).

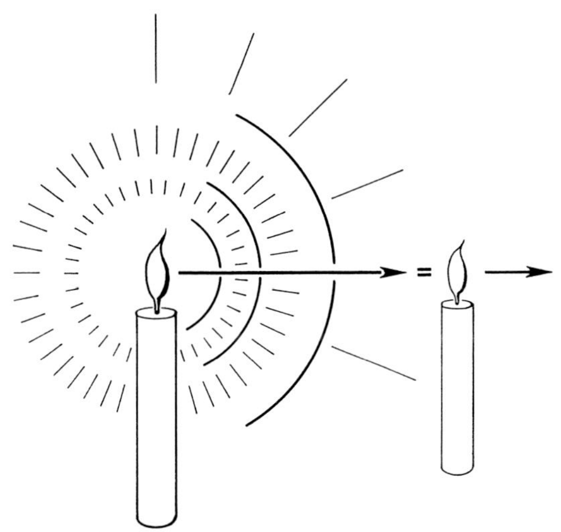

Fig. 9–1. A straight line is used to represent a ray that is perpendicular to the wave front of light.

amount of increase or decrease in vergence that a lens causes is called its *power* (expressed in diopters, D). If the lens subtracts vergence (divergence), the lens has minus power; if it adds vergence (convergence), the lens has plus power (Fig. 9–3).

From the definition of the power of the lens, we derive the fundamental *vergence formula*:

$$U + P = V$$

U represents the vergence of light entering the lens, P is the amount of vergence added or subtracted to the light by the lens (power of the lens), and V is the vergence of light leaving the lens. The location of images along the optical axis can be found by applying the vergence formula (Fig. 9–4). All units are in diopters, and all distance calculations are in meters.

$$U = 1/u \text{ (u in meters)}$$
$$V = 1/v \text{ (v in meters)}$$

Images may be real or virtual.

A *real image* is formed by light rays that are converging, that is, positive (+) vergence. A real image can be focused on a screen, although it need not be (such as the aerial image of an indirect ophthalmoscope). Although a real image is real, it may not always be clearly focused, as in ametropia.

A *virtual image* is formed by diverging rays from a point at which they appear to arise, yet the light does not physically emanate from the image point. A virtual image can be seen in a plane mirror but cannot be focused on a screen. For a virtual image to be seen, it must be acted on by an optical system. It is our eye's optical system that converts a virtual object into a real retinal image.

In summary, rays of light leave an object point in object space, traverse a lens that changes its vergence, and enter image space.

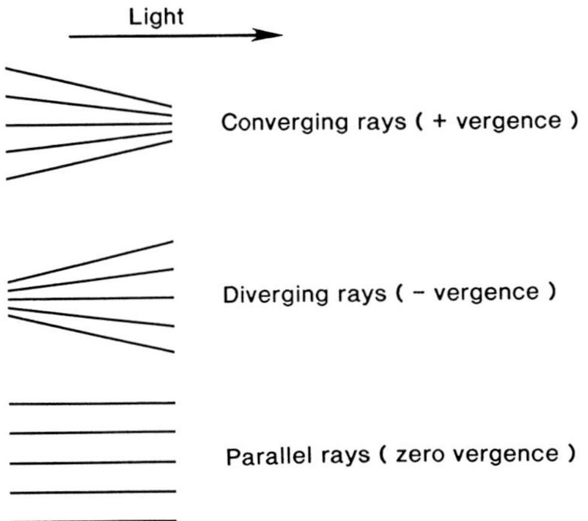

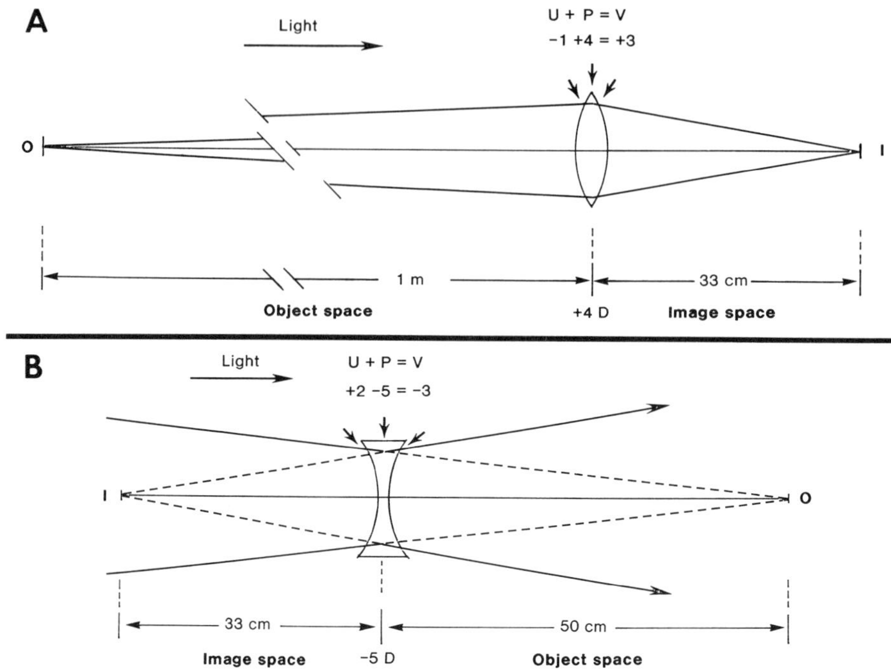

Fig. 9–4. The vergence formula (U + P = V) describes the position of images along the optical axis. *A,* A real image is formed 33 cm to the right of the lens in the image space. *B,* A virtual image is formed 33 cm to the left of the lens in the image space.

These rays may converge to a real image or diverge from an apparent or virtual image (Fig. 9–4). Optical images, real or virtual, belong to image space; optical objects, real or virtual, belong to object space.

Snell's law governs the refraction of light at any surface.

Light travels through a vacuum at a fixed velocity but travels through any other medium at a slower speed. The ratio of the speed of light in a vacuum to the speed of light in a given medium establishes the *refractive index* (n) of that medium:

$$n = \frac{\text{velocity of light in a vacuum}}{\text{velocity of light in a specific medium}}$$

The refractive index (n) is also a function of wavelength because different wavelengths of light travel at different speeds in the same media. Some typical refractive indices are shown in Table 9–1 for sodium light (wavelength, 589 nm).

When a ray strikes a new material at some angle to the normal (that is, not perpendicularly), it will bend – or be refracted – according to *Snell's law* (Fig. 9–5). Snell's law governs the refraction of light at any surface and is intimately related to the index of refraction. Accordingly, a plastic lens (n = 1.49) refracts or bends light less effectively than does a glass lens (n = 1.52) because it has a lower index of

TABLE 9–1 **Refractive Indices***

Media	Refractive index, n
Vacuum	1.00
Air	1.00
Aqueous humor	1.33
Cornea	1.38
Lens of eye	1.42
Plastic	1.49
Crown glass	1.52

* By definition, the refractive index is 1.00 in a vacuum and by convention is 1.00 for air. The index of any other medium is always greater than 1.

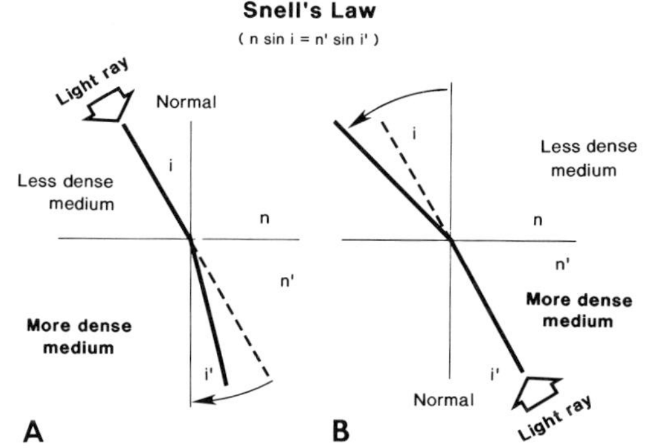

Fig. 9–5. *A,* Light traveling from a less dense medium to a more dense medium is bent toward the normal. *B,* Light traveling from a more dense medium to a less dense medium is bent away from the normal.

goniolenses. A light ray traveling from a more dense medium to a less dense medium is bent away from the normal. As the angle of incidence (i) increases, at some point the subsequent angle of refraction becomes 90° (Fig. 9–6). At this position, the angle of incidence is called the *critical angle.* If it is increased further, the light ray will not exit the medium but instead will be reflected internally. The critical angle of the cornea is 46.5°. As a result, no ray incident on the cornea at an angle of more than 46.5° can escape the anterior chamber. For this reason, a goniolens is necessary to modify the cornea-air interface to allow one to visualize the anterior chamber angle (Fig. 9–7).

refraction. As a result, a plastic lens must be thicker than a glass lens to produce the same amount of refraction.

Snell's law is important for understanding

The primary optical function of prisms is to deviate light rays.

A prism is a three-sided object made of glass or plastic whose index of refraction is greater

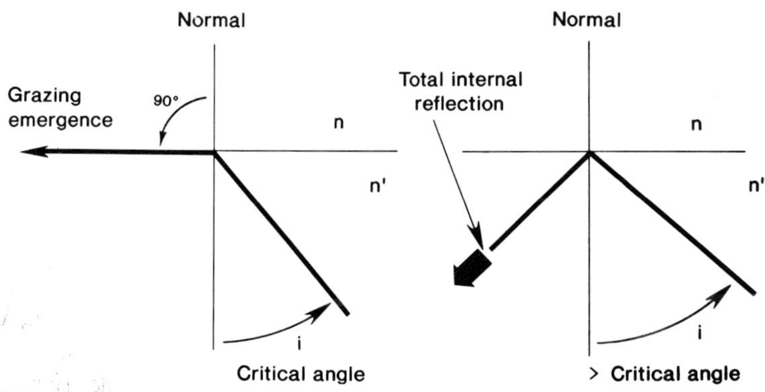

Fig. 9–6. Critical angle – total internal reflection. The index of refraction, n′, is greater than n; therefore, the incident rays at the interface between the two media are refracted away from the normal. When the critical angle is reached (which for the cornea is 46.5°), no light rays escape; all are internally reflected.

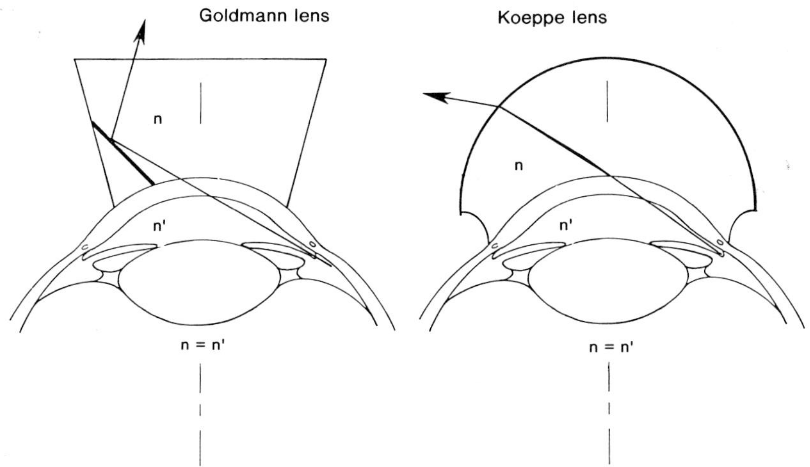

Fig. 9–7. The Goldmann and Koeppe lenses use two different strategies to overcome total internal reflection.

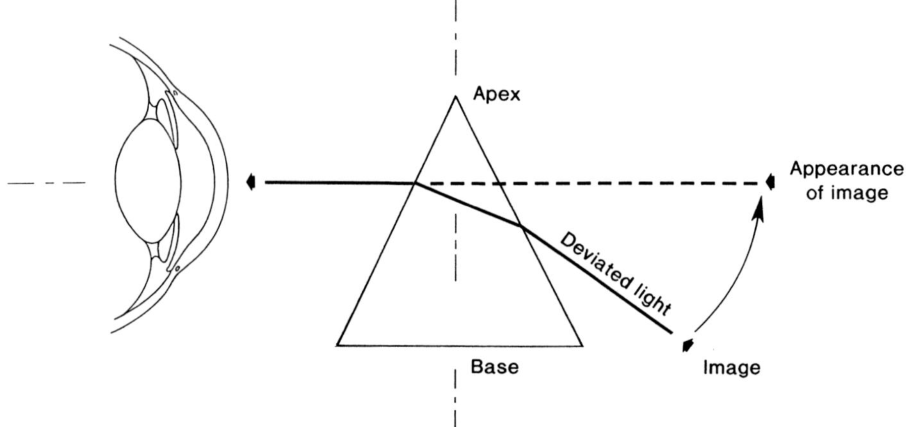

Fig. 9–8.   Displacement of images by prisms. Light is deviated toward the base of the prism, causing the image to appear to be displaced toward the apex.

than that of the surrounding medium. Incident light rays that pass through a prism are deviated toward the base of that prism. However, if one looks through a prism at an object, the image one sees is a virtual image that appears to be displaced toward the apex of the prism (Fig. 9–8).

Minimal prism deviation occurs when light rays travel symmetrically through the prism so that the angle of incidence is equal to the angle of emergence. If the prism is tilted, the deviation of the light rays will increase. Therefore, the amount of deviation is not constant but instead is dependent on the angle of incidence of light. Prisms are calibrated according to defined angles of incidence (Fig. 9–9). For practical purposes, if a prism is not held in its proper position in front of the patient's eye, the measurement will be inaccurate.

The power of a prism is defined in diopters and in terms of how much the light is deviated. One *prism diopter* (Δ) is the strength of a prism that will produce linear apparent displacement of 1 cm of an object situated 1 m away. For example, if a prism deviates light 10 cm at a distance of 1 m, it has prismatic power of 10 prism diopters (10Δ). The power of a prism is proportional to the angle (degrees) of the apex of the prism. The greater the angle, the greater the prismatic power. The relationship of prism diopter to degrees is approximately 2Δ to $1°$. This relationship can be considered nearly linear up to $45°$. Beyond $45°$, the number of prism diopters per degree increases exponentially; $90°$ is equal to an infinite number of prism diopters.

The overall size or thickness of a prism plays no role in its power, only the angular relationships of its surfaces. Therefore, a tiny wedge of prism in the apex is just as effective as are the thicker parts for deviating light. The clinical application of this principle is the *Fresnel prism*, which consists of a flat plastic surface onto which have been ground many small contiguous prisms (Fig. 9–10). It is available as an adhesive prism and is preferable to conventional prisms for temporary use because of the greater reduction in weight and bulk. Some optical clarity, however, is lost because of the ridges.

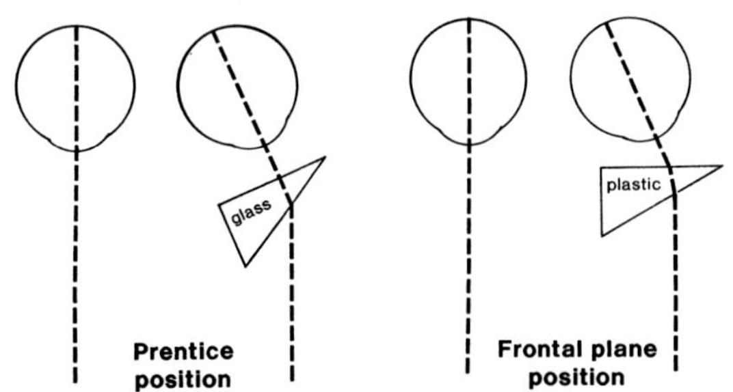

Fig. 9–9.   Glass prisms are calibrated for use in the *Prentice position* (flat surface parallel to the eye). Plastic prisms are calibrated for use in the *frontal plane position* (flat surface parallel to the patient's face).

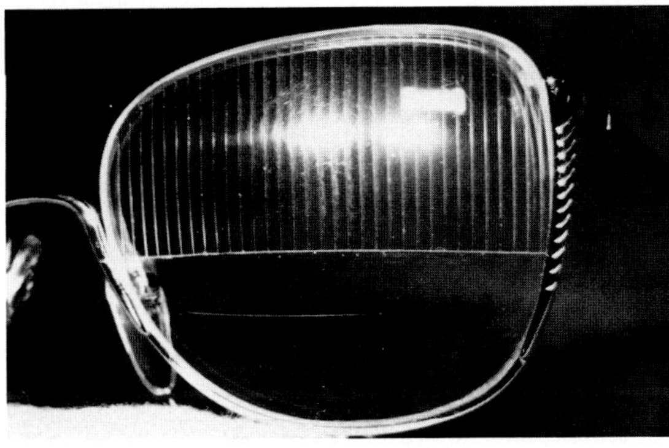

Fig. 9–10.   Fresnel prism on glasses.

A simple convex or concave lens induces a prismatic effect that can be quantitated by Prentice's rule.

Any transparent medium that refracts or alters the vergence of light is a lens. As noted previously (and as shown in Fig. 9–3), there are two types of lenses, convex and concave. A convex lens has plus (+) power because it adds convergence to incident light rays. A concave lens has minus (−) power because it diverges light.

A plus (convex) lens may be visualized as a stack of prisms with their bases facing the middle of the lens (Fig. 9–11 *A*). Light rays striking each prism are bent toward the base of the

prism, thus resulting in convergence. Similarly, a minus (concave) lens can be visualized as a stack of prisms with their bases directed away from the middle of the lens (Fig. 9–11 *B*). Because light rays are bent toward the base of a prism, a concave lens results in divergence. One should note that light traveling through the center of a lens will not be deviated. There is a point in the middle of all thin lenses called the *nodal point*, through which a ray of light can pass in a straight line.

It must be emphasized that the simple representation of a lens as a stack of prisms is useful, but one important error occurs in this approximation: the prismatic power of a lens increases as we move away from the optical center, whereas with a prism the deviation does not change.

Thus, not surprisingly, when one looks through anything but the center of the lens, the lens imparts a prismatic effect. The computation of this prismatic effect follows *Prentice's rule* (Fig. 9–12). This rule states that one finds the prismatic effect of a lens by multiplying the power of the lens (D) by the distance (in centimeters, not meters) from the central axis of the lens.

Clinically, Prentice's rule is of great importance in the use of bifocal segments. As the patient looks below the center of the lens to see through the bifocal segment, a prismatic effect is created that causes "image displacement." A "flat top" bifocal segment, in which the visual

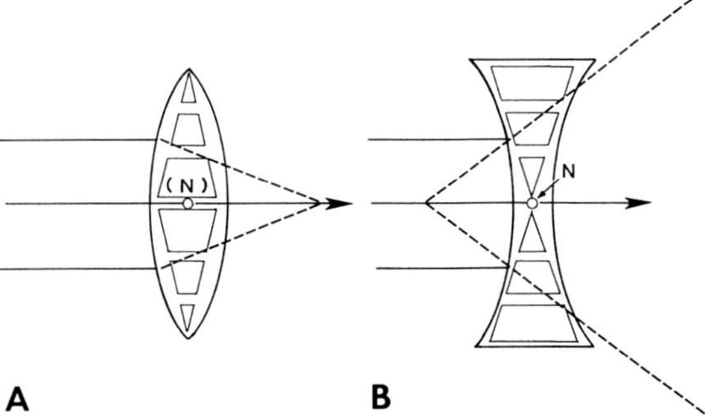

Fig. 9–11.   Simple lenses can be thought of as stacks of prisms. This concept helps one to understand the prismatic effect of lenses. The only rays that pass through the lens undisturbed are those that traverse the nodal point (N). *A*, A convex lens may be visualized as a stack of prisms with their bases facing the middle of the lens. *B*, A concave lens may be visualized as a stack of prisms with their bases directed away from the middle of the lens.

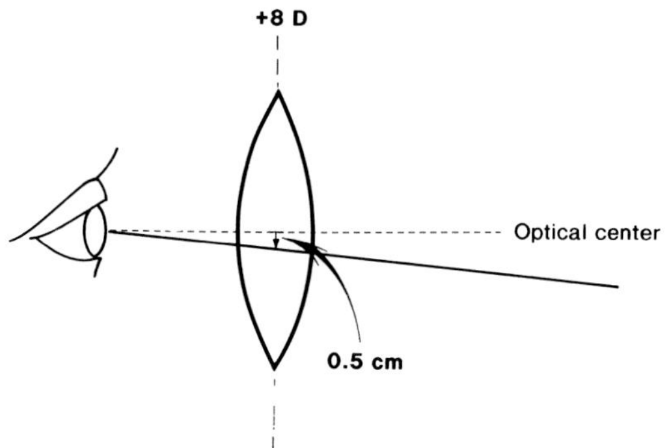

Fig. 9–12.   Prentice's rule: diopters × distance off axis (cm) = prism diopters; in this case, 8 D × 0.5 cm = 4Δ. The induced prismatic effect is base up because this is a convex lens, which can be thought of as a stack of prisms with the bases toward the center of the lens.

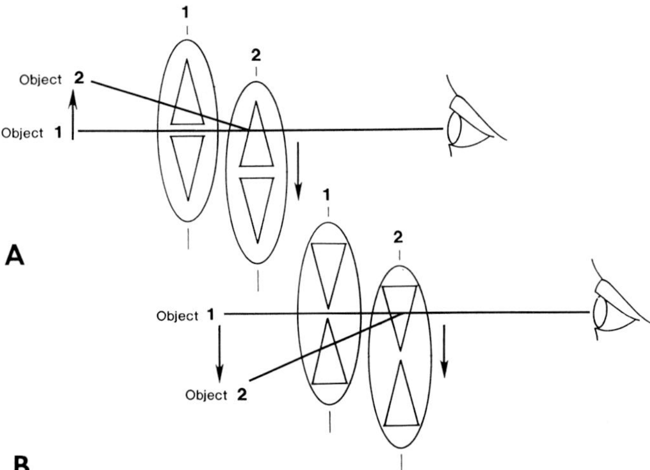

Fig. 9–13. The behavior of plus and minus lenses in producing apparent motion of objects, as in hand neutralization. *A*, The "against" motion of a plus lens. *B*, The "with" motion of a minus lens. The lenses are visualized as being composed of two prisms, base to base (*A*) and apex to apex (*B*).

axis is at the top of the bifocal component, helps reduce image displacement.

When a spherical lens is held in front of the eye and moved up and down, a virtual image seen through the lens appears to move. A plus lens will create "against" movement (the virtual image will move in the opposite direction of the lens), and a minus lens will create "with" movement. This movement, the result of prismatic effect (Fig. 9–13), is the basis of lens neutralization. The amount of movement is proportional to the power of the lens.

The focal point of a lens can be considered a measure of lens power.

When an object is in such a position on the lens axis that the rays from that object emerging from the lens are parallel (image vergence is zero), that position is called the *primary focal point* (F[1]) (Fig. 9–14). The plane containing F[1] and paralleling the lens plane is the *primary focal plane*. The distance in meters between F[1] and the lens that yields an image vergence of zero is the *focal length* (f). The focal length (f) of a

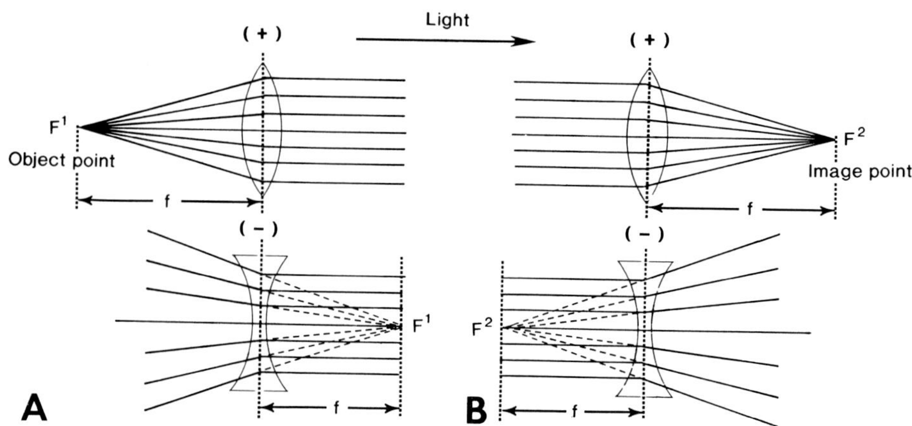

Fig. 9–14. Primary and secondary focal points. *A*, The primary focal point (F[1]) is the *object* point for which the image is at infinity. F[1] is always to the left of a (+) lens and to the right of a (−) lens. *B*, The secondary focal point (F[2]) is the *image* point for which the object is at infinity. F[2] is always to the right of a (+) lens and to the left of a (−) lens. f is the focal length of each lens.

lens can be considered a measure of lens power. The reciprocal of the focal length measured in meters equals the power of the lens in diopters: $D = 1/f$. For example, a $+5.00$ D lens has a focal length of 1/5 m, or 20 cm. The *secondary focal point* (F^2) is the image point produced when parallel light strikes the lens from an object point located at infinity. The primary and secondary focal points are equidistant from the center of the lens.

In a plus lens system, F^1 is always to the left of the lens and F^2 is to the right of the lens. In a minus lens system, F^1 is always to the right of the lens and F^2 is always to the left of the lens.

The far point is the object plane from which light emanates that will produce a sharp image on the retina without any accommodation by the eye.

To understand emmetropia (the absence of a refractive error) and the various types of ametropia (the presence of a refractive error), one must first understand the *far point plane*. By definition, the far point plane is the object plane that is conjugate with the retina when the eye is not accommodating. *Conjugate* means that the direction of light rays may be reversed, exchanging the object for the image. Therefore, an object at the far point will be focused clearly on the retina and an object on the retina will be focused clearly at the far point.

In the emmetropic eye, parallel light rays from an object at "infinity" are sharply focused on the retina without accommodation by the lens of the eye. In such an eye, the image on the retina is conjugate with the object at infinity. Therefore, the far point plane of an emmetropic eye is at infinity (Fig. 9–15).

A myopic eye either is too strong optically or has too long an axial length. In either situation, the rays from a distant object are focused in front of the retina in the vitreous. As the distant object is moved closer to the retina, eventually a point will be reached where the image will fall on the retina. This object position is the far point of the myopic eye. In myopia the

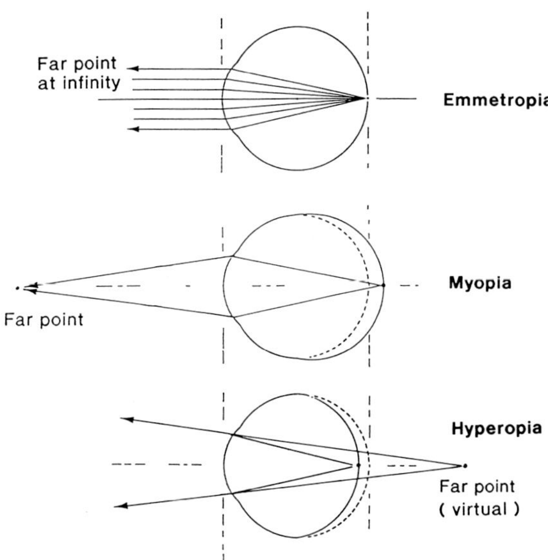

Fig. 9–15. Far points in the various refractive conditions. The far point of an emmetropic eye is at infinity. In a myopic eye, the far point is a real point in front of the eye. The far point in a nonaccommodating hyperopic eye is a virtual point behind the retina.

far point is a real point in front of the eye (Fig. 9–15).

The hyperopic eye either is too weak optically or has too short an axial length. In either case, the distant object forms a clear image behind the retina. Thus, in hyperopia, there is no object in front of the eye that can be seen clearly without accommodating. In the nonaccommodating hyperopic eye, light rays from the retina diverge as they leave the eye. Thus, the far point is "beyond" infinity, behaving as a virtual far point behind the eye (Fig. 9–15).

All that is necessary to correct myopia or hyperopia optically is a lens that will place the image of the distant object at the patient's far point (Fig. 9–16). Therefore, to correct myopia, one selects a corrective minus lens whose secondary focal point corresponds with the far point of the eye. To correct hyperopia, one selects a plus lens of such power that its secondary focal point coincides with the far point of the eye. In doing this, the corrective lens optically makes infinity appear to the eye as if it were at its far point.

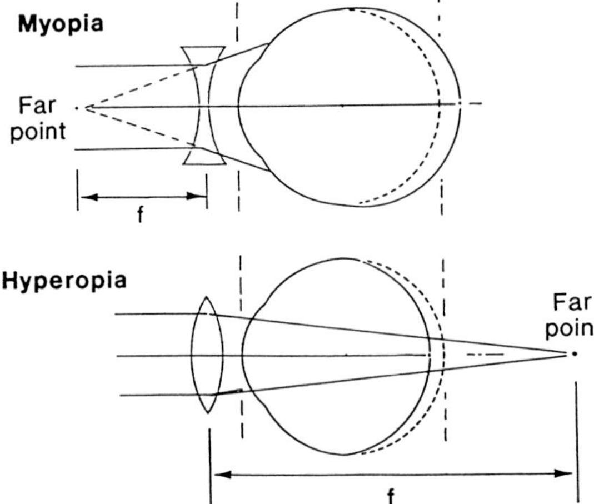

Fig. 9–16. For correction of a simple refractive error, a lens is selected whose secondary focal point coincides with the far point of the eye. From this concept one can deduce that any simple lens can be used to correct any simple refractive error, depending on where the lens is positioned in relation to the eye.

Different lenses may be effectively the same when placed at different locations.

Although the power of a lens is fixed, its effective power depends on its location with respect to the remainder of the elements in the optical system. If the position of the correcting lens is changed in relation to the eye, the secondary focal point (F^2) of the correcting lens will move away from the far point of the eye and the retinal image is then blurred unless the power of the correcting lens is changed to compensate for its altered position (Fig. 9–17). This phenomenon emphasizes the importance of *vertex distance*, or the distance of the back surface of the lens to the cornea. For any substantial refractive error (more than 5 diopters), if the vertex distance of the correcting lenses is changed, then a compensatory change must be made in the power of the lens.

Lens effectivity calculations are used mostly in determining the power of contact lenses from the patient's prescription for glasses. A useful *lens effectivity formula* is:

$$D_2 = \frac{D_1}{1 - sD_1}$$

in which D_2 equals the power of the new lens, D_1 equals the power of the original lens, and s equals the difference in location in meters. In general, two observations can be made in regard to lens effectivity.

1. A corrective lens moved closer to the eye must be more positive (or less minus).
2. The higher the power of a lens, the more significant a change in location.

Up to this point, only the power of a spherical surface with a single radius of curvature has

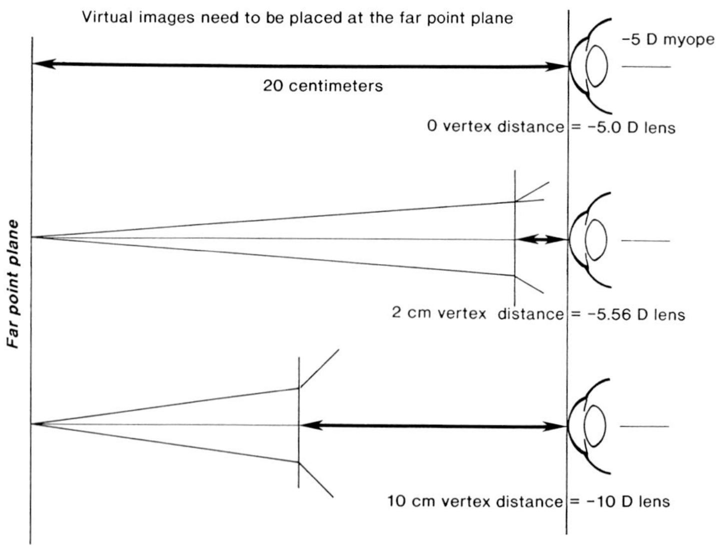

Fig. 9–17. The clinical importance of the lens effectivity formula and vertex distance (see text). If the position of the correcting lens is changed in relation to the eye, the power of the lens must also be changed.

been considered. Refraction at spherical surfaces is symmetric and point (stigmatic) images are formed. Surfaces that are *not* spherical do not form stigmatic images; such a surface is called *toroidal* or *toric*. A toric surface forms nonstigmatic images called "astigmatic" (*not* pointlike). Eighty percent of all ophthalmic lens prescriptions specify an *astigmatic correction*.

The power of a cylinder is perpendicular to its axis.

The simplest form of an astigmatic lens is the planocylinder (Fig. 9–18). Such a lens has two principal meridians: one with maximal curvature and another that is flat with no curvature. The *axis* of a planocylinder is along the meridian with no curvature. In the horizontal plane of Figure 9–18, a maximal radius of curvature is present. The power of the planocylinder is in this principal meridian, 90° from the axis meridian. The image formed by a planocylinder comes into focus along a line parallel to the cylinder's axis. The conversion of point objects into line images is the essence of astigmatic imagery.

The *Maddox rod* illustrates the principle of the planocylinder (Fig. 9–19). The Maddox rod is a series of parallel planocylinders. When positioned before the eye, a distant light spot appears as a streak perpendicular to the axis of the Maddox rod. The Maddox rod acts as a strong cylinder and forms a real image line parallel to the axis, but it is so close to the eye that it cannot be focused. Instead, the patient sees the undeviated rays, which form a virtual image of a line perpendicular to the axis of the Maddox rod at the plane of the distant light source. The Maddox rod is useful for measuring heterophorias (see Fig. 2–14 and Fig. 10–23 and 10–24).

Spherocylindric lenses should be thought of as the combination of a sphere and a cylinder.

Most lenses prescribed by ophthalmologists are combinations of spheres and cylinders called spherocylindrical (or toroidal) lenses. These lenses look like a slice from an automobile tire, having a different curvature in each meridian but having one maximal and one minimal meridian perpendicular to each other, called the *principal meridians* (Fig. 9–20). The spherocylindrical lens is specified by the orientation of the two principal meridians and the power acting in each.

The *power cross* is a convenient diagram of a spherocylinder to indicate the power in each principal meridian and the axis orientation. It is most useful when working optical problems and with retinoscopy. The arms of the power cross are drawn parallel to the principal meridians and are labeled with the total power acting in that meridian (Fig. 9–21).

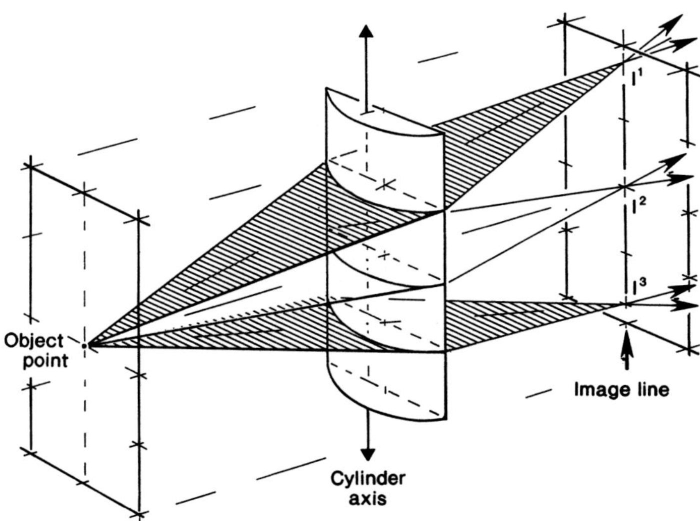

Fig. 9–18. A planocylinder lens with axis in the vertical meridian. Such a lens refracts light from an object point to an image line parallel to the cylinder axis.

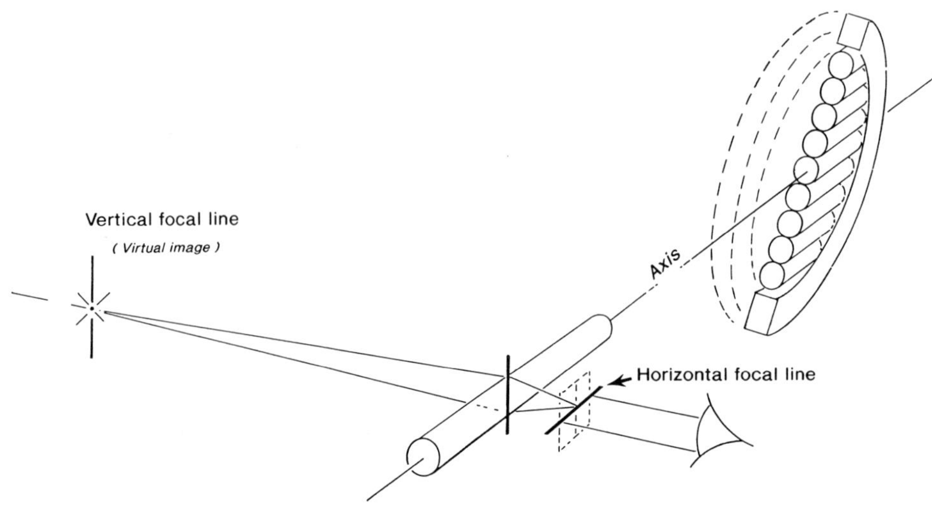

Fig. 9–19. The Maddox rod (used to measure heterophorias) is a series of very high-power cylinders. Because the eye cannot focus the real image at the horizontal focal line, it sees only the virtual image at the light source.

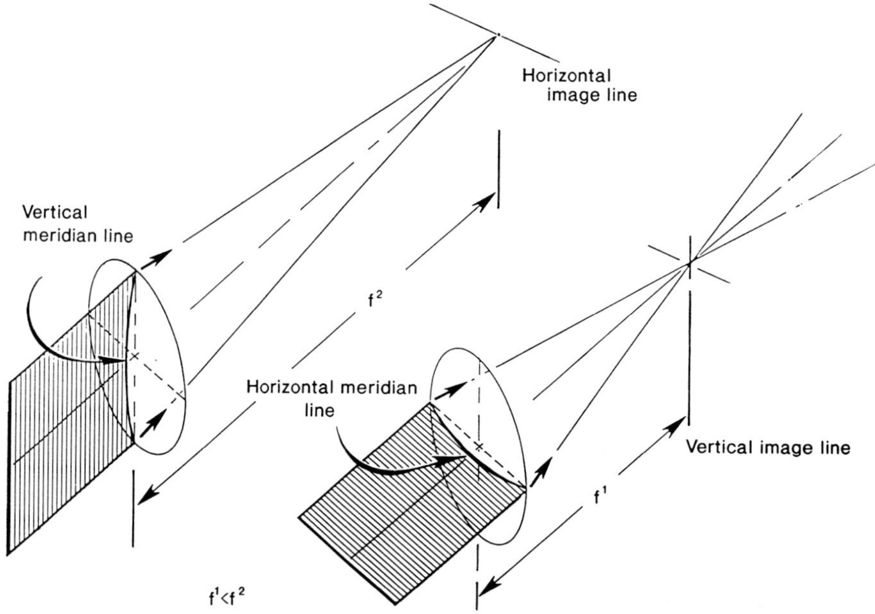

Fig. 9–20. A spherocylindrical surface. In this example, the horizontal meridian has greatest curvature (that is, power); hence, the vertical image line is focused closer to the lens. f is the focal length.

Ophthalmologists most commonly describe spherocylindrical lenses in longhand notation as a combination of a sphere and a cylinder. Unlike the power cross, this notation describes the axis of the cylinder, not the power.

> *sphere power ⊃(combined with)*
> *cylinder at axis (degrees)*

In Figure 9–22, the notation +2.00⊃+1.00 × 90° means a sphere power of +2.00 D in all axes with an additional +1.00 D of cylinder at axis 90°. One should keep in mind that the power of this cylinder is really at 180° (because the true power of a cylinder is "delivered" at 90° from the cylinder axis). In addition, the spherocylindrical form differs from the power cross diagram in that it emphasizes the power difference between the principal meridians, not the total power.

Spherocylindrical equations can be written

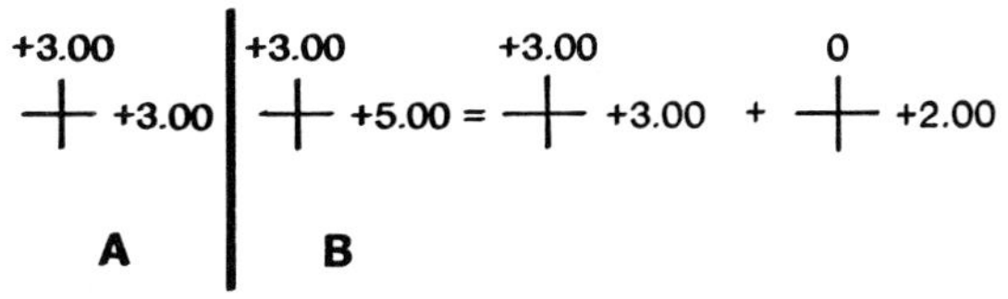

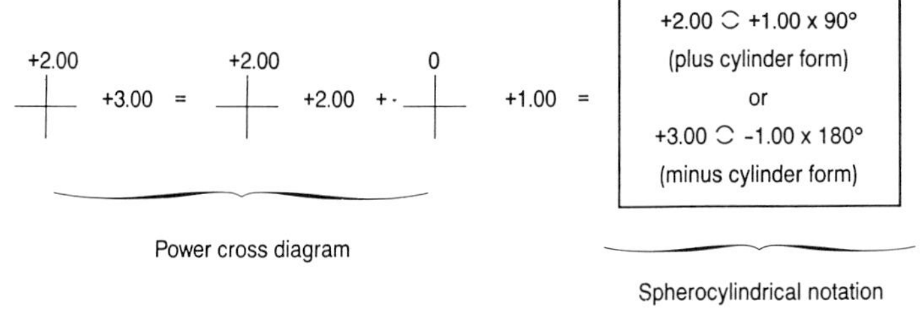

Fig. 9–21.   Power cross. *A*, A spherical lens of equal power (+3.00 D) in every axis. *B*, A spherocylindrical lens that is broken down into a spherical lens (+3.00 D) and a cylindrical lens of an additional +2.00 D power at 180°.

in plus or minus cylinder forms (Fig. 9–22). It does not matter which form is used. Nonetheless, every ophthalmologist must be able to convert one form of expression to another. To transpose one form to the other, one 1) adds the sphere and cylinder power to obtain the *new* sphere power; 2) changes the cylinder sign to the opposite sign, keeping the power the same; and 3) rotates the axis 90°. An example of this is shown in Figure 9–22.

Unlike a spherical lens, a spherocylindrical lens does not form a point image. Instead, light rays refracted by a spherocylindrical surface form a three-dimensional geometric figure called the *conoid of Sturm* (Fig. 9–23). The conoid results from the different dioptric values of the principal meridians. One can create a conoid by rolling a sheet of paper into a tube and pinching the ends off at 90° to each other. In Figure 9–23, the conoid is oriented so that the anterior end is a vertical line, followed by a vertical ellipse, a circle, a horizontal ellipse, and a horizontal line. The space between the anterior and posterior lines is called *Sturm's interval.*

Cross sections of the conoid are mostly elliptical. The smallest cross section, however, is a circle called the *circle of least confusion.* It is the clearest image that an eye with an astigmatic error or a spherocylindrical lens can produce—any other plane of focus gives a poorer image. The circle of least confusion is located at the

Fig. 9–22.   Power cross diagram and equivalent spherocylindrical notation.

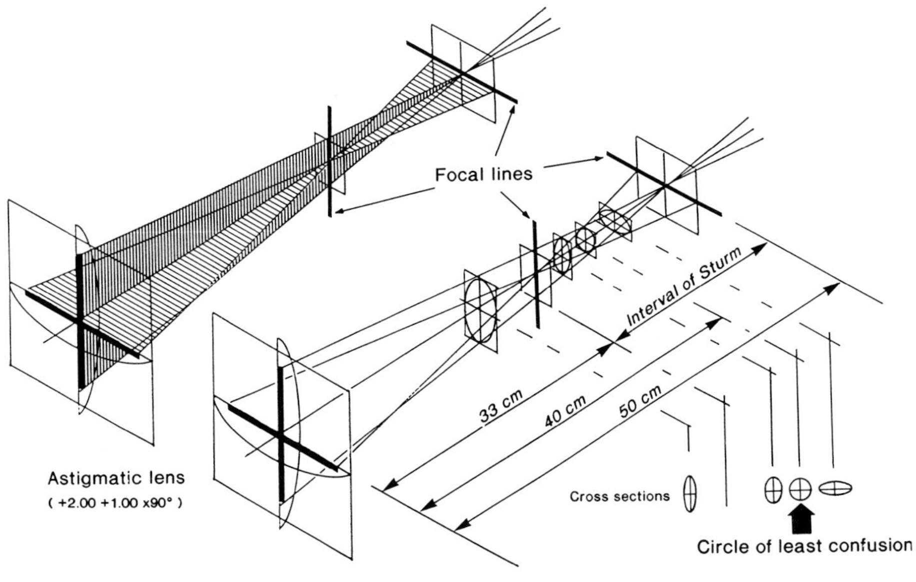

Fig. 9–23.   The conoid of Sturm.

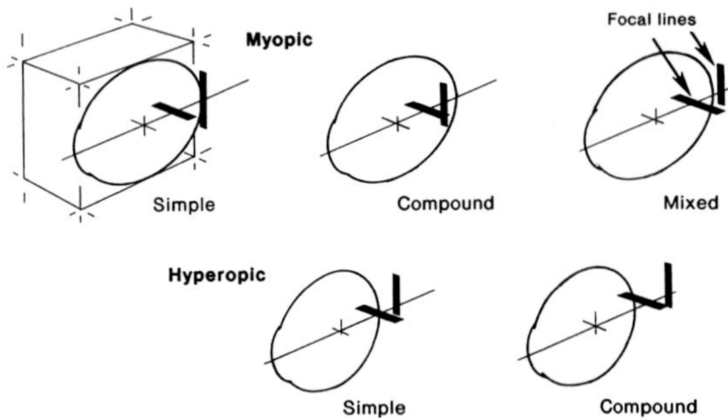

Fig. 9–24. Types of astigmatism, as determined by the positions of the two focal lines with respect to the retina.

point corresponding to the spheroequivalent of the spherocylinder. The *spheroequivalent* is the dioptric midpoint of the conoid, and when written in spherocylindrical form it equals the sphere plus one-half the cylinder. For example, $+2.00 \bigcirc +1.00 \times 90°$ has a spheroequivalent of

$$+2.50 \text{ D } \left(+2.00 + \frac{+1.00}{2} = +2.50\right)$$

or a focal length $1/2.50 = 40$ cm. Although the circle of least confusion is the dioptric midpoint of the conoid, linearly it is always closer to the anterior focal line than to the posterior focal line (Fig. 9–23).

In an astigmatic eye, the location of the image lines with respect to the retina determines the type of astigmatism (Fig. 9–24). For example, if one of the meridians in astigmatism fo-

cuses on the retina, the condition is termed *simple astigmatism.* The site at which the other meridian focuses determines the condition to be either simple myopic or simple hyperopic astigmatism.

Astigmatism is also classified on the basis of orientation of the refractive power (Fig. 9–25). An eye that is the most powerful in the vertical meridian is said to have *"with the rule"* astigmatism. It is optically corrected by plus cylinder in the vertical meridian. *"Against the rule" astigmatism* occurs when the horizontal meridian has the most power. It is optically corrected by plus cylinder in the horizontal meridian.

Magnification depends on the power of the lens and its distance from the object.

Magnification is best described by the relationship $M = U/V$. As in the vergence formula, U is the vergence power of the object and V is the vergence power of the image for any lens system. If M is positive, the image is upright. If M is negative, the image is inverted. If M is greater than 1, M describes the proportion of magnification. Conversely, if M is less than 1, M describes the proportion of minification. For example, in Figure 9–4 *A*, an object point 1 meter to the left of a $+4$ lens produces an image 33 cm to the right of the lens ($U + P = V$; $-1 + 4 = +3$). The magnification equals $U/V = -1/+3 = -0.33$. The image formed by

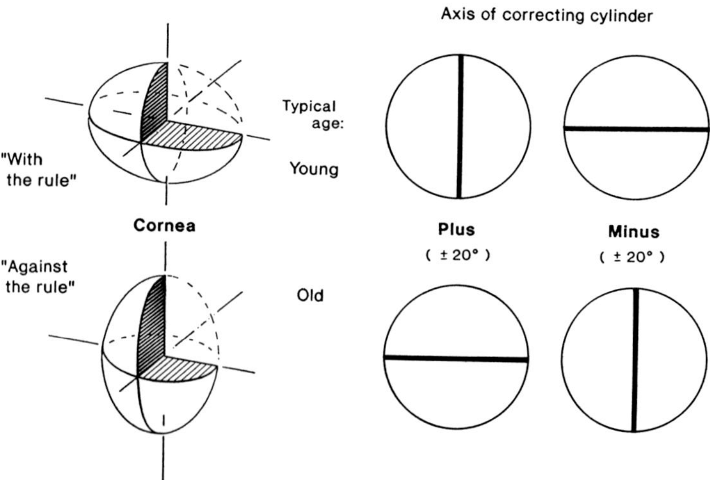

Fig. 9–25. Types of astigmatism, as determined by the orientation of the principal meridians and the orientation of the correcting cylinder axis.

such a lens would be inverted and one-third the size of the original object.

Angular magnification (ma) defines how big an image looks to an eye. To quantitate magnification, one must assume a reference distance from which to view an object. By convention, the standard reference distance is 25 cm, the focal length of a +4.00 D lens. As a result, the angular magnification of any lens equals D/4. For example, the 20-D lens used in indirect ophthalmoscopy has an angular magnification of 20/4 or 5×.

The direct ophthalmoscope can be thought of as using the patient's eye as a simple magnifier to view the patient's retina. The dioptic power of an average emmetropic eye is +60 D. Therefore, the angular magnification of the direct ophthalmoscope is 60/4 = 15×.

REFRACTION

Refractive correction for the eye is a combination of both objective and subjective measurement.

Retinoscopy is the simplest and most informative method of objective refraction, and it requires no response from the patient. There are two methods of retinoscopy. This chapter emphasizes the *neutralization method*, which uses lenses to neutralize the patient's refractive error. The *estimation method* estimates the refractive error without using lenses.

Although many refractionists would like to become so expert in retinoscopy that no reliance need be placed on other methods, the experienced clinician will seldom prescribe from retinoscopy alone if the results can be confirmed by subjective tests. Cross cylinder testing is the subjective technique most widely used today.

The retinoscope measures the far point of the patient's eye.

The streak retinoscope was first introduced in the United States by Jack Copeland in the 1920s. It is a small projector that emits a line image of the lamp filament. The lamp filament is moved up or down by a sleeve on the retino-

scope. By raising or lowering the sleeve, one can produce divergent or convergent light. Divergent light (usually the sleeve in the up position) is preferred by most retinoscopists because the image and the apparent light source move in the same direction. With convergent light, all relative movements are reversed. Some retinoscopes, however, have a reverse action, and the sleeve must be down to produce divergent light. If there is ever confusion about the correct position of the sleeve to produce divergent light, the sleeve should be moved all the way in the direction that will produce a broad, unfocused intercept on a flat surface one foot away.

As the examiner looks through the peephole of the retinoscope with the sleeve in the up (divergent) position, a band of light (called the *intercept*) is swept across the patient's pupil during retinoscopy. The patient's retina then reflects this streak of light back toward the examiner as a red, streak-shaped retinoscopic reflex (Fig. 9–26). By turning the sleeve with the index finger, the retinoscopist can rotate the projected linear streak to the desired meridian. The intercept is always swept across the patient's pupil at right angles to its length. For example, if the streak of light is oriented vertically, the intercept is swept horizontally. If it is oriented horizontally, the intercept is swept vertically (Fig. 9–27). Only small sweeps are necessary, the movement being at the wrist and not at the shoulder. As the intercept is swept across the patient's pupil, the retinoscopic reflex may move in the same direction as the intercept ("*with*" *movement*), move in the opposite direction ("*against*" *movement*), or fill the pupil with light as the intercept moves across the pupil and not move at all (*neutraliza-*

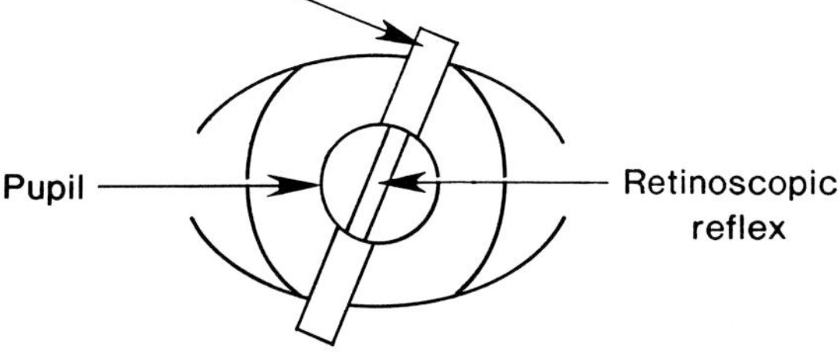

Fig. 9–26.   The retinoscopic reflex.

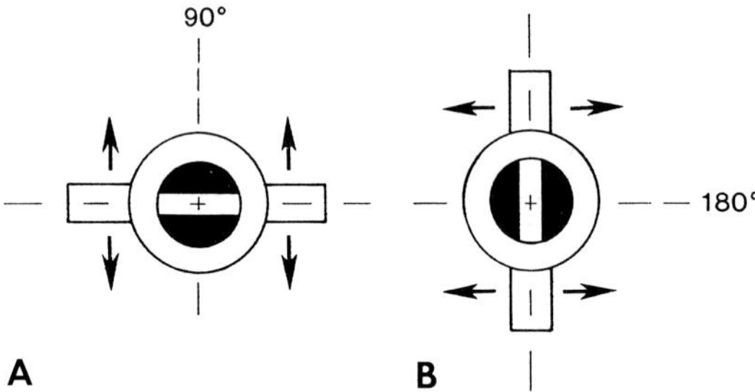

Fig. 9–27. Methods of scanning ocular meridians. *A*, The streak is horizontal to evaluate the power in the vertical meridian. *B*, The streak is vertical to evaluate the power in the horizontal meridian.

tion). The type of movement is determined simply by the position of the patient's far point with respect to the peephole of the retinoscope (Fig. 9–28). If the patient's far point is between the patient and the retinoscope, "against" movement is seen. If the far point is beyond the retinoscope, "with" movement is seen. If the patient's far point is at the peephole of the retinoscope, neutralization is seen.

The object of the neutralization method of retinoscopy is to use lenses to move the patient's far point to the peephole of the retinoscope (neutralization). Adding plus lenses in front of the patient's eye pulls the far point in toward the patient's eye (Fig. 29 *A*). Adding minus lenses pushes the far point away from the patient's eye (Fig. 9–29 *B*). These neutralizing lenses can be placed in front of the patient's eye by use of a set of trial lenses and a trial frame or of a phoroptor.

The movement and characteristics of the retinoscopic reflex indicate the location of the patient's far point.

If the retinoscopic reflex shows "with" movement, then the patient's far point is beyond the retinoscope (hyperopia), and plus lenses are added to pull the far point in toward the retinoscope. The proper amount of plus power will have been added when the retinoscopic reflex fills the pupil and no motion is seen. This is neutrality. At neutrality, the patient's retina is conjugate with the peephole.

If the retinoscopic reflex shows "against" movement, then the far point is in front of the retinoscope (myopia), and minus lenses are needed to push the far point away from the patient and toward the retinoscope. Because "with" movement is easier to see than "against" movement, it is easiest first to add enough minus power to convert the reflex to "with" movement, and then to work back by adding plus power until neutralization is reached.

Clinical experience demonstrates that neutrality is not a precise end point, but rather a zone of approximately 0.50 D power between the last of "with" movement and the beginning of "against" movement (Fig. 9–30). For practical purposes, the end point is most easily recognized at the front edge of this zone, when slight "with" movement is seen—again, because small amounts of "with" movement are easier to recognize than "against" movement.

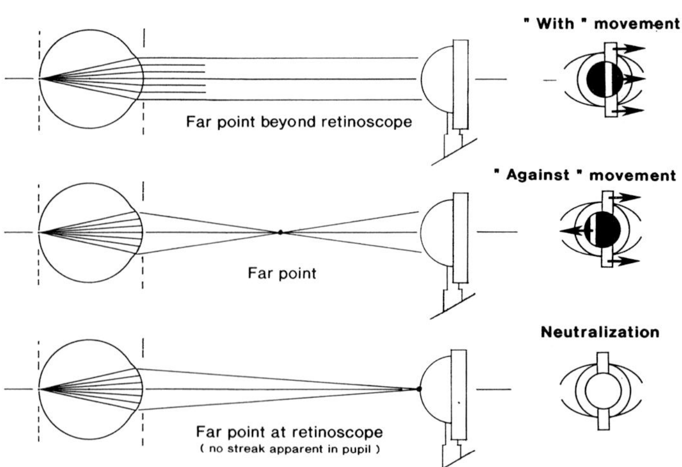

Fig. 9–28. Movement of the retinoscopic reflex.

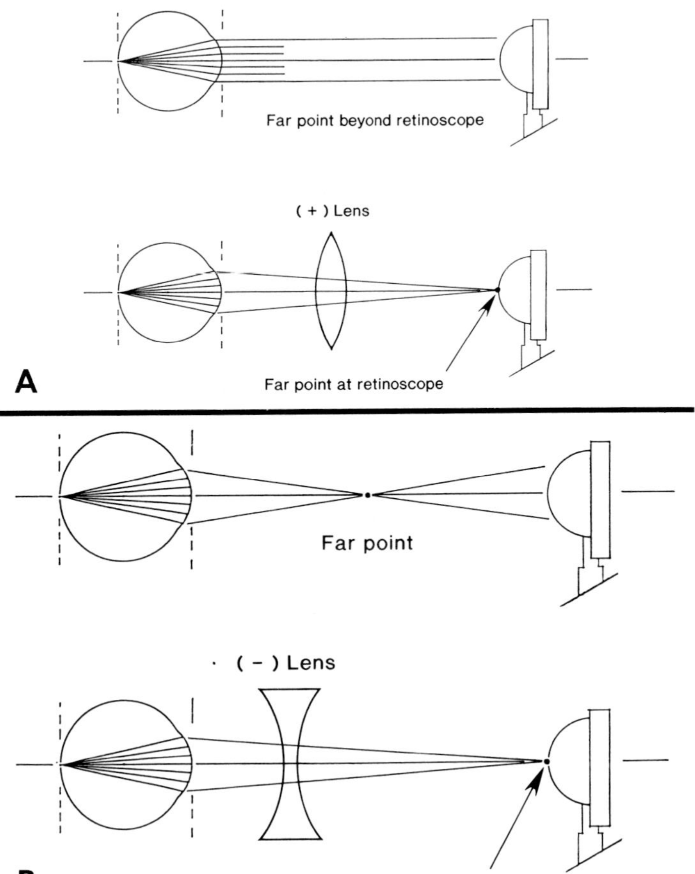

Fig. 9–29. Neutralization of the retinoscopic reflex using lenses. *A*, A plus lens pulls the far point toward the eye and the retinoscope. *B*, A minus lens pushes the far point away from the eye to the retinoscope.

The characteristics of the retinoscopic reflex also give one a clue as to the location of the far point. As the far point approaches the retinoscope (neutrality), the retinoscopic reflex becomes *faster, brighter,* and *wider.* Unfortunately, as one gets very close to neutrality the reflex becomes so large and moves so fast that it may sometimes be difficult to analyze. Errors in retinoscopy at this point are easily corrected during subjective refraction.

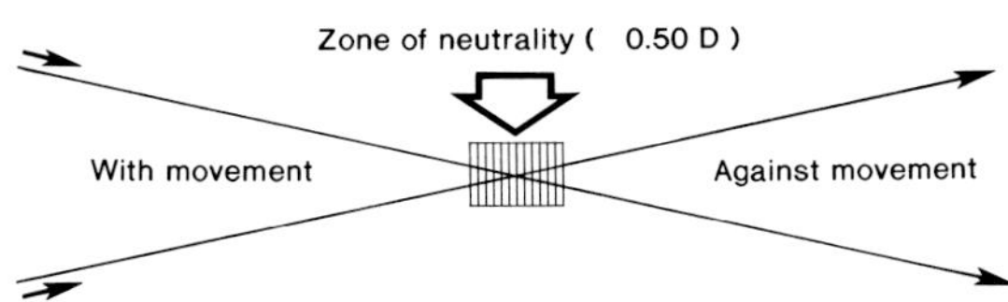

Fig. 9–30. The neutral zone. A neutral range of 0.50 D corresponds to a linear range of 50 cm at 1 m but only 13 cm at a working distance of 0.5 m; hence, the closer the working distance, the less room for error.

Accurate retinoscopy requires a consistent working distance.

When neutralization is achieved, the lens power necessary to place the patient's far point at the peephole of the retinoscope will have been determined. What is really needed, however, is the corrective lens that will move the patient's far point to the visual acuity chart on the far wall (infinity). This will always require some additional minus lens power to "push" the far point from the retinoscope farther out to infinity. The exact amount of additional minus power will depend on how far the retinoscope is from the patient's eye. This distance between the patient's eye and the retinoscope is called the *working distance*, and it is usually 66 cm (2/3 m). Thus, with a working distance of 66 cm, a 1/0.66 m or −1.5 D lens must be added to the neutralizing lenses already in place to yield the proper corrective lens for the patient's eye. The closer the working distance, the brighter the retinoscopic reflex, but the less leeway for error. The longer the working distance, the less bright the reflex, but the more sensitive retinoscopy is to small refractive error. In addition, a longer working distance makes it easier to scan close to the visual axis. Off-axis retinoscopy of more than 15° produces unwanted and erroneous astigmatism.

Astigmatic eyes exhibit different retinoscopic reflexes in the different ocular meridians.

Unfortunately for the retinoscopist, 80% of all persons with refractive error have astigmatism. Astigmatic eyes show differing motions in different ocular meridians, but there are always a maximum and a minimum representing the principal meridians. These principal meridians are at right angles to each other, and each can be thought of as having its own far point. Thus, for correction of astigmatism, each principal meridian must be neutralized separately and each far point moved to the peephole of the retinoscope. These corrections are made by use of a sphere to neutralize one meridian and a cylindrical lens to neutralize the other (spherocylindrical lens).

When retinoscopy is performed on astigmatic eyes, it is helpful to use "with" movement at all times. One should remember that it is simpler to recognize and neutralize "with" movement than "against" movement. To do this, the retinoscope sleeve is turned with the index finger to rotate the intercept from one meridian to another. If "with" movement is not seen in all meridians, minus spherical lenses are added to convert all reflexes to "with." Then, plus spherical lenses are added slowly to neutralize the least hyperopic meridian; thus, "with" movement will still be present in the remaining meridian. In other words, the first goal is to neutralize the meridian closest to neutrality (the least "with" movement). A clue to recognizing this meridian is that its streak will be the widest and have the fastest "with" movement.

Once this first meridian is neutralized, the streak is then rotated 90° to neutralize the remaining meridian. This is done by aligning the axis of a plus cylinder parallel to the reflex. The cylinder axis, the streak, and the reflex should now all be in line. The remaining "with" movement in this meridian is then neutralized by the addition of plus cylinder lenses.

The exact location of the axis of the cylinder lens is critical. Before the exact placement of the cylinder axis can be determined, the position of the principal meridians must be located. The streak retinoscope is more useful than the older spot retinoscope for locating these principal meridians. In addition, various phenomena are helpful to locate the cylinder axis: *enhancement, break phenomenon,* and *skew.*

The retinoscopist may *enhance* the reflex (make it narrower and brighter) by slowly moving the retinoscope sleeve downward. The narrower and brighter reflex helps to locate the cylinder axis with better precision. In addition, it helps to estimate the cylinder power because enhancement will occur only if there is 1 D or more of astigmatism (Fig. 9–31). If the reflex does not enhance, the sleeve should be returned to the upright position. The reflex should never be neutralized while it is enhanced.

The *break phenomenon* indicates whether the streak is off axis. The break is more easily seen if the reflex can be enhanced. If the intercept is off axis, the reflex is no longer parallel with it—there is a break or misalignment of the reflex with the intercept (Fig. 9–32). Continuity between the reflex and the streak occurs only if the streak is exactly on axis. In addition, the reflex is broader and less enhanced when off axis.

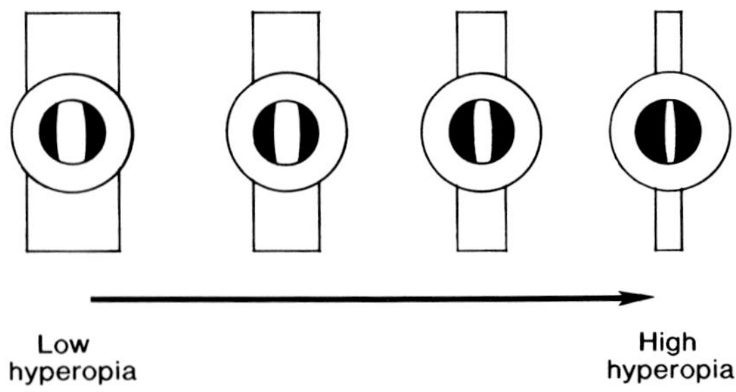

Fig. 9–31. Enhancement of the retinoscopic streak to determine the axis and power of the meridian.

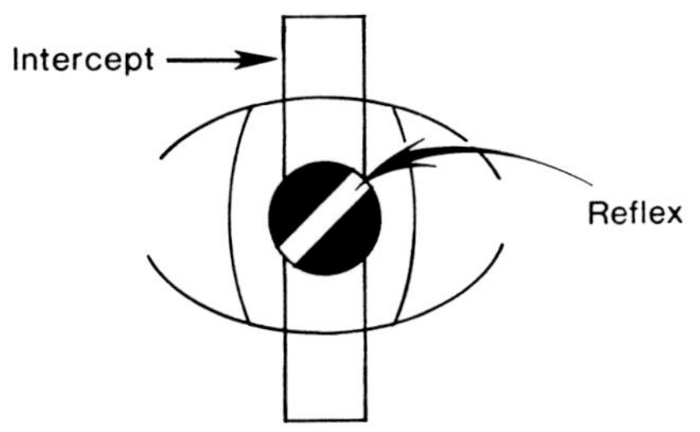

Fig. 9–32. The break phenomenon of misalignment of the reflex with the intercept.

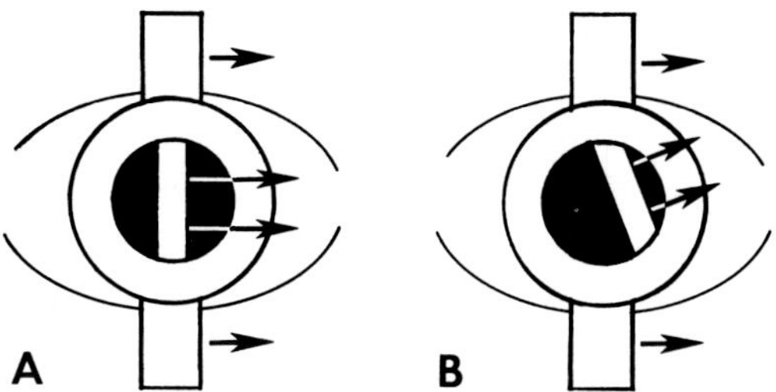

Fig. 9–33. Retinoscopic reflex. *A,* Reflex and intercept aligned. *B,* Skew deviation occurs when the streak is not aligned with the cylinder axis.

Skew tells whether the axis is off alignment. If the direction of movement of the reflex when compared with the direction of movement of the intercept is skewed (off direction), then the axis is also off alignment (Fig. 9–33). Skew is most useful in low amounts of astigmatism when break and enhancement are less evident.

"Troubleshooting" during retinoscopy can be used to the examiner's advantage.

1. *The pupil constricts during retinoscopy.* In this case, the patient is usually looking at the retinoscope light and accommodating. The patient should be reminded to look at the fixation target on the far wall. The best fixation target is a small light. Letters can induce accommodation, and large, bright lights produce annoying reflexes.

2. *The reflex changes during retinoscopy.* The patient is accommodating or relaxing accommodation. Fogging or cycloplegia may be necessary (see page 239).

3. *An irregular reflex is seen.* This is commonly seen in children under cycloplegia. Because of spherical aberration, centrally there is "with" movement and peripherally there is "against" movement. The peripheral reflex should be ignored and the center reflex neutralized.

In adults, an irregular reflex is usually due to a nuclear sclerotic cataract. The reflex is opposite to that seen in children. Centrally there is "against" movement and peripherally there is "with" movement.

4. *A scissoring movement is seen.* That is,

different portions of the pupil have different refractive errors by 4 D or more. Because one cannot neutralize the entire reflex, one should try to concentrate on the central reflex only. This can be very difficult to do, and often one has to rely heavily on subjective refinement.

5. *The reflex is dim and hard to see.* An obscure reflex suggests a high refractive error. The retinoscopist should try using high plus or minus spherical lenses to elicit a reflex. If there is no change, one should suspect a cloudy media (for example, a cataract).

Retinoscopy can be summarized in a few simple steps.

Retinoscopy follows a logical series of steps. The first step is to determine whether the eye is spherical or astigmatic. If the eye is spherical, all the meridians will appear identical and the motion will be clean. If the eye is astigmatic, the reflex differs in some meridians and a break or skew motion will be detected.

If the eye is spherical, then:

1. Enough minus lens power is added to convert all the meridians to "with" movement.
2. Plus lenses are added to neutralize the spherical error and to confirm that all meridians neutralize simultaneously.
3. Minus 1.50 D is added to compensate for the working distance.
4. The refraction is refined subjectively.

If the eye is astigmatic, then:

1. Enough minus lens power is added to

convert all the meridians to "with" movement.

2. The locations of the principal meridians are determined. The principal meridians demonstrate no break in the reflex and streak alignment and do not show skew motion. Enhancement is used for precise localization of the axis. In regular astigmatism, the primary meridians are 90° apart, with the wider band indicating the meridian nearest neutrality.

3. Plus spherical lenses are added to neutralize first the meridian with the widest band and the fastest "with" movement. This step will leave "with" movement in the remaining meridian to be neutralized second by a plus cylinder.

4. After neutralization of the first meridian with spherical lenses, the sleeve is rotated 90° and the cylinder lens axis is placed parallel to this second streak.

5. Plus cylinder power is increased until the last of the "with" movement disappears or the first "against" motion appears.

6. Minus 1.50 D is added to compensate for the working distance.

7. The refraction is refined subjectively.

Subjective refraction refines the retinoscopy result.

Although retinoscopy can often be performed accurately to within 0.50 D, subjective methods should also be used to verify and refine further any refractive error that is found by retinoscopy. Reliable responses to subjective techniques can usually be obtained by age 8 years. Cross cylinder testing is the subjective technique most widely used today.

The *cross cylinder* is a spherocylindrical lens having plus cylinder power in one principal meridian and an equal amount of minus cylinder power in the other. The strength of the cylinder is always two times and of opposite sign to the power of the sphere when expressed in spherocylindrical form, such as $-0.25 \subset +0.50 \times 90°$. The cross cylinder is named for its spherical component. Thus, in the example above, the cross cylinder is a 0.25-D cross cylinder. Finally, the spheroequivalent of a cross cylinder is zero. Therefore, if a cross cylinder is placed in front of an eye of any refractive error, the position of the circle of least confusion will not be changed.

The cross cylinder comes in a metal frame with a handle that straddles the two principal axes (Fig. 9–34). A white dot indicates the plus cylinder axis, and a red dot indicates the minus cylinder axis. When the cross cylinder is used, the patient should be looking at a Snellen target letter one to two lines larger than his or her best acuity. If the best acuity is 20/25, then the 20/30 or 20/40 line is used for the cross cylinder test.

Cross cylinders are used to verify the axis and power of astigmatism.

The axis of astigmatism is verified before the power is determined. In refining the cylinder axis, the cross cylinder straddles the correcting cylinder axis and its handle coincides with the axis of the trial cylinder. When the lenses flip, the patient reports which lens gives the sharper image. If one flip position is better, the axis is

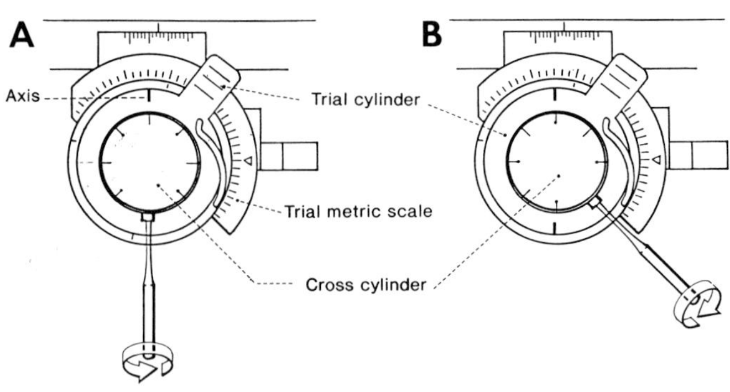

Fig. 9–34. Uses of the cross cylinder. *A*, To refine the trial cylinder axis. *B*, To refine the trial cylinder power.

modified; the direction toward which the axis is rotated depends on the type of cylinder used. If plus cylinder is used, the axis is rotated toward the white dot flip position that provides the clearer image. The cylinder axis is never rotated in increments of more than 5° to 10°. When minus cylinders are used, the red dots serve as the guide and the minus cylinder axis is rotated toward the red dot flip position that is clearer. The end point of cross cylinder testing is not maximal clarity but equal blur between the two flip positions.

Once cylinder axis is refined, cylinder power is then refined by placing the cross cylinder axis coincident with the primary axis of ocular astigmatism. In this case, the handle of the instrument straddles the principal meridians. In one flip position the red dot is coincident with the cylinder axis, and in the other position the white dot is. Once again the patient is asked which position gives the clearer image. If plus cylinder is used, cylinder power is added if the preferred position has white dots coincident with axis, and power is reduced if red dots coincide with this axis. If minus cylinder is used, the opposite is performed. As with the refining axis, the end point is not maximal clarity of acuity but equal blurriness. Changes in cylinder power are made in increments of only 0.25 D. In addition, in order to maintain the position of least confusion on the retina, 0.25 D of sphere of opposite power must be added every time 0.50 D of new cylinder is introduced.

Control of accommodation is the key to valid subjective refraction.

The purpose of clinical refraction is to determine the distance refractive correction with the eye's accommodation completely relaxed. Two methods of controlling accommodation are fogging and cycloplegia.

In adults, relaxation of accommodation can usually be achieved through the technique of *fogging*. Additional plus power is placed in front of the patient's fixating eye to pull the image of the visual acuity chart into the vitreous, thus blurring it. The idea is that if vision is artificially blurred by making the eye hyperopic, then attempts at additional accommodation

only blur the image more. Therefore, the patient's accommodation tends to relax.

In children, adequate relaxation of accommodation usually requires pharmacologic paralysis of the ciliary muscle (*cycloplegia*). A short-acting cycloplegic agent—cyclopentolate 1%—is commonly used in children, with the refraction approximately 30 minutes after administration of the drop.

A "balanced" refraction is one that equally relaxes accommodation of both eyes.

All refraction techniques described thus far are performed monocularly. With monocular refraction techniques, it is possible that accommodation is more relaxed when one eye is being refracted than when both are. The resultant accommodative imbalance is often a cause of asthenopic symptoms. Clinically, an unequal near point of accommodation is a clue that this has occurred.

To balance the manifest refraction, the vision is first fogged with +0.75 D spheres in each eye. The test chart is reduced to a single line (20/40 size), and 6 diopters of vertical prism are placed before one eye to create vertical dissociation. The patient is asked to choose which of the two 20/40 lines is clearer. If the lines are equally blurred, the refraction is already "balanced." If one line is clearer, however, plus power is added to the eye with the better vision in 0.25-D power increments until the images are equally blurred. At this point, the two eyes are "balanced" and the +0.75-D spheres are removed from each eye.

During balancing, the eye with the better vision was actually accommodating more during the initial manifest refraction. The difference in accommodation is equal to the amount of plus power added to this eye to "balance" the refraction.

A simple rule in balancing is to reduce plus power in hyperopia and to reduce minus power in myopia. In both hyperopia and myopia, one should not prescribe a lens greater in power than that found in the prebalanced refraction. The prism dissociation method described above is the most sensitive of the binocular balance techniques and yields the most consistent results.

Presbyopia requires bifocals or reading glasses.

Presbyopia is the most common refractive disorder of middle age. With the onset of presbyopia, plus power must be added to the distance refractive correction to allow adequate and comfortable reading vision. The usual method for determining the proper reading "add" is to estimate the required amount of power to add from the patient's age and to confirm the effect in trial frames (Table 9–2). After an estimated add is selected for the patient's primary near vision task, the range of clear vision—near point to far point—and the most comfortable working distance through the add are measured. As a general rule, the usual near point is 30 cm and the usual comfortable working distance is 40 cm through the add. This estimated add should be modified as necessary to satisfy the patient's true near requirements. One should not hesitate to use a tape measure to verify these distances. This is especially valuable if the patient's working conditions are somewhat unusual.

The most common error in prescribing bifocals is to make them too strong. This can be avoided by placing the planned correction in the trial frame and having the patient simulate his or her real near work and reading as accurately as possible.

CONTACT LENSES

It is estimated that more than 18,000,000 Americans wear *contact lenses*. Contact lenses correct optical defects, alter magnification, improve field of view, and enhance acuity. New types and brands of contact lenses appear and disappear so rapidly that it is difficult to remember names, much less characteristics. In addition, today's lens material often is tomorrow's relic, and any detailed description is likely to be out of date by the time it appears in print. Despite these limitations, the basic terminology, types and designs of lenses, and basic fitting guides are described below.

TABLE 9–2 Approximate Reading "Add" Needed, According to Age of Patient

Age, yr	Add
40–44	+1.25
45–49	+1.50
50–54	+1.75
55–59	+2.00
60–64	+2.25
≥65	+2.50

The two major types of contact lenses are rigid and soft contact lenses.

Contact lenses can be divided into two major groups, depending on the nature of the material composition: rigid and soft. Rigid lenses include the original polymethyl methacrylate (PMMA) lenses and the newer gas-permeable lenses made of cellulose acetate butyrate, silicone and PMMA, Fluoro-Siloxane Acrylate, or other various polymers of silicone. Most practitioners use gas-permeable lenses as their primary rigid lens because of their comfort and oxygen permeability. Advantages of gas-permeable lenses include the correction of moderate amounts of astigmatism with spherical curves, infrequent replacement, simple maintenance, and better durability and oxygen transmission than soft lenses. Disadvantages are possible prolonged adaptation and unsuitability for intermittent wear.

Soft lenses are made of various hydrogel plastics containing 40% to 70% water. They are more comfortable than rigid lenses and adaptation is so rapid that intermittent wear is practical. They seldom fall out and rarely cause spectacle blur. Disadvantages include fragility, cost, increased maintenance, and inability to correct more than minimal amounts of astigmatism without toric modifications.

The six key contact lens factors are diameter, base curve, vault, wetting angle, peripheral curve, and oxygen transmission.

From the practical standpoint of contact lens fitting, important factors that must be understood are lens diameter, central posterior curve radius (base curve), sagittal height (lens vault), wetting angle, peripheral curve design, and oxygen transmission and hydration.

The *diameter* of gas-permeable contact lenses is usually 8.0 to 9.5 mm. The diameter also determines the size of the optical zone: the larger the diameter, the larger the optical zone. A large optical zone has the advantage of avoiding optical flare. In addition, excess lens movement often can be eliminated by increasing lens diameter.

Soft contact lenses are usually 13 to 15 mm in diameter. They generally extend 1 to 2 mm beyond the limbus, and this is one reason for their comfort and rapid adaptation.

The *base curve* of a lens is the curvature of the central portion of the back surface of a lens; it is expressed in diopters or in millimeters of radius of arc. The base curve is designed to conform to the optical zone of the cornea. The curvature or refractive power of this central zone of the cornea is determined with the keratometer. K, the flattest principal meridian, needs to be determined. One usually speaks of the base curve in relation to K (that is, steeper, flatter, or on K).

Sagittal height refers to the distance between the height of a spherical arc and its chord. *Vault* refers to the sagittal height of a contact lens (Fig. 9–35) and considers the base curve and diameter simultaneously. If the base curve is increased (D) (or decreased if expressed in millimeters of arc) or the diameter is increased, the vault increases or steepens. If the base curve is decreased (D) (or increased if expressed in millimeters of arc) or the diameter is decreased, the vault decreases or flattens. If a contact lens is fit with a steep vault (steeper than K), the tear film between the cornea and the contact lens forms a tear lens having plus power; if it is fit flatter, the tear lens has minus power (Fig. 9–36). This tear lens influences the effective power of the contact lens.

The adhesion between the contact lens surface and water defines the *wetting angle*. The smaller the angle, the greater the wettability and the greater the comfort and tear distribution.

The human cornea is aspherical; its center is steeper than the periphery. Thus, contact

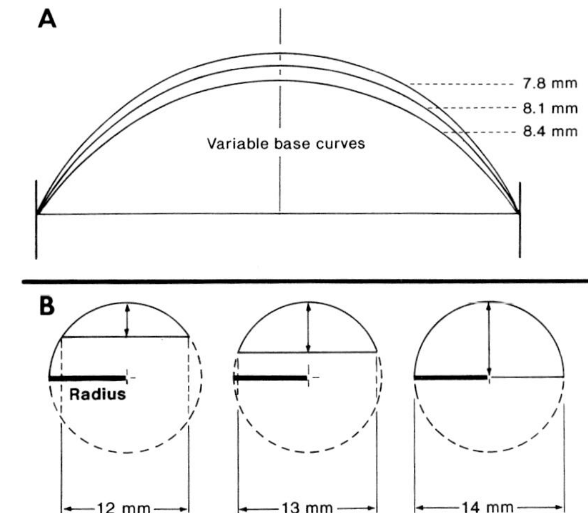

Fig. 9–35. *A,* The sagittal height or vault of the lens is increased when the radius of curvature is decreased from 8.4 to 7.8 mm, if the lens diameter is held constant. *B,* When the radius is kept constant and the diameter of the lens is increased from 12 to 14 mm, the sagittal height of the lens is increased and the lens becomes steeper.

lenses have *peripheral curves* that are flatter than the central base curve. Soft lenses have only one peripheral curve, whereas gas-permeable lenses have two or three (one or two secondary and one peripheral curve) (Fig. 9–37). Peripheral curve design is important in comfort, tear exchange, and lens movement.

Adequate *oxygen exchange* is necessary to maintain corneal integrity and prevent edema.

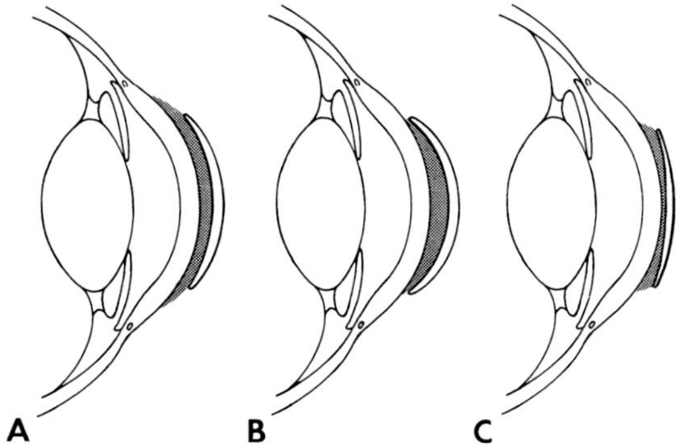

Fig. 9–36. Tear power. *A,* Plano power of tear film when the lens is fitted parallel to K. *B,* Plus power of the tear film when the lens is fitted steeper than K. The tear film is convex. *C,* Minus power of the tear film when the lens is fit flatter than K. The tear film is concave.

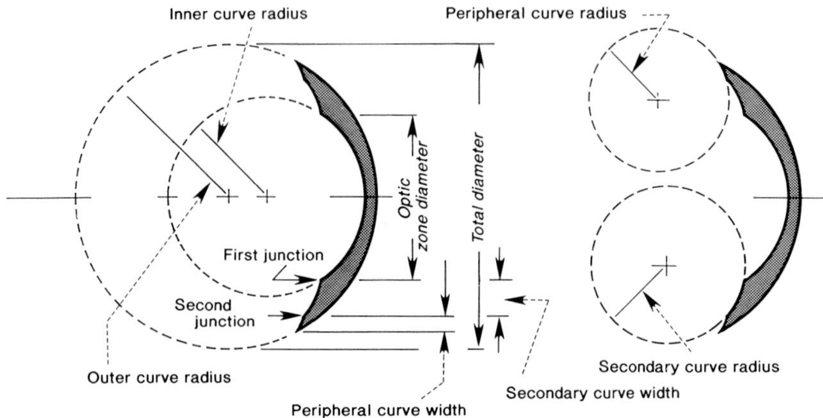

Fig. 9–37. A tricurve lens has two peripheral curve radii. A good standard peripheral curve system uses a secondary curve, which is 1.0 mm flatter than the base curve and 0.2 mm wide, and a peripheral curve, which is 0.3 mm wide and between 10.5 mm and 12.25 mm in radius depending on the base curve.

With soft lenses, there is little tear exchange and oxygen diffusion across the contact lens is the most important route for providing oxygen to the corneal epithelium. Water content determines oxygen permeability because oxygen diffuses into it independent of the components of the lens material. Thinner lenses also give better oxygen permeability. Therefore, lower-water-content lenses need to be thinner than high-water-content lenses to provide an equivalent oxygen permeability.

Gas-permeable lenses possess some oxygen permeability, but they are also highly dependent on renewal of the tear reservoir during blinking to supply adequate nutrients and oxygen to the corneal epithelium. The permeability constant (Dk) is the unofficial standard for comparing the oxygen permeability of various contact lens materials. The higher the Dk value, the higher the oxygen permeability.

Fitting of contact lenses must be individualized.

Most manufacturers suggest rules for selecting and fitting their lenses. With clinical experience, however, it soon becomes apparent that there are many rules but few certainties. If contact lenses are to be fit successfully, each patient must be individually assessed and modifications made according to the behavior of the contact lenses on the eye. Nevertheless, some basic rules provide a starting point for fitting contact lenses.

All *soft lenses* are fit with trial lenses to determine the final optimal fit. Only a small assortment of lens powers and base curves is needed because both will be modified with each individual. Below is a "rule-of-thumb" guide to fit daily-wear soft contact lenses of 38% water content. Spherical soft lenses usually correct up to 1.00 D of corneal astigmatism, although thicker lenses may mask more astigmatism.

1. The refraction is determined in minus cylinder.
2. The spheroequivalent power is calculated and modified for vertex distance if more than 4.00 D.

TABLE 9–3 Suggested Flattening Chart for Spherical and Toric Soft Contact Lens (38% Water Content)

Diameter, mm	Fit below K (D)
12.5	2.5
13.0	3.0–3.5
13.5	3.5
13.7	4.0
13.8	4.0
14.0	4.5
14.3	4.5
14.5	5.5

TABLE 9–4 Conversion of Keratometer Diopters to Millimeters

Diopters (D) to radius of curvature in millimeters (mm)

D	mm	D	mm	D	mm	D	mm	D	mm
26.00 = 12.98		36.00 = 9.37		41.00 = 8.23		46.00 = 7.33		51.00 = 6.61	
26.25 = 12.86		36.12 = 9.33		41.12 = 8.20		46.12 = 7.31		51.12 = 6.60	
26.50 = 12.73		36.25 = 9.30		41.25 = 8.18		46.25 = 7.29		51.25 = 6.58	
26.75 = 12.61		36.37 = 9.27		41.37 = 8.15		46.37 = 7.27		51.37 = 6.56	
27.00 = 12.50		36.50 = 9.24		41.50 = 8.13		46.50 = 7.25		51.50 = 6.55	
27.25 = 12.38		36.62 = 9.21		41.62 = 8.10		46.62 = 7.23		51.62 = 6.53	
27.50 = 12.27		36.75 = 9.18		41.75 = 8.08		46.75 = 7.21		51.75 = 6.52	
27.75 = 12.16		36.87 = 9.15		41.87 = 8.06		46.87 = 7.20		51.87 = 6.50	
28.00 = 12.05		37.00 = 9.12		42.00 = 8.03		47.00 = 7.18		52.00 = 6.49	
28.25 = 11.94		37.12 = 9.09		42.12 = 8.01		47.12 = 7.16		52.12 = 6.47	
28.50 = 11.84		37.25 = 9.06		42.25 = 7.98		47.25 = 7.14		52.25 = 6.46	
28.75 = 11.74		37.37 = 9.03		42.37 = 7.96		47.37 = 7.12		52.37 = 6.44	
29.00 = 11.64		37.50 = 9.00		42.50 = 7.94		47.50 = 7.10		52.50 = 6.42	
29.25 = 11.54		37.62 = 8.97		42.62 = 7.91		47.62 = 7.08		52.62 = 6.41	
29.50 = 11.44		37.75 = 8.94		42.75 = 7.89		47.75 = 7.06		52.75 = 6.39	
29.75 = 11.34		37.87 = 8.91		42.87 = 7.87		47.87 = 7.05		52.87 = 6.38	
30.00 = 11.25		38.00 = 8.88		43.00 = 7.84		48.00 = 7.03		53.00 = 6.36	
30.25 = 11.15		38.12 = 8.85		43.12 = 7.82		48.12 = 7.01		53.12 = 6.35	
30.50 = 11.06		38.25 = 8.82		43.25 = 7.80		48.25 = 6.99		53.25 = 6.33	
30.75 = 10.97		38.37 = 8.79		43.37 = 7.78		48.37 = 6.97		53.37 = 6.32	
31.00 = 10.88		38.50 = 8.76		43.50 = 7.75		48.50 = 6.95		53.50 = 6.30	
31.25 = 10.79		38.62 = 8.73		43.62 = 7.73		48.62 = 6.94		53.62 = 6.29	
31.50 = 10.71		38.75 = 8.70		43.75 = 7.71		48.75 = 6.92		53.75 = 6.27	
31.75 = 10.63		38.87 = 8.68		43.87 = 7.69		48.87 = 6.90		53.87 = 6.26	
32.00 = 10.54		39.00 = 8.65		44.00 = 7.67		49.00 = 6.88		54.00 = 6.25	
32.25 = 10.46		39.12 = 8.62		44.12 = 7.64		49.12 = 6.87		54.12 = 6.23	
32.50 = 10.41		39.25 = 8.59		44.25 = 7.62		49.25 = 6.85		54.25 = 6.22	
32.75 = 10.30		39.37 = 8.57		44.37 = 7.60		49.37 = 6.83		54.37 = 6.20	
33.00 = 10.22		39.50 = 8.54		44.50 = 7.58		49.50 = 6.81		54.50 = 6.19	
33.25 = 10.15		39.62 = 8.51		44.62 = 7.56		49.62 = 6.80		54.62 = 6.17	
33.50 = 10.07		39.75 = 8.49		44.75 = 7.54		49.75 = 6.78		54.75 = 6.16	
33.75 = 10.00		39.87 = 8.45		44.87 = 7.52		49.87 = 6.76		54.87 = 6.15	
34.00 = 9.92		40.00 = 8.43		45.00 = 7.50		50.00 = 6.75		55.00 = 6.13	
34.25 = 9.85		40.12 = 8.41		45.12 = 7.48		50.12 = 6.73		55.12 = 6.12	
34.50 = 9.78		40.25 = 8.38		45.25 = 7.45		50.25 = 6.71		55.25 = 6.10	
34.75 = 9.71		40.37 = 8.36		45.37 = 7.43		50.37 = 6.70		55.37 = 6.09	
35.00 = 9.64		40.50 = 8.33		45.50 = 7.41		50.50 = 6.68		55.50 = 6.08	
35.25 = 9.57		40.62 = 8.30		45.62 = 7.39		50.62 = 6.66		55.62 = 6.06	
35.50 = 9.50		40.75 = 8.28		45.75 = 7.37		50.75 = 6.65		55.75 = 6.05	
35.75 = 9.44		40.87 = 8.25		45.87 = 7.35		50.87 = 6.63		55.87 = 6.04	

From Conforma Laboratories, Inc. By permission.

3. The keratometry measurements are recorded in diopters.

4. A lens diameter is selected that provides 1 to 2 mm of overlap at the limbus. An average soft contact lens diameter is 14.00 mm.

5. Table 9–3 can be used to determine the initial base curve (D). Soft lenses are fit flatter than rigid lenses. According to Table 9–3, the lens usually fits 3.5 to 4.5 D flatter than K, using an average-diameter lens (13 to 14 mm). The base curve is converted from diopters to millimeters with Table 9–4. For the trial lens, it is best to err on the side of using a flatter lens.

6. After the appropriate trial lens is placed on the eye, 15 to 20 minutes should pass before the fit is assessed. An adequate fit should show at least 1 mm of movement with one complete blink before the lens glides back into position.

If there is inadequate movement, the fit is probably too tight and the contact lens will need to be flattened by decreasing the diameter or flattening the base curve (that is, increasing the radius of curvature). If there is excessive movement, the fit is probably too loose and the diameter should be increased or the base curve steepened (that is, the radius of curvature should be decreased).

7. When an adequate fit is achieved, a refraction is performed with the trial lens in place ("over-refraction") to determine the final desired power.

As an example, the fitting of a daily-wear soft contact lens with a 38% water content and 13.8-mm diameter is outlined below.

The refraction is $-3.50\bigcirc +0.50 \times 90°$; keratometry is $42.00/42.50 \times 90°$.

1. The refraction is converted to minus cylinder: $-3.00\bigcirc -0.50 \times 180°$.

2. -3.25 is used for contact lens power (spheroequivalent).

3. K = 42.00 (K is the lower keratometry reading of the two principal meridians).

4. The lens diameter in this example is 13.8 mm.

5. From Table 9–3: a 13.8-mm lens fits 4.00 D below K. Therefore, $42.00 - 4.00 = 38.00$ D = 8.88 mm (Table 9–4). One should choose the manufacturer's closest base curve, erring on the flatter side.

6. A trial lens of 13.8-mm diameter, -3.25 D power, and 8.9-mm base curve is selected. The diameter or base curve is adjusted, depending on movement and fit of the contact lens.

7. Over-refraction for final desired power.

Gas-permeable rigid lenses have better oxygen transmission than PMMA lenses and thus have increased comfort and more rapid adaptation. Although newer materials are always being developed, the "rule of thumb" fitting will be discussed for an average gas-permeable lens (35% silicone with PMMA; Dk = 16; diameter, 9.0 mm).

1. The refraction is determined in minus cylinder.

2. The sphere power only is used and modified for vertex distance if necessary.

3. The keratometry readings are recorded in diopters.

4. A diameter is selected so that the upper edge of the contact lens rides under the upper lid. An average diameter is 9.0 mm. A smaller diameter (8.5 mm) is used with steep corneas, small pupils, and narrow fissures. A larger diameter (9.5 mm) is chosen with flat corneas, large pupils, and high astigmatism (3 to 4 D).

5. The base curve is determined by taking one-third the difference between the two keratometry readings and adding this to K. All calculations are made using diopters. One must remember to take into account the power of the tear lens.

6. The appropriate trial lens is placed on the eye and assessed after 15 to 20 minutes. An adequate fit should have at least 2 mm of movement with one complete blink to allow adequate tear pumping. If movement is excessive or inadequate, the diameter or base curve is adjusted as described in step 6 on page 243. The fluorescein pattern also helps in evaluating the fit (Fig. 9–38).

7. A trial lens is over-refracted to determine the final power.

An example is outlined below. Refraction is $-3.50\bigcirc +0.75 \times 90°$; keratometry reading is $42.00/42.75 \times 90°$.

Fig. 9–38. Fluorescein is used in a trial lens diagnostic fitting procedure to better observe the relationship between the back surface of the lens and the anterior corneal surface. Darkened areas represent the green of fluorescein; the "clear" zones represent lens/cornea approximate touch relationships.

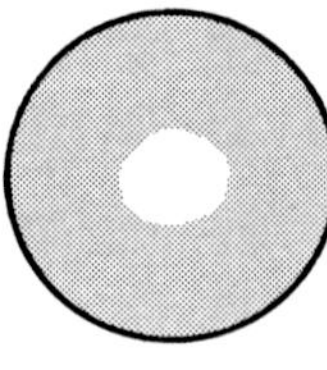

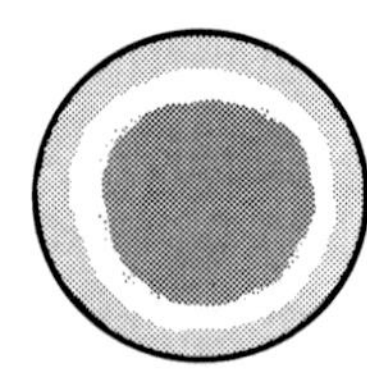

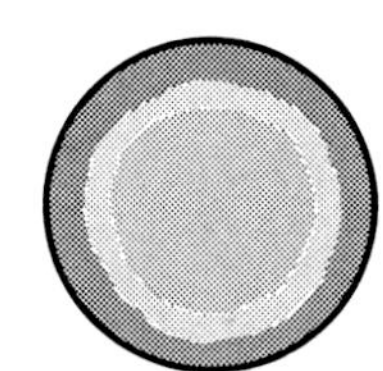

1. Refraction is converted to minus cylinder: $-2.75 \supset -0.75 \times 180°$.

2. -2.75 is used for the contact lens power (spheroequivalent).

3. Keratometry reading is $42.00/42.75 \times 90°$.

4. Lens diameter is 9.0 mm.

5. Use 42.25 for initial base curve:

$$\frac{(42.75 - 42.00)}{3} + 42.00 = 42.25$$

Because the tear lens is $+0.25$ D, one will have to compensate for this additional plus power and adjust the final trial lens power to -3.00 $(-2.75 + -0.25 = -3.00)$.

6. The trial lens is placed on the eye and modified according to its behavior on the eye.

7. Over-refraction for final desired power.

10

OCULAR MOTILITY, STRABISMUS, AND AMBLYOPIA

George G. Hohberger

The six extraocular muscles that are attached to the globe enable one to move the eyes in various directions.

Eye movements in the various directions of gaze are possible because of the six extraocular muscles that are attached to each eye (Fig. 10–1 and Table 10–1). The four *rectus muscles* (the medial, lateral, superior, and inferior) arise from a thick connective tissue ring called the *annulus of Zinn* that is located at the apex of the orbit. They pass forward along the walls of the orbit and insert into the sclera anterior to the equator of the globe at various distances from the limbus. The points of insertion of the rectus muscles are important surgical landmarks. The rectus muscles are all approximately 40 mm in length and receive their innervation at the junction of the posterior and middle one-third of the muscle. The lateral rectus is innervated by the sixth cranial (abducens) nerve. The superior rectus is innervated by the superior division of the third cranial (oculomotor) nerve. The inferior division of the third cranial nerve innervates the medial and inferior rectus muscles.

The *superior oblique* has both a muscular and a tendinous portion. The superior oblique originates from the annulus of Zinn and passes anteriorly along the superomedial wall of the orbit. It becomes tendinous approximately 10 mm before reaching the trochlea. After passing through the trochlea, the superior oblique tendon is reflected posteriorly and temporally, forming an angle of approximately 54° with the visual axis. It passes inferior to the superior rectus muscle to insert near the lateral border of the superior rectus about 13 mm from the limbus. The fourth cranial nerve (trochlear) innervates the superior oblique muscle.

The *inferior oblique* muscle originates from the periosteum of the outer crest of the lacrimal fossa located in the inferior medial aspect of the orbit. It is approximately 36 mm in length and runs posteriorly and laterally at an angle of approximately 51° to the visual axis, passing inferior to the inferior rectus muscle and inserting beneath the lateral rectus muscle approximately 12 mm posterior to the insertion of the lateral rectus. The inferior oblique muscle is innervated by the inferior division of the third cranial nerve.

The globe can rotate about its center of rotation on one of three axes: the X, Y, and Z axes of Fick.

The globe can rotate about its center of rotation on one of three axes, called the *axes of Fick* and designated as X, Y, and Z (Fig. 10–2). The

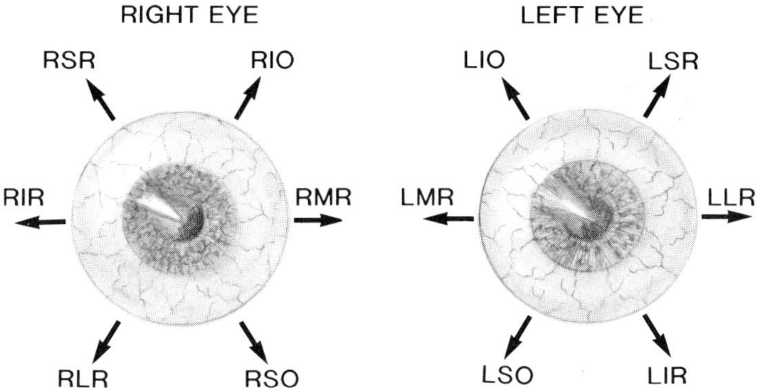

Fig. 10–1. The primary actions of the extraocular muscles. Left eye: LSR, left superior rectus; LLR, left lateral rectus; LIR, left inferior rectus; LSO, left superior oblique; LMR, left medial rectus; LIO, left inferior oblique. Right eye: RIO, right inferior oblique; RMR, right medial rectus; RSO, right superior oblique; RLR, right lateral rectus; RIR, right inferior rectus; RSR, right superior rectus.

X axis is a transverse axis, and vertical rotations of the eye take place about this axis, such as sursumduction (elevation) and deorsumduction (depression). The Y axis is a sagittal axis, and torsional rotation occurs about this axis, such as incycloduction (intorsion) and excycloduction (extorsion). The Z axis is a vertical axis, and horizontal rotations—such as adduction and abduction—take place about this axis (Fig. 10–3). The imaginary plane that passes vertically through the center of rotation and is coplanar with both the "X" and "Z" axes is called *Listing's plane.*

A single eye muscle may cause movement in more than one direction. The primary action of the superior rectus is elevation, but because of the angle at which it inserts into the sclera it has secondary actions of adduction and incycloduction (Fig. 10–4). The primary action of the inferior rectus muscle is depression, and its secondary actions are adduction and excycloduction (Fig. 10–5). The superior oblique tendon inserts into the sclera on the temporal portion of the globe, and its insertion is also behind the center of rotation (Fig. 10–6). Therefore, its primary action is incycloduction, and its secondary actions are depression and abduction. The inferior oblique muscle inserts

TABLE 10–1 Extraocular Muscles

Muscle	*Length, mm*	*Origin*	*Insertion*	*Innervation*
Medial rectus	40	Annulus of Zinn	5.5 mm posterior to medial limbus	Inferior division of third cranial nerve
Lateral rectus	40	Annulus of Zinn	6.9 mm posterior to lateral limbus	Sixth cranial nerve
Superior rectus	40	Annulus of Zinn	7.7 mm posterior to superior limbus	Superior division of third cranial nerve
Inferior rectus	40	Annulus of Zinn	6.5 mm posterior to inferior limbus	Inferior division of third cranial nerve
Superior oblique	Muscle, 30 Tendon, 30	Orbital apex above annulus of Zinn	Superotemporal quadrant posterior to equator	Fourth cranial nerve
Inferior oblique	36	Outer crest of lacrimal fossa	Inferotemporal quadrant posterior to equator	Inferior division of third cranial nerve

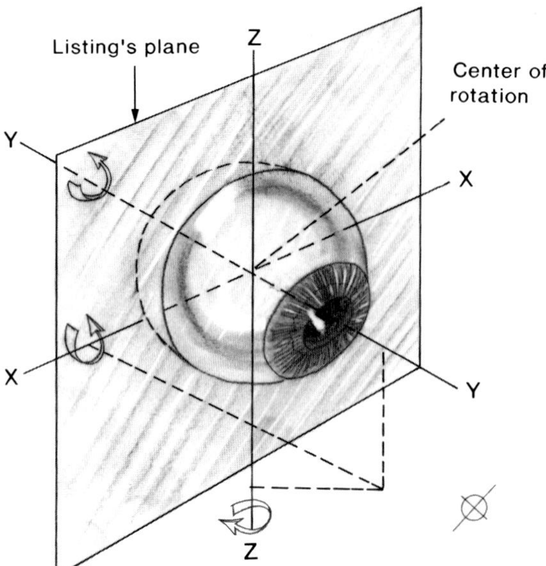

Fig. 10–2. Axes of Fick and Listing's plane.

on the temporal portion of the globe inferiorly behind the center of rotation and as a result has a primary action of excycloduction with secondary actions of elevation and abduction (Fig. 10–7). One should note that the superior muscles are intorters and the inferior muscles are extorters. In addition, the vertical rectus muscles are adductors and the oblique muscles are abductors (Table 10–2).

The term *"duction"* is used to describe movements of one eye. For example, adduction of the right eye means that the right eye rotates toward the nose. Two different terms are used to describe the movement of the two eyes together. *Versions* is used to describe conjugate movements of the eyes, that is, when the eyes move simultaneously in the same direction (for example, right gaze, left gaze, upgaze, and downgaze). *Vergence* is used to describe movements that are disconjugate, that is, when the eyes move simultaneously in opposite directions. Convergence is movement of both eyes inward (as in reading). Divergence is a movement of both eyes outward. Incyclovergence and excyclovergence are rotational vergence movements.

The finely tuned integration of agonist, antagonist, synergist, and yoke muscle activity results in smooth, steady, and coordinated eye movements. The muscle that is primarily responsible for rotating an eye in a given direction is called the *agonist*. For example, in adduction the medial rectus is the agonist. The *antagonist* is the muscle in the same eye as the agonist that rotates the eye in a direction opposite that of the agonist. For example, the medial rectus and the lateral rectus are antagonists. The muscle in the same eye as the agonist that acts with the agonist to rotate the eye in a given direction is called a *synergist*. For example, the superior oblique muscle is a synergist with the inferior rectus muscle in the depression of the eye, and the inferior oblique muscle is a synergist with a superior rectus muscle in

Right Eye Viewed From Above

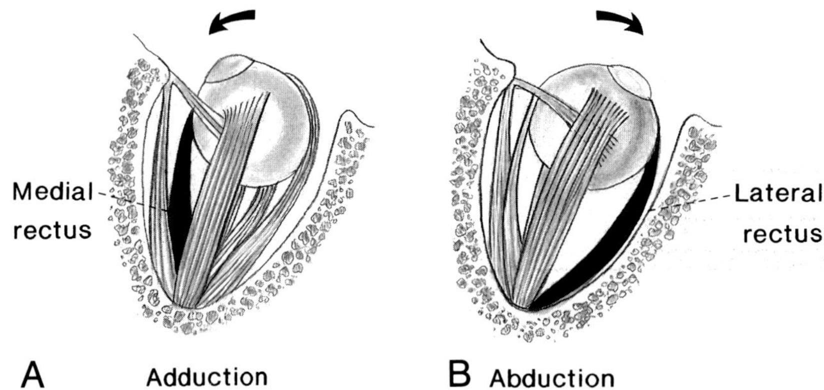

Fig. 10–3. Horizontal rectus muscles of the right eye. *A*, Contraction of right medial rectus results in adduction of the eye. *B*, Contraction of right lateral rectus results in abduction of the eye.

Right Eye Viewed From Above

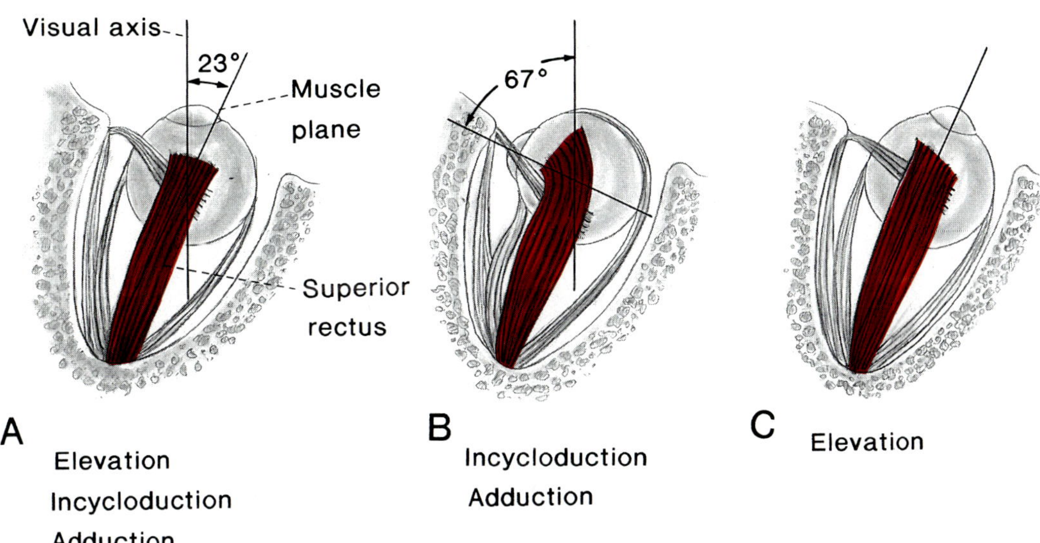

Fig. 10–4. Superior rectus muscle of right eye. *A*, With the eye in the primary position, the primary action is elevation and the secondary actions are incycloduction and adduction. *B*, With the eye in adduction, the primary action is incycloduction and secondary action is adduction. *C*, With the eye in abduction, the superior rectus is primarily an elevator. (Modified from G.K. von Noorden: Atlas of Strabismus, 4th ed. St. Louis, C.V. Mosby Company, 1983, p. 3.)

Right Eye Viewed From Below

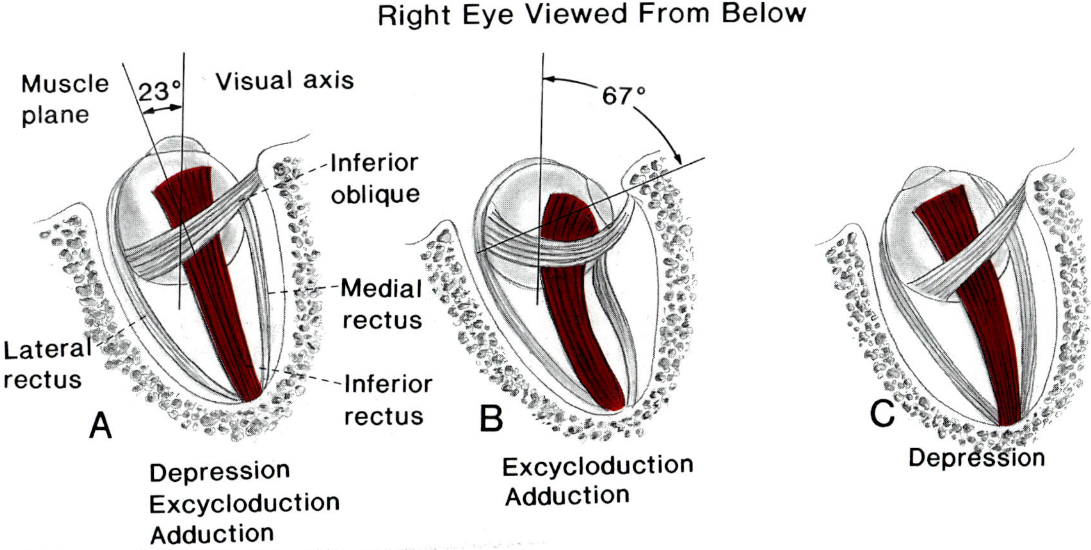

Fig. 10–5. Inferior rectus muscle of right eye. *A*, With the eye in the primary position, the primary action is depression, and the secondary actions are excycloduction and adduction. *B*, With the eye in adduction, the primary action is excycloduction and secondary action is adduction. *C*, With the eye in abduction, the inferior rectus is primarily a depressor. (Modified from G.K. von Noorden: Atlas of Strabismus, 4th ed. St. Louis, C.V. Mosby Company, 1983, p. 5.)

Right Eye Viewed From Above

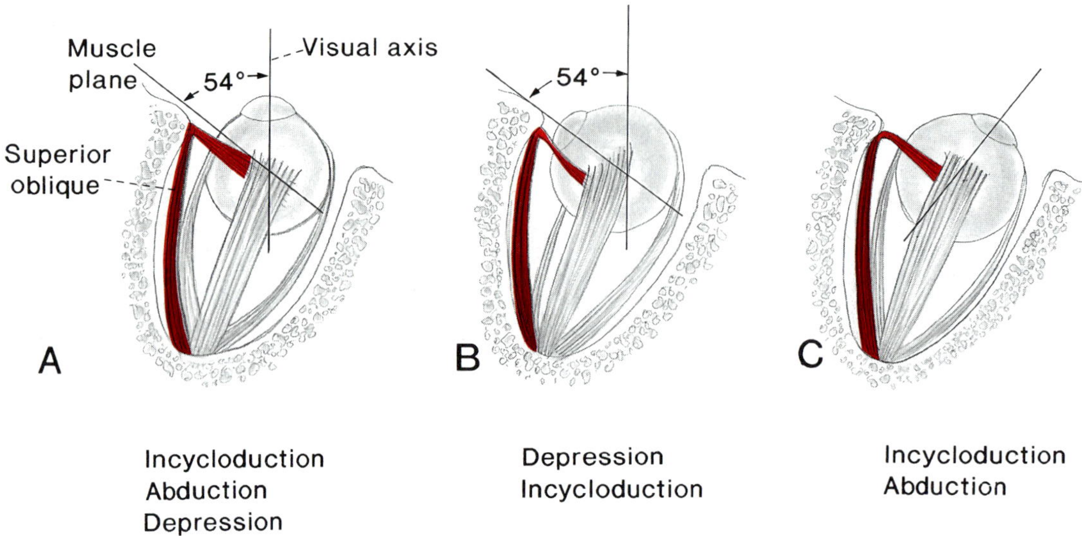

Fig. 10–6. Superior oblique muscle-tendon complex. *A*, With the eye in the primary position, the primary action is incycloduction, and the secondary actions are abduction and depression. *B*, With the eye in adduction, the primary action is depression and the secondary action is incycloduction. *C*, With the eye in abduction, the primary action is incycloduction and the secondary action is abduction. (Modified from G.K. von Noorden: Atlas of Strabismus, 4th ed. St. Louis, C.V. Mosby Company, 1983, p. 7.)

Right Eye Viewed From Below

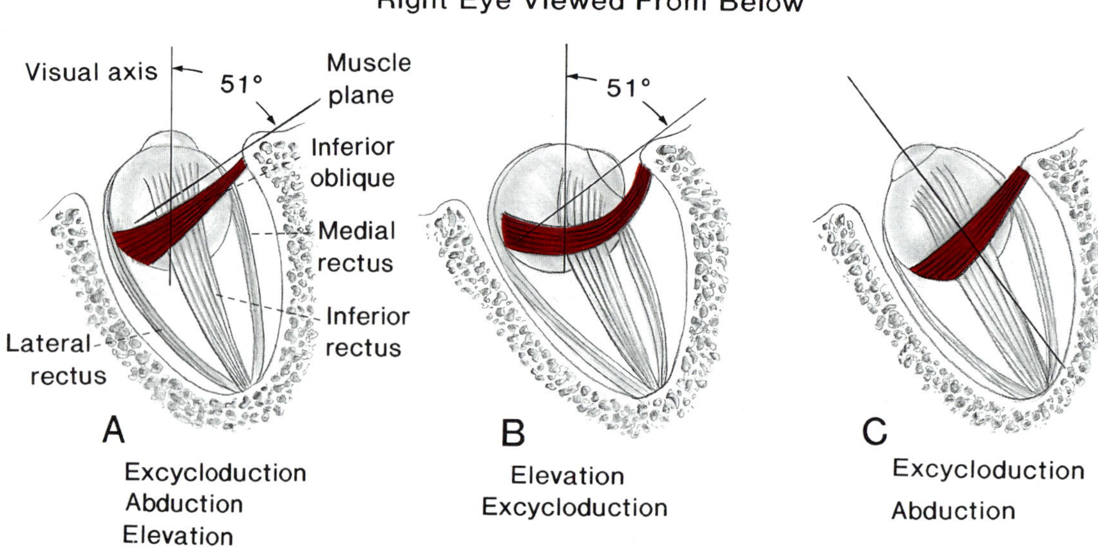

Fig. 10–7. Inferior oblique muscle of right eye. *A*, With the eye in the primary position, the primary action is excycloduction, and the secondary actions are abduction and elevation. *B*, With the eye in adduction, the primary action is elevation and the secondary action is excycloduction. *C*, With the eye in abduction, the primary action is excycloduction and the secondary action is abduction. (Modified from G.K. von Noorden: Atlas of Strabismus, 4th ed. St. Louis, C.V. Mosby Company, 1983, p. 9.)

TABLE 10–2 Action of the Extraocular Muscles in Primary Position

Muscle	Action		
	Primary	*Secondary*	*Tertiary*
Medial rectus	Adduction	—	—
Lateral rectus	Abduction	—	—
Superior rectus	Elevation	Incycloduction	Adduction
Inferior rectus	Depression	Excycloduction	Adduction
Superior oblique	Incycloduction	Depression	Abduction
Inferior oblique	Excycloduction	Elevation	Abduction

elevation of the eye. Muscles (one in each eye) that cause the two eyes to move in the same direction are known as *yoke muscles*. Each extraocular muscle in one eye has a yoke muscle in the fellow eye. For example, in right gaze the left medial rectus muscle and the right lateral rectus muscle are yoke muscles. Gaze to the left teams the right medial rectus and left lateral rectus. The yoke muscles for gaze up and to the left are the right inferior oblique and the left superior rectus; for gaze up and to the right, they are the left inferior oblique and the right superior rectus; for gaze down and to the right, they are the right inferior rectus and the left superior oblique; and for gaze down and to the left, they are the left inferior rectus and the right superior oblique. These six positions are known as the cardinal positions of gaze (Fig. 10–8).

Nerve impulses are not sent to just one extraocular muscle in isolation. Whenever a nerve impulse is sent out for the purpose of moving the eyes in a particular direction, corresponding muscles of each eye receive equal innervation to contract or relax. Whenever an agonist receives an impulse to contract, an equivalent inhibitory impulse is sent to its antagonist, which then relaxes. This inhibition of the antagonist is known as *Sherrington's law of reciprocal innervation*. Likewise, when a nerve impulse is sent to an agonist, equal and simultaneous innervation flows to the synergists and to the yoke muscles that are concerned with moving the eye or eyes in the desired direction of gaze. This equal and simultaneous innervation of synergists and yoke muscles is called *Hering's law of motor correspondence*.

Corresponding retinal points in each eye allow for stereopsis in aligned eyes and cause double vision in nonaligned eyes.

The ocular motor system provides the ability to place the image of the object of regard on the fovea and the ability to keep the image on the fovea if the object of regard should be in motion. If a person's eyes are straight, the image of the object of regard will fall on the fovea of each eye, and the image of an object in the peripheral visual field will fall on peripheral retinal points in each eye called corresponding retinal points. These *corresponding retinal points* share a common visual direction.

Each and every retinal point in one eye has a corresponding retinal point in the fellow eye. If a person has straight eyes, images that stimulate corresponding retinal points will cause similar visual sensations to be sent to the brain from each eye. The brain has the ability to take the sensation from each eye and to unify these two sensations into a single visual perception (called *sensory fusion* or *single binocular vision*). Most individuals who have sensory fusion also

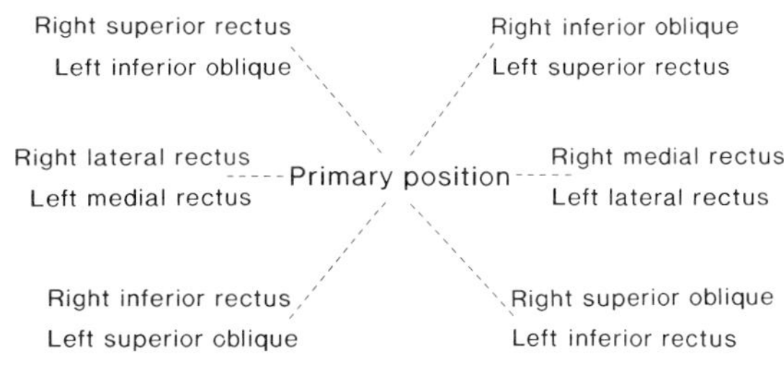

Fig. 10–8. Yoke muscles move the eyes into the cardinal positions of gaze.

have *stereopsis* (the perception that visual space has a three-dimensional quality).

If a person's eyes are not straight, the image produced by an object in the visual field will fall on noncorresponding points in each eye. When noncorresponding retinal points are stimulated, diplopia results. *Diplopia* is the perception that the same object is located in two different directions in space (double vision). Diplopia is a troublesome ocular symptom.

Children younger than 10 years whose visual system is still immature rarely complain about diplopia. Two adaptive mechanisms help them to eliminate diplopia. The first mechanism is called *suppression*. Suppression seems to occur at the level of the visual cortex. When the suppression mechanism is activated, it appears that cells in the visual cortex are able to ignore or suppress visual sensations coming from the deviating eye. The second mechanism that helps a youngster to avoid diplopia is called *anomalous retinal correspondence*. It is a complex and poorly understood concept. It is believed that it also occurs at the level of the visual cortex. In this process cortical neurons are able to change the directional value of the noncorresponding retinal points in the deviating eye so that they now have the same directional value as the retinal points in the nondeviating eye. In other words, retinal points that were at one time noncorresponding because of an ocular deviation become corresponding retinal points despite the continued presence of the deviation.

Strabismus (misalignment of the eyes) may be comitant or noncomitant.

When an individual's eyes are not straight, the image of the object of regard falls on the fovea of the fixing eye and on a nonfoveal retinal area in the deviating eye. This person is said to have *strabismus. Tropia* is a term used to indicate a manifest misalignment of the visual axes and is synonymous with strabismus. A tropia may be alternating or unilateral, intermittent or constant. A *phoria* is a tendency for the eyes to deviate but it is kept latent by the fusion mechanism of the individual. Some degree of phoria is found in almost everyone, but usually it produces no symptoms. If the amount of

heterophoria present is large it may give rise to symptoms such as asthenopia (eye strain) or intermittent diplopia.

Strabismus can be classified in several different ways. One way to classify it is according to the direction of the deviation. If the deviating eye is rotated inward toward the nose it is called *esotropia* (Fig. 10–9). If the eye deviates outward it is called *exotropia* (Fig. 10–10). *Hypertropia* is the term used to describe the situation in which there is an upward deviation of the eye (Fig. 10–11), and *hypotropia* is a downward deviation of the eye (Fig. 10–12).

Another way of categorizing strabismus is based on comitancy. *Comitant strabismus* is one in which the angle of deviation is the same in

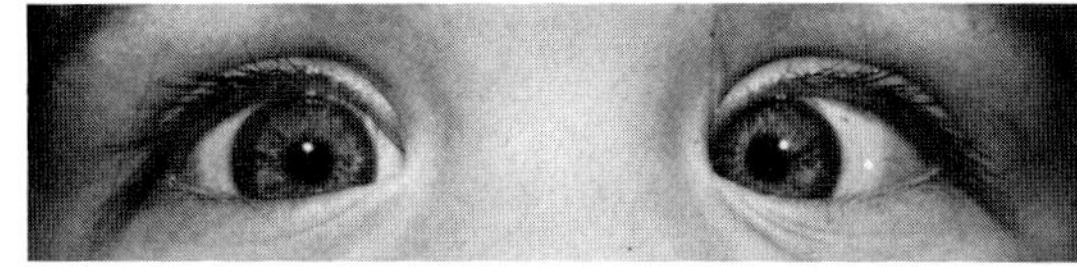

Fig. 10–9. Esotropia. The patient is fixing with the right eye and the deviating left eye is turned inward.

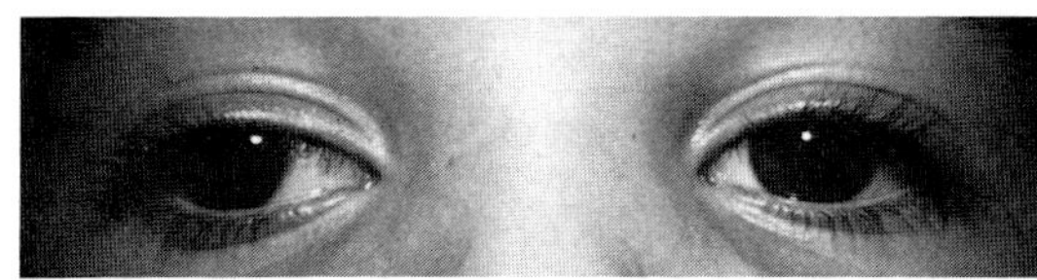

Fig. 10–10. Exotropia. The patient is fixing with the left eye and the deviating right eye is directed outward.

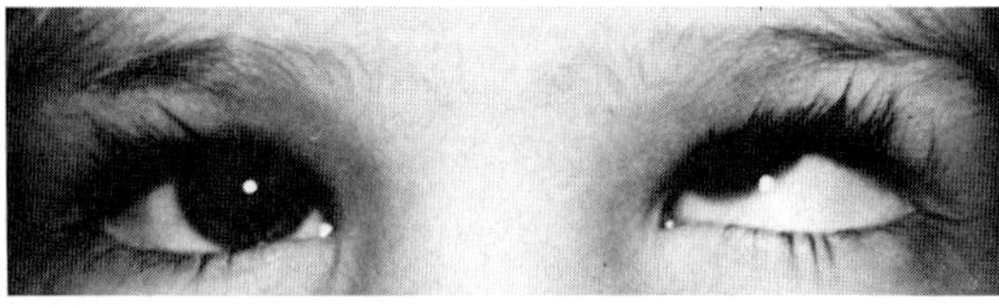

Fig. 10–11. Hypertropia. The patient is fixing with the right eye and the left eye is turned upward.

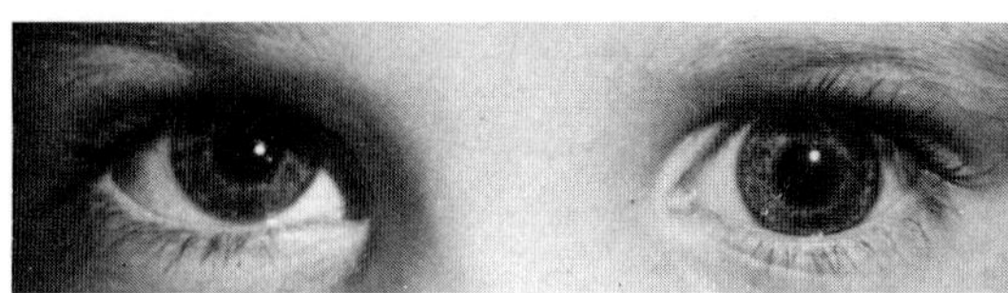

Fig. 10–12. Hypotropia. The patient is fixing with the right eye and the left eye is turned downward.

all directions of gaze. Most of the strabismus problems occurring in childhood are the comitant type. Diplopia and an abnormal head posture are rare findings in comitant strabismus, and there is usually no associated neurologic disease.

Noncomitant strabismus, however, is one in which the angle of deviation varies or changes with the direction in which the patient is looking. For example, an individual with a left sixth nerve palsy usually has an esotropia (left eye turned inward because of a weak lateral rectus) in the primary position, that is, the fixing right eye looks straight ahead (Fig. 10–13). On gaze to the left the amount of esotropia will increase because of the weak left lateral rectus muscle. However, on gaze to the right there will be no crossing of the eyes. Diplopia and abnormal head position are common in this type of strabismus. Noncomitant deviations are usually due to weakness of an extraocular muscle secondary to a cranial nerve deficit or are due to restriction of movement of the globe secondary to some local orbital abnormality, such as an orbital fracture. If an individual has had previous single binocular vision and then develops a noncomitant strabismus, it is likely that that individual will turn his or her head in whatever direction is necessary in order to re-

gain binocular function. This fact leads to an important clinical point. Any individual who consistently assumes an abnormal head position may have a noncomitant strabismus. Another important clinical point to keep in mind is that strabismus will frequently be a presenting sign in a child with organic eye disease.

Any condition that significantly reduces central visual acuity can disrupt fusion and result in an ocular deviation. Disorders such as retinoblastoma or congenital cataract frequently present with strabismus. Once a diagnosis of strabismus is made or suspected, a complete eye examination should be performed to rule out the presence of an intraocular abnormality.

In some individuals, and especially in children, certain anatomic features about the eyes and the orbits can create the appearance of strabismus when in fact there is none (*pseudostrabismus*). Factors such as a narrow interpupillary distance and prominent epicanthal folds can make a child who has straight eyes look esotropic (Fig. 10–14), and such conditions as hypertelorism or telecanthus can make a child with straight eyes look exotropic (Fig. 10–15).

The history provides valuable clues to the cause of strabismus.

The evaluation of a patient with strabismus begins with a thorough history. The examiner should attempt to characterize the deviation.

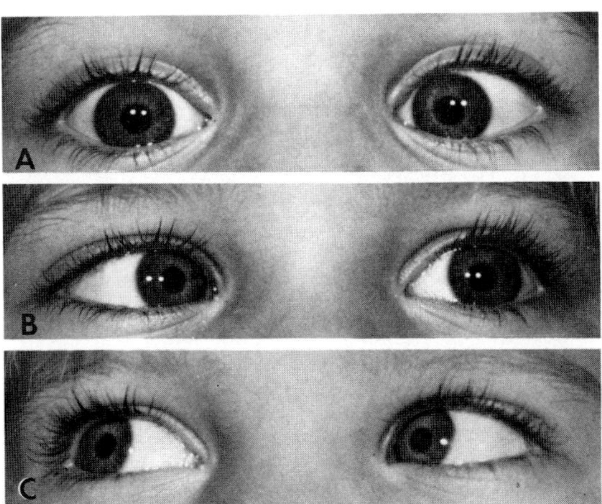

Fig. 10–13. *A*, A 3-year-old child with an acquired sixth nerve palsy of the left eye secondary to meningitis has a noncomitant esotropia. In the primary position she has a left esotropia. *B*, Gaze to the left demonstrates marked limitation of abduction of the left eye. *C*, Gaze to the right is normal.

Fig. 10–14. Patient with pseudoesotropia caused by wide nasal bridge and very prominent epicanthal folds.

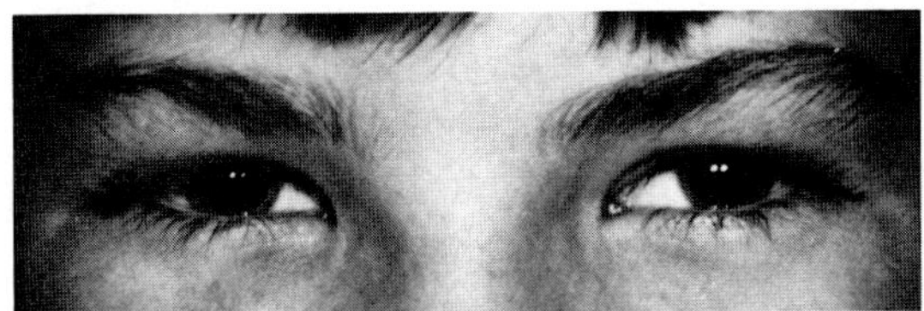

Fig. 10–15. Pseudoexotropia in a child with telecanthus.

Does the deviating eye turn in or turn out? Is there any vertical deviation? Is the deviation present constantly or only intermittently? An intermittent deviation usually indicates that the patient has some fusional ability. Does the deviation seem to occur more frequently with distance fixation or with near fixation? In patients with intermittent exotropia, the non-preferred deviating eye will become exotropic only with distance fixation. These patients usually do not demonstrate an exotropia at near fixation because accommodative convergence helps them to keep the eye from drifting out. In contrast, patients with an accommodative esotropia with a high accommodative convergence to accommodation ratio usually have little or no deviation with distance fixation, but they develop an obvious esotropia when focusing on near objects.

Is the deviation unilateral, or does it alternate between the two eyes? The nonfixing (deviating) eye may have poor vision either because of amblyopia or because of an organic ocular disease. An alternating fixation pattern between the right eye and the left eye usually indicates that the vision is essentially equal in each eye. The onset of the deviation should be documented. If it can be documented that the strabismus was congenital and not acquired, then additional diagnostic procedures such as a neurologic examination and computed tomography or magnetic resonance imaging usually are not indicated. Reviewing old photographs can be helpful, for they often show that the deviation in question has been present for a much longer time than was realized.

Previous treatment for strabismus should be documented. This would include the use of glasses, patching, orthoptic exercises, and any eye muscle operation. Heredity seems to be a definite factor in strabismus.

The examination begins with assessment of visual acuity to determine whether amblyopia is present.

The visual acuity should be measured to determine whether amblyopia is present. Amblyopia is frequently associated with strabismus, and the key to successful amblyopia therapy is early diagnosis and treatment. Strabismus may be the presenting sign in a patient with poor vision in one eye secondary to some ocular lesion (*sensory* or *secondary strabismus*). A complete dilated eye examination is necessary.

The ductions and versions should be scrutinized to determine whether there is any abnormality of ocular motility and whether the deviation is comitant or noncomitant. Assessing the deviation involves determining whether an esodeviation, exodeviation, or vertical deviation is present and then attempting to quantitate the amount of misalignment.

Determining the refractive error (with cycloplegia) is a crucial step in evaluating a patient with strabismus because accommodation plays a significant role in some types of strabismus. In a patient with accommodative esotropia, uncorrected hyperopia is a significant factor that contributes to the deviation. In a patient with an intermittent exotropia who has a significant degree of myopia, full correction of the myopia may help to control the deviation.

The tests that are used most often to determine ocular alignment are the corneal reflection tests and the cover test.

The *corneal reflection tests* make use of the fact that the anterior corneal surface acts like a highly polished convex mirror. When a light source such as a hand-held fixation light or a penlight is directed toward the cornea, it produces a virtual image of that light source. In most patients with foveal fixation, this reflected image is located slightly nasal to the center of the pupil (Fig. 10–16). The *angle kappa* is defined as the angle between the visual

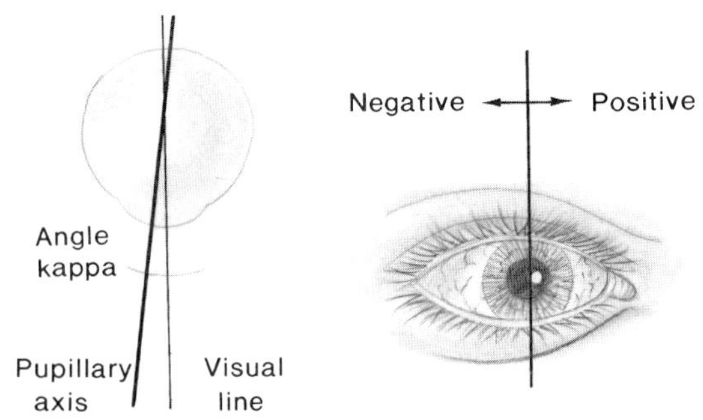

Fig. 10–16. Angle kappa.

line (the line connecting the object and the image on the fovea passing through the nodal point) and the pupillary axis (the line that goes through the center of the pupil perpendicular to the surface of the cornea). When the angle kappa is positive the light reflection is displaced nasally, whereas when the angle kappa is negative the light reflection is displaced temporally. A positive angle kappa of up to 5° is considered normal in emmetropic eyes.

The corneal reflection in the deviating eye will be displaced temporally in a patient with esotropia and nasally in a patient with exotropia. When the fixing eye is covered, the previously deviating eye will fix on the light and the light reflection will appear in the normal position. If eccentric fixation is present in the deviating eye the reflection will remain displaced when the fellow eye is covered. In some pathologic conditions such as retinopathy of prematurity and *ocular toxocariasis*, the macula may be displaced from its normal position because of retinal traction. Temporal displace-

ment of the macula results in a large positive angle kappa that simulates an exotropia.

The two reflection tests that are used most often are the Hirschberg test and the Krimsky estimate. The *Hirschberg test* attempts to quantitate the amount of deviation present (Fig. 10–17). It is based on the assumption that 1 mm of decentration of the corneal light reflection is equal to 7° or 15 Δ. If the reflection is located at the pupillary margin, which is approximately 2 mm decentration, the deviation is approximately 14° or 30 Δ. If the reflection is located at mid iris, which is about 4 mm decentration, the deviation is about 30° or 45 Δ. When the light reflection is at the limbus, a deviation of approximately 45° or 60 Δ is present. With the *Krimsky estimate*, prisms of increasing power are placed in front of the fixing eye until the light reflection is centered in the deviating eye (Fig. 10–18). The amount of prism power required to center the light is the

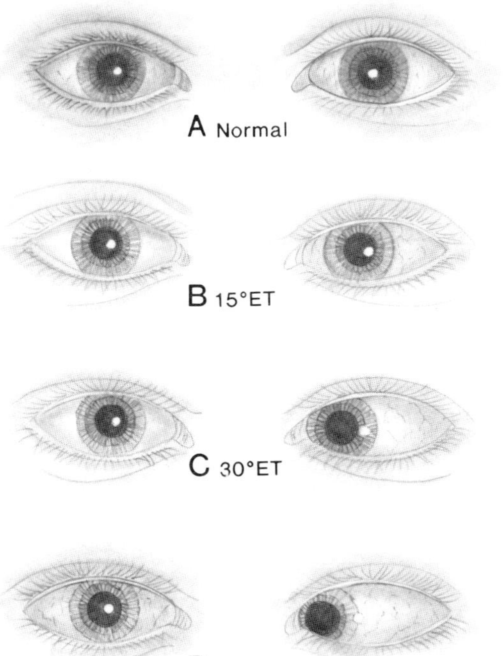

Fig. 10–17. Hirschberg test: estimation of angle of deviation by the amount of displacement of the corneal reflection in the deviating eye. ET, esotropia. (Modified from G.K. von Noorden: Atlas of Strabismus, 4th ed. St. Louis, C.V. Mosby Company, 1983, p. 45.)

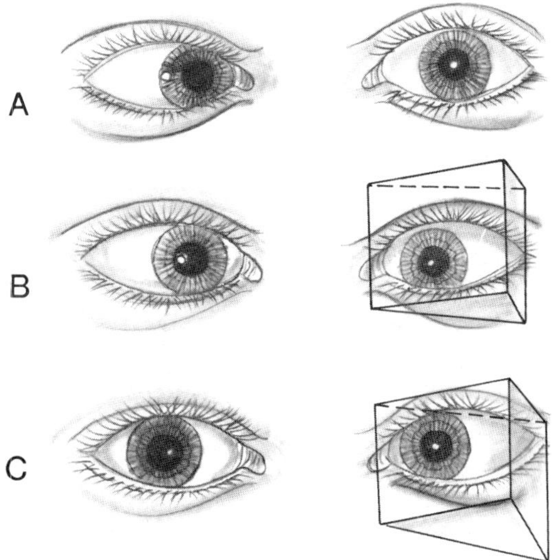

Fig. 10–18. Krimsky test. *A*, Patient with a right esotropia. *B*, Base-out prism has been placed in front of the fixing left eye. This positioning will cause the left eye to adduct and the deviating right eye to abduct (Hering's law of motor correspondence), thereby decreasing the amount of displacement of the corneal light reflection in the right eye. *C*, An increased amount of base-out prism has been placed in front of the left eye, and now the corneal light reflection in the right eye is in the normal position. The power of prism necessary to center the light reflection is equal to the amount of esotropia that is present. (Modified from G.K. von Noorden: Atlas of Strabismus, 4th ed. St. Louis, C.V. Mosby Company, 1983, p. 47.)

measure of the amount of deviation present. This test can also be performed by placing the prism in front of the deviating eye until the light reflection is centered in that eye.

The corneal reflection tests are quick and easy to perform and require only minimal cooperation on the part of the patient (Fig. 10–19). Small deviations may be missed, however, and an individual with a large positive angle kappa (but straight eyes) may be misdiagnosed as having exotropia (Fig. 10–20). These tests are performed at near fixation only. A deviation that occurs at distance fixation, such as an intermittent exotropia, will be overlooked.

The cover tests are the most accurate and most reliable tests used in the evaluation of a patient with strabismus.

The *cover tests* are performed at both near fixation (33 cm) and distance fixation (6 m), preferably with an accommodative target (Fig. 10–21 and Fig. 10–22). They require the attention and the cooperation of the patient, and they will prove valid only if the patient has central fixation. In the *cover/uncover test*, the patient fixes on a target and then one eye is covered; the examiner looks for any movement in the uncovered eye. If the uncovered eye moves outward to take up fixation, the patient has an esotropia. If the uncovered eye moves inward,

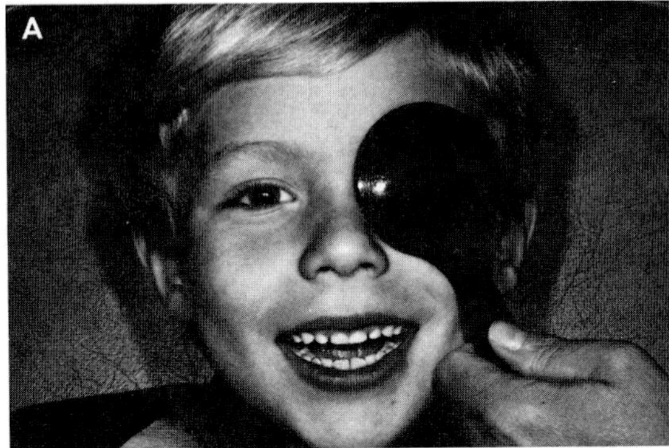

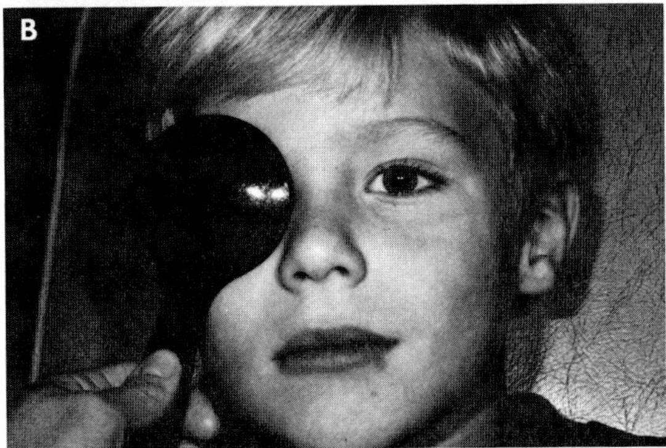

Fig. 10–21. Cover/uncover test being performed in a young child. *A,* The left eye is covered, and the examiner looks for movement of the right eye. *B,* The right eye is covered, and the left eye is observed for any movement.

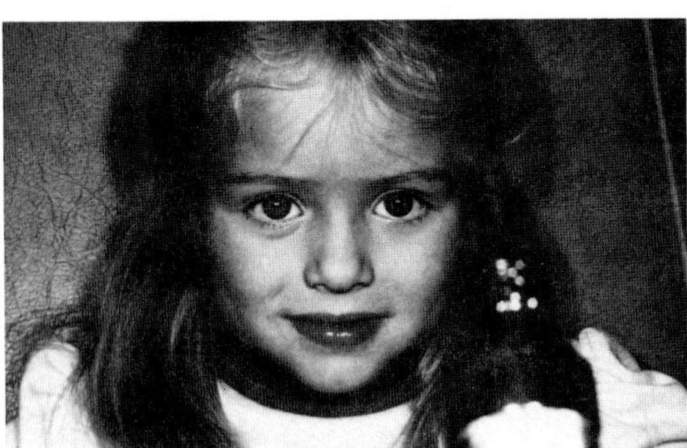

Fig. 10–19. The Hirschberg corneal reflection test. The fixation light is held one-third of a meter away from the patient in the midline and at eye level.

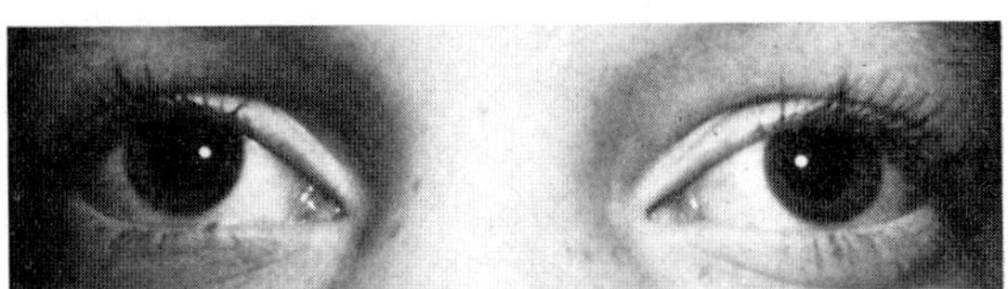

Fig. 10–20. Child with pseudoexotropia secondary to positive angle kappa.

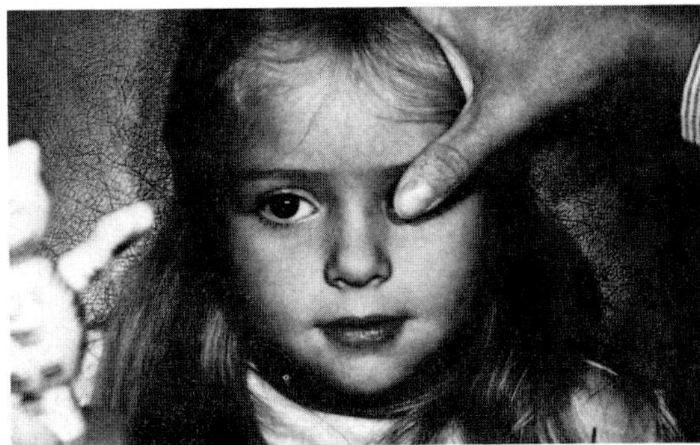

Fig. 10–22. Cover test being performed at near fixation with the examiner's thumb used as an occluder.

then the patient is exotropic; if the eye moves up or down, the patient has a vertical deviation. If the uncovered eye does not move, one can assume that that eye was fixing. The cover/uncover test is then repeated by covering the opposite eye, watching for movement in the fellow eye. If no movement is seen, the patient is said to be orthophoric.

The cover/uncover test is the only technique that can differentiate a tropia from a phoria.

In the *alternate cover test*, the occluder is placed alternately in front of each eye to dissociate the eyes and to maximize any deviation. As the cover is switched from one eye to the other, the examiner notes the movement of the uncovered eye. The alternate cover test brings out the maximal amount of deviation present, but it does not differentiate a phoria from a tropia. The cover/uncover test must be done to differentiate the phoria and tropia.

The Maddox rod and double Maddox rod tests are subjective and cannot distinguish tropia from phoria.

Two other tests that are often used in evaluating patients with strabismus are the Maddox rod and the double Maddox rod tests. These tests dissociate the eyes and produce diplopia. Horizontal, vertical, and torsional deviation can be measured. Both tests are entirely subjective (that is, they rely on patient responses), and neither test is able to differentiate a phoria from a tropia.

The *Maddox rod* consists of a series of parallel cylinders that are able to convert a point source of light into a line image. Most Maddox rods are red. When testing for a horizontal deviation (Fig. 10–23), the examiner holds the Maddox rod in front of the patient's right eye with the cylinders in the horizontal position. When the patient fixes on a point source of light, he or she will see a vertical red line with the right eye and a white light with the left eye. If the vertical line passes through the center of the white light, the patient has no deviation (orthophoric). If the red line is located to the

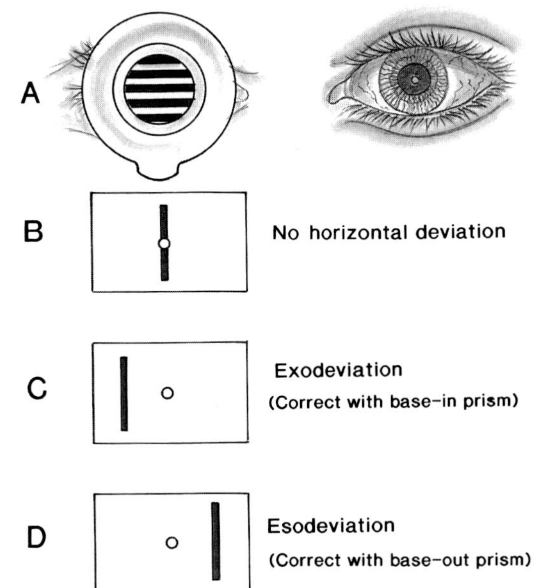

Fig. 10–23. Maddox rod test for horizontal heterophoria. (Modified from G.K. von Noorden: Atlas of Strabismus, 4th ed. St. Louis, C.V. Mosby Company, 1983, p. 53.)

right of the light, the patient has uncrossed diplopia and an esodeviation is present. If the red line is located to the left of the light, crossed diplopia is present and the patient has an exodeviation. To test for a vertical deviation (Fig. 10–24), the cylinders of the Maddox rod are oriented vertically. If the red line seen with the right eye is above the white light seen with the left eye, the right eye is lower than the left and a left hyperdeviation is present. If the red line is below the white light, a right hyperdeviation is present. The amount of deviation can be quantitated by using prisms of increasing power until the red line bisects the white light.

The *double Maddox rod* technique is used to measure torsional misalignments (cyclodeviations). The test is performed by placing a red Maddox rod in front of one eye and a white Maddox rod in front of the other. They are oriented vertically so that the patient sees a horizontal red line and a horizontal white line. A small basedown prism (4 D, for example) is placed before one eye to separate the images vertically. If a cyclodeviation is present, one of the lines will appear tilted. The patient is then asked to rotate the axis of one of the Maddox

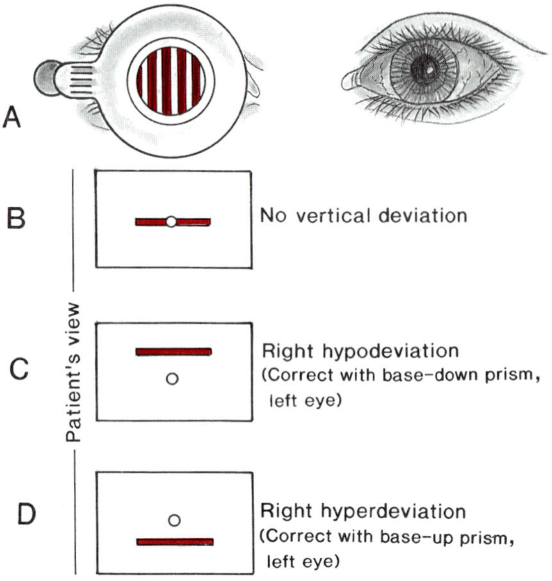

Fig. 10–24. Maddox rod test for vertical heterophoria. (Modified from G.K. von Noorden: Atlas of Strabismus, 4th ed. St. Louis, C.V. Mosby Company, 1983, p. 53.)

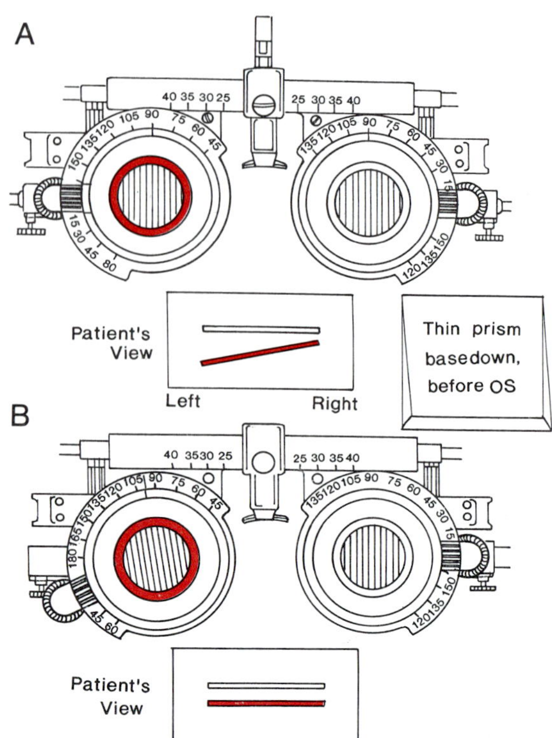

Fig. 10–25. Double Maddox rod test for cyclodeviation. *A*, Patient with a superior oblique palsy of the right eye sees the red line as being intorted. This finding indicates an excyclodeviation of the right eye. *B*, The examiner or patient rotates the axis of the red Maddox rod until the two lines are parallel. The total number of degrees that the Maddox rod is rotated away from the 90° mark on the trial frame equals the amount of cyclodeviation present. The Maddox rod has been rotated outward; this position indicates that an excyclodeviation is present. (Modified from G.K. von Noorden: Atlas of Strabismus, 4th ed. St. Louis, C.V. Mosby Company, 1983, p. 57.)

rods until the lines are horizontal and parallel. The total number of degrees that the patient rotated the Maddox rod represents the amount of cyclodeviation present (Fig. 10–25 and 10–26).

The Lancaster red-green test is most helpful for evaluating a patient with a noncomitant or paralytic strabismus.

The *Lancaster red-green test* is a subjective test and can be used only in patients with normal retinal correspondence and no suppression. The test is performed by placing red-green glasses on the patient with the red lens in front of the right eye and the green lens in front of the left eye. The patient then sits 1 m in front of a screen that contains a gridlike configuration of squares. Each square is 7 cm on a side and subtends a visual angle of 4° at a distance of 1 m. While the patient's head is held steady, the examiner uses a special hand-held projector to shine a slit of red light onto the screen. The patient is then asked to superimpose a green

slit of light, produced by the projector that he or she is holding, onto the red slit. The relative positions of the red slit and the green slit are recorded by the examiner. This process is then repeated in the cardinal positions of gaze. The patient can switch the hand-held projectors to perform the test with the left eye fixing. With the Lancaster red-green tests, one can obtain a diagrammatic record that shows the direction of gaze with the greatest amount of deviation and also shows both primary and secondary deviation. The tests can be repeated at intervals to document progression or recovery from a paralytic strabismus.

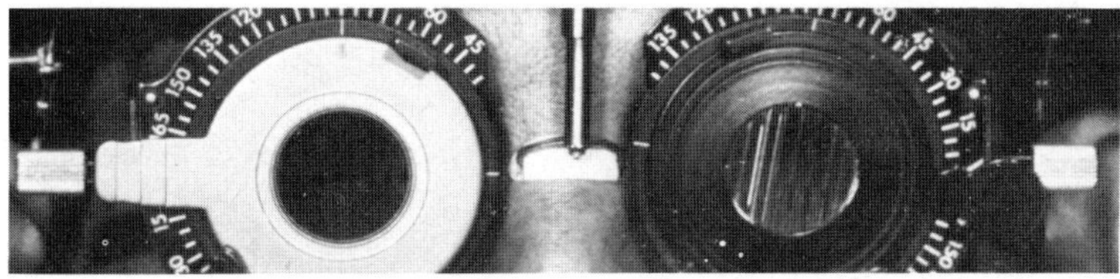

Fig. 10–26.   Double Maddox rod test in a patient with a left superior oblique palsy. Two Maddox rods, red on the patient's right and white on the patient's left, are positioned in a trial frame. Note the alignment of the Maddox rod in front of the patient's left eye. This indicates that an excyclodeviation of approximately 8° to 9° is present.

The diagnostic techniques that are most often used to evaluate a patient's sensory status are the Worth four-dot test, the Bagolini glasses, and the stereoscopic acuity test.

The *Worth four-dot test* (Fig. 10–27) is used to determine whether the patient has periph-eral fusion and whether suppression is present. Red-green glasses are worn by the patient, and a target consisting of two green lights, one red light, and one white light is then presented to the patient. With the right eye behind the red lens the patient will see two red lights, and with the eye behind the green lens the patient will see three green lights. If the patient has normal fusion, he or she will respond by saying

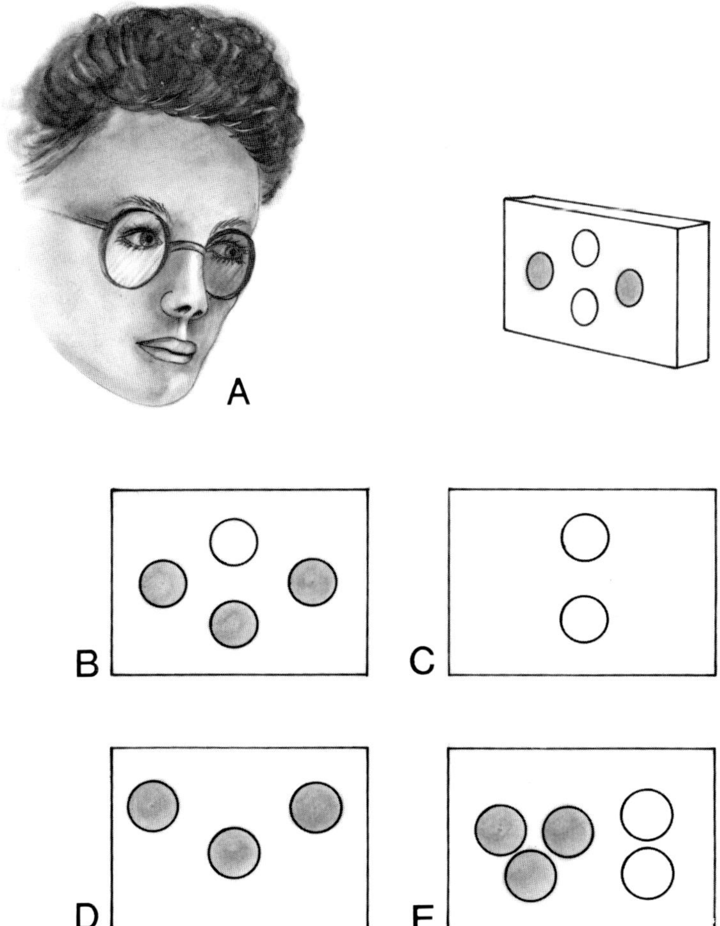

Fig. 10–27.   Worth four-dot test. *A,* Patient looking at the target with a red lens over the right eye and a green lens over the left eye. *B,* Patient sees four dots—an indication that peripheral fusion is present. *C,* Patient sees only two red dots—an indication of suppression of the left eye. *D,* Patient sees only three green dots—an indication of suppression of the right eye. *E,* Patient sees five dots simultaneously—an indication of diplopia.

that there are four lights—one red, two green, and one (the white light) that may appear to be a fluctuating mixture of red and green. If suppression is present, however, the patient will respond by saying that only two red lights are seen (indicating suppression of the left eye behind the green lens) or only three green lights are seen (indicating suppression of the right eye behind the red lens). If the patient reports seeing five lights—two red and three green—then diplopia is present.

Bagolini glasses (Fig. 10–28) are used primarily to assess retinal correspondence. They can also supply information regarding the presence of fusion or suppression. Bagolini glasses consist of plano lenses that are etched with very fine parallel striations. By convention, the stri-

ations are usually oriented at 135° in the right eye and 45° in the left eye. These striated lenses convert a point source of light into a streak of light, the axis of which is 90° to the axes of the striations. The optical principle is the same as that with the Maddox rod. The primary advantage of the Bagolini glasses is that they permit assessment of retinal correspondence under conditions that closely simulate normal seeing. With the Bagolini glasses in place, the patient looks at a fixation light either at 6 m or at 33 cm. The patient will see a streak of white light oriented at 45° with the right eye and a streak oriented at 135° with the left eye. If the two light streaks cross at their centers and form an X and if the patient has no deviation and has central fixation, then normal retinal correspon-

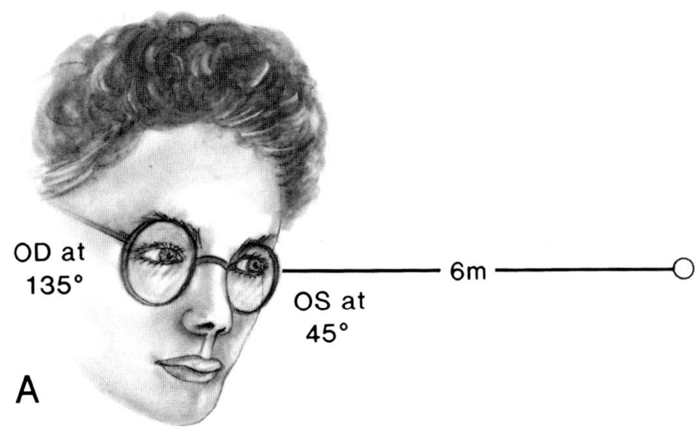

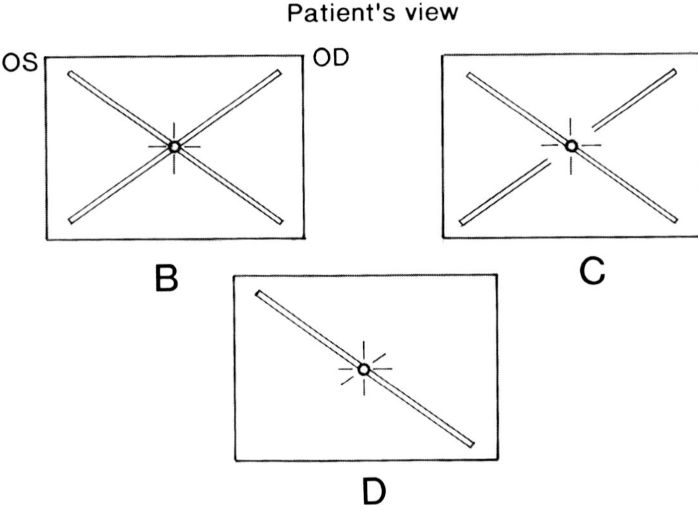

Fig. 10–28. Bagolini glasses. *A*, Patient wearing Bagolini glasses is looking at a fixation light 6 m away. *B*, If the patient has no tropia on cover test, this configuration of the two lines would indicate normal retinal correspondence. However, if the patient does have a tropia on the cover test, this same configuration would mean that anomalous retinal correspondence is present. *C*, The central gap in the line seen by the right eye indicates that foveal suppression is present in that eye. *D*, Only the line seen by the patient's left eye is present. This finding indicates both foveal and peripheral suppression of the right eye. OD, right eye; OS, left eye. (Modified from G.K. von Noorden: Atlas of Strabismus, 4th ed. St. Louis, C.V. Mosby Company, 1983, p. 95.)

dence is present. If, however, the patient does have a deviation, as demonstrated by a cover test, and still sees the two light streaks in the form of an X, then anomalous retinal correspondence is present. Inability to see all or a portion of the projected line indicates a suppression scotoma.

Measuring the stereoscopic acuity can be helpful in assessing the binocular status of a patient. The most commonly used test for stereo vision is the *Titmus stereo test*. This test uses disparate polarized pictures that, when viewed with polaroid lenses, create a stereoscopic affect. Stereopsis is measured in seconds of arc. This test is able to measure stereoacuity as gross as 3,000 seconds of arc to acuity as fine as 40 seconds of arc. Any patient who demonstrates stereoscopic acuity of 40 to 60 seconds of arc probably has little wrong with the motor or sensory part of the visual system.

Esotropia, the inward deviation of one or both eyes, is the commonest type of strabismus.

Infantile esotropia is the most common type of esodeviation (Fig. 10–29). In the past, this entity was called congenital esotropia because it was thought that most children with this problem were born with it. It is more likely, however, that the onset of this type of esotropia most often is during the first 3 months of life. By definition, infantile esotropia is an esotropia that has been documented to have been present before the age of 6 months. Although most babies with infantile esotropia will alternate fixation between the two eyes (and therefore have good vision in both eyes), it has been estimated that as many as 40% of these children may have amblyopia. *Cross fixation* is also a frequent finding; the child uses the right eye when looking to the left and uses the left eye when looking to the right. Cross fixation frequently includes a noticeable limitation of abduction of each eye on version testing, which can look much like a bilateral sixth nerve palsy. Full abduction, however, can usually be demonstrated by holding the infant at arms' length and spinning around in a circle. This

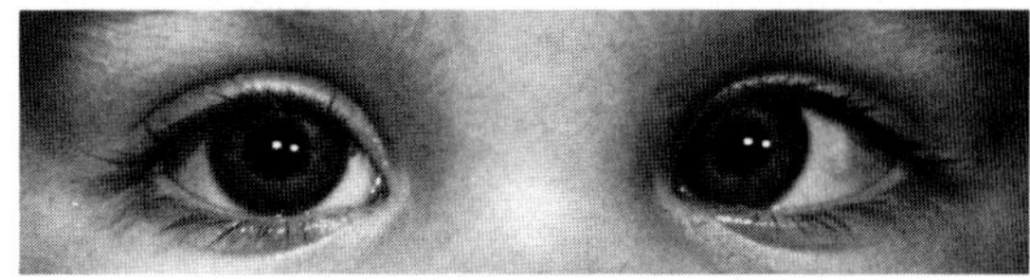

Fig. 10–29. A 1-year-old child with a moderate-angle infantile esotropia.

maneuver stimulates the vestibulo-ocular reflex and demonstrates that lateral rectus function is intact.

Children with infantile esotropia usually have large deviations (40 Δ; range, 30 to 80 Δ). The deviation is usually constant rather than intermittent and does not seem to be influenced by accommodative efforts. Most children with infantile esotropia have less than 3 D of hyperopia, which is a normal amount in infants and young children. Other eye movement abnormalities frequently associated with infantile esotropia are a dissociated vertical deviation, overaction of the inferior oblique muscles, and nystagmus. The differential diagnosis in a child with apparent infantile esotropia includes pseudoesotropia, Duane's retraction syndrome, Möbius' syndrome, congenital sixth nerve palsy, early-onset accommodative esotropia, and sensory esotropia. In infantile esotropia the goals of therapy are good vision in both eyes, straight eyes, and the development of at least some level of binocular vision. In most cases, an eye muscle operation is necessary to correct the esotropia. Preoperatively, patching therapy should be done to correct any amblyopia, and hyperopia of more than 2 D should be corrected with glasses.

Many surgical approaches have been suggested for infantile esotropia, including recession of the medial rectus muscle in each eye or recession of the medial rectus muscle and resection of the lateral rectus muscle of the same eye ("R and R"). Three or even four horizontal rectus muscles may be operated on for large deviations. Associated overaction of the inferior oblique muscle is often treated with inferior oblique weakening procedures at the time of initial operation. Reoperations for undercorrections or, less frequently, for overcorrections are common.

Esotropia may result from excess accommodation, either to focus clearly at distance (uncorrected hyperopia) or near (high accommodative convergence to accommodation ratio—AC:A ratio).

When an emmetrope (a person with no refractive error) fixes on a near object, the eyes have to increase their dioptric power in order to keep the image of that object clearly focused on the retina. The eye increases its power by changing the shape of the lens. When the ciliary muscle contracts, the lens assumes a more globular shape and thus becomes a more powerful refracting element. This process is called accommodation. In addition to the lens' changing shape, accommodative effort also causes the pupils to constrict and the eyes to converge. This combination of accommodation, pupillary constriction, and convergence is called the *near reflex*. The amount of convergence that occurs in response to the amount of accommodation generated is called the *AC:A ratio*. The normal AC:A ratio is somewhere between 3 and 5, that is, 3 to 5 Δ of accommodative convergence will occur for every diopter of accommodation used.

A child who is hyperopic (farsighted) has to use accommodation to see clearly in the distance as well as up close. This accommodative effort will stimulate convergence. A child who has a large amount of hyperopia needs to generate a large amount of accommodation to see things clearly and as a result may not be able to control the amount of convergence that results and may develop an esotropia. Likewise, a child with an average amount or even a small amount of hyperopia may develop an esotropia if the AC:A ratio is high. Esotropia that occurs as a result of accommodative effort is called *accommodative esotropia* (Fig. 10–30). The average age at onset of accommodative esotropia is 2.5 years, although it may occur as early as 6 months of age and as late as 7 years of age. This type of deviation may be genetically determined. It usually starts as an intermittent deviation, being most noticeable with near fixation. It can become a constant deviation if not

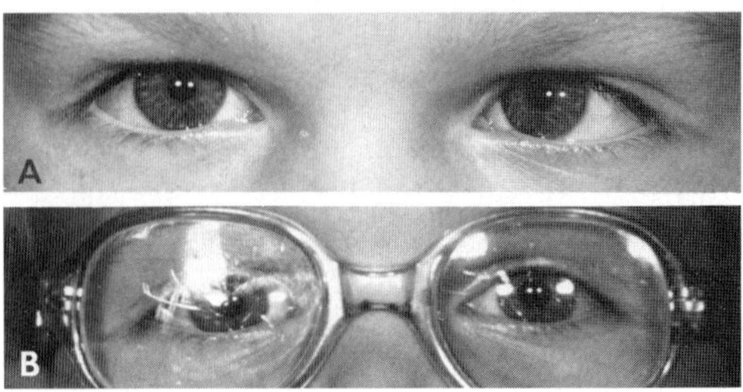

Fig. 10–30. *A*, A 3-year-old child with refractive accommodative esotropia. Without correction he demonstrates a left esotropia. *B*, With the hyperopic refractive error corrected with glasses, his eyes are straight.

treated, and amblyopia may develop if the child constantly chooses the same eye for fixation.

There are two main forms of accommodative esotropia: 1) refractive accommodative esotropia and 2) nonrefractive accommodative esotropia with a high AC:A ratio. In *refractive accommodative esotropia*, the size of the esotropia is usually between 15 and 30 Δ, and the amount of deviation is the same both at distance and at near fixation. The amount of hyperopia present is significant, usually being greater than 3 D. Children with *nonrefractive accommodative esotropia* with a high AC:A ratio usually have little or no deviation at distance fixation. However, at near fixation with accommodative targets, they develop an esotropia of moderate magnitude (20 to 30 Δ). These children usually have an average amount of hyperopia (+2 D or less).

The treatment for refractive accommodative esotropia is correction of the hyperopia with glasses. With the hyperopia corrected, the child does not need to accommodate as much; hence the stimulus for accommodative convergence will be reduced. If the patient is younger than 6 years, the full amount of hyperopic correction found on cycloplegic refraction should be prescribed. A child who is older than 6 years will probably not accept the full cycloplegic correction; therefore, the maximal amount of hyperopic correction that will not blur vision should be prescribed. If amblyopia is present, it should be treated with occlusion therapy. Youngsters with nonrefractive accommodative esotropia and high AC:A ratio (that is, a greater amount of esotropia at near and an average amount of hyperopia) should be treated with bifocal glasses. The distance segment should correct the full hyperopic error. This usually eliminates any esotropia that may be present at distance fixation. The reading segment provides additional power for near; thus the patient does not have to use very much or any accommodation at near fixation.

The role of long-acting cholinesterase inhibitors (isoflurophate or echothiophate) in the treatment of accommodative esotropia remains controversial. These topical medications are able to alter the AC:A ratio and hence can reduce or eliminate accommodative esotropia in some individuals. However, as these drugs cause pupillary constriction (miosis) and can have ocular (iris cysts and lens opacities) and systemic (reduction of plasma and erythrocyte cholinesterase) side effects, they are not recommended for long-term use.

Esotropia in a young child can be the result of poor vision in the eye.

Ocular conditions such as a cataract, optic nerve hypoplasia, and retinoblastoma that reduce central visual acuity to a significant degree can disrupt fusion and result in a *sensory deprivation esotropia*. Therefore, any child who presents with an esotropia should have an ophthalmoscopic examination performed through a dilated pupil to rule out the presence of an ocular abnormality. Once the primary problem has been taken care of, any amblyopia that is present should be treated. Surgical therapy for the residual esotropia is usually required.

Most patients with significant intermittent exotropia will require surgical correction.

Exotropia is a divergent misalignment of the visual axes. With *intermittent exotropia,* the most common type of exodeviation, the eyes are in good alignment much of the time, but for some unknown reason the patient's fusion seems to break down and one eye turns out. This is usually more pronounced when the child looks off in the distance or when the child is tired or ill. The child typically is able to bring the divergent eye back into alignment with a blink or a refixation movement. The onset of intermittent exotropia usually occurs between infancy and 4 years of age. In many cases there is a hereditary influence. A common characteristic is the tendency to close one eye outside in the bright sunlight. The reason for this behavior is not fully understood. Some practitioners think it occurs because the child has fewer near clues to stimulate convergence. Others think that bright sunlight dazzles the retina, thereby disrupting fusion and causing diplopia. Still others believe that patients with intermittent exotropia may be more photosensitive than patients with no ocular deviation.

When the eyes are straight, patients with intermittent exotropia have normal retinal correspondence and normal stereoacuity; because the eyes are straight and working together most of the time, amblyopia does not usually occur. In most patients the frequency and the magnitude of the intermittent exotropia remain unchanged with the passage of time. Others have a definite decompensation of the intermittent deviation into a constant exotropia. Nonsurgical therapy of intermittent exotropia consists of treating any amblyopia and anisometropia that may be present. Overcorrection with minus lenses may stimulate accommodative convergence, which in turn helps the patient to control the exodeviation.

Most patients with a significant intermittent exotropia will require an eye muscle operation. The indications depend on the amount of deviation present and the frequency with which it occurs. If the deviation is small and infrequent, it is reasonable just to follow the patient. If the deviation is large and occurs with increasing frequency, surgery is indicated. Surgical correction of intermittent exotropia can be accomplished either by recessing the lateral rectus muscle in each eye or by recessing the lateral rectus muscle and resecting the medial rectus muscle in the same eye. For large deviations, correction on three and sometimes four horizontal rectus muscles is necessary.

A constant exotropia can be seen in adults or children in different clinical settings.

A *constant exotropia* is encountered more often in adults manifesting a sensory exotropia or a decompensated intermittent exotropia. A sensory exotropia results because of poor vision in one eye that is most often caused by a dense cataract. After the cataract is removed and vision is restored, some patients will experience diplopia, which may resolve, depending on the amount of exotropia and the degree of fusion that is present. Constant exotropia can be seen in childhood, although it is much less common than intermittent exotropia. If an alternating fixation pattern occurs in the setting of a constant exotropia in childhood, amblyopia will not develop. When a constant exotropia develops before the age of 6 years and alternating fixation is not present, amblyopia is likely to develop in the nonfixing eye. Treatment consists of correcting any significant refractive error and amblyopia. If the exotropia is less than 15 Δ, operation is usually not required because the appearance of the eyes is usually acceptable cosmetically. For deviations of more than 15 D, operation is usually indicated. The type of procedure required is the same as that for the correction of intermittent exotropia.

A and V patterns usually result from dysfunction of the oblique muscles, and they commonly accompany horizontal strabismus.

In some patients with esotropia or exotropia, the amount of deviation changes with upgaze and downgaze. An *"A" pattern* refers to a horizontal deviation in which there is increasing convergence (or decreasing divergence) in upgaze; a *"V" pattern* indicates a horizontal deviation with increasing convergence (or decreasing divergence) in downgaze.

Approximately 20% of patients with horizontal strabismus have an associated A or V pattern (such as V pattern esotropia, A pattern esotropia, V pattern exotropia, and A pattern exotropia).

A *V pattern esotropia* is usually associated with overaction of the inferior oblique muscles; treatment consists of an inferior oblique weakening procedure in each eye along with horizontal rectus muscle operation to correct the esotropia. When a V pattern esotropia is present in the absence of overacting inferior oblique muscles, a vertical transfer of the insertions of the horizontal rectus muscles may be performed in order to eliminate the V pattern.

An *A pattern esotropia* may involve bilateral superior oblique overaction and inferior oblique underaction. If significant overaction of the superior oblique muscles is present, a weakening procedure on the superior obliques and a horizontal rectus operation for the esotropia are indicated. If there is no superior oblique overaction, the procedure of choice is supraplacement of the medial rectus muscles or infraplacement of the lateral rectus muscles in combination with appropriate horizontal surgery.

V exotropia is usually associated with overacting inferior oblique muscles, underacting superior oblique muscles, or both. This type of strabismus pattern is usually corrected by an inferior oblique weakening procedure in each eye in combination with the horizontal rectus procedure to correct the exotropia. Without inferior oblique overaction, the lateral rectus insertion should be moved upward if bilateral rectus muscle recessions are performed. If a recess/resect procedure is being done to correct the exotropia, the lateral rectus tendon should be moved upward and the medial rectus tendon downward.

In *A pattern exotropia*, the superior oblique muscles are usually overactive, and these should be weakened. If there is no superior oblique overaction, both lateral rectus muscles may be recessed and moved downward.

When horizontal rectus muscle transposition alone is used to correct A or V patterns, the horizontal rectus muscles are transposed vertically in the direction that will reduce their horizontal (adduction and abduction) effect. The medial rectus muscles are always moved in the direction of vertical gaze where the esotropia is greater and the lateral rectus muscles are always moved in the direction of vertical gaze where the exotropia is greater. In effect, the medial rectus muscles are always moved toward the apex of the pattern, and the lateral rectus muscles are always moved toward the open end of the pattern (Fig. 10–31).

Noncomitancy and secondary deviation are key features of paralytic strabismus.

A comitant deviation is one in which the magnitude of the deviation is the same in all directions of gaze. A noncomitant deviation is defined as one in which the amount of deviation changes with various directions of gaze. Paresis or paralysis of an extraocular muscle secondary to dysfunction of the third, fourth, or sixth cranial nerve is the most common cause of noncomitant strabismus. This type of strabismus is called *paralytic strabismus*. The patient with an acquired paralytic strabismus of recent onset almost always complains of diplopia and may assume an abnormal head posture in order to eliminate the diplopia and to regain binocular vision. On examination, ocular motility is limited in the field of action of the paretic muscle or muscles. In addition, a key clinical finding is that the amount of deviation in the primary position with the paretic eye fixing (secondary deviation) is greater than with the nonparetic eye fixing (primary deviation).

In a complete third nerve palsy, ptosis is present, the pupil is dilated, and the eye is exotropic and hypotropic.

A complete *third nerve palsy* results in blepharoptosis and paralysis of the medial

rectus, superior rectus, inferior rectus, and inferior oblique muscles in the involved eye (Fig. 10–32). As a result, the eye is exotropic and hypotropic. The pupil is dilated, and accommodation is absent because of paralysis of the pupillary sphincter muscle and the ciliary muscle, both of which are innervated by the parasympathetic fibers of the third nerve. Congenital third nerve palsy is the most common type seen in children, and amblyopia is common. Acquired third nerve palsy in children is usually traumatic or inflammatory, whereas in adults the most likely causes are vascular (diabetic), intracranial aneurysm, traumatic, and neoplastic.

For cases in which the blepharoptosis is severe enough to cover the pupil, diplopia is not a problem. However, in a child younger than 6 or 7 years old, this degree of blepharoptosis may cause amblyopia. In cases of acquired third nerve palsy in which diplopia is a problem, patching the paretic eye will eliminate the diplopia. The ocular deviation is usually too large for prism therapy to be of any value. If complete third nerve function has not returned after 6 to 9 months, surgery may be indicated. Because it is impossible to restore normal ocular motility to the eye with a total third nerve palsy, the goals of surgery are to make the eye straight in the primary position and to improve the ocular motility as much as possible. Surgical correction requires operation on multiple eye muscles.

Superior oblique muscle palsy is the most common paralytic strabismus encountered.

Superior oblique muscle palsy is usually caused by dysfunction of the trochlear nerve, although an abnormality of the superior oblique

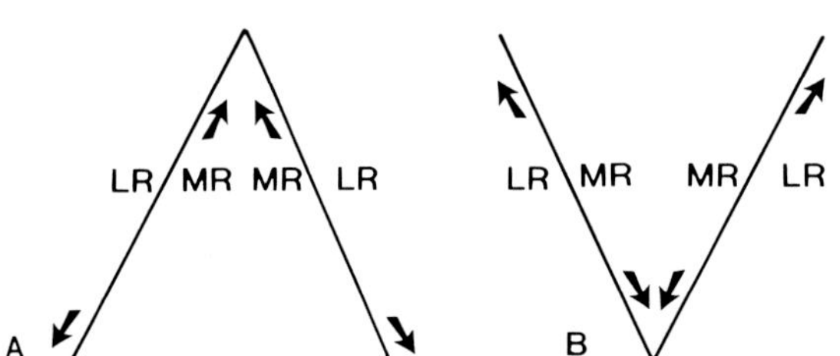

Fig. 10–31. Direction in which the horizontal rectus muscles should be moved to correct an "A" pattern (*A*) and "V" pattern (*B*) horizontal deviation. The medial rectus (MR) muscles are always moved toward the apex of the pattern, and the lateral rectus (LR) muscles are always moved toward the open end of the pattern. (Modified from G.K. von Noorden: Atlas of Strabismus, 4th ed. St. Louis, C.V. Mosby Company, 1983, p. 189.)

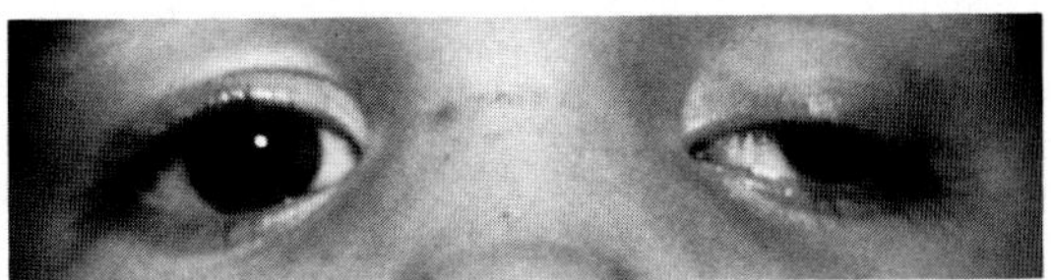

Fig. 10–32. A child with a congenital third nerve palsy on the left side. Note the blepharoptosis on the left side. The left eye is exotropic and hypotropic.

muscle or tendon itself may result in an identical clinical presentation. Fourth nerve palsies may be congenital or acquired and may be unilateral or bilateral. The congenital variety is the most common type seen in children; the presenting sign is an abnormal head posture, usually with a head tilt to the side opposite the involved eye (Fig. 10–33). The child also has a hyperphoria or a frank hypertropia of the involved eye. Patients with congenital fourth nerve palsies rarely complain of diplopia. Curiously enough, in most cases of congenital fourth nerve palsy, superior oblique function appears to be good. The most common motility abnormality seems to be a secondary overaction of the antagonist inferior oblique. This results in a noticeable upshoot of the affected eye in adduction. The hypertropia present in the affected eye will increase on gaze to the opposite side. Tilting the head to the shoulder on the same side as the involved eye will also cause the hypertropia to increase in size, and tilting the head to the opposite shoulder will cause the deviation to decrease in size (*Bielschowsky head tilt test*).

The chief presenting complaint of a patient with an acquired fourth nerve palsy is vertical diplopia. Most acquired superior oblique palsies are traumatic in origin. A superior oblique palsy is diagnosed by observing versions and ductions, using the Bielschowsky head-tilt test, and by measuring the deviation in the cardinal positions of gaze. In acquired fourth

nerve palsy, the weakness of the superior oblique is usually obvious.

If the hypertropia is not large, vertical prisms may be effective in eliminating the diplopia in the primary position and in providing the patient with comfortable vision. If an acquired fourth nerve palsy has not resolved after 6 to 9 months and prism therapy has not proved helpful, surgery is indicated. The surgical approach to superior oblique palsy can vary depending on which direction of gaze the hyperdeviation is greatest and on which muscles are overacting or underacting. Weakening of the overacting antagonist inferior oblique is probably the most common procedure performed. If there is a significant superior oblique underaction, a strengthening procedure (tuck or resection) is performed on the paretic superior oblique.

A sixth nerve palsy in an adult is usually caused by vascular disease (such as diabetes) or a neoplasm.

A *sixth nerve palsy* presents with a limitation of abduction on both versions and ductions. There is an esotropia in the primary position, and this esotropia increases on gaze toward the paretic lateral rectus muscle (Fig. 10–13). A sixth nerve palsy may be unilateral or bilateral. Congenital sixth nerve palsies do occur but are rare. Children with infantile esotropia frequently demonstrate a noticeable limitation of abduction on version testing and because of this can appear to have a bilateral congenital sixth nerve palsy. Duane's retraction syndrome is a developmental anomaly that also can be mistaken for a congenital sixth nerve palsy.

The most common causes of an acquired sixth nerve palsy in a child are inflammation, trauma, and neoplasm, and in an adult the most common causes are vascular disease (such as diabetes) or neoplasm. Recovery from an acquired sixth nerve palsy usually occurs within 3 to 6 months; in some cases the paralysis may be permanent. During the period of paralysis, secondary contracture of the antagonist medial rectus muscle can occur, resulting in an esotropia that persists even after the lateral rectus function has returned to normal. In acquired

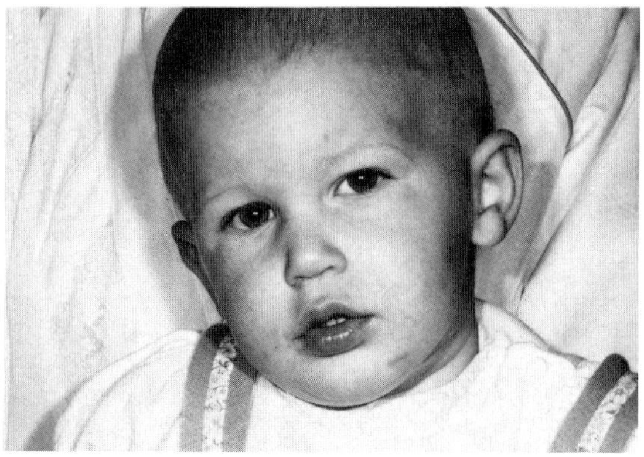

Fig. 10–33. Child with congenital superior oblique palsy of the left eye demonstrates a compensatory head tilt to the right shoulder.

sixth nerve palsy, patching will help to relieve the diplopia and the abnormal head position. In adults, patching of the nonparetic eye will also eliminate the double vision and may also help to prevent contracture of the medial rectus. Prisms can also be used to eliminate the diplopia in the primary position. In recent years, botulinum toxin has been used in the setting of an acute sixth nerve palsy. Botulinum, a nerve toxin, is injected into the antagonist medial rectus muscle, causing a complete paralysis of that muscle which lasts from weeks to months. This usually results in a decrease in the amount of esotropia that is present and in some cases eliminates the deviation altogether; it may also help to prevent contracture of the medial rectus until the paretic lateral rectus muscle regains its normal function. If the lateral rectus function has not returned after 6 to 9 months, surgery is indicated.

In Duane's syndrome, the eye retracts during attempted adduction because of simultaneous contraction of the ipsilateral medial and lateral rectus muscles—an exception of Sherrington's law.

Duane's retraction syndrome is a congenital eye movement disorder characterized by marked limitation or absence of abduction, variable limitation of adduction, and narrowing of the palpebral fissure and retraction of the globe on attempted adduction (Fig. 10–34). Most patients with Duane's syndrome demonstrate an esotropia in the primary position. The condition is bilateral in 15% to 20% of cases and seems to occur more commonly in females and in the left eye. Amblyopia occurs in approximately 20% of the patients, and in most cases it is due to anisometropia. Duane's retraction syndrome is frequently mistaken for a sixth nerve palsy. One must look closely for the retraction of the globe and narrowing of the fissure to differentiate the two. The cause of Duane's retraction syndrome is most likely a hypoplasia of the abducens (sixth nerve) nucleus or nerve. As a result, the lateral rectus muscle in the involved eye does not receive any innervation from the sixth nerve but rather

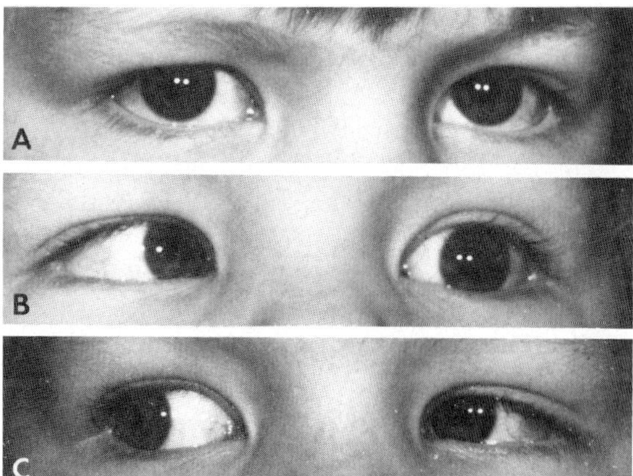

Fig. 10–34. *A*, A child with Duane's retraction syndrome of the left eye. With a slight face turn to the left, the patient's eyes are straight. *B*, On gaze left, there is marked limitation of abduction of the left eye, resulting in a large esotropia. Note also the widening of the palpebral fissure on the left with attempted abduction. *C*, Gaze to the right demonstrates normal adduction of the left eye. Note the narrowing of the palpebral fissure on the left side with adduction of the left eye.

receives partial innervation from fibers of the third nerve. Electromyographic studies in patients with Duane's syndrome have shown that there is little, if any, firing of the lateral rectus muscle on attempted abduction. However, on adduction the lateral rectus muscle paradoxically contracts instead of relaxing. This action results in a cocontraction of the lateral rectus muscle and the medial rectus muscle in the involved eye and in turn causes retraction of the globe and narrowing of the fissure.

Nonsurgical treatment of Duane's syndrome consists of correcting any anisometropia or amblyopia that may be present. Surgical treatment is indicated if there is a cosmetically unacceptable head posture or if there is a frank tropia in the primary position.

Möbius' syndrome is a congenital disorder in which there is an aplasia of the nuclei of cranial nerves VI, VII, and XII.

Möbius' syndrome is characterized by bilateral facial weakness and horizontal gaze palsies. Both of these features vary in severity and may be markedly asymmetric. In many cases an A or V esotropia is present. In most patients with Möbius' syndrome, vertical eye movements and convergence remain intact. Associated developmental anomalies include deafness, atrophy of the tongue, skeletal deformities, and mental retardation. Strabismus surgery is indicated when a noticeable esotropia is present. However, it will not improve the horizontal eye movements.

The monofixation syndrome should be suspected in patients with mild amblyopia and grossly normal ocular alignment.

The patient with *monofixation syndrome* usually has a small angle esotropia (less than 8 Δ of deviation). Monofixation syndrome may be idiopathic, but in most cases it is the result of treatment of an esotropia with glasses or operation, or it can result from anisometropia and macular lesions. *Microtropia* is a term that has been used interchangeably with monofixation syndrome. With monofixation syndrome the nonpreferred eye is usually mildly amblyopic (usually in the 20/40 to 20/60 range) with a central scotoma. Peripheral fusion is present. Stereoscopic acuity is present but is reduced usually to around 3,000 seconds of arc. Monofixation syndrome is not an uncommon condition, and it is important to recognize it as a possible cause of reduced visual acuity in one eye when no obvious strabismus is present.

Monofixation syndrome can usually be diagnosed with the *4-D baseout prism test*. When a weak baseout prism is placed in front of one eye in a normal patient with bifoveal fusion without a central suppression scotoma, the image of the fixation target will be displaced temporally from the fovea onto a parafoveal area and the patient will have diplopia. To place the image back on the fovea, the eye behind the prism will make a slight inward movement. As it does, the fellow eye will make a simultaneous and equal outward movement, in accordance with Hering's law. The eye without the prism will then make a vergence movement inward to put the image back on the fovea of that eye. In a patient with a monofixation syndrome, how-

ever, there is a central or paracentral suppression scotoma in the eye so that the 4-D baseout prism placed in front of the abnormal eye will cause no movement of either eye because the prism will have moved the image from one location to another within the suppression scotoma. As a result, there will be no diplopia and no stimulation for refixation.

Vertical ocular misalignment may be caused by neurogenic, myogenic, traumatic, or mechanical factors.

Vertical deviations are usually designated according to the position of the nonfixing eye. For example, a right hypertropia indicates that the nonfixing right eye is higher than the left eye. A left hypotropia means that the nonfixing left eye is lower than the right eye. Like horizontal deviations, vertical deviations may be comitant or noncomitant. However, unlike horizontal deviations, most of which are comitant, most vertical deviations tend to be noncomitant. Noncomitant vertical deviations are produced by weakness of one or more vertically acting muscles or by mechanical restriction of vertical movement.

Muscle weakness may be neurogenic, myopathic, or neuromuscular in origin. Neurogenic muscle weakness is due to an abnormality or injury to the nerve that innervates the muscle, for example, a third or fourth nerve palsy. Myopathic weakness results from intrinsic muscle disease such as chronic progressive external ophthalmoplegia. The prime example of neuromuscular weakness is that produced by myasthenia gravis. Mechanical restriction of vertical movement occurs in disease processes such as Graves' ophthalmopathy, in which there are fibrosis and contracture of some of the extraocular muscles, and with orbital floor fracture, in which the inferior rectus muscle or surrounding tissue is caught in the fracture site, which tethers the globe and prevents full elevation. Patients with noncomitant vertical deviations sometimes assume an abnormal head posture in order to maintain some degree of binocularity. Some may tilt their head to one side; others may depress or elevate their chin.

Brown's syndrome (poor elevation of the eye during adduction) is due to mechanical restriction of the superior oblique tendon.

The chief clinical feature of *Brown's syndrome*, also called *superior oblique tendon sheath syndrome*, is the inability to elevate the affected eye in adduction (Fig. 10–35). The ability to elevate the eye improves as the eye moves into a more abducted position. Usually there is full or almost full elevation in abduction. There may be a slight downshoot of the involved eye on adduction because of the mechanical effect of a tight superior oblique tendon that cannot relax on adduction. Occasionally there is a widening of the palpebral fissure on adduction, and a V pattern may be present. The forced duction test is positive with very noticeable resistance to passive elevation in adduction. It is bilateral in about 10% of cases.

Brown's syndrome may be congenital or acquired. The cause of congenital Brown's syndrome is thought to be a short or tight superior oblique tendon. The most common cause of acquired Brown's syndrome is probably superior oblique strengthening procedures (tuck and resection) performed for superior oblique palsy. Brown's syndrome has also been reported after orbital trauma, scleral buckling procedures, and sinus operation, and it has been reported in association with frontal sinusitis and rheumatoid arthritis. Surgical treatment is indicated if there is an abnormal head position that is unacceptable on a cosmetic basis or if there is a significant hypotropia in the primary position. The surgical procedure that is used is a tenotomy or tenectomy of the superior oblique tendon.

Dissociated vertical deviation is a common but poorly understood entity in which the eye drifts upward when sensory input is decreased.

Dissociated vertical deviation is an eye movement abnormality in which the affected eye drifts slowly upward when it is occluded or drifts upward spontaneously during a period of visual inattention (Fig. 10–36). This upward drift is followed by a slow downward movement of the eye when occlusion is removed or a refixation stimulus occurs. Dissociated vertical deviation is not a true vertical deviation in that there is no associated hypotropia of the fellow eye. Dissociated vertical deviation is usually bilateral and is frequently associated with other types of strabismus, most commonly infantile esotropia and occasionally intermittent exotropia. The cause of dissociated vertical

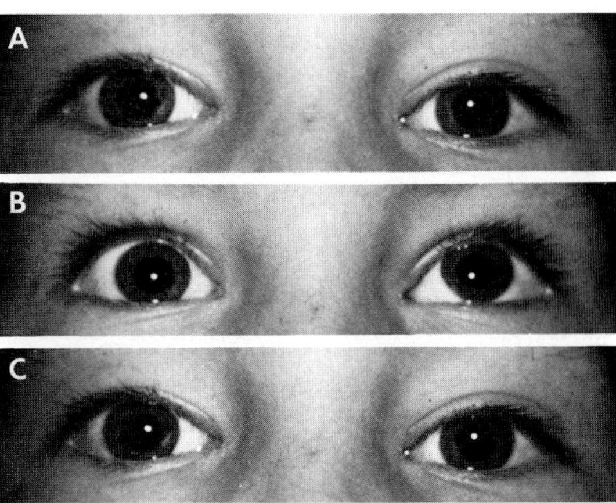

Fig. 10–36. *A,* Child with dissociated vertical deviation of the left eye. In the primary position the eyes are in good horizontal and vertical alignment. *B,* After momentary occlusion of the left eye, the left eye becomes hypertropic. *C,* With refixation, the left eye returns to the primary position without any associated hypotropia of the right eye.

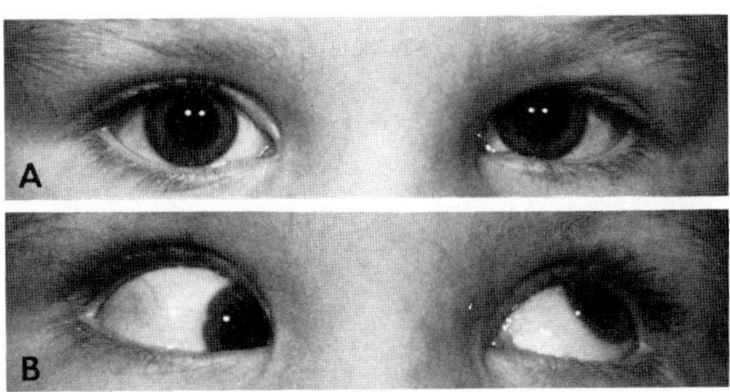

Fig. 10–35. *A,* A 2-year-old child with congenital Brown's syndrome of the right eye. The eyes are straight in the primary position. *B,* Gaze up and to the left demonstrates marked limitation of elevation of the right eye.

deviation is unknown. Surgical treatment is indicated if the deviation is manifesting with a frequency and a magnitude of deviation that are cosmetically unacceptable. The surgical approaches used most often are bilateral superior rectus recessions. Some surgeons prefer inferior rectus resections either alone or in combination with superior rectus recessions.

Weakness of both the superior rectus and the inferior oblique muscles of the same eye is a double elevator palsy.

A patient with a *double elevator palsy* is unable to elevate the involved eye in either adduction or abduction (Fig. 10–37). It is as if both a superior rectus palsy and an inferior oblique palsy are present in the same eye. There is usually a large hypotropia in the involved eye causing the patient to assume a chin-up position. Frequently, there is an associated horizontal deviation, and a true ptosis is often present on the involved side. Amblyopia in the involved eye is present in about half the patients with double elevator palsy. Most cases of double elevator palsy are congenital and thought to be due to a supranuclear lesion in the pretectal area on the contralateral side. The indication for surgi-

cal intervention is an abnormal head posture or a significant hypotropia in the primary position.

Amblyopia is decreased vision in one or both eyes secondary to refractive, sensory, or strabismic causes.

The visual system of a newborn child is not fully developed, and in order for the visual system to reach its full potential both eyes must receive adequate and equal visual stimulation from birth to 8 or 9 years of age. Any ocular condition that prevents adequate and equal visual stimulation during this crucial period of development can result in visual loss that is called *amblyopia*. In amblyopia, the reduction in visual acuity is usually unilateral, although in some rare cases it can be bilateral. It is estimated that 2% to 3% of the population of the United States has amblyopia; it is the most common cause of visual loss during the first 45 years of life. Amblyopia is potentially correctable if treated appropriately in early childhood. Treatment in adults is generally ineffective.

Amblyopia in and of itself produces no detectable changes in the eye. However, it always develops in association with some other abnormality that is usually apparent on clinical examination. Amblyopia can occur in any of the following settings: strabismus, anisometropia, ametropia, and visual stimulus deprivation.

Strabismic amblyopia is characterized by unilateral visual loss that develops as a result of a strong preference to fix with just one eye (dominant eye) while continually suppressing images in the deviating eye. Approximately half of children with strabismus will develop amblyopia. *Anisometropia* is a condition in which the refractive error in one eye is significantly different from that in the fellow eye. In this situation the child has a relatively sharp retinal image in one eye and a relatively blurred image in the other eye. This disparity in retinal image clarity can result in amblyopia, with the amblyopia occurring in the more ametropic eye.

Ametropic (iso-ametropic) *amblyopia* is bilateral and associated with large hyperopic, myopic, or astigmatic refractive errors that are approximately the same in the two eyes. In any of these cases the patient's visual acuity is equally blurred

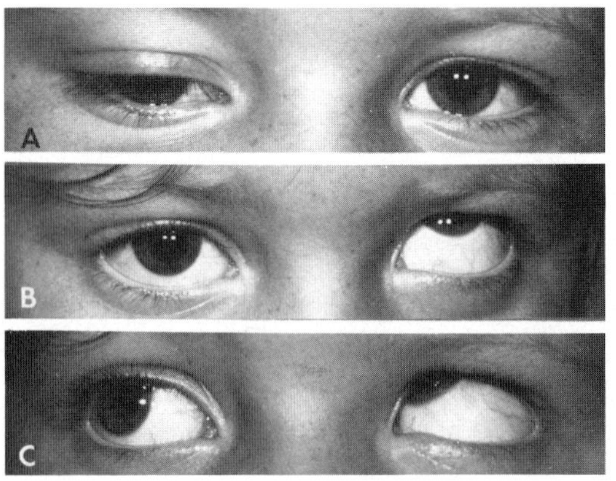

Fig. 10–37. *A*, Child with double elevator palsy of the right eye. In the primary position the patient is fixing with the normal left eye, and there is a large hypotropia of the right eye. Note the pseudoptosis that accompanies the hypotropic right eye. *B*, Marked limitation of elevation of the right eye on upgaze. *C*, Gaze up and to the right demonstrates moderate limitation of elevation of the right eye in abduction. Elevation of the right eye in adduction was similarly limited.

in the two eyes and may not be correctable to 20/20 at the time of the initial refraction. However, if the refractive error is corrected early when the visual system is still developing, gradual improvement in the visual acuity of the two eyes can be anticipated. *Stimulus deprivation amblyopia* occurs in an infant who is born with or who develops in the first few years of life any ocular problem that precludes the production of a good, sharp retinal image. Conditions such as lid tumors, corneal opacities, cataracts, and vitreous hemorrhage are the main causes of stimulus deprivation amblyopia. Some patients may have more than one type of amblyopia present at the same time (that is, anisometropia plus strabismus or visual stimulation deprivation plus strabismus). These patients will require concurrent treatment for each type of amblyopia.

Little is known about the changes that occur in the visual system of humans with amblyopia.

An enormous amount of data about amblyopia has been collected from animal experiments in kittens and young monkeys. Form vision deprivation has been induced in these animals by suturing the eyelids together or by the use of an opaque contact lens. Strabismus has been induced in these animals by disinserting one of the horizontal rectus muscles. These studies show that abnormal visual experiences (form vision deprivation or abnormal binocular interaction) early in life can lead to profound changes in the "wiring pattern" and processing abilities of the visual centers in the brains of these animals. Morphologic changes have been observed in the cells of the lateral geniculate nucleus and in the cells of the visual cortex, which are driven by the deprived or deviating eye. If the abnormal visual experience is not corrected at a sufficiently early stage, the abnormalities in the visual system are usually irreversible. Extrapolation of these data to humans implies that there is a critical period during which humans are susceptible to developing amblyopia as a result of form vision deprivation or abnormal binocular interaction. The critical period seems to be from birth to approximately 8 or 9 years of age. The susceptibility to develop amblyopia appears to be greatest in the first 3 months of life and decreases as the child gets older. Once the visual system matures (age 8 to 9 years), amblyopia no longer occurs.

Amblyopia must be detected early for therapy to be effective.

If amblyopia is not detected and treated early, it may be irreversible, resulting in reduced visual acuity in one eye for the rest of a person's life. Amblyopia affects only the central form vision of the eye; other visual functions such as peripheral vision, color vision, and dark adaptation are normal. The degree of visual loss depends on the type of abnormal visual experience and the age at which it occurs. The amblyopia that results from form vision deprivation in an infant or young child has a much poorer prognosis than that which results from strabismus or anisometropia. A newborn with a dense congenital cataract in one eye, for example, may end up with visual acuity in that eye of less than 20/800 even after the removal of the cataract and correction with a contact lens. Other patients, such as those with a mild degree of anisometropia, may have visual acuity as good as 20/25 in the involved eye without correction.

The *crowding phenomenon* is another characteristic that is frequently seen in patients with amblyopia. An individual with amblyopia has more difficulty identifying Snellen test letters when they are presented in a full line than when they are presented as single isolated letters; this phenomenon is thought to be due to contour interaction.

Another clinical feature of the amblyopic eye is the effect of reduced illumination. If the amount of light entering the normal eye is gradually reduced by placing a series of neutral density filters in front of it, the visual acuity will be reduced proportional to the density of the filter. In the amblyopic eye, however, there is little if any further reduction in visual acuity as the illumination is decreased. In an eye with organic disease, the visual acuity will be decreased even more than in a normal eye as illumination is decreased.

Determining the visual acuity in children is the best method of detecting amblyopia.

Amblyopia is diagnosed by determining the visual acuity in each eye. Most children between the ages of 3 and 4 years can be tested successfully with symbols such as Allen picture cards. Children between the ages of 4 and 6 usually perform well with the Snellen E game. Youngsters 6 years or older usually can be tested with the regular Snellen chart. Because children with amblyopia frequently demonstrate the crowding phenomenon, vision testing should be performed with a full line of letters. If only single optotypes are used, amblyopia may not be detected. In infants and preverbal children, determining the visual acuity becomes more problematic. In these children, the examiner has to compare the fixation pattern of each eye in order to come to some conclusions about the level of visual acuity. In young children with strabismus, the presence of spontaneous alternating fixation is a good sign and suggests that equal vision is present. Amblyopia may be suspected when the examiner occludes the fixing eye and the deviated eye does not fix well or when the child strenuously objects to having the fixing eye covered but does not object when the deviated eye is covered.

A technique called *forced preferential looking* shows promise as an assessment of the subjective visual acuity of infants and preverbal children. If it proves reliable, it will be a valuable tool for the early detection of amblyopia.

The earlier the treatment of amblyopia, the more successful the outcome.

The treatment rationale in amblyopia is directed into two areas. The first is the correction of any significant refractive error that may be present in the amblyopic eye. The second and more important aspect of amblyopia therapy is occlusion of the better eye. The initial treatment should be full-time occlusion of the good eye with an adhesive patch (Fig. 10–38). Full-time *occlusion therapy* is continued until the vision of both eyes becomes equal or until no improvement has been demonstrated after a 3-month period of treatment.

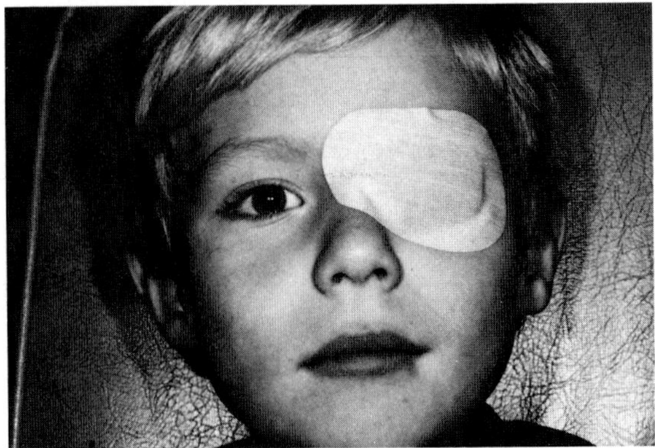

Fig. 10–38. An adhesive patch is used to occlude the preferred left eye in a child with amblyopia of the right eye.

If the vision in the amblyopic eye has improved with full-time occlusion, it must be maintained until the child's visual system reaches maturity (at age 8 or 9 years). Treatment may involve the use of part-time occlusion with regular follow-up visits.

In children with mild amblyopia who have latent nystagmus or allergic skin problems or who resist patching, a useful alternative to occlusion is the concept of *penalization*. With this technique, the nonamblyopic eye is optically undercorrected and atropinized and the refractive error in the amblyopic eye is fully corrected. The goal of this technique is to blur the vision in the nonamblyopic eye enough to cause the individual to switch fixation to the nondominant, amblyopic eye.

As a general rule, amblyopia therapy takes priority over strabismus surgery. Surgery should probably wait until amblyopia has been treated and maximal visual acuity obtained.

Treatment of infants and young children with form vision deprivation, such as that occurring with a congenital cataract, includes the removal of the cataract, correction of the refractive error, and occlusion of the good eye.

Surgery for strabismus involves changing the position of one or more muscles on the globe to improve ocular alignment and function.

Strabismus surgery is performed to provide the patient with some level of binocular vision, to eliminate diplopia, to improve the movement of one or both eyes, to correct an abnormal head posture, or to improve the cosmetic appearance of the patient. In most strabismus cases, the deviation is not caused by any abnormality of the extraocular muscles but rather by abnormal innervation to the extraocular muscles. Apparently this innervation is not of sufficient quality or quantity to balance the forces of the extraocular muscles and to keep the eyes in alignment. Ocular alignment can be predictably altered in most cases by changing the position and tension of the extraocular muscles. Three basic procedures can be performed on the extraocular muscles: weakening, strengthening, and transposition.

The primary weakening procedure is a recession.

In a muscle *recession* the muscle is detached from its insertion on the globe and then reattached at a predetermined point to put slack into the muscle and reduce its tension.

Other weakening procedures consist of a *myotomy* or *tenotomy*, in which the extraocular muscle or tendon is partially or completely transected; a *myectomy*, in which a piece of muscle is removed; a *disinsertion*, in which the muscle is released at its insertion; and a *marginal myotomy*, in which multiple incomplete incisions are made across the muscle.

A muscle resection is the most commonly performed strengthening procedure.

In a muscle *resection* the muscle is usually detached at its insertion, a predetermined length of muscle or tendon is excised from the distal end, and the muscle is then reattached to the globe at the original insertion. This procedure increases muscle tension and tends to enhance the pulling action of the muscle. A muscle advancement is a strengthening procedure that is usually reserved for previously recessed muscle. The previously recessed muscle is detached from the globe and reattached at or near the original insertion. In some cases, advancement is combined with a resection to enhance the strengthening effect.

A *tuck* is performed by creating a fold or a loop in the muscle or tendon. This loop or fold is secured at its base with nonabsorbable suture. This technique shortens the muscle or tendon and increases the tension. A tuck is not usually performed on a rectus muscle because it creates extra bulk beneath the conjunctiva that can appear unsightly. A tuck is most commonly used to strengthen a weak superior oblique muscle.

Muscle transposition procedures are most often performed for a motility abnormality or ocular misalignment secondary to a paralyzed rectus muscle.

In the *muscle transposition* technique, other rectus muscles or parts of rectus muscles with normal function in the same eye are detached at their insertions and then reattached at or near the insertion of the paralyzed muscle. This repositioning of the muscles supplies forces that help to improve the ocular alignment and to restore some of the pulling power that was originally supplied by the paralyzed muscle. In the case of a sixth nerve palsy, the tendons (total or partial) of the superior rectus and the inferior rectus in the same eye are transposed to the insertion of the paralyzed lateral rectus muscle in order to provide some abducting force. In a double elevator palsy, the tendons of the medial rectus and the lateral rectus are moved to the insertion of the superior rectus to provide some elevating force. In procedures performed to correct horizontal strabismus with A and V patterns, transposition of the horizontal rectus muscles inferiorly or superiorly is often combined with a recession or resection procedure.

Adjustable sutures may decrease the overcorrections and undercorrections in muscle operations.

Overcorrections and undercorrections are inevitable consequences of strabismus operations. They are an undesirable yet expected complication in a certain percentage of cases. The *adjustable suture technique* was developed in an attempt to decrease the number of unwanted overcorrections and undercorrections. In this technique, a recession or resection procedure is performed in the usual fashion. The suture used for the recession or resection procedure is brought out through the conjunctiva and tied with a temporary cinch or bow knot instead of being tied permanently, and the procedure is concluded. The patient's ocular alignment is then evaluated later on the day of operation or on the first postoperative morning. If a significant overcorrection or undercorrection is present, the suture, which is readily accessible, can be used to adjust the position of the muscle or muscles and thereby improve the alignment of the eyes. This adjustment is performed with topical anesthesia with the patient fully awake. The adjustable suture technique can be used only with cooperative adult and young adult patients. Most children are not suitable candidates for this technique.

11

EVALUATION AND CARE OF INJURIES TO THE EYE AND OCULAR ADNEXA

David C. Herman

Among the more challenging aspects of eye care is the treatment of traumatic injuries of the globe and ocular adnexa. Familiarity with examination techniques and preparation for emergency procedures are vital for adequate emergency care. Although specialized care may be needed for definitive treatment, the immediate history, examination, and treatment of the traumatic injury often determine the final visual and cosmetic outcome. A prepared, systematic approach to the care of ocular trauma will help to achieve the best possible result.

Emergency ophthalmic care starts with a thorough history.

The history taken from the patient and family must be very detailed and include pertinent negative and positive responses (Table 11–1). Minor details that seem unimportant in the excitement immediately surrounding the presentation of a patient with trauma may prove to be very important later. The time and place of the injury should be recorded. This information is particularly important if the patient was injured at work. What the patient was doing at the time of injury and whether ocular protection was worn should be noted. The visual status before ocular injury should also be investigated; in particular, the presence of amblyopia

or other visually significant disease should be documented.

The nature of the injury should be recorded with as much detail as possible. Major classifications of injury are 1) projectile, 2) blunt trauma, 3) explosion injuries, and 4) chemical burns. The most common projectile injuries result from hammering of metal or other solid objects. The so-called metal-on-metal injuries are the result of high-velocity metal or stone fragments that penetrate the globe. Projectiles of organic material that enter the globe cause special problems with an increased probability of infection or intraocular irritation resulting in intense inflammation. Blunt trauma may cause injury to the globe in the form of ocular hemorrhage, disruption of intraocular contents, and, in severe cases, rupture of the globe. Fractures of the bony orbit frequently occur with blunt trauma. Explosion injuries may cause any combination of the aforementioned injuries as well as injury to the orbit and lids. Chemical burns may be extremely damaging and require immediate therapy.

The patient's recollection of his or her vision immediately after the injury can be helpful for predicting the integrity of the posterior structures of the eye if they are not visible on examination because of media opacities. The time of the last meal or oral intake is important in pa-

275

TABLE 11-1 Important Questions to Ask During Evaluation of Ophthalmic Trauma

Have the "ABCs" (*a*irway, *b*reathing, *c*irculation) been addressed?

What was the vision in the affected eye before the injury and immediately after the injury?

Is there a past history of amblyopia or ophthalmic disease?

Did the injury occur at the patient's place of employment?

Was eye protection, such as goggles, worn?

Was there exposure to any type of chemical and, if so, was the eye irrigated?

Are there any areas of paresthesia around the eyes?

When was the patient's last oral intake?

---

tients whose injuries are sufficiently severe to require immediate operation. This information will be useful to the anesthesiologist if sedation or general anesthesia is planned. If an emergency operation is a possibility, oral intake should be withheld until a decision is made.

The most important element of a careful examination is the measurement of visual acuity.

In situations of severe trauma, *general medical stabilization* of airway, circulation, spinal trauma, and other life-threatening conditions always takes precedence over ocular care. Once the patient's condition is stable, ocular examination and treatment should be done as soon as possible.

The first examination to be performed in any patient with trauma is evaluation of the *visual acuity* in each eye. This should be done before any other diagnostic procedures are attempted. The only exception to this is the patient who presents with a history of ocular exposure to caustic substances. In this case, the ocular tissues should be copiously irrigated with large volumes of water or sterile saline even before a complete history is taken. An eye chart may not be readily available, but it is not required to determine an adequate visual acuity. Visual acuity can be tested with any available printed material such as newspaper, magazine, or book; the vision should be

recorded by stating the exact source and size of the printed material. The reactivity and symmetry of the pupils should be checked in every patient, in addition to confrontation fields, ocular rotations, and alignment. Pressure on the globes should be avoided whenever the possibility of ocular perforation is present. Therefore, applanation tensions should be determined only after a complete examination of the anterior segment.

The bony structure of the orbit should be evaluated for displacement.

The external examination is important in orbital and lid trauma. Gross inspection of the symmetry of the features of the face may give a good indication of the extent of injury. Any exophthalmos or enophthalmos should be measured with an exophthalmometer. Vertical or horizontal displacement of the globe should also be measured. The bony structures of the orbit should be evaluated, including a check for displacement of the maxillary or zygomatic processes and the superior orbital rim. If signs or symptoms of trauma are present, a careful sensory examination of the skin surrounding the eye should be performed to document areas of anesthesia. Any swelling of the periocular tissues should be lightly palpated to determine whether crepitus is present; this is an indication of orbital-sinus continuity secondary to an orbital wall fracture.

A blowout fracture of the orbit often accompanies blunt ocular trauma.

Fractures of the medial or inferior walls of the orbit are most common with blunt trauma; the orbital volume increases and the orbital contents may prolapse through or become incarcerated in the bony defect (see Fig. 8–26 and 8–27). The most common signs are enophthalmos and restricted motility. Eye positions should be measured with an exophthalmometer to document either enophthalmos or exophthalmos. The ocular rotations should be carefully evaluated and recorded. Radiographic studies are required to delineate the location and extent of the orbital fractures. Anteriorposterior, lateral, and Waters' views are the most helpful views on plain radiography. If available, computed tomography of the orbits with axial, coronal, and sagittal views is the best method of showing the site of fracture and the amount of prolapsed tissue. In the acute setting, the administration of broad-spectrum antibiotics is advised to prevent microorganisms in the sinus from causing orbital cellulitis.

Orbital fractures may accompany more severe periocular trauma. The first priority is to evaluate the globe. If collapse of the orbit is severe, the orbital tissues may impinge on the globe and raise intraocular pressure to the point of damage. Optic nerve compression and compromise may be present, although the intraocular pressure is normal. Progressive compressive optic neuropathy in orbital trauma is an indication for immediate intervention. Plain radiography and computed tomography can be used to evaluate the extent of bony and soft tissue damage. After the patient's condition is stabilized and the integrity of the globe is ensured, the patient should be referred to the appropriate specialist for repair.

The *eyelids* should be carefully evaluated, with particular attention to the lid margins, medial and lateral canthal tendons, and the lacrimal drainage system. The orbicularis oculi is a sphincter, and an interrupted tendon will pull away from the point of insertion when forced closure is attempted. In patients in whom interruption of the canthal tendons is suspected, asking the patient to perform forced closure of the eye will allow evaluation of these structures. The puncta and canaliculi should be evaluated by inspection only. Probing should be done only by persons with experience in the procedure to avoid further damage to the lacrimal drainage system. As a rule, any incision extending through the lid margin nasal to either the superior or the inferior punctum should be assumed to involve the canaliculus and should be repaired (Fig. 11–1).

If perforation of the globe is suspected, the subconjunctival space should be explored.

After the external examination is complete, slit-lamp biomicroscopy should be performed. Examination of the globe should be systematic

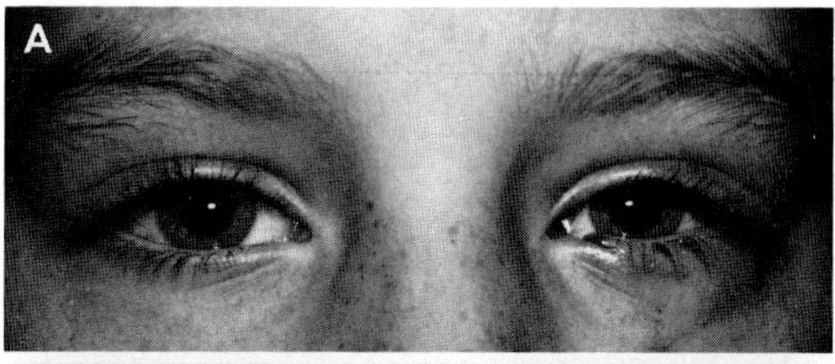
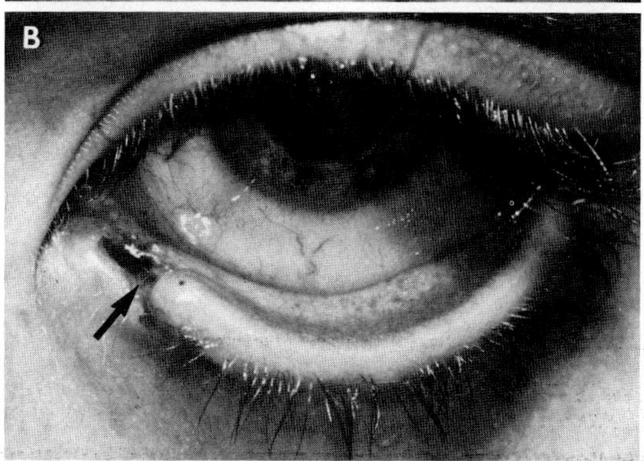

Fig. 11–1. Medial eyelid laceration involving the canaliculus. *A,* On external inspection, the subtle findings of a small lid laceration belie the severity of injury. *B,* Eversion of the lid shows the full extent of injury with severed canaliculus (*arrow*).

and thorough. Because ocular hemorrhage or rapid development of a cataract may obscure the view into the eye, the first look into the patient's eye may be the only chance. A good method to examine the globe is to evaluate each layer as it is encountered. Such a systematic approach will help to avoid inadvertent omissions. All findings, negative as well as positive, should be recorded.

The most external layer of the globe to be examined is the conjunctiva, and careful examination may give clues of serious ocular damage. A *subconjunctival hemorrhage* (blood beneath the conjunctiva on the surface of the globe) is common in patients with ocular trauma (Fig. 11–2). The nature of the trauma is the key to the management of subconjunctival hemorrhage. For any circumstance in which violation of the globe is suspected, the subconjunctival space must be surgically explored in search of the site of penetration. Subconjunctival hemorrhage may mask the site of entry in projectile injuries. In explosion injuries in which multiple small fragments are involved (such as an automobile accident with small fragments of glass), careful examination of the conjunctiva is

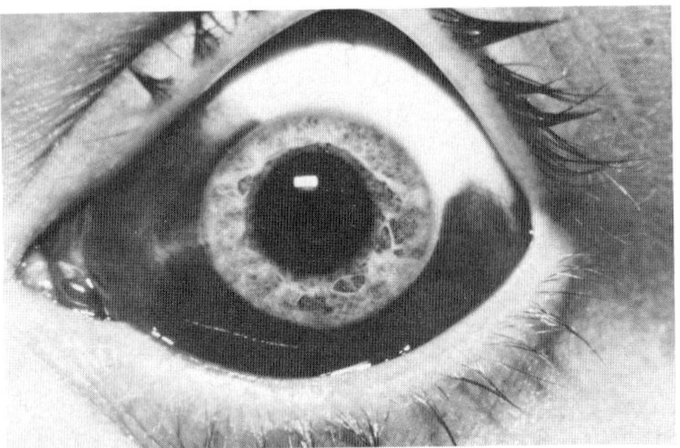

Fig. 11–2. Posttraumatic subconjunctival hemorrhage obscures the inferior globe.

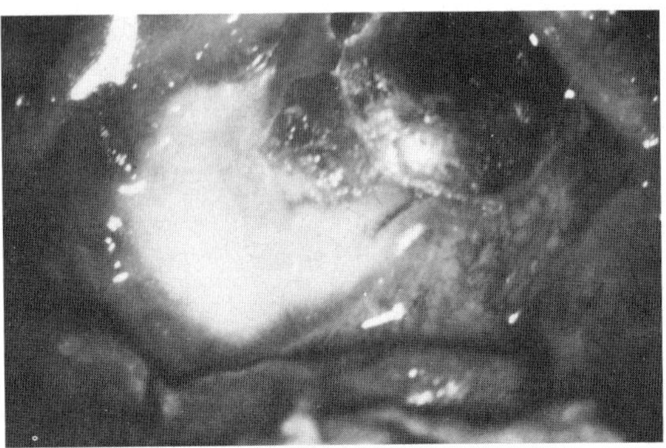

Fig. 11–4. Avascular "porcelain-white" conjunctiva and sclera after alkali exposure.

required to identify any foreign bodies. Isolated conjunctival lacerations are uncommon. Most heal well without surgical repair, but it is important to determine that an underlying laceration of the globe is not present (Fig. 11–3).

Injuries to the globe and ocular adnexa from strong acids or alkali are often blinding.

Tissue damage from caustic substances leads to scarring of the lids, conjunctiva, and cornea. In general, *injuries from strong alkalis are worse than those from acids.* The application of a strong acid to tissue causes a denaturation of the proteins that prevents further diffusion of the acid into the tissues. Strong alkalis, however, do not cause denaturation of proteins and continue to diffuse deeply into the tissues for long periods.

Eyes are often quiet-appearing and "porcelain white" from destruction of the scleral and conjunctival blood vessels by the caustic substances (Fig. 11–4).

Prompt, copious irrigation of all tissues exposed to strong acids or alkalis must be performed in any patient in whom exposure to caustic substances is suspected (Fig. 11–5). At least 1 liter of sterile water or saline must be used. After irrigation, the eyes should be examined carefully, with particular attention to epithelial defects of the cornea and conjunctiva. Destruction of the accessory lacrimal glands, scarring and cicatrization of the lids and conjunctiva, and opacification and vascularization of the cornea are common mechanisms of blindness in these patients.

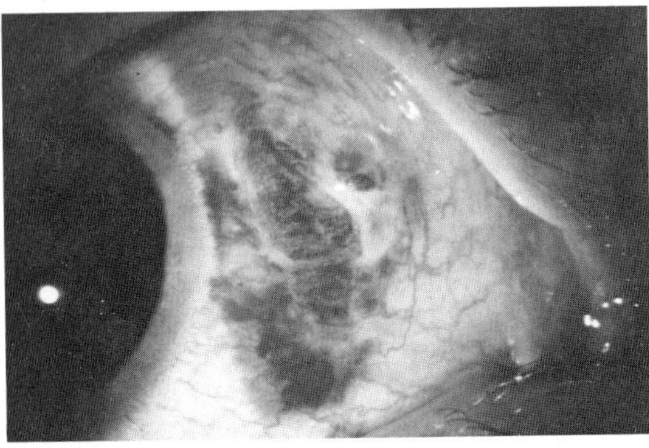

Fig. 11–3. Conjunctival lacerations with hemorrhage should always lead one to suspect a deeper laceration of the sclera.

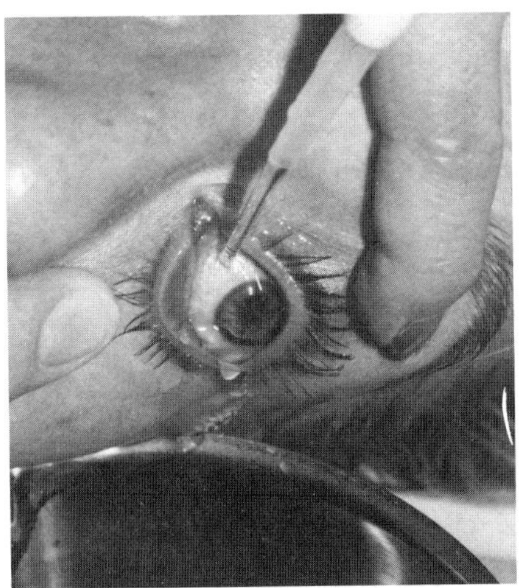

Fig. 11–5. Proper method of ocular irrigation after caustic chemical exposure.

Corneal abrasion is probably the most common traumatic injury to the globe.

A careful corneal examination is important because most traumatic insults to the globe involve the cornea. One should determine first whether the cornea is clear and whether there are any irregularities in the epithelium. Staining of the epithelium with fluorescein will help to delineate the site and extent of epithelial abrasions. After careful examination to determine the extent of the *corneal abrasion*, the conjunctiva under the eyelids should be inspected to determine whether any foreign bodies are present. Often the pattern of the corneal abrasion will indicate where the foreign body can be found (Fig. 11–6). Multiple foreign bodies can be present. After the foreign body is removed and the remainder of the ophthalmic examination is completed, a cycloplegic and antibiotic ointment should be instilled in the cul-de-sac and the eye should be patched. The patient should be reexamined in 12 to 24 hours to determine the extent of epithelial regrowth and should be examined daily until the epithelium is healed.

Foreign bodies that are imbedded in the cornea (Fig. 11–7) should be removed only after careful slit-lamp examination has determined that the foreign body is no deeper than 25% of the corneal thickness, unless facilities and sur-

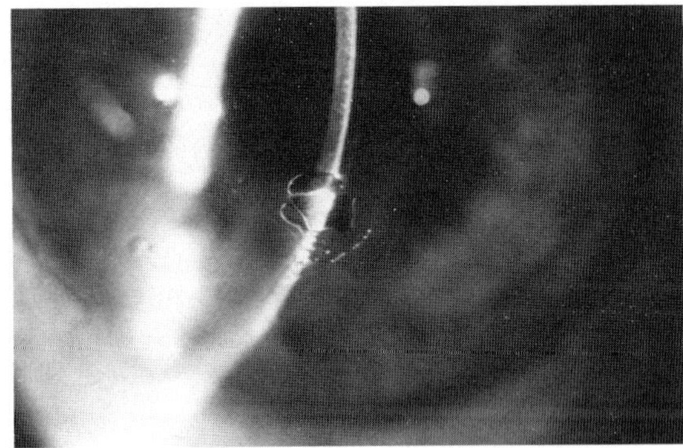

Fig. 11–7. Corneal foreign body and abrasion.

gical expertise are readily available for surgical repair. Superficial corneal foreign bodies can be removed with a cotton-tipped applicator or a 30-gauge needle tip. After the foreign body is removed, the eye is treated for a corneal abrasion.

Corneal perforations require immediate repair.

Corneal trauma accompanied by a shallow anterior chamber or an eccentrically shaped pupil is aposematic of a *corneal perforation* (Fig. 11–8). When the site of perforation is not obvious, *Seidel's test* should be performed to identify the site of perforation. Fluorescein 2% eyedrops are instilled and the eye is examined with a blue cobalt light by slit-lamp biomicroscopy. If a corneal leak is present, a disturbance or "wave" is seen in the tear film from escaping aqueous humor. In some corneal perforations,

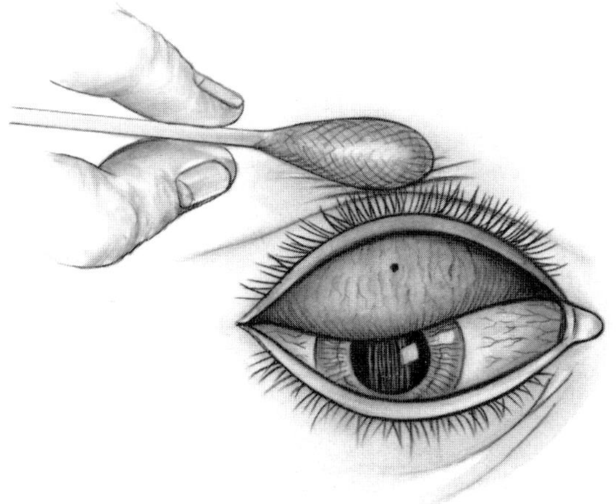

Fig. 11–6. Linear, vertically oriented corneal abrasions should raise suspicion of a foreign body on the upper eyelid tarsal plate.

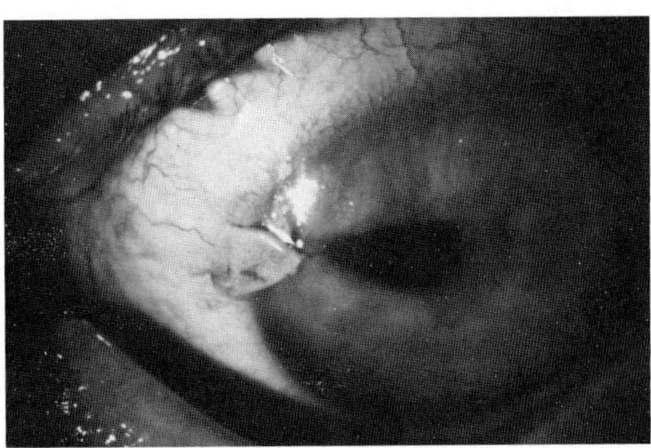

Fig. 11–8. Corneal laceration with iris prolapse and eccentric pupil. Notice that the pupil "points" toward the perforation.

the iris will often come forward and plug the wound. This condition usually causes the pupil to become eccentrically shaped.

A perforated globe should be repaired with the patient under general anesthesia. Induction should be done without succinylcholine to avoid an increase in intraocular pressure from extraocular muscle contraction during induction. If facilities are not available to repair the laceration, a shield (not an eye patch) should be placed over the eye to protect it from further injury (Fig. 11–9), and the patient should be referred to the appropriate specialist for repair. The patient should take no food or drink by mouth to avoid unnecessary delays before surgical repair. These same guidelines should be followed any time the globe is perforated or ruptured.

Blunt injury to the globe can cause corneal edema with or without tears in Descemet's membrane. This is not uncommon in injuries caused by a fist or a small ball or in an infant after forceps delivery.

The most common cause of a hyphema is a partial avulsion of the iris root.

Examination of the anterior chamber should determine whether erythrocytes, leukocytes, fibrin, pigment, or foreign bodies are present. A *hyphema* is a collection of erythrocytes in the anterior chamber and often follows blunt injury. The hyphema may be microscopic, with the cells circulating freely in the anterior chamber and visible only through the slit lamp, or it may be layered inferiorly or across the surface of the iris and visible on gross

inspection (Fig. 11–10). The most common cause of bleeding is partial avulsion of the iris from the iris root, but it may come from any site on the iris. Eyes with hyphema from blunt trauma should be evaluated very carefully to avoid further trauma to the globe with additional bleeding.

There has been much controversy regarding the appropriate care of hyphema, particularly whether the patient should be treated as an inpatient or an outpatient or whether the antifibrinolytic aminocaproic acid should be administered. It is reasonable, however, to treat a patient with a hyphema with a strong cycloplegic and bed rest for the first 3 to 5 days. The eye should be examined at a slit lamp if possible for the first 3 days and the intraocular pressure should be carefully monitored. If a total hyphema is present with a high pressure, an anterior chamber washout should be considered. This will help to prevent future corneal staining, and the reduction in intraocular pressure will preserve the optic nerve. The severe nature of the eye injury should be explained thoroughly to the patient, and potential future complications, such as glaucoma or cataract, should be discussed to emphasize that long-term follow-up is necessary.

If chronic inflammation persists after trauma, an intraocular foreign body should be considered.

Trauma is often followed by intraocular inflammation, which may be manifested by leu-

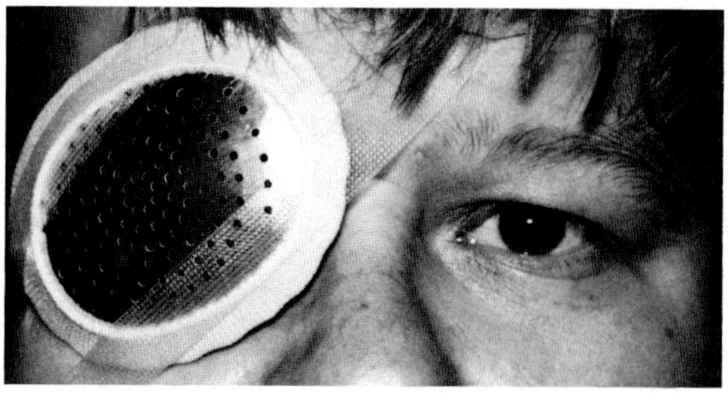

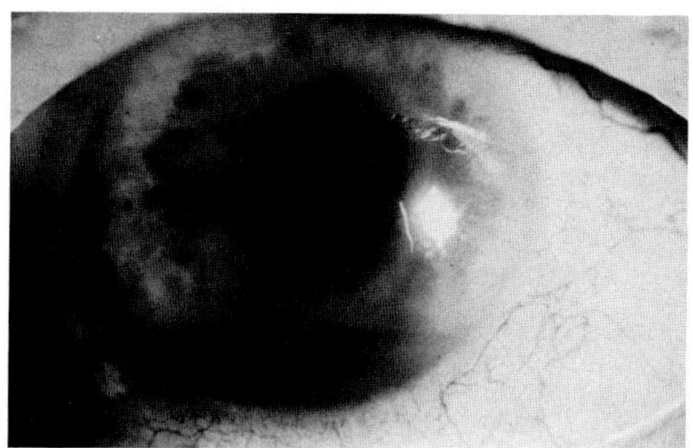

Fig. 11–9. A shield, not a patch, should be placed over a traumatized, "open" eye until it can be repaired.

Fig. 11–10. A large hyphema with layering of erythrocytes.

kocytes in the anterior chamber. The severity of inflammation may range from mild, with the presence of only a few cells, to severe, with a hypopyon and a fibrin clot. Before *posttraumatic inflammation* is diagnosed, however, a careful search should be performed to rule out ocular perforation with or without the presence of an intraocular foreign body. Intraocular foreign bodies in the anterior chamber or elsewhere can also elicit a severe inflammatory response and must always be considered in patients with posttraumatic ocular inflammation. As a rule, anterior chamber foreign bodies are usually associated with findings of a corneal perforation. Seidel's test and radiography should be included in the evaluation of every patient with moderate to severe posttraumatic inflammation.

Careful examination of the iris is important. Transillumination defects can give clues to the location of intraocular foreign bodies. Occasionally, a foreign body pierces the cornea and may lodge in the iris and not reach the posterior segment of the eye. An abnormal fluttering movement of the iris called *iridodonesis* may be seen when there is posterior displacement of the lens due to blunt trauma. Traumatic tears of the iris sphincter can cause mydriasis and posttraumatic anisocoria. A small localized rupture of the iris sphincter may cause an irregularly shaped, poorly reactive pupil.

Blunt trauma may cause rupture of zonules with instability of the lens (phacodonesis) or a cataract.

The lens of the eye should be evaluated for clarity and stability. The blunt or penetrating trauma can cause local or generalized cataract formation. Occasionally the track of an intraocular foreign body can be seen passing through the lens. Ocular trauma may rupture the zonular fibers, with resultant lens instability and movement (*phacodonesis*). This sign can best be elicited by asking the patient to look from side to side while the lens is viewed through the slit lamp. Phacodonesis after blunt trauma to the globe may or may not require operation to remove the lens. If the degree of phacodonesis is small, careful observation alone may suffice.

Cataracts may be caused by perforating eye injuries or foreign bodies.

An opaque lens caused by ocular perforation or foreign body injury is usually managed surgically. The location of the missile in the posterior segment of the globe can sometimes be determined by ultrasonography, but this examination should be avoided in a globe that is not intact. Occasionally after foreign body injury, the lens may develop a small sectoral opacity. If the remainder of the lens remains clear, the lens need not be removed at the time of foreign body removal (Fig. 11–11). Although in many patients the sectoral cataract will progress to a completely opaque lens, in some the opacity may not worsen and may even improve.

A traumatic vitreous hemorrhage may obscure the view of the fundus.

The vitreous should be examined to evaluate the presence of cells or intraocular foreign bodies. *Vitreous hemorrhage* can accompany ocular trauma and may range from a few scattered erythrocytes in the vitreous cavity to a massive vitreous hemorrhage that obscures the retina. Any type of ocular trauma may cause vitreous hemorrhage. Avulsion of retinal vessels associated with retinal tears and hemorrhage due to intraocular foreign bodies are two common examples.

Vitreous hemorrhage that appears to arise from the peripapillary vessels is sometimes seen after severe head trauma. This is known as *Terson's syndrome* and is thought to be caused by an

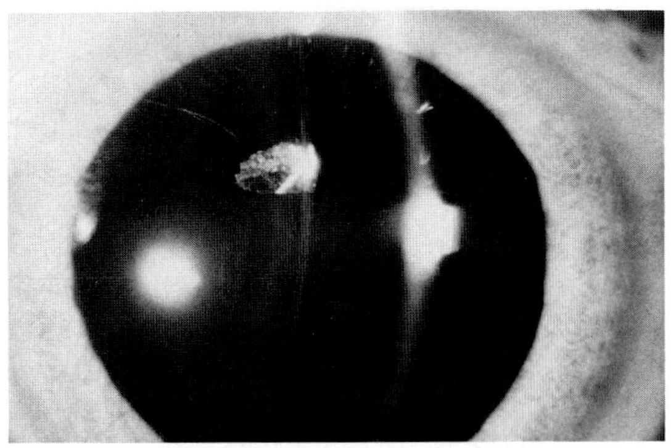

Fig. 11–11. Metallic foreign body in lens.

abrupt increase in intracranial pressure that is transmitted through the optic nerve sheath to the lamina cribrosa with bleeding from the central retinal vessels.

Vitreous hemorrhage after blunt trauma may resolve spontaneously. In the meantime, if the globe is intact, the posterior pole should be scanned with ultrasonography to evaluate for a retinal detachment or an unsuspected intraocular foreign body.

In subacute ocular trauma, leukocytes may be seen in the vitreous. These can be due either to posttraumatic inflammation or to inflammation induced by an intraocular foreign body. Foreign bodies of organic matter often cause a severe intraocular reaction with a sufficient number of leukocytes to obscure the ocular fundus. If the clarity of the media permits, the vitreous should be carefully examined for intraocular foreign bodies. If identified, their location should be carefully documented because subsequent hemorrhage or inflammation may obscure them from later view. Hemorrhages that do not clear spontaneously or that are associated with an intraocular foreign body should be managed surgically.

Trauma to the retina may cause hemorrhage, edema, or tears.

The retina often shows manifestations of ocular injury. Some of the more common findings are retinal hemorrhage, retinal foreign body, commotio retinae (Berlin's edema), choroidal tears, retinal tears, or retinal dialysis.

Retinal hemorrhage may be intraretinal or subhyaloid. Intraretinal hemorrhage is an extravasation of blood within the retinal substance itself. It manifests as flame-shaped hemorrhages that follow the contour of the nerve fiber layer. *Purtscher's retinopathy* is a term used to describe intraretinal hemorrhages after trauma and is generally reserved for cases in which no direct injury to the globe is suspected. Postulated causes for the retinal hemorrhage have been fat emboli and increased dynamic intravascular pressure. Subhyaloid hemorrhages arise from retinal vessels and collect under the hyaloid face of the vitreous. These are often sharply delineated and may show a layering of erythrocytes. Subhyaloid

hemorrhages may be caused by the avulsion and tearing of retinal vessels or from increased intracranial pressure in Terson's syndrome.

Intraocular foreign bodies should be removed as soon as possible, with very few exceptions.

Organic foreign bodies are the most troublesome because they are generally contaminated. Even if the foreign body is sterile, there is usually severe inflammation that can rapidly lead to disorganization of the globe with loss of all visual potential. Organic foreign bodies should be removed within 12 to 24 hours if at all possible.

Projectile metallic foreign bodies nearly always result from metal striking metal and are usually sterile. Severe intraocular inflammation, however, may be produced by intraocular foreign bodies containing iron (*siderosis*) or copper (*chalcosis*). Therefore, most metallic foreign bodies should be removed as soon as possible. Intraocular and periocular antibiotics should be given at the time of operation. The role of systemic antibiotics in the treatment of intraocular foreign bodies is controversial.

Most intraocular foreign bodies that enter the vitreous progress posteriorly to the retina. The impact site of the foreign body usually appears as a whitish area in the retina itself. The foreign body may be found overlying this area (Fig. 11–12). If the foreign body has passed through the retina into the choroid, there usually is surrounding hemorrhage. Careful documentation of the position of an intravitreal or intraretinal foreign body is important because subsequent cataract or other clouding of the media may occur.

Commotio retinae (Berlin's edema) is a whitish discoloration of the retina that occurs after blunt ocular trauma (Fig. 11–13). The whitish area is due to disruption of the outer retina with intraretinal edema. Acutely, scotomas corresponding to the involved area may occur, but they usually resolve within several weeks.

Choroidal tears generally result from blunt trauma and are seen as linear lesions through which the underlying sclera can be visualized (Fig. 11–14). The overlying retina is usually intact. Choroidal tears are not treatable, but late

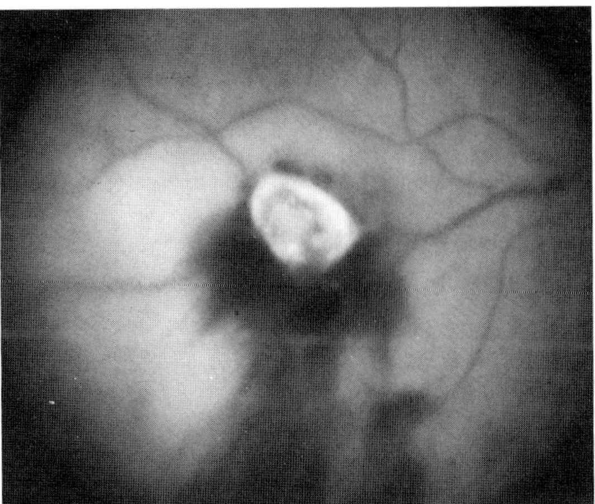

Fig. 11–12. Metallic intraocular foreign body suspended in the vitreous. Behind the foreign body is the impact site with hemorrhage.

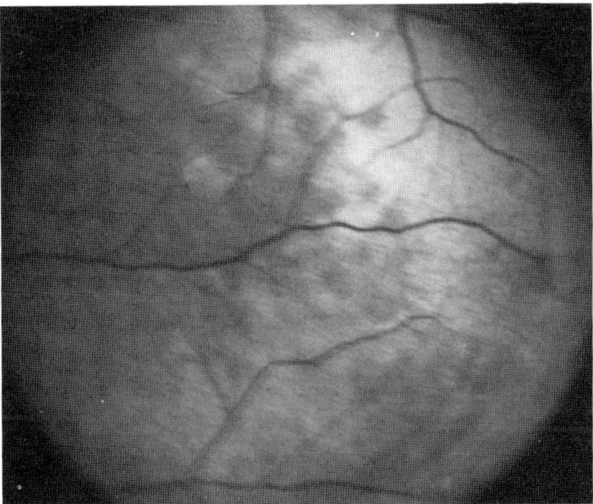

Fig. 11–13. The whitish discoloration of the retina peripherally after blunt ocular trauma is commotio retinae. When it involves the macula, it is sometimes referred to as "Berlin's edema."

complications such as serous or serosanguineous retinal detachment or subretinal neovascular vessel formation may require therapy.

Trauma can cause *retinal tears*. Indirect ophthalmoscopy is essential for diagnosis because traumatic retinal tears generally are found at the area of the vitreous base. This is the area of the vitreous most firmly attached to the retina, and ocular trauma may cause the vitreous

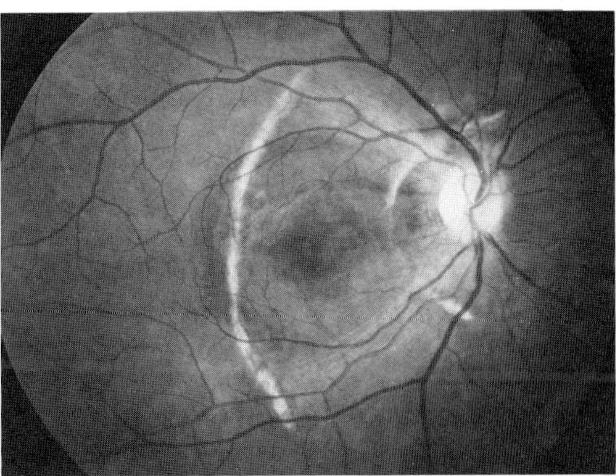

Fig. 11–14. Choroidal tears, one near the disc and one temporal to the macula, after blunt ocular trauma.

to try to pull away from the retina in these areas. If the vitreous cannot free itself, the retina may tear. Horseshoe tears and retinal dialysis are the usual types of retinal tears in trauma. Retinal dialysis is a tear of the retina along the margin where the retina meets the pars plana and is most common in the superior nasal quadrant. Retinal detachment resulting from retinal tears or retinal dialysis should be referred to the appropriate specialist for repair.

Progressive optic nerve dysfunction necessitates intervention.

Ocular or periocular trauma can result in optic nerve injuries. Trauma to the brow may cause a fracture of the optic canal leading to optic nerve compression and injury. Severe trauma may even lead to complete avulsion of the optic nerve from the posterior surface of the globe. A high-resolution computed tomographic scan of the orbit with canal views is the most sensitive examination for optic canal and optic nerve damage. Serial visual field examination can be useful for documenting possible progression of optic nerve injury. If progression of a defect is noted or vision is decreasing, neurosurgical consultation should be obtained. Systemic corticosteroids may be indicated to decrease optic nerve swelling after injury, but their use is controversial.

12

MANAGEMENT OF OPHTHALMIC SPECIMENS FOR PATHOLOGIC EXAMINATION

R. Jean Campbell

The purpose of this chapter is to guide the ophthalmologist in the handling of surgical specimens for submission to the laboratory. These include eyelid and conjunctival specimens; corneal buttons; evisceration specimens; enucleation and exenteration specimens; orbital tissue; ocular fluids; and, rarely, extraocular muscle specimens and decompression specimens from patients with Graves' ophthalmopathy. Preoperative photographs may be helpful for teaching purposes and as documentation for medicolegal matters.

Communication between the surgeon and the pathologist is essential.

If the maximal amount of information is to be obtained from the specimen, a pertinent *history*, particularly with regard to previous surgical procedures, is of paramount importance. Before further procedures, the original microscopy slides and the pathology report of the previous operations must be available for review.

Consideration must be given to whether special examinations of the fresh surgical specimen are needed because careful organization will be required. The questions that must be asked are: 1) will the specimen need to be cultured? 2) should part of the specimen be frozen

for immunohistochemistry or other studies? and 3) will electron microscopic examination be required? Verbal communication with the pathologist in such instances is necessary, is courteous, and is ultimately of great benefit to the patient.

Each tissue specimen to be examined must be sent to the pathology laboratory in a suitable container that is clearly labeled with the patient's name, code number, age, and sex; date of operation; and the *exact anatomic site*. It must be accompanied by a request form that, in addition to the information that is on the container, gives the surgeon's name and the suspected clinical diagnosis. A diagram of the specimen, particularly of epithelial lesions, is helpful.

Special tissue studies require special preparation.

The pathologist and the surgeon must determine whether special studies are indicated, and the first issue to be addressed is whether *infection* is present. Handling of infected tissues always requires special care and is of particular importance when the patient has acquired immunodeficiency syndrome (AIDS) or hepatitis. These concerns must be made known to the microbiologist and pathologist, and the

284

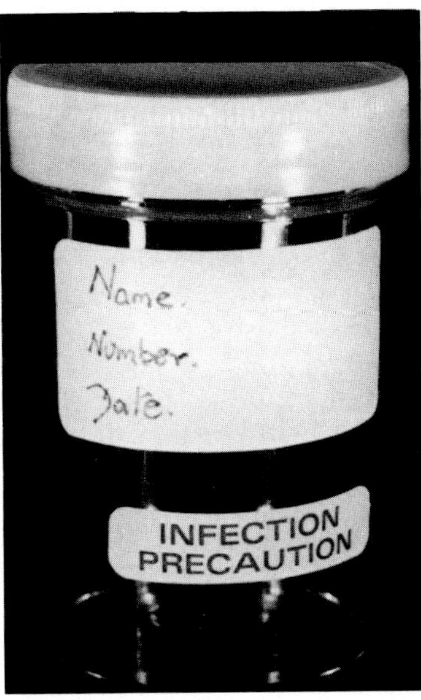

Fig. 12–1. Container for infected material, suitably marked "Infection Precaution."

container must be suitably marked (Fig. 12–1). For reasons of confidentiality, the word "AIDS" should not appear on the container or the form.

Communication with the microbiologist ensures that slides for smears and appropriate transport media will be available in the operating room. It is important that viable tissue is submitted for culture. In certain circumstances, the microbiologist may be present in the operating room to handle the tissues appropriately. If *Acanthamoeba* or other protozoa are suspected, the microbiologist will take smears for calcofluor or trichrome stains and will plate the appropriate media in the operating room. The request form should be completed in advance and should clearly state the suspected organism(s).

Once cultures have been obtained, the next concern is whether tissue should be frozen for studies such as immunohistochemistry, gene rearrangement, or tissue diagnosis. *Immuno-histochemical studies* require that fresh, viable tissue be mounted on a viscous medium and snap-frozen in liquid nitrogen. The laboratory must be notified so that a technician, with a kit that includes a vacuum flask, is present when the tissue is removed. Such studies are needed for lymphoid lesions, suspected pemphigoid, and the identification of cytoskeletal markers in the determination of the cell origin of tumors. Examination of fresh tissue may be more sensitive than that performed on formalin-fixed specimens. Immunopathologic profiles may be obtained by flow cytometry; fresh tissue is preferred, although the studies can also be performed on paraffin-embedded tissues.

Frozen-section histopathologic analysis is necessary when an immediate diagnosis will alter the course of operation.

Optimal resection of a malignant tumor requires that the margins of excision be clear. The edges of the specimen—that is, temporal, nasal, inferior, and superior—require identification (Fig. 12–2). A marker pen or suitable labeling on the mount is helpful. If orientation of the

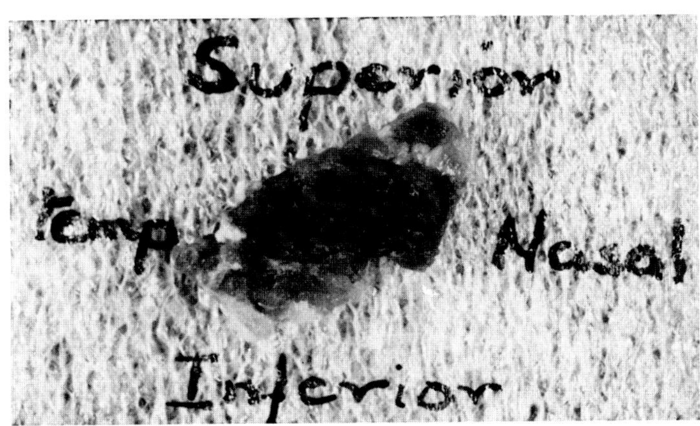

Fig. 12–2. Tissue mounted on sponge that is clearly marked for orientation purposes.

tissue is particularly difficult, the surgeon needs to be present when the pathologist performs the gross examination. Frozen section then confirms complete tumor removal.

Special consideration is required if sebaceous carcinoma or malignant melanoma is suspected. *Sebaceous carcinoma* may require frozen section of fresh tissue to demonstrate the lipid within the tumor cells with oil red O stain. Tissue placed in alcohol cannot be evaluated properly because the alcohol dissolves the lipid. The entire specimen, however, should NEVER be submitted for frozen section because freezing produces irreversible artifact. It is not possible to make an accurate diagnosis on frozen section of densely pigmented tissue, such as *melanoma*, because bleaching is required so that the cells can be seen.

A frozen section is prepared by mounting the fresh tissue specimen on a viscous medium and then snap-freezing. The specimen is then cut on a cryostat and the iced section is mounted on a slide and stained so that a diagnosis can be determined within a few minutes. The material is subsequently submitted for routine processing together with a representative portion of unfrozen tissue. The remainder of the tissue is preserved in fixative or is totally embedded in paraffin. When a biopsy specimen is being obtained, it is important to remember that necrotic tissue is often nondiagnostic. The sample should include the abnormal tissue together with a rim of normal tissue. The tissue must be handled very gently; crushing with forceps renders tissues noninterpretable. Once the tissue is removed, it must not be allowed to dry out because this process produces further artifact and complicates interpretation. It is important that the paramedical staff within the operating room is aware of these issues so that they, when necessary, can handle the tissues gently and appropriately. Thus, after the needs for microbiologic analysis and for freezing have been addressed, the tissue must be placed *promptly* in a fixative.

The choice of tissue fixative is crucial.

The most commonly used tissue fixative for routine examination is 10% neutral buffered *formalin*. It is not, however, a universal fixative.

For example, cystine, oxalate, and urate crystals are soluble in formalin, and fixation in absolute alcohol is required for their demonstration. The recommended volume of fixative is at least 10 times the volume of the tissue. An enucleated eye, for instance, should be submerged in approximately 100 mL of fixative solution.

Electron microscopic examination requires fresh *glutaraldehyde* or *Trump's solution* for optimal fixation. The specimen must be promptly transported to the laboratory for refrigeration. If a portion of the interior of an eye such as retina or uvea is required for electron microscopic examination, it is advisable that the globe be opened by the pathologist immediately upon its removal so that the fixative has prompt contact with the tissue that is to be examined. Orbital and other tumors that do not lend themselves to immediate diagnosis by frozen section or light microscopy may require electron microscopic examination. However, it is important to remember that electron microscopy may not be as efficient in the determination of tumor type as are immunopathologic profiles performed on frozen tissues.

The ocular tissues need to be submitted on an appropriate base to permit orientation and sectioning.

Small specimens, such as *conjunctiva*, need to be placed on a suitable support mount before immersion in the fixative. If this is not done, the tissue will curl and the margins of resection may be difficult to assess. At our institution, a dehydrated cucumber slice with albumin "glue" is the preferred support mount for conjunctival specimens. Another convenient mount is a moistened Weck cell sponge. A small portion of sponge is dampened in the fixative, excess moisture dried, and the tissue carefully laid on the surface, cut edge down. On no account must the tissue be placed on dry sponge because the sponge will swell on immersion in the fixative and cause stretching and distortion of the tissue. It is important that the tissue sample is submerged in the fixative and does not adhere to the lid or walls of the container above the solution.

Corneal epithelial scrapings that are removed with a Beaver blade should be left on the blade. The blade with cells is then detached from the handle and placed in the appropriate fixative.

Enucleation specimens should be rinsed quickly in saline to remove excess blood before immersing in 10 times the volume of fixative. If blood is left on the specimen, it coagulates and the presence of extrascleral tumor is then difficult for the pathologist to assess. The container should have a wide neck so the specimen can be removed easily (Fig. 12–3).

If the eye cannot be processed in the laboratory of the hospital, it should be allowed to fix for 48 hours before it is sent to a reference laboratory. The eye should be wrapped in a formalin-soaked gauze, placed in a container that is resistant to pressure, and be accompanied by a letter or form with the pertinent clinical history and other significant data. A preliminary telephone communication with the pathologist is always helpful.

Exenteration specimens require a large tub of fixative. Fat absorbs fixative solution rapidly and at the expense of more vital structures that are needed for examination. On no account should the specimen be "stuffed" into a small container.

Examination of *ocular fluids* includes those of the aqueous and vitreous. Taps of the anterior chamber are performed for identification of inflammatory and malignant cells. Vitrec-

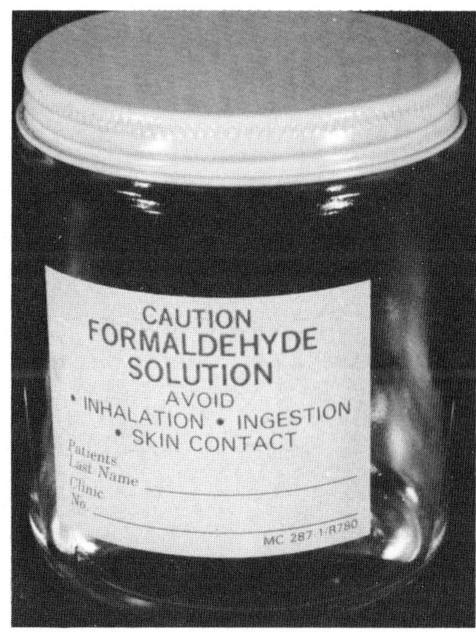

Fig. 12–3. Suitable container, appropriately labeled, with wide neck for enucleation specimen.

tomy specimens are useful for suspected tumor or mesenchymal membranes. Two specimens should be obtained, one for cytology and one for culture.

In summary the surgeon plays an important role in ophthalmic pathology. Communication with the pathologist before, during, and after the operation is essential to optimize the preparation, handling, and interpretation of tissue specimens, especially if special studies are required.

13

OPHTHALMOLOGISTS FAMOUS FOR OTHER ACHIEVEMENTS

John D. Bullock

Ophthalmologists are an amazing lot! They have excelled in many different fields of endeavor, including, among others, literature, athletics, physics, chemistry, language, business, politics, and religion.

Sir Arthur Conan Doyle received his M.B., C.M., and M.D. degrees from the University of Edinburgh. He was in general medical practice in South Sea, Portsmouth, England, for 8 years before going to Vienna to study ophthalmology. After going to London, he became affiliated with the Westminster Eye Infirmary and established an ophthalmology office at 2 Devonshire Place, at the top of Wimpole Street, near Harley Street. Sir Arthur Conan Doyle is best known as the creator and author of the Sherlock Holmes stories (Fig. 13–1).

Robin Cook received a B.A. degree from Wesleyan University and his M.D. degree from Columbia University. After a surgical internship and residency at Queen's Hospital in Honolulu, Hawaii, Cook did his residency in ophthalmology at the Massachusetts Eye and Ear Infirmary and was an instructor in ophthalmology at Harvard Medical School. Robin Cook is the author of numerous popular novels, in-cluding *Year of the Intern*, *Sphinx*, *Brain*, *Fever*, *God Player*, *Mindbend*, and *Harmful Intent*. He is probably best known for *Coma*, which was a huge commercial success, both as a book and as a movie (Fig. 13–2).

Henry B. Stallard received his M.D. degree from St. Bartholomew's Hospital Medical College, where he also did his residency in ophthalmology. He was a pathologist at the Moorfield's Eye Hospital and served in the Middle East and Normandy during World War II. Stallard invented numerous eye surgical instruments and was the author of the textbook *Eye Surgery*. As the author of more than 100 articles in ophthalmology, he made important contributions across the breadth of the specialty with his work on filtration surgery for glaucoma, radiation therapy for retinoblastoma, and the lateral orbitotomy approach for tumors. Academic honors included service as the president of the Ophthalmological Society of the United Kingdom and as Associate Editor of the *British Journal of Ophthalmology*. Henry Stallard was also an internationally recognized middle-distance runner. He helped set the world's record in the 2-mile relay in 1920, won the Bronze Medal in the 1924 Paris Olympics in the 1,500-meter run, and also ran fourth in the 800-meter run. The 1924 Paris Olympics were immortalized by the film *Chariots of Fire*, in which the character of Henry B. Stallard appears in numerous scenes (Fig. 13–3).

This chapter is based on two previously published articles: J.D. Bullock: Ophthalmologists: setting new sights. Harvard Med Alumni Bull, Summer 1989, pp 50–54; J.D. Bullock: Alex Trebek, Jeopardy, and ophthalmologists famous for other activities. Dayton Med 45:149–152, 1989.

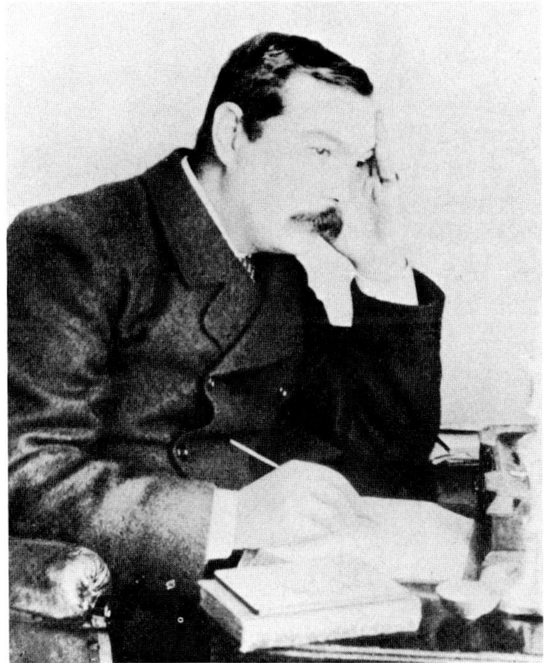

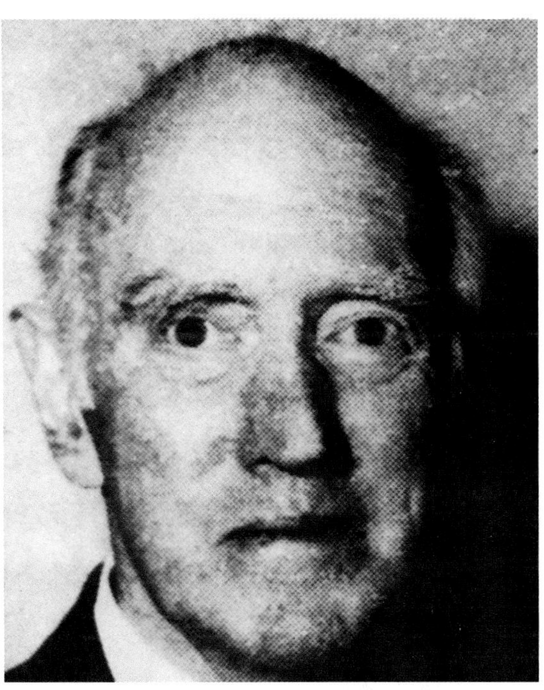

Fig. 13–1. Sir Arthur Conan Doyle. (From A.E. Rodin, J.D. Key: Medical Casebook of Doctor Arthur Conan Doyle: From Practitioner to Sherlock Holmes and Beyond. Malabar, Florida, Robert E. Krieger Publishing Company, 1984. By permission of the publisher.)

Fig. 13–3. Henry B. Stallard. (From H.B. Stallard. Br Med J 4:302, 1973. By permission of the British Medical Association.)

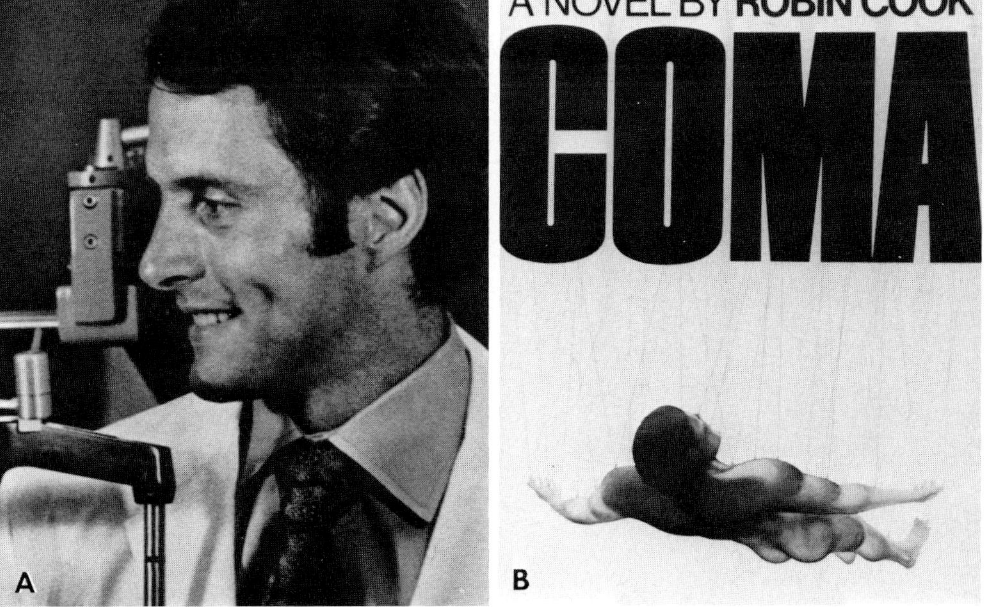

Fig. 13–2. *A*, Robin Cook. *B*, Book cover of *Coma*, a novel written by Robin Cook. (*B* from R. Cook: Coma. Boston, Little, Brown & Company, 1977. By permission of the publisher.)

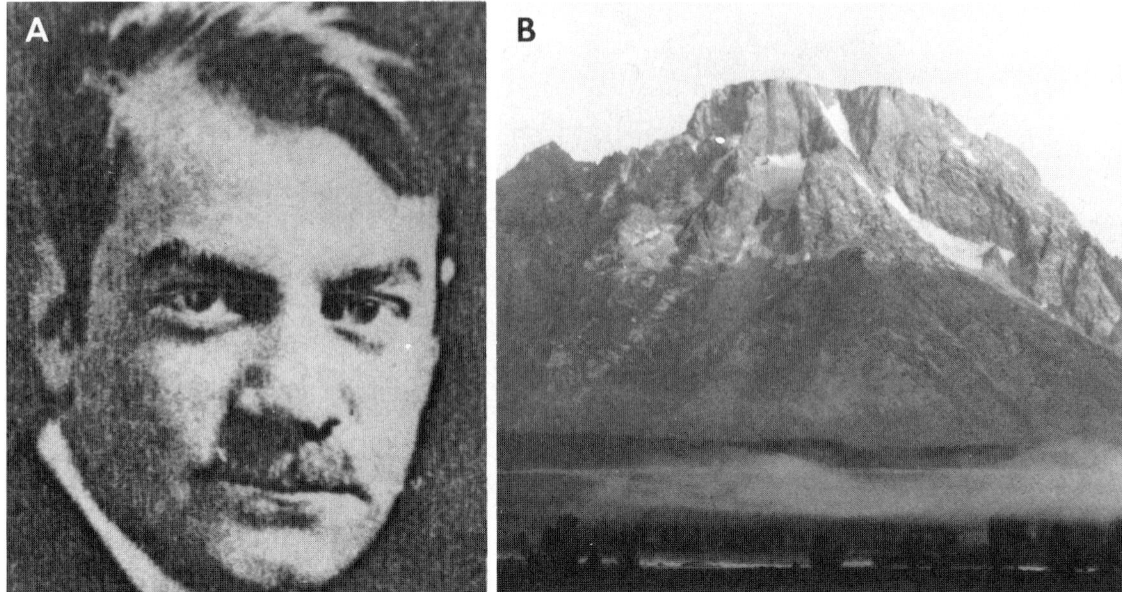

Fig. 13–4.   *A*, LeGrand H. Hardy. *B*, Mount Moran, in the Grand Tetons, Grand Teton National Park, Wyoming. This 12,594-foot mountain was first ascended by LeGrand H. Hardy in 1922. (*A*, from M.C. Wheeler: The Eye Institute in New York: An Intimate History. New York, Cooper Square Publishers, 1969, pp. 151–152. By permission of The Edward S. Harkness Eye Institute.)

LeGrand H. Hardy received an A.B. degree from Brigham Young University and B.S. and M.D. degrees from Columbia University. He was an intern at New York City Hospital, did his residency in ophthalmology at Bellevue Hospital, and was on the staff of the Harkness Eye Institute. Important contributions to ophthalmology include the development of the Hardy-Rand-Rittler color plates and founding the American Orthoptic Council. Hardy was also a mountain climber, and in 1922 he was the first to ascend the highest summit (12,594 feet) of Mount Moran, in the Grand Tetons, Grand Teton National Park, Wyoming (Fig. 13–4).

David W. Sime received his B.A. and M.D. degrees from Duke University. He was a surgical intern at Duke, completed his residency in ophthalmology at the Bascom Palmer Eye Institute, and currently practices ophthalmology in Miami, Florida. Sime gave up professional baseball and football contracts for his medical

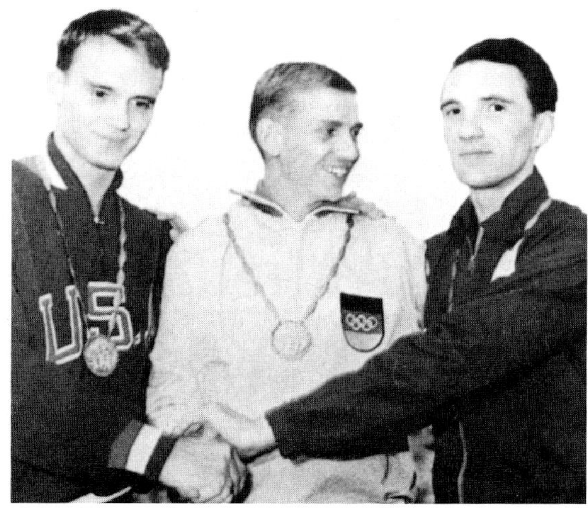

Fig. 13–5.   David W. Sime (left), Silver Medalist in the 100-meter dash in the 1960 Rome Olympics, together with Armin Hary (center) of West Germany, Gold Medalist, and Peter F. Radford (right) of Great Britain, Bronze Medalist. (From J.D. Bullock: Ophthalmologists: setting new sights. Harvard Med Alumni Bull, Summer 1989, pp. 50–54. By permission of the Harvard Medical School Alumni Association.)

education. He later became "The World's Fastest Human." In 1956 Sime set five world records in track, including the 100-yard dash, which he ran in 9.3 seconds. Sime won a Silver Medal at the Rome Olympics in 1960, running the 100-meter dash in 10.2 seconds (Fig. 13–5).

Thomas H. Casanova III received a B.A. degree from Louisiana State University and his M.D. degree from the University of Cincinnati College of Medicine. He was an intern at the Good Samaritan Hospital in Cincinnati, did his residency in ophthalmology at Louisiana State University, and was a fellow in oculoplastic surgery at the University of Utah. He currently practices in Crowley, Louisiana. Casanova was a three-time all-American football player at Louisiana State University. He played professional football with the Cincinnati Bengals while attending medical school and was an all-pro safety and punt returner (Fig. 13–6).

Judith E. Melick received her M.D. degree from Harvard Medical School. She was an intern at the Pennsylvania Hospital and a resident in ophthalmology at the Wills Eye Hospital and she currently practices in Philadelphia. Melick placed fifth in the 1972 Munich Olympics in the 100-meter breast stroke and helped set an Olympic record in the 400-meter medley relay (Fig. 13–7).

Hermann von Helmholtz obtained his M.D. degree from the Friedrich Wilhelm Medical Institute and served as a physician to the Potsdam Army Regiment. In 1851, he invented the ophthalmoscope and a refraction device. In 1856, he wrote the *Handbook of Physiological Optics*. Helmholtz was also a famous physicist who made monumental discoveries in electricity, magnetism, and sound. His most important discovery, however, was the first law of thermodynamics—conservation of energy (Fig. 13–8).

Fritz Pregl received his M.D. degree from the University of Graz and practiced ophthalmology for 2 years, performing eye surgery. Pregl then left ophthalmology to study biochemistry for 1 year. He later became professor and chairman of the Medical/Chemical De-

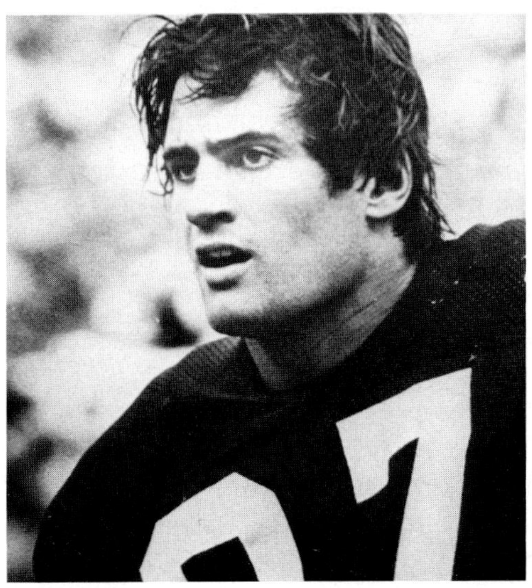

Fig. 13–6. Thomas H. Casanova III, professional football player with the Cincinnati Bengals. (From J.D. Bullock: Ophthalmologists: setting new sights. Harvard Med Alumni Bull, Summer 1989, pp. 50–54. By permission of the Harvard Medical School Alumni Association.)

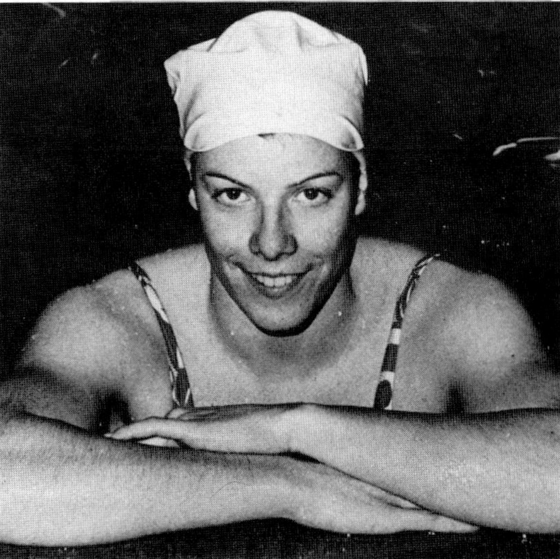

Fig. 13–7. Judith E. Melick, swimmer who helped set an Olympic record in the 400-meter medley relay at the 1972 Munich Olympics. (From J.D. Bullock: Ophthalmologists: setting new sights. Harvard Med Alumni Bull, Summer 1989, pp. 50–54. By permission of the Harvard Medical School Alumni Association.)

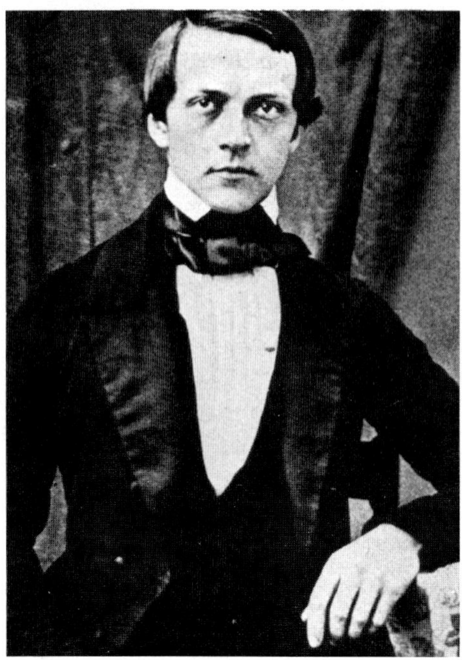

Fig. 13–8.   Painting of Hermann von Helmholtz, a famous physicist who discovered the first law of thermodynamics. (From J.D. Bullock: Ophthalmologists: setting new sights. Harvard Med Alumni Bull, Summer 1989, pp. 50–54. By permission of the Harvard Medical School Alumni Association.)

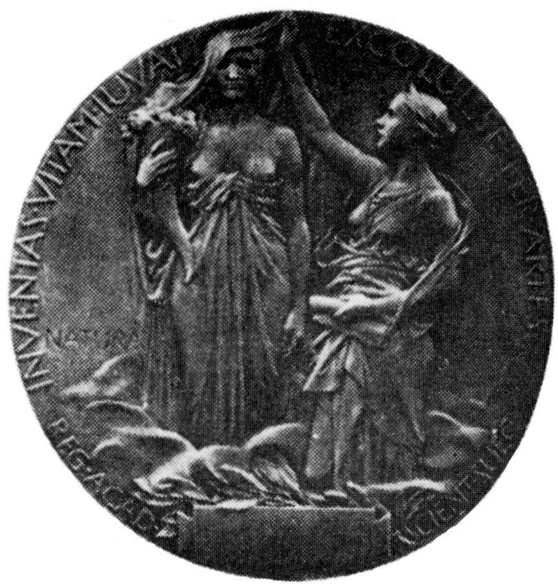

Fig. 13–9.   Nobel Prize in chemistry, won by Fritz Pregl for his pioneering work in quantitative organic microanalysis. (Copyright the Nobel Foundation. By permission.)

partment at the University of Graz. He won the Nobel Prize in chemistry in 1923 for his pioneering work in quantitative organic microanalysis (Fig. 13–9).

Thomas Young attended the Hunterian School of Anatomy and St. Bartholomew's Hospital School of Medicine in London, the University of Edinburgh, and the University of Göttingen. He received M.B. and M.D. degrees from Cambridge University. Young made many brilliant contributions to ophthalmology, discovering astigmatism, accommodation, light interference, and the wave nature of light. He was the first to calculate the wavelengths of seven colors, and he developed the concept of a continuous light spectrum. Young also was the first person to measure visual fields and the blind spot, he provided the first geometric construction of refracted rays, and he developed equations of geometric optics.

Thomas Young was also a famous linguist

with knowledge of 12 languages (English, Greek, Latin, French, Italian, German, Spanish, Arabic, Hebrew, Syriac, Persian, and Chaldee). Young began to study the texts of the Rosetta stone in 1814 (8 years before Champollion), and he provided the key that unlocked the secrets of hieroglyphics–namely, that in the transliteration of non-Egyptian names, hieroglyphic symbols and phonetic values were used. He realized that the demotic texts were a mixture of symbolic and alphabetical characters (Fig. 13–10).

Ludwick Lejzer Zamenhof studied medicine in Moscow and Warsaw, received his ophthalmology training at the Jewish Hospital in Warsaw and at the University of Vienna, and practiced in Warsaw, Kherson, and Grodno, Poland. He was fluent in eight languages, including Polish, French, German, Russian, Yiddish, Latin, Greek, and English. Zamenhof is best known for his creation of the international language Esperanto (Fig. 13–11).

Jules Stein received his M.D. degree from Rush Medical College in Chicago and studied ophthalmology at the University of Vienna. He completed his residency at the Cook County Hospital and practiced ophthalmol-

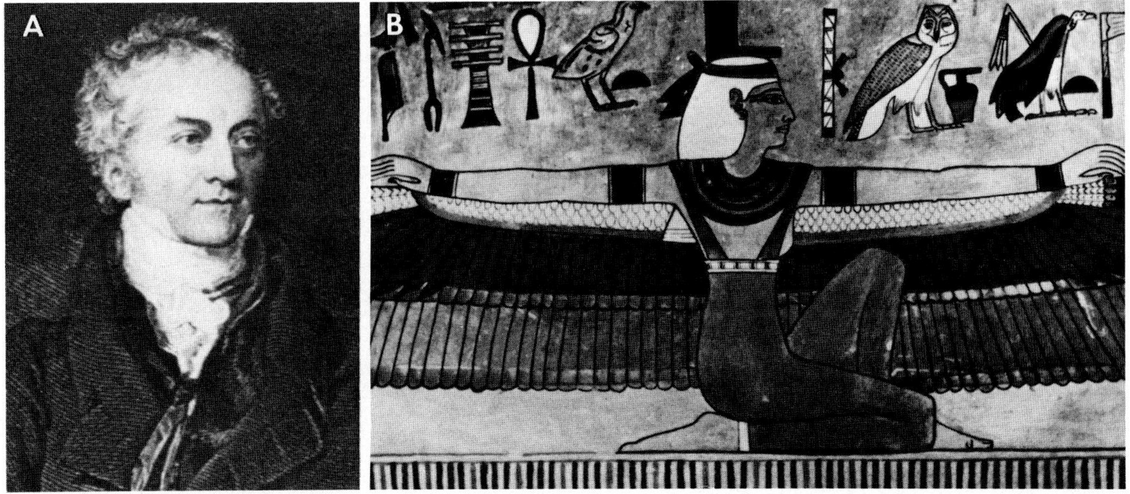

Fig. 13–10. *A*, Thomas Young. *B*, Examples of hieroglyphics, the Egyptian language deciphered by Thomas Young. (*A*, from F. Oldham: Thomas Young. Br Med J 4:150–152, 1974. By permission of the British Medical Association. *B*, from J.D. Bullock: Ophthalmologists: setting new sights. Harvard Med Alumni Bull, Summer 1989, pp. 50–54. By permission of the Harvard Medical School Alumni Association.)

ogy for 3 years in Chicago. Stein founded the Music Corporation of America (MCA), the parent company of the Leeds Music Company, Decca Records, and Universal Pictures-Television. A great philanthropist, he founded Research to Prevent Blindness and the Jules Stein Eye Institute at the University of California, Los Angeles, and was influential in the establishment of the National Eye Institute (Fig. 13–12).

Jose Rizal received his B.A. degree from the University of Santo Tomas, in the Philippines, and his M.D. and Ph.D. degrees from the Central University of Madrid. He studied ophthalmology in Paris, Berlin, Heidelberg, the United States, London, and Japan. (A plaque commemorating his ophthalmology training hangs at the University Eye Clinic in Heidelberg, Germany.) After completing his medical studies, he returned to the Philippines and established an eye clinic in his hometown of Calamba. His first patient was his mother,

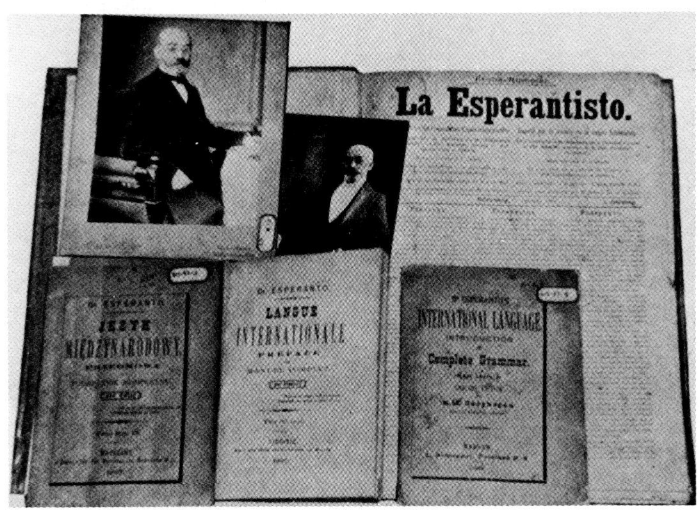

Fig. 13–11. Photographs of Ludwick Lejzer Zamenhof and examples of Esperanto, the international language that he devised.

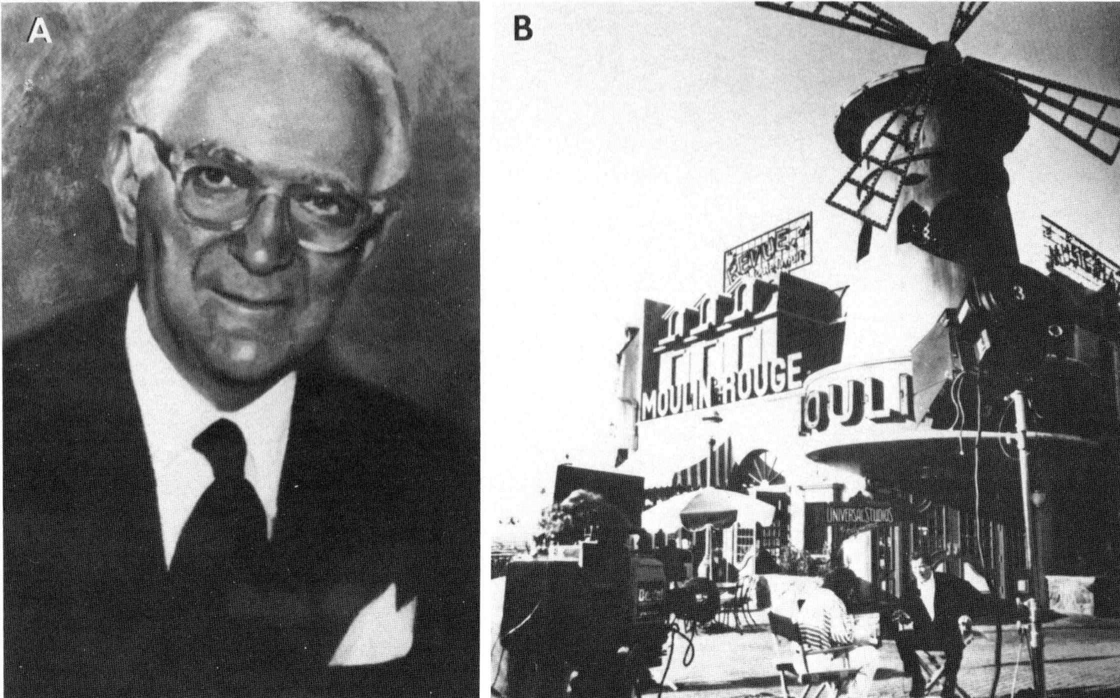

Fig. 13–12. *A*, Jules Stein. *B*, Movie set from Universal Studios, a subsidiary of Music Corporation of America (MCA), founded by Jules Stein. (*A*, by permission of the Jules Stein Eye Institute. *B*, by permission of Universal City Studios.)

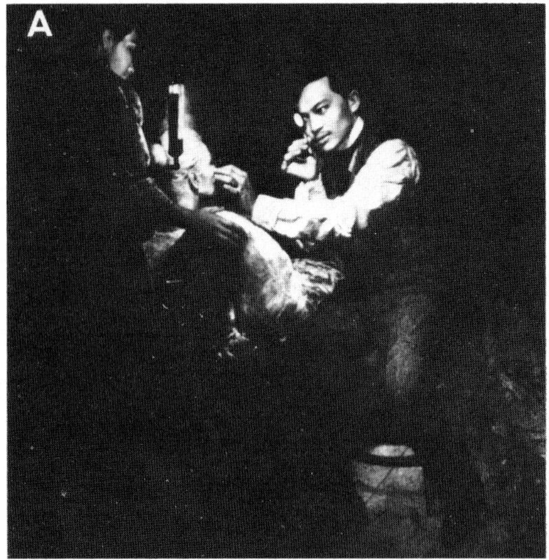

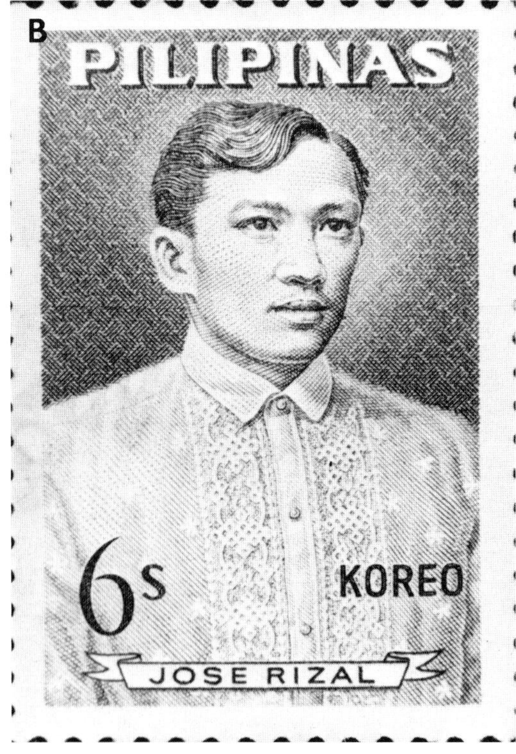

Fig. 13–13. *A*, *Dr. Rizal Treating His Own Mother*, by Romeo Enriquez. *B*, Philippine stamp, depicting her national hero, Jose Rizal. (*A*, by permission of the National Historical Institute, Manila, Philippines. *B*, from J.D. Bullock: Ophthalmologists: setting new sights. Harvard Med Alumni Bull, Summer 1989, pp. 50–54. By permission of the Harvard Medical School Alumni Association.)

whose sight was restored by successful cataract surgery (Fig. 13–13 *A*).

Jose Rizal is the national hero of the Philippines, and the love, respect, and admiration afforded him there are comparable to that for George Washington and Abraham Lincoln in American national heritage. His life was dedicated to rebellion against the Spanish, who ruled his homeland. He was also a poet and novelist. He organized the Filipino League and was eventually arrested and executed (at the age of 35) for conspiracy against Spain (Fig. 13–13 *B*).

Peter Juliani was a distinguished ophthalmologist in the thirteenth century. He received his M.D. degree from the University of Paris in 1247 and became professor of medicine at the University of Siena, Italy. He was the author of twelve books on medicine, the most famous of which was *Liber de Oculo* (*Book on the Eye*). Juliani gave up medicine in 1262 to become dean of the cathedral and superintendent of schools in Lisbon, Portugal. He later became Bishop of Mondonedo, Archbishop of Portugal, and finally chaplain to Pope Urban IV. Under Pope Gregory X, Peter was appointed cardinal in 1274. He was elected Pope John XXI in September 1276 and died in May 1277 (Fig. 13–14).

To be a truly successful ophthalmologist today, one must be multitalented, possessing the best attributes of each of the individuals described above: intelligence, a methodical attention to detail, a logical and analytical mind, physical stamina, dedication, concern for others, high ethical standards, a willingness to make sacrifices, imagination, versatility, political savvy, a success-oriented personality, and an ability to be stimulated by new challenges and to take risks. An examination of this small group of people, like studying the rays of light at a focal point, reflects the impressive breadth of interest and ability that all excellent ophthalmologists share and can marshal in the care of their patients.

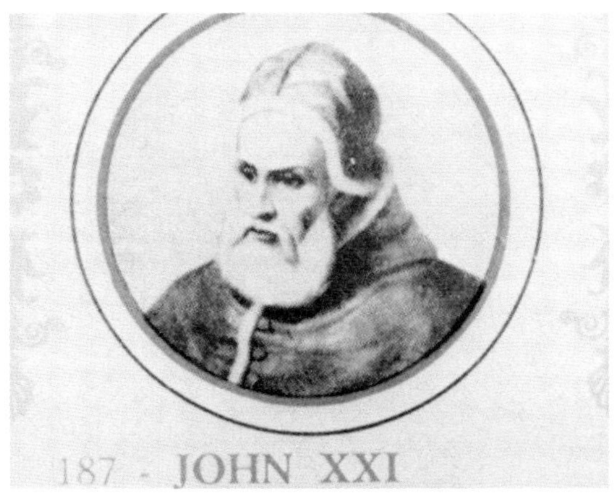

Fig. 13–14. Painting of Peter Juliani, who became Pope John XXI. (From J.D. Bullock: Ophthalmologists: setting new sights. Harvard Med Alumni Bull, Summer 1989, pp. 50–54. By permission of the Harvard Medical School Alumni Association.)

ABBREVIATIONS

Abbreviations, much more than the language from which they are derived, change over time. In the interest of accurate communication, therefore, their use is discouraged. The abbreviations and definitions listed below are included not as an imprimatur but to assist the student new to the field in deciphering the oftentimes cryptic ophthalmic record.

AC	anterior chamber
AC/A	accommodative convergence/accommodation ratio
ACT	alternate cover test
AION	anterior ischemic optic neuropathy
ALT	argon laser trabeculoplasty
AMPPE	acute multifocal placoid pigment epitheliopathy
AO–HRR	American Optical's Hardy-Rand-Rittler color vision plates
APD	afferent pupillary defect (see RAPD)
ARC	abnormal retinal correspondence
ARMD	age-related macular degeneration
ASC	anterior subcapsular cataract
BCC	basal cell carcinoma
BD	base-down prism
BDR	background diabetic retinopathy
BI	base-in prism
BMR	bilateral medial rectus recession
BO	base-out prism
BRAO	branch retinal artery occlusion
BRVO	branch retinal vein occlusion
BSS	balanced salt solution
BU	base-up prism
BUT	break-up time (of tear film)
Bx	biopsy
CAI	carbonic anhydrase inhibitor
CBB	ciliary body band
c.c.	with correction (*cum correctio*)
C/D	cup-to-disc ratio
CDCR	conjunctivodacryocystorhinostomy
C&F	cell and flare
CF	confrontation field
CF	count fingers vision
CL	contact lens
CME	cystoid macular edema
CMV	cytomegalovirus
COAG	chronic open-angle glaucoma
CPEO	chronic progressive external ophthalmoplegia
CRAO	central retinal artery occlusion
CRVO	central retinal vein occlusion
CSM	central, steady, and maintained fixation
CT	cover test
D	diopter
D-15	Farnsworth Panel D-15 color vision test
D-100	Farnsworth Panel D-100 color vision test
DCG	dacryocystography
DCR	dacryocystorhinostomy
DSG	dacryoscintigraphy
DVD	dissociated vertical deviation
DWSCL	daily-wear soft contact lens
Dx	diagnosis
ECCE	extracapsular cataract extraction
EKC	epidemic keratoconjunctivitis
EOG	electro-oculogram
EOM	extraocular muscles
EPI	epinephrine
ERG	electroretinogram
ESR	erythrocyte sedimentation rate
Et	esophoria

ET	esotropia at distance
ET'	esotropia at near
E(T)	intermittent esotropia at distance
E(T)'	intermittent esotropia at near
EUA	examination under anesthesia
EWCL	extended-wear soft contact lens
FA	fluorescein angiography
FB	foreign body
FTC	full to confrontation visual fields
FTFC	full to finger counting (confrontation visual fields)
F_3T	trifluorothymidine
Fx	fracture
GPC	giant papillary conjunctivitis
gtts	drops (guttae)
HCL	hard contact lens
HM	hand motion
HSV	herpes simplex virus
hT	hypotropia at distance
hT'	hypotropia at near
HT	hypertropia at distance
HT'	hypertropia at near
H(T)	intermittent hypertropia at distance
H(T)'	intermittent hypertropia at near
Hx	history
HZ	herpes zoster
ICCE	intracapsular cataract extraction
ICE	iridocorneal epitheliopathy
IDU	idoxuridine
INO	internuclear ophthalmoplegia
IO	inferior oblique
IOFB	intraocular foreign body
IOL	intraocular lens
ION	ischemic optic neuropathy
IOP	intraocular pressure
IPD	interpupillary distance
IR	inferior rectus
IRMA	intraretinal microvascular abnormalities
KP	keratic precipitates
K's	keratometric readings
K sicca	keratoconjunctivitis sicca
LCT	lateral canthal tendon
LE	left eye
LL	lower lid
LP	light perception
LR	lateral rectus
MCT	medial canthal tendon
MEWDS	multifocal evanescent white dot syndrome
MG	Marcus-Gunn pupil
MG	myasthenia gravis
MLF	medial longitudinal fasciculus
MM	malignant melanoma
MR	medial rectus
NFL	nerve fiber layer
NLD	nasolacrimal duct
NLP	no light perception; total blindness
NPA	near point of accommodation
NPC	near point of convergence
NPDR	nonproliferative diabetic retinopathy
NS	nuclear sclerosis
NVD	neovascularization of the disc
NVE	neovascularization – elsewhere
OA	overactive muscle
OAG	open-angle glaucoma
OA IO	overactive inferior oblique
OA SO	overactive superior oblique
OD	right eye (*oculus dexter*)
OKN	optokinetic nystagmus
ON	optic nerve
Ortho.	orthophoria
OS	left eye (*oculus sinister*)
OU	both eyes (*oculi uterque*)
P_1	pilocarpine 1% eyedrops
PAM	potential acuity meter
PAS	peripheral anterior synechiae
PBK	pseudophakic bullous keratopathy
PC	posterior chamber
PD	prism diopter (symbol: Δ)
PD	pupillary distance
PDR	proliferative diabetic retinopathy
PERRLA	pupils equal, round, reactive to light, accommodation
PF	Pred Forte
PH	pinhole visual acuity
PHNH	pinhole no help
PHPV	persistent hyperplastic primary vitreous
PI	peripheral iridectomy or iridotomy
PI	Phospholine iodide
PK	penetrating keratoplasty
pl	plano lens
POAG	primary open-angle glaucoma
POHS	presumed ocular histoplasmosis syndrome
PPRF	pontine paramedian reticular formation

PRP	panretinal photocoagulation
PSC	posterior subcapsular cataract
PSP	progressive supranuclear palsy
PVC	posterior vitreous collapse
PVD	posterior vitreal detachment
PVR	proliferative vitreoretinopathy
PXF	pseudoexfoliation
RAP	retinal artery pressure (ophthalmodynamometry)
RAPD	relative afferent pupillary defect
RD	retinal detachment
RE	right eye
RK	radial keratotomy
RLF	retrolental fibroplasia
ROP	retinopathy of prematurity
RPE	retinal pigment epithelium
R & R	recess and resect (recess-resect)
s.c.	without correction (*sine correctio*)
SCC	squamous cell carcinoma
SCL	soft contact lens
SLE	slit-lamp examination
SO	superior oblique
SPK	superficial punctate keratopathy
SR	superior rectus
SRNVM	subretinal neovascular membrane
SS	scleral spur
$T_{1/2}$	timolol maleate (Timoptic) 0.5% eyedrops
Ta	applanation tonometry
TBUT	tear breakup time
TM	trabecular meshwork
T_{MM}	tension by Mackay-Marg tonometry
T_s	tension by SchiSchiøtz tonometry
T_t	tension by finger palpation (tactile)
UGH	uveitis-glaucoma-hyphema syndrome
Va	visual acuity
VEP	visual-evoked potential
VER	visual-evoked response
VF	visual fields
X	exophoria at distance
X′	exophoria at near
XT	exotropia at distance
XT′	exotropia at near
X(T)	intermittent exotropia at distance
X(T)′	intermittent exotropia at near

INDEX

ISBN 0-397-51142-6
90000
9 780397 511426